Nurse as Educator

THE JONES AND BARTLETT SERIES IN NURSING

Nurse as Educator

Principles of Teaching and Learning

Susan B. Bastable, Ed.D., M.Ed., R.N.

Associate Professor and Chair
Undergraduate Program, College of Nursing
State University of New York
Health Science Center at Syracuse

Jones and Bartlett Publishers
Sudbury, Massachusetts

Boston   London   Singapore

Editorial, Sales, and Customer Service Offices
40 Tall Pine Drive
Sudbury, MA 01776
508-443-5000
800-832-0034
info@jbpub.com
http://www.jbpub.com

Jones and Bartlett Publishers International
Barb House, Barb Mews
London W6 7PA
UK

Library of Congress Cataloging-in-Publication Data

Nurse as Educator: principles of teaching and learning / [edited by]
    Susan B. Bastable.
            p.   cm. — (The Jones and Bartlett series in nursing)
    Includes bibliographical references and index.
    ISBN 0-7637-0310-9
    1. Health education.   2. Teaching.   3. Learning.   I. Bastable,
Susan Bacorn.   II. Series.
    [DNLM: 1. Education, Nursing—methods.   2. Learning—nurses'
instruction.   3. Teaching—nurses' instruction.   WY 18 N9715 1997]
RT90.N86   1997
613—dc21
DNLM/DLC
for Library of Congress   97-7066
                                                                        CIP

Production Editor: Marilyn E. Rash
Manufacturing Manager: Dana L. Cerrito
Editorial Production Service: Pre-Press Company, Inc.
Design/Typesetting: Pre-Press Company, Inc.
Cover Design: Hannus Design Associates
Cover Printing: Coral Graphic Services, Inc.
Printing and Binding: Hamilton Printing Company

Printed in the United States of America
01 00 99 98 97   10 9 8 7 6 5 4 3 2 1

To the past, present, and future students
in my Nurse As Educator course

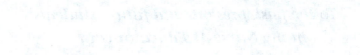

CONTENTS

FOREWORD

The role of nurses in educating the community for health has been an essential theme since the inception of public health nursing in the United States at the turn of the century. At that time, waves of immigrants who were attempting to establish lives in a strange land underscored the pressing need for community-based health care. Soon it was realized that education was a significant ingredient for successfully delivering care that could be continued in the home by family members. Education was also recognized as an essential element of preventive services delivered in clinics, milk stations, schools, and factories. Nurses assumed the role with ease, and in some parts of the country, community agencies were called Instructive Visiting Nursing Associations.

In the advent of the next turn of the century, the kaleidoscope of American health care has come to rely on the nurse as a primary health-care educator. Nurses have encouraged their patients to become educated health-care consumers and more self-reliant in matters of health that affect them. The role of the nurse in patient teaching is central and critical to improving the health of individuals and the population at large. It is important in both institutional and community-based settings. *Nurse as Educator: Principles of Teaching and Learning* is an important book that comes at a propitious time in the history of American health care. As we approach the year 2000, formal preparation of nurses for their ever-increasing role in patient teaching, health education, and health promotion has become part of the curricula in undergraduate and graduate nursing programs. Therefore, the value and relevance of this book take on even greater significance because it contains approaches to patient teaching that are seminal to both nursing practice and nursing education arenas.

Nurse as Educator: Principles of Teaching and Learning is a substantive book that combines theoretical and pragmatic content with balance. It is designed to teach nurses about the developmental, motivational, and sociocultural differences that affect teaching and learning. Additionally, it provides for the application of theory in chapters devoted to development of educational objectives, instructional methods, and strategies for evaluation of the educational process. The book has broad application in patient education as well as in providing valuable information to the practice field in general and to nursing education in particular.

Nurse as Educator: Principles of Teaching and Learning is a timely and needed addition to the professional literature. Its value to the field will increase as we confront the challenges of a rapidly changing health-care system and the increasingly sophisticated needs of the American public for education that serves to promote and maintain health. The role of nurses as educators will be supported and enhanced as a result of this scholarly contribution to the professional body of knowledge. It addresses a compelling component of professional activity that will become even more prominent in the twenty-first century.

M. Louise Fitzpatrick, Ed.D., R.N., F.A.A.N.
Dean and Professor, College of Nursing
Villanova University

PREFACE

The impetus for writing this textbook arose from a perceived need for a comprehensive text covering the basic principles of teaching and learning that could be used by nurses involved in educating patients and their families as well as in educating nursing and allied health-care staff and nursing students. Encouragement came from undergraduate and graduate students in my "Nurse as Educator" class, who desired a text that adequately addressed the essential components of the teaching and learning process. Years of fruitless and frustrating search for a book that fulfilled this need only made the effort to write one all the more imperative. Although over the past few decades numerous articles have been published in the nursing literature on issues related to patient and staff education, no one text has existed to date that considers all important attributes of the learner and the many aspects of the teaching role.

Nurses are information brokers, and teaching is a competency expected of all registered nurses. A sound knowledge base of teaching and learning principles is an essential prerequisite for nursing practice, whether nurses serve as direct patient care providers, whether they participate in in-service and continuing education programs to assist nursing colleagues and other health-care practitioners to deliver quality services to the consumer, whether they function as faculty members in preparing nursing students for future practice, or whether they be students in colleges of nursing across the country who will be the nursing professionals of tomorrow. Whoever the learner may be, the nurse as educator must have a sound understanding of the teaching and learning process, including consideration of learner characteristics as well as the techniques and strategies for educating others.

The importance of client as well as staff and student education has never been greater than it is today. In the rapidly changing health-care environment, it is mandatory that nurses in the role of educators be proficient at teaching patients and their families self-care management skills through an understanding of the basic techniques of instruction to satisfy federal and state mandates as well as institutional expectations and professional standards in the delivery of nursing care, teaching being one important aspect of their professional role.

There are multiple variables currently operating in the health-care arena that necessitate professional nurses to be competently and confidently prepared to assume responsibility for educating different population groups in a variety of settings. An upsurge in consumer demand for more participation in health promotion and disease prevention measures, increased efforts at cost-containment of health-care resulting in early patient discharges and higher patient acuity levels in institutional and community settings, and a greater number of chronically ill persons as the population ages are just a few reasons why clients must be better educated for independence in self-care. So, too, must staff and student nurses be better prepared through education to meet the increased demands for nursing care and to function in advanced practice roles as they face new professional opportunities and the many complex challenges of the future.

The purpose of this textbook is to serve as a primary resource for professional nurses and nursing students who need to know more about the essential aspects of teaching and learning. It will help them to become proficient as educators, taking into consideration first and foremost the needs and characteristics of the learner and then using proper instructional approaches that will not only fulfill the learner's needs but also match the resources and requirements of the settings in which they practice. In general, nurses recognize their legal and ethical responsibilities to teach others, and many acknowledge that they devote much of their time to the education of their clients, but most nurses will admit they have had little formal preparation to successfully and securely carry out this role expectation.

This textbook has been sequentially divided into three main parts for logical organization and readability of the content. Part I consists of an overview of the principles of teaching and learning, highlighting the historical and current trends in education for health care; addressing the ethical, legal, and economic foundations of the education process; and reviewing the learning theories generic to the nurse's understanding of how someone acquires cognitive, affective, and psychomotor behaviors. Part II examines attributes of the learner, such as learning needs and styles, developmental stages, motivation and compliance factors, literacy levels, special needs, and sociocultural characteristics that the nurse educator must assess prior to teaching others. Part III focuses on the techniques and strategies useful for the planning, implementation, and evaluation of teaching and learning.

A strength of this publication is the amount of theoretical material on relevant topics related to teaching and learning that is contained in each chapter. Examples are used throughout to help the reader understand the link between theory and application. This text is unique in giving attention to special population groups, gender and sociocultural attributes of the learner, adult literacy levels, instructional settings, assessment of motivation, characteristics of the creative teacher, and outcome evaluation.

Initially, I planned to undertake single-handedly the responsibility for preparing this text in its entirety. However, it became clearly evident when I first conceived of the idea to write this manuscript what an enormous effort it would take to complete such a large project. Therefore, I wisely sought the help of contributors whose expertise as educators has given this final product the scope, depth, and quality that was so desired. Although the chapters are written by various authors, the language and format of each chapter are consistent with one another.

The major audiences for which this text is intended are upper-division-level baccalaureate and masters-level nursing students preparing for professional and advanced practice roles. In addition, the information contained herein will be most helpful to staff nurses and those who are in-service, staff development, or continuing-education coordinators. This text is also useful for faculty involved in and graduate students anticipating a teaching career in a formal educational setting of a school of nursing. Although the content of all chapters is designed specifically for application to patient education, most of the chapters contain theory relevant and applicable to teaching a diverse audience of learners. It is my sincere hope that readers will find this book a useful tool that contributes significantly to nursing practice and nursing education for the benefit of the consumers we serve.

CONTRIBUTORS

Susan B. Bastable, Ed.D., R.N.
Associate Professor and Chair of Undergraduate Program
College of Nursing
State University of New York
Health Science Center at Syracuse
Syracuse, New York

Margaret M. Braungart, Ph.D.
Professor of Psychology
Chairperson of the Department of Health Sciences and Human Studies
College of Health Professions
State University of New York
Health Science Center at Syracuse
Syracuse, New York

Richard G. Braungart, Ph.D.
Professor of Sociology and International Relations
Maxwell School
Syracuse University
Syracuse, New York

Kathleen Fitzgerald, M.S., R.N., C.D.E.
Patient Educator
St. Joseph's Hospital Health Center
Syracuse, New York

Diane S. Hainsworth, M.S., R.N.
Clinical Nurse Specialist, Surgery/Neurology
Crouse Hospital
Syracuse, New York

Sharon Kitchie, M.S., R.N.C.S.
Patient Education Coordinator
University Hospital
State University of New York
Health Science Center at Syracuse
Syracuse, New York

M. Janice Nelson, Ed.D., R.N.
Professor Emeritus
College of Nursing
State University of New York
Health Science Center at Syracuse
Syracuse, New York

Virginia E. O'Halloran, Ed.D, R.N., C.
Associate Professor
Department of Nursing
College of Mount Saint Vincent
Riverdale, New York

Eleanor Richards, Ph.D., R.N., C.S.
Associate Professor
Department of Nursing
State University of New York at New Paltz
New Paltz, New York

Cynthia D. Sculco, Ed.D., R.N.
President, Nurse Ed. Communications, Inc.
132 East 95th St.
New York, New York

Kay Viggiani, M.S., R.N., C.N.S.
Associate Professor
Nursing Division
Keuka College
Keuka Park, New York

Priscilla Sandford Worral, Ph.D., R.N.
Coordinator for Nursing Research
University Hospital
State University of New York
Health Science Center at Syracuse
Syracuse, New York

ACKNOWLEDGMENTS

A special thanks to my husband, Jeffrey, to my two children, Garrett and Leigh, and to my parents, Robert and Dorrie Bacorn, and to Stephen and Gerry Bastable, for all their love, support, understanding, and encouragement during the many months of writing and editing.

In sincere appreciation to all of my contributors for their untiring efforts, patience, and professional expertise and to my nursing colleagues and staff at the College of Nursing at SUNY Health Science Center at Syracuse for their loyal assistance through this process of publication.

A tribute to my students for their constant enthusiasm and inspiration and for the sharing of their ideas and experiences.

To the faculty at Allegheny University of the Health Sciences (formerly Hahnemann University), Syracuse University, and Teachers College, Columbia University for giving me the foundational knowledge and skills to pursue my professional career in nursing.

And, in grateful recognition of the New York State/United University Professions Affirmative Action Committee for the Dr. Nuala McGann Drescher Affirmative Action Leave Program award, which partially funded this project.

PART I
Principles of Teaching and Learning

CHAPTER 1

Overview of Education in Health Care

Susan B. Bastable

CHAPTER HIGHLIGHTS

Historical Foundations for the Teaching Role of Nurses

Social and Economic Trends Impacting on Health Care

Purpose, Benefits, and Goals of Patient and Staff Education

The Education Process Defined

Role of the Nurse as Educator

Barriers to Education and Obstacles to Learning

Perspectives on Research in Patient and Staff Education

Questions to Be Asked Regarding the Delivery of Educational Services

KEY TERMS

education process   teaching
instruction   learning
patient education   staff education

OBJECTIVES

After completing this chapter, the reader will be able to

1. Discuss the evolution of the teaching role of nurses.
2. Recognize the trends impacting on nursing practice in particular and on the health-care system in general.
3. Identify the purpose, benefits, and goals of patient and staff education.
4. Compare and contrast the education process to the nursing process.
5. Define the terms *teaching* and *learning*.
6. Identify the reasons why patient and staff education is an important role for professional nurses.
7. Discuss barriers to education and obstacles to learning.
8. Formulate questions that nurses in the role of educator should ask about the teaching-learning process.

Education in health care today, both patient education and nursing staff/student education, is a topic of utmost interest in every setting in which nurses practice. The current trends in health care are making it imperative that patients and their families be prepared to assume responsibility for self-care management and that nurses in the workplace be accountable for the delivery of high-quality care. The focus is on outcomes—whether it be that the patient and family have learned essential knowledge and skills for independent care or that staff nurses and nursing students have acquired up-to-date knowledge and skills to competently and expertly render care to the consumer in a variety of settings. The need for nurses to teach others will continue to increase in this era of health-care reform. With changes rapidly forthcoming in the system of health care, nurses will find themselves in increasingly demanding, constantly fluctuating, and highly complex positions (Jorgensen, 1994). It is necessary for nurses in the role of educators to understand the forces, historical and present day, that have impacted and continue to impact on their responsibilities in practice, with teaching being a major aspect of the nurse's professional role.

The purpose of this chapter is to shed light on the historical evolution of teaching as part of the professional nurse's role; offer a perspective on the current trends in health care making patient teaching a highly visible and required function of nursing care delivery; address continuing educa-

tion efforts to ensure ongoing practice competencies of nursing personnel; and clarify the broad purposes, benefits, and goals of the teaching-learning process. In addition, this chapter focuses on the philosophy of the nurse-patient partnership in teaching and learning, compares the education process to the nursing process, identifies barriers to teaching and learning, and highlights the status of research in the field of patient as well as staff education. The focus is on the overall role of the nurse in teaching and learning, no matter who the audience of learners may be. Nurses must have a basic prerequisite understanding of the principles, practice, and process of teaching and learning to carry out their professional responsibilities with efficiency and effectiveness.

HISTORICAL FOUNDATIONS FOR THE TEACHING ROLE OF NURSES

Health education has long been considered a major component in the repertoire of standard caregiving by the nurse. The role of the nurse as educator is deeply entrenched in the heritage and development of the profession. For decades, patient teaching has been recognized as an independent nursing function, and likewise for decades, nurses have been educating other nurses for professional practice. Florence Nightingale not only developed the first school of nursing but also devoted a large portion of her career to educating physicians, health officials, and nurses about the importance of proper conditions in hospitals and homes to assist patients in maintaining adequate nutrition, fresh air, exercise, and personal hygiene to improve their well-being. Nurses have always educated others—patients, families, and colleagues—and it is from these roots that nurses have expanded their practice to include the broader concepts of health and illness (Chow et al.,1984).

As early as 1918, the National League of Nursing Education (NLNE) in the United States, now known as the National League for Nursing (NLN), observed the importance of health teaching as a function within the scope of nursing practice, including responsibility for the promotion of health and the prevention of illness in such settings as schools, homes, hospitals, and industries. Two decades later, the NLNE declared that a nurse was fundamentally a teacher and an agent of health regardless of the setting in which practice occurred (National League of Nursing Education, 1937). By 1950, the NLN identified course content dealing with teaching skills, developmental and educational psychology, and principles of the educational process of teaching and learning as areas in the curriculum common to all nursing schools (Redman, 1993). The implication was that nurses were to be prepared, on graduation from their basic nursing program, to assume the role as teacher of others. The American Nurses' Association has for years promulgated statements on the functions, standards, and qualifications for nursing practice, of which patient teaching is an integral aspect. In addition, the International Council of Nurses has long endorsed health education as an essential requisite of nursing care delivery.

Today, state Nurse Practice Acts (NPAs) universally include teaching within the scope of nursing practice responsibilities. Nurses are expected to provide instruction to consumers for them to maintain optimal levels of wellness, prevent disease, manage illness, and develop skills to give supportive care to family members. Nursing career ladders often incorporate teaching effectiveness as a measure of excellence in practice (Rifas et al.,1994). The recent development of clinical pathways, synonymously referred to as critical pathways, has become a popular, multidisciplinary approach to delineating predetermined client outcomes that are used to measure patient adherence to pathway expectations. Nurses are in the forefront of this innovative strategy for the delivery of patient care, and the teaching of patients and families as well as health-care personnel is the means to accomplish the goals of providing cost-effective, safe, and high-quality care.

In recognition of the importance of patient education by nurses, as recently as 1993 the Joint Commission on Accreditation of Healthcare Organizations (JCAHO) delineated nursing standards for patient education. These standards, in the form of mandates, are based on descriptions of positive outcomes of patient care dependent on nursing care teaching activities that are patient and family oriented. Required accreditation standards have provided the impetus for nursing service managers to put greater emphasis on unit-based clinical education activities and to improve nursing interventions relating to patient education for the purpose of achieving client outcomes (McGoldrick et al.,1994). In addition, the Patient's Bill of Rights issued by the American Hospital Association and adopted by hospitals nationwide has established the rights of patients to receive complete and current information concerning diagnosis, treatment, and prognosis in terms they can reasonably be expected to understand. Most recently, the PEW Health Professions Commission (1995), influenced by the dramatic changes currently surrounding health care, has published a broad set of competencies that it believes will mark the success of the health professions in the 21st century. Seventeen recommendations to the health professions have been proposed by the commission. Over one-half of them pertain to the importance of patient and staff education and to the role of the nurse as educator. Among the recommendations, the commission addresses the need to provide clinically competent and coordinated care, involve patients and their families in the decision-making process regarding health interventions, provide education and counseling on ethical issues, expand access to effective care, ensure cost-effective and appropriate care, and provide for prevention of illness and promotion of healthy lifestyles.

Accomplishing the goals of all these organizations calls for a redirection of education efforts on "training the trainer," that is, preparing nursing staff through continuing education, in-service programs, and staff development to maintain and improve their clinical skills and teaching abilities. Presently, the demand for educators of patients and the general public is rapidly accelerating, and the demand for educators of nursing students is at an all-time high. Also, nurses are the primary educators of their fellow colleagues and other health-care staff personnel. It is essential that professional nurses be prepared to effectively perform teaching services that meet the needs of individuals and groups in different circumstances across a variety of practice settings (Bell, 1986).

SOCIAL AND ECONOMIC TRENDS IMPACTING ON HEALTH CARE

In addition to the standards put forth by professional nursing organizations, the mandates by health-care institutions and accrediting bodies, and the regulations by federal and state agencies, there has arisen an increasing emphasis on nurses' potential role in teaching activities as a result of social and economic trends nationwide affecting the public's health. The following are some of the significant forces impacting on nursing practice in particular and on the health-care system in general (Jorgensen, 1994; Luker & Caress, 1989; McGinnis, 1993; Latter et al., 1992; Goldsmith, 1986; and Kellmer-Langan et al., 1992):

1. The federal government, through health-care reform initiatives, has established national health-care goals and objectives for the near future as outlined in *Healthy People 2000: National Promotion and Disease Prevention Objectives* (Department of Health and Human Services, 1990). This document describes national needs in relation to health promotion and disease prevention. Objectives include the development of effective health education programs to assist individuals to recognize and change risk behaviors, to adopt or maintain protective health practices, and to make appropriate use of health-care delivery systems. Achievement of these national objectives would dramatically cut health-care costs, prevent the premature onset of disease and disability, and help all Americans lead healthier and more productive

lives. Nurses, as the largest body of health-care professionals who embody the professional philosophy of holistic care, are being looked on as capable of making a real difference in educating people to attain and maintain healthy lifestyles.

2. The growth of managed care, the shifts in payor coverage, and the issue of reimbursement for the provision of health care have led to an increasing emphasis on outcome measures, achievable primarily through success of patient education efforts.

3. Health providers are beginning to recognize the economic and social values in practicing preventive medicine through health education initiatives.

4. Political emphasis is on productivity, competitiveness in the marketplace, and cost-containment measures to restrain health-service expenses. Politicians and health-care administrators acknowledge the importance of health education as a requisite to accomplishing these goals in today's society.

5. The health-care reform movement is opening up new avenues for expansion of preventive and promotion education efforts directed at communities, schools, and workplaces in addition to the traditional care settings.

6. There is concern on the part of health-care professionals regarding legal pressures of malpractice and disciplinary action for incompetency. Continuing education, either by legislative mandate or as a requirement of the employing institution, has come to the forefront in recent years as the answer to the challenge of ensuring the competency of practitioners. Continuing education has emerged as a response to the change and expansion of knowledge in the nursing profession. It is a means to transmit new knowledge and skills as well as reinforce or refresh previously acquired knowledge and abilities to guarantee the continuing growth of staff nurse competencies.

7. The interest that continues to be exhibited by nurses in defining their own role, body of knowledge, and expertise has focused on patient education as central to the practice of nursing.

8. Consumers are demanding increased knowledge and skills about how to care for themselves and how to prevent disease. A rise in consumerism in health-service provision is paralleling the interest exhibited in other aspects of consumer involvement in the marketplace. As people are becoming more aware of and more knowledgeable about health-care matters, they are questioning the nature of their impairments and needs and are demanding a greater understanding of treatments and goals. The health-care trends of the 1990s, emphasizing consumer rights and responsibilities, have increased the demand for patient and consumer information services, and these demands are expected to intensify in the future.

9. Demographic trends are requiring an emphasis to be placed on self-reliance and maintenance of a healthy status over the longer lifespan that most people can now expect to enjoy. The percentage of the U.S. population older than 65 years will climb dramatically in the next 20 to 30 years as the baby boom generation of the post–World War II era will reach the late adulthood years and become victims of degenerative illnesses.

10. Among the major causes of morbidity and mortality are those diseases now recognized as being lifestyle related and preventable through educational interventions.

11. The proportionate increase in the incidence of chronic and incurable conditions necessitates that individuals and families participate in their care and manage their own illnesses.

12. Advanced technology is increasing the complexity of care and treatment as well as diverting large numbers of patients from the inpatient health-care setting. Life support and maintenance technologies are enabling patients to carry on with their lives away from the acute, direct caregiving arenas, necessitating patient education to help them independently follow through with self-management activities.

13. Earlier hospital discharge is forcing patients and their families to be more self-reliant on managing their own illnesses. Patient teaching can facilitate an individual's adaptive responses to illness.

14. There is a belief on the part of nurses and other health-care providers, which is supported by research, that patient education improves compliance and, hence, health and well-being. Under-

standing by clients of their treatment plans can lead to increased cooperation with therapeutic regimens and may enable them to independently solve problems encountered outside the protected care environments of hospitals, thereby increasing their independence.

15. There is an increased proliferation in the number of self-help groups established to support clients in meeting their physical and psychosocial needs. Success of these support groups and behavioral change programs, such as Weight Watchers, has led to an upsurge in public interest as well as nurse involvement and advocacy for these educational endeavors.

These examples are indicative of the major trends operating in this country to create a climate that is forcing nurses to recognize the need to develop their expertise in teaching to keep pace with the demands of patient and staff education. Nurses are in a key position to carry out health education. Since nurses are the health-care providers who have continuous contact with patients and families and are usually the most accessible source of information for the consumer, patient teaching is likely to become an even more important function within the scope of nursing practice (Woody et al., 1984).

PURPOSE, BENEFITS, AND GOALS OF PATIENT AND STAFF EDUCATION

Current and continuously improving patient and staff education programs are an integral part of today's system of health-care delivery to the public. In light of cost-containment measures by health-care agencies and despite the sometimes scarce resources available, nurses continue to pursue the goals of involving patients in exploring and expanding their self-care abilities through interactive patient education efforts (McGoldrick et al., 1994). Patient education has demonstrated its potential to increase consumer satisfaction, improve quality of life, ensure continuity of care, effectively reduce the incidence of complications of illness, promote adherence to health-care treatment plans, decrease patient anxiety, and maximize independence in the performance of activities of daily living. In addition, education energizes and empowers consumers to become involved in the planning of teaching sessions. In turn, the educator role of nurses enhances their job satisfaction when they recognize that their teaching actions have the potential to forge therapeutic relationships with patients, allow for greater patient-nurse autonomy, and create change that really makes a difference in the lives of others.

Because it has been estimated that 80% of all health needs and problems are handled at home, there truly does exist a need to educate people on how to care for themselves—both to get well and to stay well (Health Services Medical Corporation, Inc., 1993). As Robin Orr (1990) noted, illness is a natural life process, but so is mankind's ability to learn. Along with the ability to learn is a natural curiosity that allows people to view new and difficult situations as challenges rather than as defeats. "Illness can become an educational opportunity . . . a 'teachable moment' when ill health suddenly encourages them to take a more active role in their care" (Orr, 1990, p. 47). Numerous studies have documented the fact that informed patients are more likely to comply with medical treatment plans and find innovative ways to cope with illness, are better able to manage symptoms of illness, are less likely to experience complications, and are more satisfied with care when they receive adequate information about how to care for themselves. One of the most frequently cited complaints by patients in litigation cases is that they were not adequately informed.

Just as the need exists for teaching clients to help them become participants and informed consumers to achieve independence in self-care, the need also exists for staff nurses to be exposed to up-to-date and ongoing information with the ultimate goal of enhancing their practice so they can play a key role in improving the nation's health.

THE EDUCATION PROCESS DEFINED

The *education process* is a systematic, sequential, planned course of action consisting of two major interdependent operations, teaching and learning, which form a continuous cycle. This process also involves two interdependent players, the teacher and the learner. Together they jointly perform teaching and learning activities, the outcome of which is a mutually desired behavior change that fosters growth in the learner and, it should be acknowledged, growth in the teacher as well. Thus, the education process should always be a participatory approach to teaching and learning.

The education process has always been compared to the nursing process and rightly so, because the steps of each process run parallel to one another, but with a different slant. The education process, like the nursing process, consists of the basic elements of assessment, planning, implementation, and evaluation. The nursing process, which begins with assessment, is a logical, scientifically based framework for nursing. It provides a rational basis for nursing practice rather than an intuitive one. It is a method for diagnosing, planning, implementing, and evaluating nursing interventions and thus is a means for monitoring and judging the overall quality of those interventions based on objective data and scientific criteria. Whereas the nursing process focuses on the planning and implementation of care based on the assessment and diagnosis of the physical and psychosocial needs of the patient, the education process identifies instructional content and methods based on the assessment and prioritization of the client's learning needs, readiness to learn, and learning styles. Both processes are ongoing, with assessment and evaluation perpetually redirecting the planning and implementation phases of the processes. If mutually agreed on behavioral outcomes for the learner are not achieved, as determined by evaluation, then the education process can and should begin again through reassessment, replanning, and reimplementation (Figure 1–1).

It should be noted that the actual act of teaching is subsumed as one component of the education process. Education, as the broad umbrella process, includes the acts of teaching and instruction. *Teaching* is a deliberate intervention that involves the planning and implementation of instructional activities and experiences to meet intended learner outcomes according to a teaching plan. *Instruction*, a term often used interchangeably with teaching, is in fact one aspect of teaching that involves the communicating of information about a specific skill in the cognitive, psychomo-

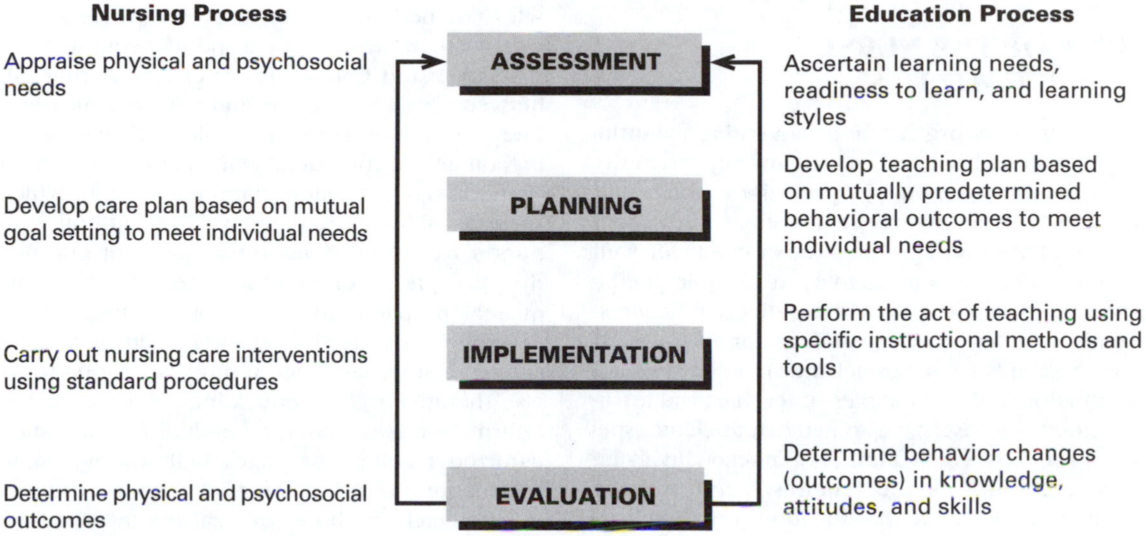

Nursing Process   **Education Process**

Appraise physical and psychosocial → ASSESSMENT ← Ascertain learning needs,
needs   readiness to learn, and learning
                                                                                      styles

                                                                                      Develop teaching plan based
Develop care plan based on mutual   PLANNING   on mutually predetermined
goal setting to meet individual needs   behavioral outcomes to meet
                                                                                      individual needs

                                                                                      Perform the act of teaching using
Carry out nursing care interventions IMPLEMENTATION specific instructional methods and
using standard procedures   tools

                                                                                      Determine behavior changes
                                                                                      (outcomes) in knowledge,
Determine physical and psychosocial   EVALUATION   attitudes, and skills
outcomes

FIGURE 1–1. Education Process Parallels Nursing Process

tor, or affective domain with the objective of producing learning. Teaching and instruction are often formal, structured, organized activities prepared days in advance, but they can be performed informally on the spur of the moment during conversations or incidental encounters with the learner. Whether formal or informal, planned well in advance or spontaneous, teaching and instruction are nevertheless deliberate and conscious acts. The fact that teaching and instruction are intentional does not necessarily mean that they have to be lengthy and complex tasks, but it does mean that they are conscious actions on the part of the teacher in responding to an individual's need to learn (Narrow, 1979). The cues that someone has a need to learn can be communicated in the form of a verbal request, a puzzled or confused look, or a gesture of defeat or frustration. In the broadest sense, teaching is a highly versatile strategy that can be applied in preventing, promoting, maintaining, or modifying a wide variety of behaviors in a learner who is receptive (Redman, 1971).

Learning, on the other hand, is defined as a change in behavior (knowledge, skills, and attitudes) that can occur at anytime or in any place as a result of exposure to environmental stimuli. Learning is an action by which knowledge, skills,

and attitudes are consciously or unconsciously acquired such that behavior is altered in some way that can be observed or measured (see Chapter 3).

The success of the nurse educator's endeavors at teaching is measured not by how much content has been imparted, but by how much the person has learned. Specifically, *patient education* is a process of assisting people to learn health-related behaviors in order to incorporate them into everyday life with the purpose of achieving the goal of optimal health and independence in self-care (Smith, 1989; Bell, 1986). *Staff education* is the process of influencing the behavior of nurses by producing changes in knowledge, attitudes, values, and skills required to maintain and improve their competencies for the delivery of quality care to the consumer. Both patient and staff education involves a relationship between learner and educator for the purpose of having the learner's information needs (cognitive, psychomotor, and affective) met by the health-care provider through education. A useful paradigm to assist nurses to organize and carry out the education process is the ASSURE model (Rega, 1993). The acronym stands for *A*nalyze learner, *S*tate objectives, *S*elect instructional methods and tools, *U*se teaching materials, *R*equire learner performance, and *E*valuate/revise the teaching and learning process.

ROLE OF THE NURSE AS EDUCATOR

For many years, organizations governing and influencing nurses have encouraged and supported the view that nurses should play a major role in health education. Teaching has been seen as an essential component of nursing practice in caring for well and ill clients. For nurses to act in the role of educator, no matter whether their audience is patients, family members, nursing students, or nursing staff and other agency personnel, they must have a solid foundation in the principles of teaching and learning. Educationalists have argued that teaching, especially the teaching of adults, is a function involving complex concepts and requires special training in instructional skills if education programs conducted by nurses are to be successful.

Luker and Caress (1989), in particular, have challenged the wisdom of involving all nurses in patient education as an unrealistic and undesirable goal of the profession. Luker and Caress suggest that it is unreasonable to expect every nurse to take responsibility for teaching patients when the majority of nursing practitioners have had only a basic nursing education background from diploma or associate's degree–level programs. Patients, by virtue of their illnesses, may have special learning difficulties that require teaching interventions to be carried out by nurses who are well grounded in the principles of teaching and learning.

As the American system of nursing education now stands, the multiple-entry, unstandardized approach to educating nurses for practice leaves little room in the diploma and associate's degree–level curriculum for including the breadth and depth of information on teaching and learning principles necessary to adequately prepare nurses to function in the role of educator. Nevertheless, legal and accreditation mandates as well as professional nursing standards of practice have made patient education an integral part of high-quality care to be delivered by all registered nurses, regardless of their level of nursing school preparation. One solution, albeit controversial, is to make teaching the sole responsibility of, at minimum, baccalaureate-degree graduates. Ideally, the educator role should be delegated to master's-prepared nurses, particularly the advanced practice nurses such as clinical nurse specialists and nurse practitioners,

who have both the interest and the knowledge base to make them expert patient and staff educators.

Luker and Caress (1989) clearly distinguish between patient teaching and patient education. They say patient teaching "implies a didactic information giving approach," while patient education "implies something more comprehensive, for which specialist skills are required" (p. 714). Although all nurses are able to function as givers of information, the question they pose is, are all nurses adequately prepared to assess for learning needs, determine whether information given is received and understood, and take appropriate action to revise the approach to educating the client if the information is not comprehended? Because standardized teaching packages help to overcome these potential deficits in nurses' ability to function as teachers, there still remains the need for them to be able to assess the suitability of the standardized material for the learner and to adapt it accordingly if necessary. To ensure that patient education programs are clinically accurate and educationally sound, these two authors advocate that nurses with minimal basic education be excluded from the education process. Nevertheless, as of today, patient education is a mandated responsibility of all registered nurses licensed in the United States. Given this fact, it is imperative to examine the present role expectations of nurses, regardless of their preparatory background, with respect to teaching.

Certainly the role of the nurse as teacher of patients and families, nursing staff, and students should stem from a partnership philosophy. The provision of information to the learner, whoever the learner may be, should stress the fact that teaching and learning are participatory processes. A learner cannot be made to learn. However, an effective approach in educating others is to actively involve learners in the education process. There is growing evidence that effective education and learner participation go hand in hand. The nurse should act as a facilitator, creating an environment conducive to learning—one that motivates individuals to want to learn and makes it possible for them to learn. The assessment of learning needs, the planning and designing of a teaching program, the implementation of instructional methods and materials, and the evaluation of teaching and learning should involve both the educator and the learner. In the case of patient education, the approach to be used that is more in keeping with ideals of self-care would be to transfer the responsibility for learning from the nurse to the patient. The emphasis should be on the facilitation of learning from a nondirective rather than a didactic teaching approach (Luker & Caress, 1989).

The nurse also needs to serve as coordinator of teaching efforts and as client advocate in helping to lend consistency of care amid a fragmented care delivery system involving many providers. Certainly patient education requires a collaborative effort among health-care team members, all of whom play a more or less important role in teaching. But nurses, with their holistic approach to care delivery as well as the respect and trust traditionally bestowed on them by consumers of health care, can and should capture the educator role as a professional domain and position themselves as client advocates, helping to clarify information and support the patients and family members in their efforts to achieve the goal of optimal health.

BARRIERS TO EDUCATION AND OBSTACLES TO LEARNING

It has been said by many educators that adult learning takes place not by the teacher's initiating and motivating the learning process, but rather by the teacher's removing or reducing obstacles to learning and enhancing the process after it has begun. The educator should not limit learning to the information that is *intended* but should clearly make possible the potential for informal, *unintended* learning that can occur each and every day with each and every teacher-learner encounter (Redman, 1975).

Unfortunately, there are numerous barriers confronting nurses in carrying out their responsibilities for educating clients as well as obstacles that interfere with learning. *Barriers* to education are those factors impeding the nurse's ability to deliver educational services. *Obstacles* to learning are those factors that negatively impact on the ability of the learner to attend to and process information. It is impossible to cite them all, but Cohen (1981), Close (1988), Gilroth (1990), Rifas et al. (1994), Walker (1987), Redman (1975), Ruzicki (1989), Honan et al. (1988), and Lipetz et al. (1990), in particular, have addressed some of the

major factors negatively influencing the teaching-learning process. For a thorough review of organizational, environmental, and clientele factors impacting on the delivery of education in health care, see Chapters 4, 6, and 13.

Barriers to Education

The following are the major barriers interfering with the ability of nurses to carry out their roles as educators:

1. Many nurses as well as other health-care personnel are traditionally ill prepared to teach. Studies have revealed that the principles of teaching and the concepts of learning are unclear to a large number of practicing nurses. Many nurses admit that they do not feel competent or confident with regard to their teaching skills. As cited previously, nursing education has for years failed to adequately prepare nurses for the role as educator, either during basic training or afterward. Although nurses are expected to teach, content in teaching and learning principles in nursing school curricula has been neglected, glossed over, or watered down as a result of its being integrated into and throughout programs of study. As early as the mid 1960s, Pohl (1965) found that one-third of the 1500 nurses questioned reported that they had no preparation for the teaching they were doing, while only one-fifth felt they had adequate preparation. More recently, Kruger (1991) surveyed 1230 nurses in staff, administrative, and education positions regarding their perceptions of the extent of nurses' responsibility for and level of achievement of patient education. Although all three groups strongly believed that patient education is a primary responsibility of nurses, in contrast, this author also found that patient education activities by nurses overall were rated as not being satisfactorily achieved. The findings of this research study indicate that the role of the nurse as patient educator needs to be strengthened.

2. There are a multitude of health-care providers covering much of the same content, but not necessarily with consistency. There seems to be a "malfunction" of the health-care team as a result of inadequate coordination and delegation of responsibility so that health teaching can proceed in a timely, smooth, organized, and thorough fashion. Content needs to be standardized, teaching responsibilities need to be made clear, and lines of communication must be strengthened among a wide variety of health-care providers.

3. Personal characteristics of the nurse educator play an important role in determining the outcome of a teaching-learning interaction. Motivation to teach is a prime factor in determining the success of an educational endeavor (see Chapter 11). Teaching by nurses sometimes is relegated to a low-priority status because of the physical, task-oriented nature of nursing care, the relatively minor importance assigned to teaching, and the lack of confidence on the part of practitioners in performing the teaching role.

4. Until recently, low priority was often assigned to patient and staff education by administration and supervisory personnel. With the new JCAHO mandates, the level of attention to the educational needs of consumers and health-care personnel is likely to change dramatically. However, budget allocations for educational programs still remain tight and can interfere with the adoption of innovative and timesaving teaching strategies and techniques.

5. Lack of time to teach is a major ongoing barrier. Very ill patients are hospitalized for only short periods of time; nurses' schedules and responsibilities are very demanding; and the movement toward community-based care often results in nurses and patients having fleeting contact with one another in emergency, outpatient, and other ambulatory care settings. The textbook approach to teaching has been the ideal but is no longer realistic. Nurses must know how to adopt an abbreviated, efficient, and expeditious approach to patient and staff education by using appropriate instructional methods and tools at their disposal. Discharge planning will play an ever more important role in ensuring continuity of care across settings.

6. The type of documentation system used by health-care agencies has an effect on the quality and quantity of patient teaching recorded. Both formal and informal teaching is often done but not documented because of the lack of ease of and inattention to documentation. Inadequate recording of teaching efforts impedes communication between health-care providers regarding what has been taught and raises the real possibility of legal liability of professionals.

Obstacles to Learning

The following are the major obstacles interfering with the learner's ability to attend to and process information:

1. The stress of acute and chronic illness, anxiety, sensory deficits, and low literacy in patients are just a few reasons that dampen learner motivation and interfere with the process of learning.

2. The negative impact of the hospital environment itself, resulting in loss of control, lack of privacy, and social isolation, can interfere with a client's active role in health decision making and involvement in the teaching-learning process.

3. Lack of time to learn due to rapid patient discharge from care can discourage and frustrate the learner, impeding the ability and willingness to learn.

4. Personal characteristics of the learner have a major impact on the degree of achieving predetermined behavioral outcomes. Readiness to learn, motivation and compliance, and learning styles are some of the prime factors influencing the success of educational endeavors.

5. The extent of behavioral changes needed, both in number and complexity, can overwhelm learners and dissuade them from attending to and accomplishing learning objectives and goals.

6. Lack of support and ongoing positive reinforcement from the nurse and significant others serves to block the potential for learning.

7. Denial of learning needs, resentment of authority, and lack of willingness to take responsibility (locus of control) are some psychological obstacles to accomplishing behavioral change.

8. The inconvenience, complexity, inaccessibility, fragmentation, and dehumanization of the health-care system often result in frustration and abandonment of efforts by the learner to participate in and comply with the goals and objectives for learning.

PERSPECTIVES ON RESEARCH IN PATIENT AND STAFF EDUCATION

The literature on patient and staff education is extensive from both a research- and nonresearch-based perspective. If one attempts to conduct a computer literature search in the library, for example, there are literally thousands of articles on teaching and learning available from the general to the specific. Luker and Caress (1989) reported that the nonresearch literature on patient education is prescriptive in nature and tends to give tips on "how to do" patient teaching, promoting individualized approaches to teaching and learning. In addition, the literature reveals that the psychological advantages of patient education are given more attention than the physiological outcomes. An increasing number of articles report pertinent research on teaching specific population groups, focusing on the needs of learners with short-term conditions as opposed to the learning needs of those suffering with long-term chronic illness. Studies from acute-care settings usually focus on preparing a patient for a procedure, with emphasis on the benefits of information to alleviate anxiety and promote psychological coping. Much more research must be conducted on the benefits of reducing stress by preparing patients for procedures as well as for managing independently at home through anticipatory teaching approaches. Evidence suggests that patients cope much more effectively when taught exactly what to expect (Smith, 1989).

More research is definitely needed on the availability of teaching methods and tools for both patient and staff education using the new technologies of computer-assisted instruction, distance learning, video- and audiotapes for home use, and cable television. Given the significant incidence of low literacy rates among patients and their family members, much more investigation needs to be done on learner comprehension of printed versus visual materials as well as written versus verbal instruction. Research on gender issues, the impact of socioeconomics on learning, and the strategies of teaching cultural groups and special populations is definitely in order. This text has attempted to address these subjects in much more detail than is typically found in other patient education resources. However, primary sources of information from nursing literature on the issues of gender and socioeconomic attributes of the learner are scanty, to say the least, and the findings from interdisciplinary research on the impact of gender on learning are still quite inconclusive.

In addition, further investigation should be undertaken to document the cost-effectiveness of educational efforts in reducing hospital stays, decreasing readmissions, improving the personal quality of life, and minimizing complications of illness and therapies. Furthermore, given the number of variables that potentially interfere with the teaching-learning process, additional studies must be conducted to examine the effects of environmental stimuli, the factors involved in readiness to learn, and the influences of learning styles on learner motivation, compliance, comprehension, and the ability to apply knowledge and skills once they are acquired. One particular void is the lack of information in the research database on how to assess motivation (Luker & Caress, 1989). The author of Chapter 6 proposes parameters to assess motivation but notes the paucity of information specifically addressing this issue.

Oberst (1989) delineated the major issues in patient education studies pertinent to the evaluation of the existing research base and the design of future studies. She identified four broad problem categories:

1. Selection and measurement of appropriate dependent variables (educational outcomes).
2. Design and control of independent variables (educational interventions).
3. Control of mediating and intervening variables.
4. Developing and refining the theoretical basis for research in education.

QUESTIONS TO BE ASKED REGARDING THE DELIVERY OF EDUCATIONAL SERVICES

In examining the elements of the education process and the role of the nurse as teacher, there are many questions that can be posed with respect to the principles of teaching and learning. Listed below are some of the important questions that the following chapters address:

- How can teaching be tailored to specific clientele?
- What determinants influence the learners' behaviors?
- What instructional methods and materials are available to support teaching efforts?
- How can the health-care team work together to coordinate educational efforts?
- What are the common mistakes made in the teaching of others?
- Under what conditions should certain teaching methods and materials be used?
- What can be done about the inequities (in quantity and quality) in the delivery of education services?
- What resources are available for education in various health-care settings?
- What are the theories and principles that support the education process?
- What are the ethical, legal, and economic issues involved in patient and staff education?
- What are the factors that negatively and positively influence patient and staff education efforts?
- What elements need to be taken into account when developing and implementing teaching plans?

SUMMARY

Nurses are considered information brokers—educators who can make a significant difference in how patients and families cope with their illnesses, how the public benefits from education directed at prevention of disease and promotion of health, and how staff nurses gain competency and confidence in practice through continuing education activities. There are many challenges and opportunities ahead for nurse educators in the delivery of health care as this nation moves into the twenty-first century. The foremost challenge for nurses is to be able to demonstrate, through research and action, that there is a definite link between education and positive behavioral outcomes of the learner. In this era of cost containment, government regulations, and health-care reform, the benefits of education must be made clear to the public, to health-care employers, as well as to other health-care providers, the insurance companies, and all employers as payors of health-care benefits. To be effective and efficient, nurses must be willing and able to work collaboratively with other members of the health-care team to provide consistently high-quality care to the consumer. The responsibility of nurses for the delivery of care to the consumer can be accomplished, in part, through education based on solid principles of teaching and learning. The key to effective education for patients, families, and nursing staff is the nurse's ongoing concern of and commitment to the role of educator.

References

Bell, J.A. (1986). The role of microcomputers in patient education. *Computers in Nursing, 4*(6), 255-258.

Chow, M.P., Durrand, B.A., Feldmann, M.N., & Mills, M.A. (1984). *Handbook on pediatric primary care*, 2nd ed. New York: Wiley.

Close, A. (1988). Patient education: A literature review. *Journal of Advanced Nursing, 13*, 203-213.

Cohen, S.A. (1981). Patient education: A review of the literature. *Journal of Advanced Nursing, 6*, 11-18.

Department of Health and Human Services. (1990). *Healthy people 2000: National health promotion and disease prevention objectives.* DHHS publication [PHS] 91-50212. Washington, DC: U.S. Government Printing Office.

Gilroth, B.E. (1990). Promoting patient involvement: Educational, organizational, and environmental strategies. *Patient Education and Counseling, 15*, 29-38.

Goldsmith, J.C. (1986). The U.S. health care system in the year 2000. *J.A.M.A., 256*(24), 3371-3375.

Health Services Medical Corporation, Inc. (1993). Wealth in wellness begins "Selfwise." *Worksite Wellnews, 1*(3), 1.

Honan, S., Krsnak, G., Petersen, D., & Torkelson, R. (1988). The nurse as patient educator: Perceived responsibilities and factors enhancing role development. *Journal of Continuing Education in Nursing, 19*(1), 33-37.

Jorgensen, C. (1994). Health education: What can it look like after health care reform? *Health Education Quarterly, 21*(1), 11-26.

Kellmer-Langan, D.M., Hunter, C., & Nottingham, J.P. (1992). Knowledge retention and clinical application after continuing education. *Journal of Nursing Staff Development, 8*(1), 5-10.

Kruger, S. (1991). The patient educator role in nursing. *Applied Nursing Research, 4*(1), 19-24.

Latter, S., Clark, J.M., Wilson-Barnett, J., & Maben, J. (1992). Health education in nursing: Perceptions of practice in acute settings. *Journal of Advanced Nursing, 17*, 164-172.

Lipetz, M.J., Bussigel, M.N., Bannerman, J., & Risley, B. (1990). What is wrong with patient education programs? *Nursing Outlook, 38*(4), 184-189.

Luker, K., & Caress, A.L. (1989). Rethinking patient education. *Journal of Advanced Nursing, 14*, 711-718.

McGinnis, J.M. (1993). The role of patient education in achieving national health objectives. *Patient Education and Counseling, 21*, 1-3.

McGoldrick, T.K., Jablonski, R.S., & Wolf, Z.R. (1994). Needs assessment for a patient education program in a nursing department: A delphi approach. *Journal of Nursing Staff Development, 10*(3), 123-130.

Narrow, B. (1979). *Patient teaching in nursing practice: A patient and family centered approach.* New York: Wiley.

National League of Nursing Education. (1937). *A curriculum guide for schools of nursing.* New York: The League.

Oberst, M.T. (1989). Perspectives on research in patient teaching. *Nursing Clinics of North America, 24*(2), 621-627.

Orr, R. (1990). Illness as an educational opportunity. *Patient Education and Counseling, 15*, 47-48.

PEW Health Professions Commission. (1995). *Critical challenges: Revitalizing the health professions for the twenty-first century*, The Third Report of the PEW Health Professions Commission. San Francisco: University of California.

Pohl, M.L. (1965). Teaching activities of the nursing practitioner. *Nursing Research, 14*(1), 4-11.

Redman, B.K. (1971). Patient education as a function of nursing practice. *Nursing Clinics of North America, 6*(4), 573-580.

Redman, B.K. (1975). Guidelines for quality of care in patient education. *The Canadian Nurse, 71*(2), 19-21.

Redman, B.K. (1993). *The process of patient education*, 7th ed. St. Louis: Mosby-Year Book.

Rega, M.D. (1993). A model approach for patient education. *MEDSURG Nursing, 2*(6), 477-479, 495.

Rifas, E., Morris, R., & Grady, R. (1994). Innovative approach to patient education. *Nursing Outlook, 42*(5), 214-216.

Ruzicki, D.A. (1989). Realistically meeting the educational needs of hospitalized acute and short-stay patients. *Nursing Clinics of North America, 24*(3), 629-636.

Smith, C.E. (1989). Overview of patient education: Opportunities and challenges for the twenty-first century. *Nursing Clinics of North America, 24*(3), 583-587.

Walker, A. (1987). Teaching the illiterate patient. *Journal of Enterostomal Therapy, 14*(2), 83-86.

Woody, A.F., Ferguson, S., Robertson, L.H., Mixon, M.L., Blocker, R., & McDonald, M.R. (1984). Do patients learn what nurses say they teach? *Nursing Management, 15*(12), 26-29.

CHAPTER 2

Ethical, Legal, and Economic Foundations of the Educational Process

M. Janice Nelson

CHAPTER HIGHLIGHTS

A Differentiated View of Ethics, Morality, and the Law

Evolution of Ethical and Legal Principles in Health Care

Application of Ethical and Legal Principles to Patient Education
   Autonomy
   Veracity
   Nonmalfeasance
   Confidentiality
   Beneficence
   Justice

Legality of Patient Education and Information

Documentation

A Graphic Summation

Economic Factors of Patient Education: Justice and Duty Revisited
   Financial Terminology
      Direct Costs
      Indirect Costs
   Cost Savings, Cost Benefit, and Cost Recovery
   Program Planning and Implementation
   Cost-Effectiveness and Cost-Benefit Analysis

Future Directions in Patient Education

KEY TERMS

ethical, legal, and moral rights and duties
cost recovery

cost savings
cost-benefit ratio

OBJECTIVES

After completing this chapter, the reader will be able to

1. Identify the six major ethical principles.
2. Distinguish between ethical and legal dimensions of the health-care delivery system, including patient education.
3. Describe the importance of nurse practice acts.
4. Describe the legal and financial implications of documentation.
5. Delineate the ethical, legal, and economic importance of federal, state, and accrediting body regulations and standards in the delivery of health-care services.
6. Differentiate among financial terms associated with development, implementation, and evaluation of patient education programs.
7. Identify trends in patient education.

Today as never before in the evolution of the health-care field, there is a critical consciousness of individual rights stemming from both natural and constitutional law. Health-care organizations are laden with laws and regulations insuring patients' rights to a quality standard of care, to the right of informed consent, and subsequently to the right of self-determination. Consequently, it is crucial that the providers of care be equally proficient in matters of educating the public as well as in matters of educating students or staff who are or will be the practitioner educators of tomorrow. Although the physician is primarily held legally accountable, it is a known fact that patient education generally falls to the nurse or some other appointed designee. Indeed, given the close relationship of nurse to patient, the role of the nurse in this educational process is absolutely essential and mandated as such through the varying state nurse practice acts.

We are indeed living in an age of an enlightened public that is more than aware of individual constitutional rights regarding freedom of choice and rights to self-determination. Thus it may seem curious to some that the federal government, state governments through their respective departments of health, professional organizations such as the American Hospital Association (AHA) and the

American Nurses' Association (ANA), and private sector organizations such as the Hastings Center and the Kennedy Institute for Bioethics find it necessary to legislate, regulate, or provide standards and guidelines to insure the protection of human rights when it comes to matters of health care. The answer of course is that the federal government abandoned its historical "hands-off" policy of physicians and the health professions in the wake of serious breaches of public confidence and shaking revelations of abuses of human rights in the name of biomedical research.

These issues of human rights are fundamental to the delivery of quality health-care services; they are equally fundamental to the education process in that the intent on the part of the educator should be one of freeing the student or the client to make informed choices and to be in control of the consequences of those choices regardless of the outcome. Thus, in explicating the role of the nurse in the teaching-learning process, it would be remiss to omit the ethical and legal foundations of that process. Also, in the interest of justice, which refers to equal distribution of benefits and burdens, it is important to include the relationship of cost to the provider institution in the provision of such services.

It is readily acknowledged that teaching and learning principles with their inherent legal and ethical dimensions apply to any situation where the educational process is occurring. However, the purpose of this chapter is to provide the ethical, legal, and economic foundations that justify the patient education initiative on the one hand and rights and responsibilities of the provider on the other. This chapter explores the differences between the concepts of ethical, moral, and legal; it explores the ethical and legal foundations of human rights; it reviews the ethical and legal dimensions of health care; it examines the importance of documentation of patient teaching efforts; and it analyzes the economic factors that must be considered in the delivery of patient education in health-care settings.

A DIFFERENTIATED VIEW OF ETHICS, MORALITY, AND THE LAW

Although ethics as a branch of classical philosophy has been studied across the centuries, by and large these studies were left to domains of the philosophical and religious thinkers. However, in these modern times of increased complexity of living in general, coupled with heightened awareness of an educated public, ethical issues related to health care have surfaced as a major concern of both health-care providers and recipients of these services. In the end, the deontological posture of Kant, or individual rights of clients prevail, whether this refers to diagnosis, treatment, and modalities of intervention or educating clients about their condition so that informed choices relative to that condition can be made—not by health professionals alone, but in concert with or by clients.

Ethical principles of human rights are rooted in natural laws, which, in the absence of any other, are binding on human society. Inherent in these natural laws are the principles of respect for parents, respect for others, truth telling, honesty, respect for life, purity of heart, and so on. Ethics as a discipline interprets these basic principles of behavior in broader terms and assumes argumentative discourse in favor of particular postures. Although there are multiple perspectives on the rightness or wrongness of human acts, the most commonly referenced are the writings of the sixteenth century philosopher Immanuel Kant, who promulgated the *deontological* notion of the "Golden Rule," and John Stuart Mill of the nineteenth century, who purported a *teleological* approach to ethical decision making, that is, that given alternatives, choices should be made that result in the greatest good for the greatest number of people.

Likewise, the legal system and its laws are based on ethical and moral principles that, through experience and over time, society has accepted as behavioral norms (Lesnick & Anderson, 1962). This accounts in part for the fact that the terms *ethical, moral,* and *legal* are so often used in synchrony. However, it should be clear that while these terms are certainly interrelated, they are not necessarily synonymous. *Ethical* refers to norms or standards of behavior. Although the term *moral* or *morality* is generally used interchangeably with *ethics,* one might differentiate by positing that *moral* refers to an internal value system (a certain "moral fabric") that is expressed externally in ethical behaviors. Ethical principles deal with moral values and are thus not enforceable by law, nor are these principles laws in and of themselves. What is *legal,* on the other hand, refers to rules governing behavior or conduct that are enforceable under threat of punishment or penalty, such as a fine, imprisonment, or both. The intricate relationship between ethics and the law explains why ethics terminology, such as informed consent, confidentiality, nonmalfeasance, or justice, can be found within the language of the legal system. In keeping with this train of thought, while nurses may cite professional commitment or moral obligation as the justification for patient education as one dimension of their role, in reality legitimation for this role stems from the nurse practice act in force in the particular state where the nurse resides, is licensed, and is employed. In essence, the nurse practice act not only is legally binding but also is protected by the police authority of the state in the interest of protecting the public.

EVOLUTION OF ETHICAL AND LEGAL PRINCIPLES IN HEALTH CARE

Just as in the past ethics was relegated to the philosophical and religious domains, so too, from a historical vantage point, medical and nursing care was considered a humanitarian if not charitable endeavor often provided by religious orders and others considered to be generous of spirit, caring in nature, and magnanimous, dedicated, and self-sacrificing in their service to others. Public sentiment was so strong in this regard that for many years, health-care organizations, considered as charitable institutions, were largely immune from legal action "because it would compel the charity to divert its funds for a purpose never intended" (Lesnik & Anderson, 1962, p. 211). In the same manner, health-care practitioners in the past—who were primarily physicians and nurses—were usually regarded as "Good Samaritans" who acted in "good faith."

Although there are numerous court records of lawsuits involving hospitals, physicians, and nurses dating back to the early 1900s, those numbers pale in contrast to the volumes being generated on a daily basis in today's world. Further, despite the horror stories that have been handed down through the years regarding inhumane and often torturous treatment of prisoners, the mentally infirm, the disabled, and the poor, there was limited focus in the past on ethical aspects of that "care," much less any thought of legal protection for the rights of such unfortunate human beings. Clearly all of this has changed. *Informed consent,* for example, which is a basic tenet of ethical thought, was established in the courts as early as 1914 by Justice Benjamin Cardozo. Cardozo determined that every adult of sound mind has a right to protect his or her own body and to determine how it shall be treated (Boyd, 1992). Although the Cardozo decision was of considerable magnitude, governmental interest in bioethical underpinnings of human rights in the delivery of health-care services did not really surface until after World War II.

Over the years, legal authorities such as federal and state governments maintained a hands-off posture when it came to issues of biomedical research or physician-patient relationships. However, human atrocities committed by the Nazis in the name of biomedical research during World War II shocked the world into critical awareness of gross violations of human rights. Nor were these abuses confined to wartime Germany. On American soil, the nontreatment of syphilitic blacks in Alabama, the injection of live cancer cells into nonconsenting elderly adults at the Brooklyn Chronic Disease Hospital, and the use of institutionalized mentally retarded children to test hepatitis vaccines at Willowbrook Developmental Center on Long Island, New York, shocked the nation and raised a critical consciousness of disturbing breaches in the physician-patient relationship (Weisbard & Arras, 1984).

Stirred to action by these disturbing phenomena, in 1974 Congress moved with all due deliberation to create the National Commission for the Protection of Human Subjects of Biomedical and Behavioral Research. From this unprecedented act, Institutional Review Boards for the Protection of Human Subjects (IRBPHS) were rapidly established at the local level. With primary emphasis on informed consent, confidentiality, and truth telling, and with specific concern for vulnerable populations such as infants, children, prisoners, and the mentally ill, every proposal for biomedical research today that involves human subjects must be submitted to a local IRBPHS for intensive review and approval in order to proceed with a study. Further, in its concern about the range of ethical issues associated with medical practice and a perceived need to regulate biomedical research, Congress established the President's Commission for the Study of Ethical Problems in Medicine and Biomedical and Behavioral Research (Weisbard & Arras, 1984).

Interestingly enough, as early as 1950, the ANA developed and adopted *Code for Nurses with Interpretative Statements*, which was revised in 1976 and again in 1985. This code represents an articulation of professional values and moral obligations in relation to the nurse-patient relationship and in support of the profession and its mission.

Whether coincidental or deliberate, in 1975 the AHA followed suit through the dissemination of a document entitled *Patient's Bill of Rights* (Boyd, 1992; Aleksandrowicz & Norcross, 1984). A copy of these patient rights are framed and posted in a public place in every hospital across the United States. Furthermore, federal standards of the Health Care Financing Administration (HCFA) require that the patient is provided with a personal copy of these rights either at the time of admission to the hospital or long-term care facility or prior to the initiation of care of treatment when admitted to an HMO, home care, or a hospice. As a matter of fact, many states have adopted the statement of patient rights as part of the state health code, which in turn places these rights under the jurisdiction of the law and are therefore legally enforceable under threat of penalty.

APPLICATION OF ETHICAL AND LEGAL PRINCIPLES TO PATIENT EDUCATION

In considering the ethical and legal responsibilities inherent in the patient education process, the six major ethical principles intricately woven through the ANA *Code for Nurses* and the AHA *Patient's Bill of Rights* are the same principles that encompass the very issues that precipitated federal intervention into health-care affairs. These principles are autonomy, veracity, confidentiality, nonmalfeasance, beneficence, and justice.

Autonomy

In considering the principle of *autonomy,* for example, laws have been enacted to protect the patient's right to self-determination. Federal mandates regarding informed consent are evident in every application for federal funding to support biomedical research. The local IRBPHS assumes the role of judge and jury to ascertain adherence to these enforceable regulations. The Patient Self-Determination Act (PSDA) enacted by Congress, which became effective December 1, 1991, is a second example of autonomy enacted into law. Any health-care facility, including acute- and long-term care, HMOs, hospice, home care, and so on, that is receiving Medicare and/or Medicaid funds is subject to adherence to the PSDA. The law requires, either at the time of hospital admission or prior to the initiation of care or treatment in an HMO, hospice, or home-care program, "that every individual receiving health care be informed in writing of the right under state law to make decisions about his or her health care, including the right to refuse medical and surgical care and the right to initiate advance directives" (Mezey et al., 1994, p. 30). Mezey et al. (1994) readily acknowledge the nurse's responsibility to ensure informed decision making by patients, which includes but is certainly not limited to advance directives (e.g., living wills, durable power of attorney). Documenta-

tion of such instruction must appear in the patient record, which is the legal document validating that such instruction took place.

A principle worth noting in the ANA *Code for Nurses* (1985, p. 16) is that addressing collaboration "with members of the health professions and other citizens in promoting community and national efforts to meet the health needs of the public." Although not so specified in the ANA document, this principle certainly provides a justification for patient education both within and external to the health-care organization. It provides an ethical rationale for health education classes open to the community such as childbirth education courses, smoking cessation classes, weight reduction sessions, discussions on women's health issues, positive interventions for child abuse, and many more. While health education per se is not an interpretive part of the principle of autonomy, it certainly lends credence to the ethical notion of assisting the public to attain greater autonomy when it comes to matters of health promotion and high-level wellness. In fact, consistent with the *Model Nurse Practice Act,* published by the ANA in 1978, most contemporary nurse practice acts contain a statement identifying *health education* as a *legal duty or responsibility* of the registered nurse.

Veracity

Veracity, or truth telling, is closely linked with informed decision making and informed consent. The Cardozo landmark decision (*Schloendorff v. Society of New York Hospitals*) regarding an individual's fundamental right to make decisions about his (or her) own body provides a basis in law for patient education or instruction regarding invasive medical procedures including the truth regarding risks or benefits involved in these procedures (Whitman et. al., 1992). Nurses are often confronted with issues of truth telling, as was exemplified in the *Tuma* case (Rankin & Stallings, 1990), which emerged from issues surrounding the concept of full disclosure of information to the patient. Tuma was eventually exonerated from professional misconduct charges, but the case emphasized a significant point of law to be found in the *New York State Nurse Practice Act* (1972), for one, that states, "A nursing regimen shall be consistent with and shall not vary any existing medical regimen." In some instances, this creates a double bind for the nurse. This is so because Creighton (1986) is very emphatic in making the point that failure or omission to properly instruct the patient relative to invasive procedures is tantamount to battery.

Yet another dimension of the legality of truth telling lies in the role of the nurse as expert witness. Professional nurses who are recognized for their skill or expertise in a particular area of nursing practice may be called on to testify in court on behalf of either the plaintiff (one who initiates the litigation) or the defendant (the one being sued). The concept of expert testimony speaks for itself—to tell the truth.

Nonmalfeasance

Nonmalfeasance, the principle of "do no harm," is the ethical fabric of legal determinations encompassing malpractice or negligence. According to Lesnik and Anderson (1962), "The term *negligence* is intended to refer to the doing or nondoing of an act, pursuant to a duty, that a reasonable person in the same circumstances would or would not do and the acting or the nonacting is the proximate cause of injury to another person or his property" (p. 234). The term *malpractice*, on the other hand, "refers to a limited class of negligent activities committed within the scope of performance by those pursuing a particular profession involving highly skilled and technical services" (Lesnik & Anderson, 1962, p. 234). It can be said, then, that malpractice is limited in scope to those whose life work requires special education and training as dictated by specific educational standards, whereas negligence embraces all improper and wrongful conduct by anyone arising out of any activity.

The concept of *duty* is closely tied to the concepts of malpractice and negligence. Nurses' duties are spelled out in job descriptions at places of employment. Policy and procedure manuals of a particular facility exist certainly to protect the patient, but they also exist to protect the employee (nurse) and the facility against litigation. Policies are more than guidelines. Policies and procedures

determine standards of behavior (duties) expected of employees of a particular employing institution and can be used in court in the determination of negligence. Expectations of professional nursing performance are also measured against the nurse's level of education and concomitant skills, standing orders and protocols, standards of care promulgated by the profession (ANA), and standards of care promulgated by the various clinical specialty organizations of which the nurse may be a member (Yoder Wise, 1995). If the nurse is certified in a clinical specialty or identifies herself as a "specialist" although not certified, he or she will be held to the standards of that specialty (Smith, 1987).

In the instance of litigation, the key operational principle is that the nurse is not measured against the optimal or maximum of professional standards of performance; rather, the yardstick is laid against the prevailing practice of what a prudent and reasonable nurse would do under the same circumstances in a given community. Thus, the nurse's duty of patient education (or lack thereof) is measured not only against prevailing policy of the employing institution but also against prevailing practice in the community. In the case of clinical nurse specialists (CNSs), nurse practitioners (NPs), or clinical education specialists (CESs), for example, the practice is measured against institutional policies for this level of worker as well as against prevailing practice of nurses performing at the same level in the community or in the same geographic region.

Confidentiality

Confidentiality refers to privileged information or to a social contract or covenant in legal terms. The nurse-patient relationship is considered as privileged in most states. This means that the nurse may not disclose information acquired in a professional capacity from a patient without the consent of the patient ". . . unless the patient has been the victim or subject of a crime, the commission of which is the subject of legal proceeding in which the nurse is a witness" (Lesnik & Anderson, 1962, p. 48). In recent years, the diagnosis of aquired immune deficiency syndrome (AIDS) has been protected as privileged and confidential by state laws, regardless of the fact that AIDS is a communicable disease. It is a fairly recent development in some states that under certain conditions, such as death or impending death, members of the family or a spouse can be apprised of the patient's condition if this were previously unknown. The question of the moral obligation of the person with AIDS to divulge his or her condition remains largely unresolved.

Beneficence

The principle of *beneficence* (do good) is legalized through adherence to critical tasks and duties contained in job descriptions, adherence to policies, procedures, and protocols set forth by the health-care facility, and adherence to standards and codes of ethical behaviors established and promulgated by professional nursing organizations. Adherence to these various professional performance criteria and principles, including adequate and current patient education, speaks to the nurse's commitment to acting in the best interest of the patient. Such behavior emphasizes patient welfare and deemphasizes the provision of quality care under threat of litigation.

Justice

Justice speaks to fairness and equal distribution of goods and services. The law *is* the "Justice System." The focus of the law is the protection of society; the focus of health law is the protection of the consumer. As noted earlier, adherence to the *Patient's Bill of Rights* is legally enforced in most states. This means that the nurse or any other health professional can be subjected to penalty or to litigation for *discrimination* in provision of care because of, for example, a lack of proper instruction regarding risks and benefits of invasive medical procedures or a lack of proper instruction regarding self-care activities related to healthy well-being (such as home dialysis) that are beyond normal activities of daily living of normal, healthy human beings.

Furthermore, when a nurse is employed by a particular health-care facility, he or she enters into a contract, written or tacit, to provide nursing services in accordance with the policies of the facility. Failure to provide nursing care (including educational services) based on patient diagnosis (e.g., AIDS) or persistence in providing substandard care based on patient diagnosis, culture, na-

tional origin, sexual preference, and the like can result in liability for *breach of contract* with the employing institution.

LEGALITY OF PATIENT EDUCATION AND INFORMATION

The patient's right to adequate information regarding his or her physical condition, medications, risks, and access to information regarding alternative treatments is clearly spelled out in the AHA's *Patient's Bill of Rights* (1975). As stated earlier, many states have adopted these rights as part of their health code, thus rendering the rights legal and enforceable by law. Patients' rights to education and instruction are also regulated by way of *standards* promulgated by accrediting bodies such as the Joint Commission on Accreditation of Healthcare Organizations (JCAHO). Although these standards are not enforceable in the same manner as law, lack of organizational conformity can lead to loss of accreditation, which in turn jeopardizes the facility's eligibility for third-party reimbursement, as well as loss of Medicare and Medicaid reimbursement. Secondly, *state regulations* pertaining to patient education are published and enforced under threat of penalty (fine, citation, or both) by the Department of Health in many states. New York, for one, is heavily regulated in this regard. Thirdly, *federal regulations,* enforceable as laws, mandate patient education in those health-care facilities receiving Medicare and Medicaid funding. As discussed earlier, the federal government also mandates full patient disclosure in cases of participation in biomedical research in any setting or for any federally funded project or experimental research involving human subjects.

Although federal authorities have generally tended to hold physicians responsible and accountable for proper patient education, particularly as this pertains to issues of informed consent (*Scakia v. St. Paul Fire and Marine Ins. Co.,* 1975 [Smith, 1987]), it is a well-known fact that at least in hospitals this task usually falls to the nurse or some other facility-appointed designee. Physicians' responsibility notwithstanding, from a professional and legal vantage point, nurses are fully legitimized in their role of patient educator by virtue of their respective nurse practice acts. The issue regarding patient education is not usually one of omission on anyone's part; rather, at the heart of the matter is the issue of proper documentation or lack thereof that education occurred.

DOCUMENTATION

The 89th Congress enacted the Comprehensive Health Planning Act in 1965 (Public Law 89-97, 1965). The entitlements of Medicare and Medicaid—which revolutionized health-care provision for the elderly and the poor—were established through this act. One of the acknowledgments in the act was the importance of preventive and rehabilitative dimensions of health care. Thus, to qualify for Medicare and Medicaid reimbursement, "a hospital has to show evidence that patient education has been a part of patient care" (Boyd, 1992, p. 21). For at least the past 20 years, the JCAHO (formerly JCAH) has reinforced the federal mandate by requiring evidence (documentation) of patient and/or family education in the patient record. Pertinent to this point is the doctrine of *respondeat superior*, or the "master-servant" rule. *Respondeat superior* provides that the employer may be held liable for negligence, assault and battery, false imprisonment, slander, libel, or any other tort committed by an employee (Lesnik & Anderson, 1962). The landmark case supporting the doctrine of *respondeat superior* in the health-care field was the 1965 case of *Darling v. Charleston Memorial Hospital.* In essence, while the *Darling* case dealt with negligence in the performance of professional duties of the physician, it brought out, possibly for the first time, the professional obligations or duties of nurses to ensure the well-being of the patient.

Haggard (1989) points out that of all omissions in documentation, patient teaching "is probably the most undocumented skilled service because nurses do not recognize the scope and depth of the teaching they do" (p. 144). Lack of documentation also reflects negligence in adhering to the mandates of the particular nurse practice act. This is unfortunate when considering that patient records can be subpoenaed for court evidence. Appropriate documentation can be the determining factor in the outcome of litigation. Pure and sim-

ple, if the instruction isn't documented, instruction didn't occur! Further, documentation is a vehicle of communication that provides critical information to other health-care professionals involved with the patient's care. Failure to document not only renders other staff potentially liable but also renders the facility liable and in jeopardy of losing JCAHO accreditation, as well as possibly losing appropriate Medicare and Medicaid reimbursement to the institution. In any litigation where the doctrine of *respondeat superior* is applied, outcomes can hold the organization liable for damages (monetary retribution). Thus, it behooves the nurse as both employee and professional not only to provide patient education but also to document it appropriately and be critically conscious of the legal and financial ramifications to the health-care facility in which he or she is employed.

A GRAPHIC SUMMATION

In consideration of the amount of material presented in this section, a visual representation of the linkages between ethical principles and the law is displayed in Table 2–1. It should be noted that the *Patient's Bill of Rights* is linked to or associated with every ethical principle. The *Patient's Bill of Rights* (1975) is rooted in the conditions of participation in Medicare set forth under federal standards of the Health Care Financing Administration (HCFA), which are further emphasized by corresponding accreditation standards promulgated by JCAHO. All serve to insure the fundamental rights of every person as a consumer of health-care services.

ECONOMIC FACTORS OF PATIENT EDUCATION: JUSTICE AND DUTY REVISITED

Some might consider the parameters of health-care economics and finances as objective information that can be utilized for any number of purposes, for example, fiscal solvency and/or forecasting of economic growth of an organization. Others would agree that in addition to the legality of adherence to regulations in health care regardless of the economics involved, there is also an ethical dimension

TABLE 2–1.   Linkages between ethical principles and the law

Ethical Principles	Legal Actions/Decisions
Autonomy (self-determination)	Cardozo decision regarding informed consent Institutional review boards Patient Self-Determination Act *Patient's Bill of Rights* JCAHO/HCFA standards
Veracity (truth telling)	Cardozo decision regarding informed consent *Patient's Bill of Rights* *Tuma* decision JCAHO/HCFA standards
Confidentiality (social contract)	Privileged information *Patient's Bill of Rights* JCAHO/HCFA standards
Nonmalfeasance (do no harm)	Malpractice/negligence rights and duties Nurse Practice Acts *Patient's Bill of Rights* *Darling v. Charleston Memorial Hospital* State health codes JCAHO/HCFA standards
Beneficence (do good)	*Patient's Bill of Rights* State health codes Job descriptions Standards of Practice Policy and procedure manuals JCAHO/HCFA standards
Justice (equal distribution of benefits and burdens)	*Patient's Bill of Rights* Antidiscrimination/Affirmative Action laws Americans with Disabilities Act JCAHO/HCFA standards

that speaks certainly to quality of care, but also to justice. Justice refers to equal distribution of goods and services. In the interest of patient care, the client as human being has a right to quality care regardless of economic status, national origin, race, and the like, and health professionals have a duty to see to it that such services are provided. In like manner, the health-care organization has the right to expect that it will receive its fair share of reimbursable revenues for services rendered. Thus, as an employee of the provider organization, the nurse has a duty to carry out organizational policies and mandates by acting in an accountable and responsible manner. This includes assuming fiscal accountability for patient education activities,

whether these are offered on an inpatient basis or offered as a service to the larger community.

The principle of justice is a critical consideration within the discourse on patient education. The rapid changes and trends so evident in the contemporary health-care arena are described as chaotic by some and are, in many ways, defying the humanistic and charitable underpinnings that have characterized health-care services in this country across the decades. Indeed, health-care organizations are caught between the horns of a dilemma. On the one hand, the realities of capitation and managed care mean shrinking revenues, which in turn dictate shorter patient stays in hospitals and doing more with less while concomitantly expanding clinical services into outpatient and home care.

On the other hand, these same organizations are held to the exact standards of care that are underwritten by the *Patient's Bill of Rights* (AHA, 1975), which are regulated as a contingency of Medicare and Medicaid participation by the federal HCFA and for agency accreditation by the JCAHO. In turn, although there are some exceptions (e.g., home health-care agencies), hospital accreditation in particular dictates eligibility for third-party reimbursement in both the public and private sectors.

Over and above the financial facts, these same "charitable," not-for-profit organizations no longer enjoy the legal immunity that existed in yesteryear. The doctrine of *respondeat superior* is alive and well. Embedded in a Supreme Court decision stemming from *Abernathy v. Sisters of St. Mary's* in 1969, "the court held that a 'non-governmental charitable institution is liable for its own negligence and the negligence of its agents and employees acting within the scope of their employment'" (Strader, 1985, p. 364). The court further declared that this ruling would apply to all future cases as of November 10, 1969. Thus the regulated right of clients to health education carries a corresponding duty of health-care organizations to provide that service. In an environment of shrinking health-care dollars, shrinking nursing staffs, and shortened lengths of stay, the organization is challenged to ensure the competency of nursing staff to provide educational services and to do so in the most efficient and cost-effective manner possible. This is an interesting dilemma when considering the fact that patient health education is invariably identified as a legal responsibility of registered nurses in the respective nurse practice acts of most states, yet few pre-baccalaureate education programs can adequately prepare nursing students for this critical function—if the respective programs prepare them at all. Consequently, it seems important here to provide an overview of fiscal terminology that directly impacts both staff and patient education.

Financial Terminology

First of all, *no* health-care service is provided (education or otherwise) without an accompanying cost of human and material resources. Thus, it is important to know that costs are divided into two categories: *direct* and *indirect*.

Direct Costs

Chief among direct costs are *personnel salaries* and *employment benefits*. This portion of an organizational budget is always the largest and usually accounts for 70% to 80% of the total predictable expenditure of any health-care facility. Within this framework, because of its labor-intensive function, the division of nursing is apportioned the largest budgetary amount—usually 50% of the total or better. And, of course, the higher the educational level of nursing staff, the higher the cost.

Equipment is also categorized under direct cost. Regardless of individual ingenuity, health-care organizations obviously cannot function without equipment and its necessary replacement when indicated. In the same manner, educational functions cannot generally be operationalized without proper audiovisual equipment, such as overhead projectors, slide projectors, blackboards, copying machines, computer terminals, and the like. Coupled with this is the need for supplies with which to operate the equipment or simply to function in accordance with one's job responsibilities. Although there may be times when rental or leasing of equipment is less expensive than purchase, rental and leasing costs are still categorized as direct costs.

Time is a direct cost. Although in a technical sense the purpose of salary is to buy employee time along with the benefit of his or her particular expertise, it is often difficult to predict the amount of time it will actually take to plan, implement, and evaluate various educational programs. If planning, for example, exceeds the allocated time allowed and the employee gets into "overtime," although the employee sees an increase in his or her paycheck, the extra cost may not have been anticipated or planned for in the budget planning process. Time then becomes one of the major factors considered in a cost-benefit analysis. In other words, if the cost of salaries and the time it takes to prepare and offer patient education programs is greater than the equivalent financial gain to the institution (e.g., no change in patient length of stay), the facility may look to other ways of providing the educational offering, such as programmed instruction via computer or a patient television channel.

Direct costs are also fixed or variable. *Fixed costs* are those that are predictable and remain the same over time. Fixed costs are controllable. Salaries, for example, are fixed costs, and they are also controllable. The facility usually makes an annual determination to give employee raises; by the same token, a decision can be made not only to freeze salaries but also to cut positions and thereby cut costs. Utilities such as heat, light, and air-conditioning are fixed costs, as are mortgages, loan repayments, and the like.

Variable costs are those that, in the case of health-care organizations, depend on volume. The number of meals prepared, for example, depends on the patient census. From an educational vantage point, the demand for diabetic instruction depends in large part on the volume of diabetic patients. If volume is low in a particular facility, cost may be high due to the fact that the request may be so rare that a new program needs to be redesigned or readapted each time a diabetic patient is admitted to the facility. Likewise, if the volume of diabetic patients is high, it is less costly to standardize programs of instruction for the diabetic clientele. Although a direct cost, requirements for supplies can also vary depending on volume. Variable costs can become fixed costs when volume remains consistently high over time, which may warrant the addition of personnel and possibly volume purchasing.

Indirect Costs

Indirect costs are those that may be fixed but are not directly related to the actual delivery of an educational program. These include but are certainly not limited to institutional overhead such as heating or cooling, light, space, and support services of maintenance, housekeeping, security, and equipment.

Hidden costs are those that can neither be anticipated nor accounted for until after the fact. Low employee productivity can produce hidden costs. Organizational budgets are prepared on the basis of what is known and predictable, with projections for variability included. Personnel budgets are based on division of labor (e.g., *x* number of RNs, *x* number of LPNs, and *x* number of nursing assistants) to accommodate the predicted patient

volume, as determined by the predicted number of patient days and the number and classification of patient-care hours. There is an underlying assumption of employee productivity that is commensurate with the predicted workload. Low productivity of one (or more) on a nursing unit, for example, can have a direct impact on the workload of others. This in turn can affect morale, which has the potential of precipitating turnover. Turnover has an inherent ripple effect of increasing recruitment and new employee orientation costs. In this respect, the costs are appropriately identified as "hidden."

Cost Savings, Cost Benefit, and Cost Recovery

Although mandated by laws and standards, for all intents and purposes, patient education costs are generally not recoverable. Although the cost of educational programs is a legitimate expense to the institution, unless specifically ordered by the physician, patient education is not recoverable under third-party reimbursement as a separate entity. Rather, the cost is subsumed under the room rate and is therefore technically absorbed by the health-care facility. Additionally, under DRGs (diagnosis-related groups: reimbursement based on diagnosis), managed care, and capitation (reimbursement tied to number of "heads," i.e., number of patients), the effectiveness of patient education becomes critical to the ability of the patient to understand and carry out what is required of him or her in order to be discharged safely within the time frame allocated for a cost savings to the agency.

Cost savings are realized when hospital stays are shortened or fall within the DRG length of stay, when patients sustain fewer complications, and when utilization of expensive services decrease, thus reducing hospital costs. In an ambulatory setting such as an HMO, cost savings are realized when patient education keeps people healthy longer, thus controlling or preventing high utilization of expensive diagnostic testing or inpatient services.

Cost benefit is a result of increased patient satisfaction stemming from educational programs. In this era of "capturing" a patient population for lifetime coverage, patient satisfaction is critical to his or her return for future health-care services.

Cost recovery results when either the patient or insurer pays a fee for service for the educational services provided.

To offset the dilemma of striving for cost containment and solvency in an environment of shrinking fiscal resources, health-care organizations have developed alternative strategies for patient education to realize cost savings, cost benefit, or cost recovery. Kosik and Reynolds (1986), for example, describe a preoperative teaching program for scheduled surgical patients prior to admission to the hospital. Reported outcomes or cost savings as well as cost benefit to the institution are decreased patient anxiety, increased patient satisfaction, and decreased nursing hours. Wasson and Anderson (1993) describe other innovative programs designed for cost benefit such as the "Teddy Bear Clinic" operated at Flint (Michigan) Osteopathic Hospital. Children were invited to bring their teddy bears in for a "checkup," which provided the opportunity for some health education for the children. The children were subsequently toured through the pediatric unit, with the overall goal of reducing their fears by acquainting them with common hospital equipment as well as the general design of the pediatric unit, should any of the children eventually require hospitalization.

Cost recovery is realized through the marketing of health education programs offered for a fee (fee for service). Haggard (1989) provides a lengthy description of how and under what circumstances costs can be recovered for patient education. Under Medicare and Medicaid guidelines, for example, reimbursement may be made for programs "furnished by providers of services to the extent that the programs are appropriate, integral parts in the rendition of covered services which are reasonable and necessary for the treatment of the individual's illness or injury"(*Medicare and Medicaid Guide,* 1986, p. 9023). Haggard (1989) further explains that in some states Blue Cross/Blue Shield will allow for outpatient diabetic education if such programs follow guidelines or standards set by reputable organizations such as the Association of Diabetic Educators. The key to success in obtaining third-party reimbursement is the ability to demonstrate that the patients take better care of themselves and consequently experience fewer hospitalizations (Haggard, 1989).

The final suggestion for cost recovery is the development and marketing of a cadre of health education programs that are open to all consumers in the community such as childbirth education, smoking cessation, or weight control classes. The critical element, of course, is not only the recovery of costs but also the *generation of revenue.*

Program Planning and Implementation

The key elements to consider when planning a patient education offering intended for generation of revenue include an accurate assessment of material costs such as paper supplies, duplication or printing of program brochures, publicity, and rental space in which to offer the program, should this be required. It is essential that the time of professional personnel required to prepare and offer the program be included. If an hourly rate of annual salary is unknown, a simple rule of thumb is to divide the annual base salary by 2080, which is the standard number of hours worked by most people in the course of a year. If the program is to be offered on the premises of the institution, there may be no need to plan for a space rental fee; however, indirect costs such as housekeeping and security should be prorated as a bona fide cost of the program. (Such a practice is not only good fiscal management, but it also provides an accounting of the contributions of other departments to the educational efforts of the facility.)

Fees for the program should be set at a level high enough to cover the aggregate costs of program preparation and delivery. If the interest is of cost benefit to the facility, such as provision of diabetic education classes for diabetics in the community to reduce the number of costly hospital admissions, then the goal may be to cover costs only. The fee is set by dividing the number of anticipated attendees into the calculated cost. On the other hand, if the intent is to offer a 7-week program for smoking cessation or a 6-week childbirth education program in the interest both of improving the wellness of the community and of revenue generation for the facility, then the fee is set higher than cost in order to realize a profit.

Over the course of a year, it is usually necessary to give an accounting of how the time of educational personnel was spent and whether such time allocation was of benefit to the institution.

Cost benefit to the institution can be measured, for example, by increased patient satisfaction as determined by patient satisfaction questionnaires, decreased hospitalizations of the diabetic population, or an increase in utilization of obstetrical services.

Cost-Effectiveness and Cost-Benefit Analysis

In the majority of health-care organizations, the department of staff development bears the major responsibility for staff education and training and for patient education programs that exceed the boundaries of bedside instruction. Total budget preparation for these departments is best explained by the experts in the field (Abruzzese, 1992; Kelly, 1985; del Bueno & Kelly, 1980).

There is no one single best method to determine the effectiveness of patient education programs. Most experts in the field tend to differentiate between cost benefit and cost-effectiveness (Kelly, 1985). *Cost benefit* refers to the relationship between costs and outcomes. Outcomes can be actual revenue generated as a result of an educational offering, or outcomes can be expressed in terms of shorter patient stays or reduced hospitalizations for particular diagnostic groupings of patients. Under DRGs or capitation methods of reimbursement, the institution realizes a cost savings that can be expressed in monetary terms. If the cost of an educational offering is less than the revenue generated, if costs are recoverable under third-party reimbursement, or if costs are less than savings to the facility, the program is categorized as a cost benefit. The measurement of costs against monetary benefits is commonly referred to as the *cost-benefit ratio.*

Cost-effectiveness, on the other hand, refers to the efficiency of an educational offering. If program objectives are achieved and there is a *reliable measure of positive change in behavior* of the participants and *reliable evidence of maintenance of these behaviors,* the program is determined to be cost-effective. Although behavioral changes are highly desirable, they are in many respects less tangible. For example, reduction in patient anxiety cannot be measured in real

dollars. Therefore, a comparative analysis of behavioral outcomes should be made between two or more programs to determine the one that is most cost-effective. Changes in the philosophical posture of many health-care organizations would dictate that those programs that realize a cost benefit are the most desirable. Thus, as difficult as it may be from the standpoint of justice, it behooves the nurse educator to attempt to interpret behavioral changes in terms of cost savings to the institution.

FUTURE DIRECTIONS IN PATIENT EDUCATION

It is a known fact that hospitals and other health-care organizations have had a long-standing commitment to patient education. This process as we have known it has usually occurred at the bedside, in clinic waiting rooms, or in groups on the hospital premises. Some of this familiar educational process will certainly continue because it plays an important role in discharge planning for the patient and in the long run is cost-effective for the institution. At the same time, in the interest of conservation of time and resources, patient educators have utilized newer technologies to accomplish tasks associated with patient education. Closed-circuit television is one good example. Although it has its limitations, this modality has become a common, useful tool to disseminate patient information. Patients can remain in their rooms during the presentation, and it releases nursing personnel for other duties when they might otherwise be involved with live demonstrations of baby baths or preparation of insulin for injection. Drawbacks of closed-circuit TV include the fact that it is usually fixed; that is, the programs are usually offered at a specified time of day or evening, which may not be conducive to particular patient learning. Also, if there is no follow-up, it is near impossible to determine whether the programmed instruction is effective.

Meanwhile, experts in the field (Wasson & Anderson, 1993; Abruzzese, 1992; Anderson, 1990; Haggard, 1989; Smith, 1987) all predict that patient education will take on new dimensions in one way or another. These dimensions include but are not limited to the following:

- Most teaching will occur in the outpatient setting.
- Use of computerized instruction for hospital, ambulatory care settings, physicians' offices, or home will increase.
- Utilization of interactive video programs will increase.
- Wellness screening programs will increase.
- Emphasis on nutrition, diet, and exercise, with various accompanying educational offerings will increase.
- Interorganizational linkages to enhance cooperative endeavors in the patient education enterprise will increase.
- Third-party reimbursement will increase as cost-benefit ratios demonstrate cost-effectiveness of consumer education.

SUMMARY

Ethical and legal dimensions of human rights provide the justification for patient education, particularly as this relates to issues of self-determination and informed consent. These rights are enforced through federal and state regulations and through performance standards promulgated by accrediting bodies for implementation at the local level. The nurse's role as educator is legitimized through the definition of nursing practice as set forth by the prevailing nurse practice act in the state where the nurse is licensed and is employed. In this respect, patient education is a nursing *duty* that is grounded in *justice;* that is, the nurse has a *legal responsibility* to provide patient education, and regardless of culture, race, ethnicity, and so forth, all clients have a *right* to health education relevant to their physical aberration or condition. Justice also dictates that education programs should be designed to be consistent with organizational goals while meeting the needs of patients to be informed, self-directed, and in control of their own health-care needs.

References

Abernathy v. Sisters of St. Mary's, 446 SW2d 559 (MO 1969).

Abruzzese, R.S. (1992). *Nursing staff development: Strategies for success.* St. Louis: Mosby.

Aleksandrowicz, L.I., & Norcross, S. (1984). *Nurse administrator's desk reference.* Owings Mills, MD: Rynd Communications.

Anderson, C. (1990). *Patient teaching and communicating in an information age.* Albany, NY: Delmar.

Boyd, M.D. (1992). Policies, guidelines, and legal mandates for health teaching. In N.I. Whitman, B.A. Graham, C.J. Gleit, & M.D. Boyd (Eds.), *Teaching in nursing practice: A professional model* (pp. 17-30). Norwalk, CT: Appleton & Lange.

Code for Nurses with Interpretative Statements (1976, 1985). Kansas City, MO: American Nurses' Association.

Creighton, H. (1986). Informed consent. *Nursing Management, 17*(10), 11-13.

Darling v. Charleston Memorial Hospital, 211 NE2d 253 (IL 1965).

del Bueno, D., & Kelly, K. (1980). How cost-effective is your staff development program? *Journal of Nursing Administration, 10*(4), 31.

Haggard, A. (1989). *Handbook of patient education.* Rockville, MD: Aspen.

Kelly, K.J. (Spring 1985). Cost-benefit and cost-effectiveness analysis: Tools for the staff development manager. *Journal of Nursing Staff Development, 6*(2), 9-15.

Kosik, S.L., & Reynolds, P.J. (Winter 1986). A nursing contribution to cost containment: A group preoperative teaching program that shortens hospital stay. *Journal of Nursing Staff Development, 5*(1), 18-22.

Lesnick, M.J., & Anderson, B.E. (1962). *Nursing practice and the law.* Philadelphia: Lippincott.

Medicare and Medicaid Guide. (1986). Washington, DC: U.S. Government Printing Office (p. 9023).

Mezey, M., Evans, L.K., Golub, Z.D., Murphy, E., & White, G.B. (1994). The patient self-determination act: Sources of concern for nurses. *Nursing Outlook, 42*(1), 30-38.

Model Nurse Practice Act (1978). Kansas City, MO: American Nurses' Association.

New York State Nurse Practice Act. (1972). Albany, NY: New York State Nurses' Association.

Patient's Bill of Rights. (1975). Chicago: American Hospital Association.

Rankin, S.H., & Stallings, K.D. (1990). *Patient education: Issues, principles, practices.* Philadelphia: Lippincott.

Smith, C.E. (1987). *Patient education: Nurses in partnership with other health professionals*. Philadelphia: Saunders.

Strader, M.K. (1985). Malpractice and nurse educators: Defining legal responsibilities. *Journal of Nursing Education, 24*(9), 363-367.

Wasson, D., & Anderson, M.A. (1993). Hospital-patient education: Current status and future trends. *Journal of Nursing Staff Development, 10*(3), 147-151.

Weisbard, A.J., & Arras, J.D. (1984). Commissioning morality: An introduction to the symposium. *Cardozo Law Review, 6*(4), 223-241.

Whitman, N.I., Graham, B.A., Gleit, C.J., & Noyd, M.D. (1992). *Teaching in nursing practice: A professional model*. Norwalk, CT: Appleton & Lange.

Yoder Wise, P.S. (1995). *Leading and managing in nursing*. St. Louis: Mosby.

CHAPTER 3

Learning Theory and Nursing Practice

Margaret M. Braungart
Richard G. Braungart

CHAPTER HIGHLIGHTS

KEY TERMS

learning	behaviorist learning
respondent conditioning	operant conditioning
cognitive learning	gestalt perspective
information-processing perspective	cognitive development perspective
social cognition perspective	social learning
psychodynamic learning	humanistic learning

OBJECTIVES

After reviewing the five learning theories summarized in this chapter, the reader will be able to

1. Differentiate among the basic approaches to learning relative to each of the five learning theories.
2. Define the principal constructs of each learning theory.
3. Give an example of how to apply each theory to a specific situation with respect to changing the attitudes and behavior of learners.
4. Outline alternative strategies for learning in a given situation using at least two different learning theories.
5. Identify the differences and similarities in the learning theories specific to (a) the basic procedures of learning, (b) the assumptions made about the learning, (c) the task of the educator, (d) the sources of motivation, and (e) how transfer of learning is facilitated.

Learning is the lifelong, dynamic process by which individuals acquire new knowledge or skills and alter their thoughts, feelings, and behavior. Despite the significance of learning in human development, disagreement exists over how learning occurs, what kinds of experiences facilitate or hinder the learning process, and what ensures that learning becomes relatively permanent.

These are the kinds of debates that stimulated the growth of educational psychology—an area of specialization within the field of psychology devoted to the scientific study of learning, teaching, and assessment. Challenging popular notions about learning (e.g., "Spare the rod and spoil the child," "Males are more intelligent than females," "You can't teach an old dog new tricks"), the growing body of literature that has developed in educational psychology over the past century provides useful pedagogical tools to guide the teaching and learning process. Rather than offering a single or simple answer, educational psychology provides diverse theoretical perspectives on learning—alternative descriptions and explanations about how learning occurs and what motivates people to learn and change (Gage & Berliner, 1992; Gagné, 1985; Hilgard & Bower, 1966; Hill, 1990).

Why do nurses need to know learning theories? Professional accountability and personal growth are two reasons. Increasingly, health practitioners are required to demonstrate that they regularly employ sound methods and clear ratio-

nales in their patient education and interaction, staff management and training, as well as community and continuing education. Given the structure of health care in the United States, nurses are often responsible for designing and implementing plans and procedures for improving health education. A solid grounding in learning theory is essential for effective nursing practice. Beyond one's nursing profession, however, knowledge of the learning process relates to nearly every aspect of daily life. Learning theories can be applied at the individual, group, and program levels to change unhealthy habits, build constructive relationships, develop effective behavior, and become more adept at comprehending and teaching new material.

In this chapter, the principal learning theories are reviewed. In nursing education, behaviorist, cognitive, and social learning theories are most frequently discussed and applied to professional practice (Redman, 1993). Although primarily developed by psychiatrists and therapists, psychodynamic and humanistic theories also are included in this review. These latter two theories contribute much to the understanding of human motivation and emotions, which have a significant influence on the learning process. While this chapter's focus is on learning theory in relation to nursing practice, readers are encouraged to think about ways to use these principles of learning in their personal lives as well.

The chapter is organized as follows. First, five leading learning theories—behaviorist, cognitive, social learning, psychodynamic, and humanistic theories—are summarized and illustrated with examples from nursing and health care. The theories are then compared with regard to (1) their fundamental procedures for changing behavior, (2) the assumptions made about the learner, (3) the role of the educator in encouraging learning, (4) sources of motivation, and (5) how learning is transferred to new situations and problems. Finally, some common features of learning are identified in relation to the issues raised earlier about how learning occurs, the kinds of experiences that promote the learning process, and ways to ensure that learning is relatively permanent. The goal of this review is to provide a conceptual framework for subsequent chapters in this book as well as to suggest alternative approaches that nurses can use in a variety of health-care roles to enhance learning and change in patients, staff, themselves, and other people in their lives. After completing the chapter, it is hoped that readers will be able to identify the essential principles of learning, describe various ways the learning process can be approached, and develop alternative strategies to change attitudes and behavior in different settings.

LEARNING THEORIES

In this section, the basic principles and related concepts of the behaviorist, cognitive, social learning, psychodynamic, and humanistic learning theories are summarized. Questions to consider while reading include the following:

Is the impetus for learning and change largely derived from environmental experiences or from the internal dynamics of the learner?

Is the learner viewed as relatively passive or more active?

What is the educator's task in the learning process?

What motivates individuals to learn?

Is the transfer of learning more strongly influenced by the structure of the situation or by the learner's understanding and emotional feelings?

Behaviorist Learning Theory

Focusing mainly on what is directly observable, the behaviorists view learning as the product of the stimulus conditions (S) and the responses (R) that follow—sometimes termed the S-R model of learning. Whether dealing with animals or people, the learning process is similar and relatively simple. Generally ignoring what goes on inside the individual—which, of course, is always difficult to ascertain—the behaviorists closely observe responses and then manipulate the environment to bring about the intended change (Bigge & Shermis, 1992; Henton & Iverson, 1978).

To modify people's attitudes and responses, the behaviorists recommend either altering the stimulus conditions in the environment or changing what happens after a response occurs. Motivation is explained as the desire to reduce some drive (drive-reduction); hence, satisfied, complacent, or satiated individuals have little motivation to learn and change. Getting behavior to transfer from the initial learning situation to other settings is largely a matter of practice (strengthening habits) and a similarity in the stimuli and responses between the learning situation and future situations where the response is to be performed. Much of behaviorist learning is based on respondent conditioning and operant conditioning procedures.

Respondent conditioning (also termed classical or Pavlovian conditioning) emphasizes the importance of stimulus conditions and the associations formed in the learning process (Hilgard & Bower, 1966; Klein & Mowrer, 1989). According to this basic model of learning, a neutral stimulus (NS)—a stimulus that has no particular value or meaning to the learner—is paired with a naturally occurring unconditioned or unlearned stimulus (UCS) and unconditioned response (UCR) (Figure 3-1). After a few such pairings, the neutral stimulus alone, without the unconditioned stimulus, elicits the same response. Often occurring without thought or awareness, learning takes place when the newly conditioned stimulus (CS) now becomes associated with the conditioned response (CR).

As an illustration from health care, someone without much experience with hospitals (hospitals are neutral stimuli [NS]) may go to visit a sick relative (see Figure 3-1). While in the relative's

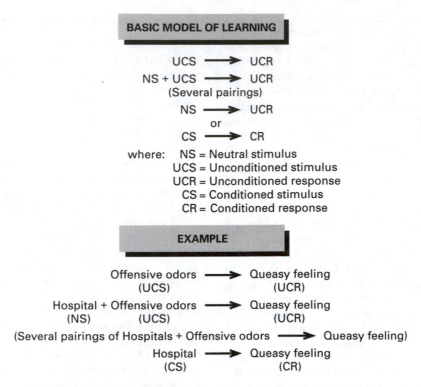

FIGURE 3–1.   Respondent Conditioning Model of Learning

room, the visitor may smell offensive odors (UCS) and feel queasy and light-headed (UCR). After this initial and repeated visits, hospitals (now the CS) may become associated with feeling anxious and nauseated (CR), especially if the visitor smells odors similar to the first experience. Respondent conditioning highlights the importance of the "atmosphere" and staff morale in health care. Often without thinking or reflection, these are the associations that patients and visitors formulate as a result of their hospital experiences, providing the basis for long-lasting attitudes toward medicine, health-care facilities, and health professionals.

Besides influencing the acquisition of new responses to environmental stimuli, principles of respondent conditioning may be used to extinguish a previously learned response. Responses are decreased if the presentation of the conditioned stimulus is not accompanied by the unconditioned stimulus over time. Thus, if the visitor who became dizzy in one hospital subsequently goes to other hospitals to see relatives or friends without smelling offensive odors, then her discomfort and anxiety about hospitals may lessen after several such experiences.

Systematic desensitization is a technique based on respondent conditioning that is used by psychologists to reduce fear and anxiety in their clients (Wolpe, 1982). The assumption is that fear of a particular stimulus or situation is learned, and therefore, it can be "unlearned" or extinguished. Fearful individuals are first taught relaxation techniques, and while in a state of relaxation, the fear-producing stimulus is gradually introduced at a nonthreatening level so that anxiety and emotions are not aroused. After repeated pairings of the stimulus under relaxed, nonfrightening conditions, the individual learns that no harm will come to him from the once-fearful stimulus. Finally, he is able to confront the stimulus without being anxious and afraid. Taking the time to help patients relax and reduce their stress when applying some medical intervention—even a painful procedure—lessens the likelihood that patients will build up negative and anxious associations about medicine and health care.

Certain respondent conditioning concepts are particularly useful in nursing practice. *Stimulus generalization* is the tendency of initial learning experiences to be easily applied to other similar stimuli. For example, when listening to friends and relatives tell about a hospital experience, it becomes apparent that a highly positive or negative personal encounter may color patients' evaluations of their hospital stay as well as their subsequent feelings about having to be hospitalized again. With more and varied experiences, individuals learn to differentiate among similar stimuli, and *discrimination learning* occurs. Much of nursing education and clinical practice involves discrimination learning. *Spontaneous recovery* is another useful concept for nurses to know. Although a response may appear to be extinguished, it may "recover" and reappear at any time (even years later), especially when stimulus conditions are similar to the initial learning experience. Spontaneous recovery helps us understand why it is so difficult to truly eliminate unhealthy habits and addictive behaviors such as smoking, alcoholism, or drug abuse.

Operant conditioning, developed largely by B. F. Skinner (1974, 1989), focuses on the behavior of the organism and the *reinforcement* that occurs after the response (Gagné, Briggs, & Wagner, 1988; Modgil & Modgil, 1987). A reinforcer is a stimulus or event applied after a response that strengthens the probability that the response will be performed again. When specific responses are reinforced on the proper schedule, behaviors can be either increased or decreased. Table 3–1 summarizes ways to increase and decrease responses using the contingencies of operant conditioning. The two ways to increase the probability of a response are to apply positive reinforcement or negative reinforcement after a response occurs. According to Skinner (1974), using *positive reinforcement* or reward greatly enhances the likelihood that a response will be repeated in similar circumstances. As an illustration, although a patient moans and groans as he attempts to get up and walk for the first time after an operation, praise and encouragement (reward) for his efforts (response) will improve the chances that he will continue struggling toward independence.

A second way to increase a behavior is by applying *negative reinforcement* after a response is made, which involves the removal of an unpleasant stimulus through either *escape conditioning* or *avoidance conditioning*. The difference between the two types of negative reinforcement is timing. In escape conditioning, as an unpleasant stimulus is being applied, the individual responds in some way that causes the uncomfortable stimulation to

---

TABLE 3–1.   Operant conditioning model: Contingencies to increase and decrease the probability of an organism's response

I. To *increase* the probability of a response:

    A. *Positive reinforcement:* application of a pleasant stimulus

       Reward conditioning: a pleasant stimulus is applied following an organism's response

    B. *Negative reinforcement:* removal of an aversive or unpleasant stimulus

       Escape conditioning: as an aversive stimulus is applied, the organism makes a response that causes the unpleasant stimulus to cease

       Avoidance conditioning: an aversive stimulus is anticipated by the organism, who makes a response to avoid the unpleasant event

II. To *decrease* or extinguish the probability of a response:

    A. *Nonreinforcement:* an organism's conditioned response is not followed by any kind of reinforcement (positive, negative, or punishment)

    B. *Punishment:* following a response, an aversive stimulus is applied which the organism cannot escape or avoid

cease. For example, suppose as a young student nurse is being chastised by her instructor, she says something humorous, and her instructor stops criticizing and laughs. Because the use of humor has allowed the student to escape an unpleasant situation, chances are she will employ humor again to alleviate a stressful encounter.

In avoidance conditioning, the unpleasant stimulus is anticipated rather than being directly applied. Avoidance conditioning has been used to explain the tendency of some people to become ill in order to refrain from doing something they do not want to do. For example, a child fearing a teacher or test may tell her mother that she has a stomachache. If allowed to stay home from school, the child increasingly may complain of sickness to avoid an unpleasant situation. If a person becomes truly ill when fearful events are anticipated, sickness is the behavior that has been increased through negative reinforcement.

According to operant conditioning principles, behaviors may be decreased through either *nonreinforcement* or *punishment*. Skinner (1974) maintained that the simplest way to extinguish a response is not to provide any kind of reinforcement for some action. For example, offensive jokes in the workplace may be handled by showing no reaction, and after several such experiences, the joke teller, who more than likely wants attention—and negative attention is preferable to no attention—may decrease the use of abrasive humor. Keep in mind too that desirable behavior that is ignored may lessen as well.

If nonreinforcement is ineffective, then punishment may be employed as a way to decrease responses, although there are risks in using punishment. Under punishment conditions, the individual cannot escape or avoid an unpleasant stimulus. Suppose, for example, the young student nurse's attempt at humor was met by the instructor's curt remark, "Right now, we are talking about the need for you to change your behavior, and if you continue to make the same mistake, the records will document your errors, and undoubtedly your grade will suffer." The problem with using punishment as a technique for teaching is that the learner may become highly emotional or deflect attention away from the behavior that needs to be changed. One of the cardinal rules of operant conditioning is to "punish the behavior, not the person."

If punishment is employed, it should be administered immediately after the response with no distractions or means of escape. Punishment must also be consistent and at the highest "reasonable" level (e.g., nurses who apologize and smile as they admonish the behavior of a staff member or patient are sending out mixed messages and are not likely to be taken seriously or to successfully decrease the behavior they intend). Moreover, punishment should not be prolonged (bringing up old grievances or complaining about a misbehavior at every opportunity), but there should be a "timeout" following punishment to make certain there is no opportunity for positive reinforcement. The purpose of punishment is not to do harm or to serve as a release for anger; the goal is to decrease a specific behavior and to instill self-discipline.

The use of *reinforcement* is central to the success of operant conditioning procedures. For operant conditioning to be effective, it is necessary to assess what kinds of reinforcement are likely to increase or decrease behaviors for each individual. Not every patient wants lots of attention from nurses or finds terms of endearment rewarding. A second issue involves the timing of reinforcement. Through experimentation with animals and humans, it has been demonstrated that the success of operant conditioning procedures partially depends on the schedule of reinforcement (Hill, 1990). Initial learning requires a continuous schedule, reinforcing the behavior quickly every time it occurs. If the behavior is not emitted, then responses that approximate or resemble the desired behavior can be reinforced, gradually shaping behavior in the direction of the goal for learning. As an illustration, for geriatric patients who appear lethargic and unresponsive, nurses might begin by rewarding small gestures such as eye contact or a hand that reaches out, then build on these friendly behaviors toward greater human contact and connection with reality. Once a response is well established, however, it becomes ineffective and inefficient to continually reinforce; reinforcement then can be administered on a fixed (predictable) or variable (unpredictable) schedule after a given number of responses have been emitted or after the passage of time.

Operant conditioning techniques provide relatively quick and effective ways to change behavior. Carefully planned programs using *behavior modification* procedures can be applied to health care (Bootzin, 1975; Taylor, 1986). For example, the families of chronic back pain patients have been taught to minimize their attention to the patients whenever they complain and behave in dependent, helpless ways, but to pay a lot of attention when the patients attempt to function independently, express a positive attitude, and try to live as normal a life as possible. Some patients respond so well to operant conditioning that they report experiencing less pain as they become more active and involved.

The behaviorist theory is simple, easy to use, and encourages clear, objective analysis of observable environmental stimulus conditions and learner responses. There are, however, some criticisms and cautions to consider. According to this model, learners are assumed to be relatively passive and easily manipulated, which raises the crucial issue of ethics: "Who" is to decide "what" the "desirable" behavior should be? Too often the desired response is conformity and cooperation to make someone's job easier or more profitable. In addition, the theory's emphasis on extrinsic rewards and external incentives reinforces and promotes materialism rather than self-initiative, a love of learning, and intrinsic satisfaction. Another shortcoming of behavior modification programs is that clients' changed behavior may deteriorate over time, especially once they are back in their former environment—an environment with a system of rewards and punishments that may have gotten them into trouble in the first place. We now move from focusing on responses and behavior to the role of mental processes in learning.

Cognitive Learning Theory

While behaviorists generally ignore the internal dynamics of learning, cognitive learning theorists stress the importance of what goes on "inside" the learner (Farnham-Diggory, 1992; Flavell, 1977; Hill 1990; Puckett & Reese, 1993). The key to learning and changing is the individual's *cognition* (perception, thought, memory, and ways of processing and structuring information). According to this perspective, in order to learn, individuals must change their cognitions. A highly active process largely directed by the individual, learning involves perceiving the information, interpreting the informa-

tion based on what is already known, and then reorganizing information into new insights or understanding.

According to cognitive theorists, the individual's goals and expectations are the sources of motivation that create disequilibrium, imbalance, tension, and the desire to act. Educators and those trying to influence the learning process must recognize the variety of perceptions, ways of thinking about information, and diverse goals and expectations brought to any learning situation. To promote transfer, the learner must mediate or "act on" the learning in some way. Similar patterns in the initial learning situation and subsequent situations also facilitate transfer. From a cognitive perspective, however, rather than rote memory and drill, the key factor is understanding (including considerations of learner readiness, knowledge of one's learning style, and ability to reorganize information).

The *gestalt* perspective of cognitive learning emphasizes the importance of perception in learning (Hilgard & Bower, 1966; Kohler, 1947, 1969; Notterman & Drewry, 1993). Rather than focusing on discrete stimuli, gestalt refers to the configuration or organization of a pattern of cognitive elements, reflecting the maxim that "the whole is greater than the sum of the parts." A basic gestalt principle is that the structuring of perception is directed toward simplicity, equilibrium, and regularity. For example, look at the bewildered faces of some patients listening to a detailed, evasive explanation about the disease they have, when what they desire most is a simple, clear explanation that settles their uncertainty and relates directly to them and familiar experiences.

Another gestalt principle is that perception is selective, which has several ramifications. First, since no one can attend to all the surrounding stimuli at any given time, individuals *orient* themselves to certain features of an experience while screening out or *habituating* to other features. Patients in severe pain or worried about their hospital bills may not attend to some well-intentioned patient education information. Second, what individuals choose to attend to and ignore is influenced by a host of factors: past experiences, needs, personal motives and attitudes, reference groups, and the particular structure of the stimulus or situation (Sherif & Sherif, 1969; Sherif, 1976). Assessing these internal and external dynamics has a direct bearing on how a nurse approaches any learning situation with an individual or group. Moreover, because individuals vary widely with regard to these and other characteristics, they will perceive, interpret, and respond to the same event in different ways, perhaps distorting reality to fit their goals and expectations. This helps explain why an approach that is effective with one patient may not work with another patient.

Some of the psychological tendencies used to organize the perceptual world that have been identified by gestalt psychologists are of special interest to health professionals (Taylor, Peplau, & Sears, 1994). For example, consider *figure-ground* relations. Although the staff may think that the central requirement of a patient's treatment is taking all the medication prescribed (the figure), the patient may view this requirement as unimportant (the ground)—"As long as I feel somewhat better, why take medication?"

Another perceptual tendency is to strive for *closure*. Closure involves the psychological desire to complete, end, or conclude a gestalt or situation that is unfinished. There are some corollaries to the principle of closure. The more unclear or uncertain the perceived situation, the more people will (1) grasp at alternative patternings, (2) be influenced by external suggestions, and (3) be affected by their internal needs and motivations. For example, patients left unclear and uncertain while awaiting medical test results and a physician's diagnosis are likely to be in a state of imbalance and tension. Some patients may construct their own diagnosis and scenario based on deeper psychological desires and goals. Recognizing that some people have a greater need for closure than others, a minority of individuals may resort to extreme behaviors to reduce uncertainty (i.e., spending a fortune on medical quackery, denying medical treatment, and perhaps even attempting suicide).

Because individuals perceive, interpret, and respond to the same situation in different ways, it is no wonder that communication problems abound in the health-care system. Health professionals need to provide as much structure as possible, based on what is known about a patient's condition. If a diagnosis is unclear, it may be wiser to tell patients this information than to leave them wondering. Patients with extreme needs for closure in an uncertain disease condition may benefit from

counseling and therapy to help them accept what they view as a very difficult, anxiety-producing situation.

Cognitive and information-processing perspectives emphasize thinking processes: thought, reasoning, the way information is encountered and stored, and memory functioning (Bigge & Shermis, 1992; Hilgard & Bower, 1966). Taking issue with the behaviorists, to cognitive theorists, reward is not necessary for learning; more important are the learner's goals, expectations, and experiences. Experience, in fact, is the key to learning: by exploring and discovering the environment, individuals formulate their unique *cognitive map* about how the world operates. For example, some patients who have never been in a hospital have little idea what to expect and are baffled and irritated by the staff's coded language and invasive procedures. Staff members, on the other hand, have highly developed, detailed cognitive maps about hospital care and may view as routine what the patient perceives as bizarre, bewildering, frightening, or insulting. Also, cognitive theorists make an important distinction between learning and performance. Just because a behavior is not performed does not mean that learning has not occurred; the learning may be demonstrated at a later time.

How information is processed, stored, and retrieved is useful for nurses to know (Sternberg, 1991). An information-processing model of memory functioning is illustrated in Figure 3–2. While looking at the diagram, consider the model's implications for patient education. The first stage in the memory process involves attention to environmental stimuli. As an example, if a patient is not attending to what a nurse is saying, perhaps because he is weary or distracted, it would be prudent to try the explanation at another time when the patient is more receptive and attentive.

In the second stage, the information is attended to by sensory processing. Questions for nurses to ask themselves include (1) what is the patient's preferred mode of sensory processing (visual, auditory, or motor manipulation), and (2) are there sensory deficits? In the third stage, the information is briefly *encoded* (transforming and incorporating information into memory in a particular form) into short-term memory, after which it is either disregarded and forgotten or stored in long-term memory. Long-term memory involves

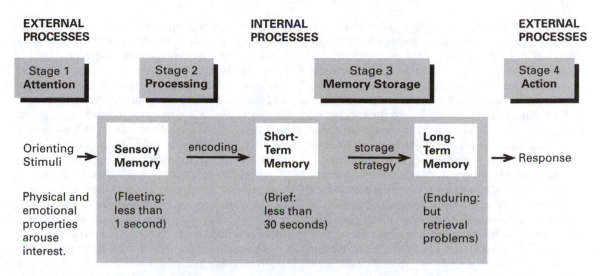

FIGURE 3–2.   Information-Processing Model of Memory

organizing the information by using a preferred strategy for storage (e.g., imagery, association, rehearsal, breaking the information into units). While long-term memories are enduring, a central problem is remembering and retrieving the stored information at a later time. The last stage involves the action or response that the individual makes on the basis of how information was processed and stored. An important implication for nursing is that if patients are unable to remember or reproduce information accurately, nurses should examine closely how the patient attends to, processes, and stores the information that is presented and then help the patient "reprocess" what needs to be learned.

Memory processing and the retrieval of information are enhanced by organizing information and making it meaningful. Forgetting or difficulty in retrieving information from long-term memory may occur because the information has faded from lack of use, other information interferes with retrieval (what comes before or after a learning session may well interfere with storage and retrieval), or individuals are motivated to forget for a variety of conscious and unconscious reasons. This material on memory processing and functioning is highly useful in nursing practice—whether developing health education brochures, engaging in one-to-one patient education, giving a staff development work-

shop, preparing community health lectures, or studying for one's courses and examinations.

Cognitive development is a third perspective that focuses on qualitative changes in perceiving, thinking, and reasoning as individuals grow and mature (Flavell, 1977; Flavell & Markman, 1983). Cognitions are based on how external events are conceptualized, organized, and represented within each person's mental framework or *schema*—a framework that is partially dependent on the individual's stage of cognitive development. From infancy through adolescence, marked changes occur in the way youngsters perceive, reason, and represent the world around them, largely as a function of their growth, maturation, and experience. Readiness to learn is an important consideration, which is based partially on the learner's stage of cognitive development.

How learning occurs and characteristic stages of cognitive development have been identified by theorists such as Jean Piaget (Piaget & Inhelder, 1969) and Jerome Bruner (1966). These theorists concur that learning is an active process that transpires as the child interacts with the environment. Piaget's theory is perhaps the best known and posits that dual processes are involved in learning, as learners (1) *assimilate* information to make it fit their cognitive schema (e.g., a three-year-old child may think that the moon is following her around) and (2) *accommodate* information by changing their cognitive structures (e.g., although fearful of doctors because of a bad experience, several encounters with a friendly, nonthreatening doctor may lead a small child to conclude that not all doctors are scary people). Adults also assimilate and accommodate information into their schemas, and nurses need to ascertain how patients are interpreting and storing (assimilating or accommodating) their health experiences and education.

Through his observations of children's perception and thought processes at different ages, Piaget identified and described four stages of cognitive development (sensorimotor, preoperational, concrete operations, and formal operations) over the course of infancy, childhood, and adolescence.[1] However, researchers have reported that while the cognitive stages develop sequentially, some adults never reach the formal operations stage (Huyck & Hoyer, 1982). These adults may learn better from highly concrete approaches to health education. Developmental psychologists have also proposed advanced stages of reasoning in adulthood beyond formal operations. For example, it may not be until middle age that adults are able to deal with contradictions, synthesize information, and more effectively integrate what they have learned (Kramer, 1983; Riegel, 1973). Assessing each patient's level of cognitive functioning is a first step in communicating effectively and accomplishing health education.

The *social cognition* perspective within the cognitive theory highlights the influence of social factors on perception, thought, and motivation. A host of scattered explanations can be found under the rubric of social cognition (Fiske & Taylor, 1991). One of the most popular in education is the *attribution theory*, which concerns the cause-effect relationships and explanations that individuals formulate to account for their own and others' behavior and how the world operates. Many of these explanations are unique to the individual and tend to be strongly colored by cultural values and beliefs. For example, patients with certain religious views or a particular parental upbringing may believe that their disease is some kind of punishment for their sins; other patients may blame their disease on the actions of others. From this perspective, the patients' attributions may or may not promote wellness and well-being, and additional work may be necessary to try to change some unhealthy attributions. The medical staff's attributions need to be considered as well.

A significant contribution of the cognitive theory is its recognition and appreciation of the rich diversity in teaching and learning experiences (Farnham-Diggory, 1992). Consider, for example, the wide variation in the ways in which learners actively structure their perceptions, approach a learning situation, and encode-process-store-retrieve information. The challenge to educators is to foster insight, creativity, and problem solving. Difficulties lie in ascertaining exactly what is going on inside the mind of each individual and in designing learning activities that encourage people to restructure their perceptions, reorganize their thinking and behavior, and originate solutions. The next learning theory to be discussed combines principles of both behaviorist and cognitive theories.

Social Learning Theory

Most learning theories assume the individual must have direct experiences in order to learn. The social learning theory contends that much of learning occurs by observation—watching other people and seeing what happens to them (Rosenthal & Zimmerman, 1978). Learning is often a social process, and other individuals, especially "significant others," provide compelling examples or role models for how to think, feel, and act. While Miller and Dollard (1941) viewed social learning as a mixture of behaviorist and psychodynamic influences, Bandura (1977, 1986) is credited with outlining the behaviorist and cognitive dimensions of the theory as well as designing experiments to demonstrate the extraordinary power of the social learning theory. Figure 3–3 illustrates the dynamics of social learning based on Bandura's work.

---

[1] Piaget (Piaget & Inhelder, 1969) identified four sequential stages of cognitive development: (1) the *sensorimotor stage* during infancy, where infants explore their environment and attempt to coordinate sensory information with motor skills; (2) the *preoperational stage* during early childhood, where youngsters are able to mentally represent the environment, regard the world from their own egocentric perspective, and come to grips with symbolization; (3) the *concrete operations stage* during the elementary school years, where children are able to attend to more than one dimension at a time, conceptualize relationships, and operate on the environment; and (4) the *formal operations stage* during adolescence, where teenagers begin to think abstractly, are able to deal with the future, and can see alternatives and criticize.

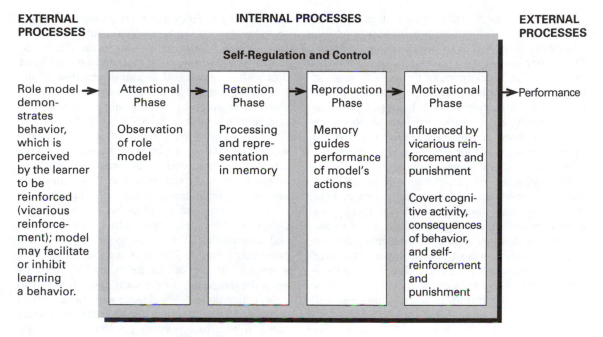

FIGURE 3–3.   Social Learning Theory

SOURCE: Based on Bandura (1977).

Role modeling is a central concept of the theory. As an example from nursing education, a more experienced nurse who demonstrates desirable professional attitudes and behavior sometimes is used as a mentor for a less experienced nurse. *Vicarious reinforcement* is another concept from the social learning theory and involves viewing other people's emotions and determining whether role models are rewarded or punished for their behavior. The behavior of a role model may be imitated, even when no reward is involved for either the role model or the learner. In many cases, however, whether the model is perceived by the observer to be rewarded or punished may have a direct influence on learning. This may be one reason why it is difficult to attract nurses to specialize in geriatric care; although some highly impressive role models work in the field, geriatric nurses are often accorded low status within the profession and may be paid less than nurses in other specialties.

While much of the social learning theory is based on behaviorist principles, the self-regulation and the control that the individual exhibits in the learning process reflect cognitive principles. Bandura (1977) outlined a four-step, largely internal process that directs social learning. As seen in Figure 3–3, the first phase is the attentional phase, a necessary condition for any learning to occur. Research indicates that role models with high status and competence are more likely to be observed, although the learner's own characteristics (needs, self-esteem, competence) may be the more important determiner of attention. Second is the retention phase, which involves the storage and retrieval of what was observed. Third is the reproduction phase, where the learner copies the observed behavior. Mental rehearsal, immediate enactment, and corrective feedback strengthen the reproduction of behavior. Fourth is the motivational phase, involving whether the learner is motivated to perform a certain type of behavior or not. Reinforcement or punishment for a role model's behavior, the learning situation, and the appropriateness of subsequent situations where the behavior is to be displayed affect a learner's performance (Bandura, 1977; Gage & Berliner, 1988). Well suited to conducting patient education and staff development, this organized approach to learning requires attention to the social environment, the behavior to be performed, and the individual learner.

The social learning theory extends the learning process beyond the educator-learner relationship and direct experiences to the larger social world. The theory helps explain the socialization process as well as the breakdown of behavior in society. Responsibility is placed on the educator or leader to be an exemplary role model and to choose socially healthy experiences for individuals to observe and repeat (requiring the careful evaluation of learning materials for stereotypes, mixed or hidden messages, and negative impacts). However, simple exposure to competent role models correctly performing a behavior that is rewarded (or performing some undesirable behavior that is punished) does not ensure learning. Attention to the learner's individuality and the dynamics of self-regulation may help sort out the varying effects of the social learning experience. The final two theories to be reviewed focus on the importance of emotions and feelings in the learning process.

Psychodynamic Learning Theory

Although not usually treated as a learning theory, some of the constructs from the psychodynamic theory (based on the work of Sigmund Freud and his followers) have significant implications for learning and changing behavior (Hilgard & Bower, 1966; Field, Cohler, & Wool, 1989; Notterman & Drewry, 1993). Largely a theory of motivation stressing emotions rather than cognition and responses, the psychodynamic perspective emphasizes the importance of conscious and unconscious forces in guiding behavior, personality conflicts, and the enduring impact of childhood experiences.

A central principle of the theory is that behavior may be conscious or unconscious—that is, individuals may or may not be aware of their motivations and why they feel and act as they do. According to the psychodynamic view, the most primitive source of motivation comes from the id and is based on libidinal energy (the basic instincts, impulses, and desires we are born with), which includes *eros* (the desire for pleasure and sex, sometimes called the "life force") and *thanatos* (aggressive and destructive impulses, or "death wish"). Patients who survive or die, despite all predictions to the contrary, provide illustrations of such primitive motivations. The

id, according to Freud, operates on the basis of the *pleasure principle*—to seek pleasure and avoid pain. Dry, dull health education lectures given by nurses who go through the motions of the presentation without much enthusiasm or emotion inspire few patients to listen or to heed the advice. This does not mean, however, that only pleasurable presentations will be acceptable.

The id (primitive drives) and superego (internalized societal values and standards, or the "conscience") are mediated by the ego, which operates on the basis of the *reality principle*—rather than insisting on immediate gratification, people learn to take the long road to pleasure and weigh the choices or dilemmas in the conflict between the id and superego. Healthy ego (self) development, emphasized by Freud's followers, is an important consideration in the health fields, as indicated by several examples. Patients with ego strength can cope with painful medical treatments because they recognize the long-term value of enduring discomfort and pain to achieve a positive outcome. Patients with weak ego development, on the other hand, may miss their appointments and treatments or may engage in short-term pleasurable activities that work against their healing and recovery. Helping patients develop ego strength and adjust realistically to a changed body image or lifestyle brought about by disease and medical interventions is a significant aspect of the learning and healing process. Health professionals themselves require personal ego strength to cope with the numerous predicaments in the everyday practice of medicine, as they face conflicting values, ethics, and demands. Nursing burnout, for example, is rooted in an overly idealized concept of the nursing role and unrealistic expectations for the self in performing the role.

When the ego is threatened, as can easily occur in the medical setting, *defense mechanisms* may be employed to protect the self. The short-term use of defense mechanisms is a way of coming to grips with reality. The danger is in the overuse or long-term reliance on defense mechanisms, which allows individuals to avoid reality and may act as barriers to learning and transfer. Table 3–2 describes some of the more commonly used defense mechanisms. Employing defense mechanisms is not limited to patients; medical staff also resort to their use. Since health-care provision and working in hospitals are likely to be stressful

TABLE 3–2.   Ego defense mechanisms: Ways of protecting the self from perceived threat

Denial: ignoring or refusing to acknowledge the reality of a threat

Rationalization: excusing or explaining away a threat

Displacement: taking out hostility and aggression on other individuals rather than directing anger at the source of the threat

Repression: keeping unacceptable thoughts, feelings, or actions from conscious awareness

Regression: returning to an earlier (less mature, more primitive) stage of behavior as a way of coping with threat

Intellectualization: minimizing anxiety by responding to threat in a detached, abstract manner without feeling or emotion

Projection: seeing one's own unacceptable characteristics or desires in other people

Reaction formation: expressing or behaving the opposite of what is really felt

Sublimation: converting repressed feelings into socially acceptable action

Compensation: making up for weaknesses by excelling in other areas

---

experiences, knowledge of defense mechanisms is essential.

As an example of defense mechanisms in health care, Elizabeth Kübler Ross (1969) pointed out that patients' initial reaction to being told they have a serious illness is to employ the defense mechanism of *denial*. It is too overwhelming for patients to process the information that they are likely to die. While most patients gradually accept the reality of their illness, the dangers are that if they remain in a state of denial, they may not seek treatment and care, and if their illness is contagious, they may not protect others against infection. A common defense mechanism employed by medical staff is to intellectualize rather than deal realistically at an emotional level with the significance of disease and death. Dehumanization and treating patients as body parts rather than as whole individuals (with spiritual, emotional, and physical needs) are occupational hazards in the health professions.

Another central assumption of the psychodynamic theory is that personality development occurs in stages, with much of adult behavior derived from earlier childhood experiences and conflicts. One of the most widely used models of personality development is Erikson's (1968) eight stages of life, organized around a psychosocial "crisis" to be resolved at each stage.[2] Treatment regimens, communication, and health education need to include considerations of the patient's stage of personality development. For example, in working with 4- and 5-year-old patients, where the crisis is "initiative versus guilt," health professionals

should encourage these children to offer their own ideas and to make and do things themselves; staff also must be careful not to make these children feel guilty for their illness or misfortune. As a second example, the adolescent's desire to have friends and to find an identity requires special attention in health care. Adolescent patients may need help and support adjusting to a changed body image and addressing their fears of weakness, lack of activity, and social isolation. One danger is that they may treat their illness or impairment as a significant dimension of their identity and self-concept.

According to the psychodynamic view, personal difficulties arise and learning and perception are limited when individuals become *fixated* or stuck at an earlier stage of personality development. They then must work through the previously unresolved crisis to develop and mature emotionally. For example, some staff members and patients

---

[2]Erikson's (1968) eight stages in life and their respective crises are outlined as follows: During infancy the psychosocial crisis to be resolved is *trust versus mistrust*. The early childhood years involve issues of *autonomy versus doubt*, followed by *initiative versus guilt*. The school-age child comes to terms with *industry versus inferiority*. Adolescence involves the crisis of *identity versus identity diffusion* or confusion. Young adults attempt to resolve the crisis of *intimacy versus isolation*. Middle-age adults focus on *generativity versus stagnation*. Older adults struggle with *integrity versus despair*. Erikson noted that the two most significant periods of personality growth occur during adolescence and older adulthood—an important observation for nurses to consider when working with these two age groups.

feel an inordinate need to control the self, other people, and certain social situations. This behavior may have been rooted in their inability to resolve the crisis between "trust versus mistrust" at the earliest stage of life. It is essential in working with these individuals to build a trusting relationship and to encourage them gradually to relinquish some control.

Past conflicts, especially during childhood, may interfere with the ability to learn or to transfer learning. What people resist talking about or learning, termed *resistance*, is an indicator of underlying emotional problems, which must be dealt with for them to move ahead emotionally and behaviorally. For instance, the young, pregnant teenager who refuses to engage in a serious conversation about sexuality (e.g., changes the subject, giggles, looks out into space, expresses anger) indicates underlying emotional conflicts that need to be addressed.

Serious problems in miscommunication can occur in health care as a result of childhood learning experiences. As an illustration, some physicians and nurses themselves may have had the experience as a child of standing helplessly by watching someone they love and once depended on endure disease, suffering, and death. Although they could do little as children to improve the situation, they may be compensating for their childhood feelings of helplessness and dependency as adults by devoting their careers to fending off and fighting disease and death. These motivations, however, may not serve them well as they attempt to cope, communicate, and educate dying patients and their families.

Emotional conflicts are not always due to internal forces; society exerts pressures on individuals that promote emotional difficulties as well. The reluctance of health professionals to be open and honest with a terminally ill patient partially may be derived from American culture, which encourages medical personnel to "fix" their patients and extend life. Staff may or may not be conscious of these pressures, but either way they are likely to feel guilty and "a failure" when dealing with a dying patient.

The concept of transfer has special meaning to psychodynamic theorists. *Transference* occurs when individuals project their feelings, conflicts, and reactions—especially those developed during childhood with significant others such as parents—onto authority figures and other individuals in their lives. The danger is that the patient-nurse relationship may be distorted and unrealistic because of the biases inherent in the transference reaction. For example, because patients are sick, they may feel helpless and dependent and then regress to an earlier stage in life when they relied on their parents for help and support. Their childhood feelings and relationship with a parent—for better or worse—may be transferred to a nurse taking care of them. While sometimes flattering for nurses, the "love" and dependency that patients feel may operate against the autonomy and independence needed to "get back on their feet." Patients may also remind a nurse of someone from their past, creating a situation of countertransference.

The psychodynamic approach reminds us to pay attention to emotions, unconscious motivations, and the psychological growth and development of all those involved in health care and learning. One problem with this approach is that much of the analysis is speculative and subjective. Individual nurses' biases, emotional conflicts, and needs may distort their evaluation of other persons and situations. Another caution is that the psychodynamic theory may be used inappropriately; it is not the job of the nurse to probe into the private lives and feelings of patients to uncover deep, unconscious conflicts. A third danger is that health professionals may use the many psychodynamic principles as a way of explaining away rather than dealing with people as individuals who need emotional care. As an illustration, researchers found that rather than using Kübler Ross's model of death and dying to help terminally ill patients and their families discuss their fears and emotions, some health professionals used it to categorize, label, and dismiss dying patients (Dunkel-Schetter & Wortman, 1982; Pattison, 1977).

Humanistic Learning Theory

Underlying the humanistic perspective on learning is the assumption that each individual is unique and that all individuals have a desire to grow in a positive way. One difficulty is that society's values and expectations (e.g., males are less emotional than females, some ethnic groups are "inferior" to others, making money is more important than caring for people) and adults' mistreatment of their children and each other (e.g., inconsistent or harsh discipline, humiliation and belittling, abuse and neglect) may retard positive psychological growth. Spontaneity, the importance of emotions and feelings, the right of individuals to make their own choices, and human creativity are the cornerstones of a humanistic approach to learning (Gage & Berliner, 1992; Pine, 1977).

Motivation is derived from each person's needs, subjective feelings about the self, and the desire to grow. The transfer of learning is facilitated by curiosity, a positive self-concept, and open situations where people respect individuality and promote freedom of choice. Under such conditions, transfer is likely to be widespread, enhancing flexibility and creativity.

Like the psychodynamic theory, the humanistic perspective is largely a motivational theory. Maslow (1954), a major contributor to humanistic theory, is perhaps best known for identifying the *hierarchy of needs* (Figure 3–4), which he says plays such an important role in human motivation. At the bottom of the hierarchy are physiological needs (food, warmth, sleep); then come safety needs; next is the need for belonging and love, followed by self-esteem, cognitive, and aesthetic needs. At the top of the hierarchy are self-actualization needs (maximizing one's potential). An assumption is that basic level needs must be met before individuals can be concerned with learning and self-actualizing. Thus, patients who are hungry, tired, and in pain will be motivated to get these biological needs met before being interested in learning about their medications, rules for self-care, and health education. While intuitively appealing, research has not been able to support Maslow's hierarchy of needs with much consistency. For example, although some people's basic needs may not be met, they may nonetheless engage in creative activities, extend themselves to other people, and enjoy learning (Pfeffer, 1985; Wahba & Bridwell, 1976).

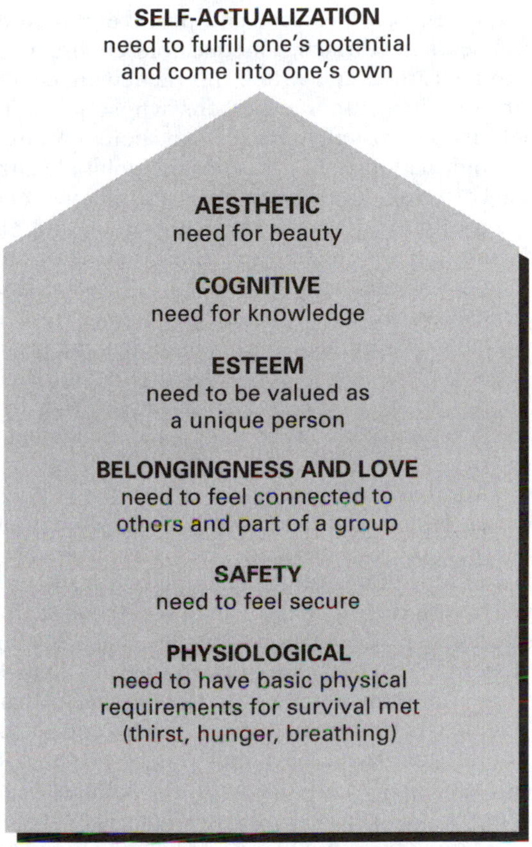

Besides personal needs, the humanists contend that self-concept and self-esteem are necessary considerations in any learning situation. The therapist Carl Rogers (1961, 1994) argued that what people want is *unconditional positive self-regard* (the feeling of being loved without strings attached). Experiences that are threatening, coer-

SELF-ACTUALIZATION
need to fulfill one's potential
and come into one's own

AESTHETIC
need for beauty

COGNITIVE
need for knowledge

ESTEEM
need to be valued as
a unique person

BELONGINGNESS AND LOVE
need to feel connected to
others and part of a group

SAFETY
need to feel secure

PHYSIOLOGICAL
need to have basic physical
requirements for survival met
(thirst, hunger, breathing)

FIGURE 3–4.   Hierarchy of Needs
SOURCE: Adapted from Maslow (1954).

cive, and judgmental undermine the ability and enthusiasm of individuals to learn. It is essential that those in positions of authority convey a fundamental respect for the people with whom they work. If a nurse is prejudiced against AIDS patients, then little will be healing or therapeutic in her relationship with them until she is genuinely able to feel respect for the patient as an individual.

Rather than acting as an authority, according to the humanists, the role of any educator or leader is to be a *facilitator* (Buscaglia, 1982). Listening rather than talking is the skill needed. Since the uniqueness of the individual is fundamental to the humanistic perspective, much of the learning experience requires a direct relationship between the educator and the learner, with instruction tailored to the needs, self-esteem, and positive growth of each learner. Learners, not educators, choose what is to be learned, and within this framework educators serve as resource persons whose job is to help guide learners to make wise choices. Mastering information and facts is not the point of learning. Fostering curiosity, enthusiasm, initiative, and responsibility are much more important and enduring and should be the primary goals of any educator. Rather than inserting health education videos into television sets for patients to view or routinely distributing piles of pamphlets and pages of small-print instructions to patients and their families to read, the humanist perspective has much to contribute in the design and implementation of health education.

Another humanistic principle is that feelings and emotions are the keys to learning, communication, and understanding. The humanists worry that in today's stressful society people easily lose touch with their feelings, which sets the stage for emotional problems and difficulties in learning (Rogers, 1961). "Tell me how you feel" is a much more important statement to the humanists than "tell me what you think," since thoughts and admonitions (the latter of which Rogers calls "the shoulds") may be at odds with true feelings. Consider the implications of the following statements: (1) a young person who says, "I know I should go to medical school and become a doctor because I am smart and that is what my parents want, but I don't feel comfortable with sick people—I don't even like them!" or (2) the dying patient who says, "I realize that I am going to die, but I feel so sad that I am losing my family, my friends, and my self; frankly, I am afraid of dying—all the pain and suffering, being a burden—I'm scared!" In both cases, the humanists would argue, the overriding factor that will affect the behavior of the young person and the dying patient is their feelings, not their cognitions.

The humanistic learning theory has modified the approach to education and changing behavior by giving primary focus to the subjective needs and feelings of the learner and by redefining the role of the educator. The theory has its weaknesses as well. Research has not been able to substantiate some of the theory's strongest claims, and the theory has been criticized for promoting self-centered learners who cannot take criticism or compromise

their deeply felt positions. Charged with being more of a philosophy—or a cult—than a science, the "touchy-feely" approach of the humanists makes some learners and educators feel truly uncomfortable. Moreover, information, facts, memorization, drill, practice, and the tedious work sometimes required to master knowledge, which the humanists minimize and sometimes disdain, have been found to contribute to significant learning, knowledge building, and skill development (Gage & Berliner, 1992; Giaconia & Hedges, 1982).

COMPARISON OF LEARNING THEORIES

A comparative summary of the five learning theories outlined in this chapter can be seen in Table 3-3. Generalizations can be made about the differences as well as the similarities in what the theories say about acquiring knowledge and changing feelings, attitudes, and behavior.

With regard to some of the differences among the theories, each theory has its own assumptions, vocabulary, and way of conceptualizing the learning process. The theories differ in their emphasis on the relative influence of external or internal factors in learning, whether the learner is viewed as more passive or active, the task of the educator, how motivation is explained, and how transfer of learning is accomplished. A logical question is which of these five theories "best" describes or explains learning—which theory, in other words, would be the most helpful to nurses interested in increasing knowledge or changing the behavior of patients, staff, or themselves? The answer to this question is that each theory makes an original contribution to understanding the learning process and can be used singly and in combination to help practitioners acquire new information and alter existing thoughts, feelings, and behavior.

Relative to the unique contributions of the learning theories, each theory gives focus to important considerations in any learning situation. For example, the behaviorists urge us to pay attention to and change stimulus conditions and provide reinforcement to alter behavior. While criticized for being reductionistic, the behaviorists' emphasis on manipulating the environment and reinforcements is admittedly simpler and easier than trying to undertake a massive overhaul of an individual's internal dynamics (perceptions, cognition, feelings, and personality history and conflicts). Moreover, getting someone first to behave in a more appropriate way (abstaining from bad habits and engaging in healthy behavior) may not be as threatening or daunting to the learner as it would be to suggest the need for internal personality changes. Desired responses are modified and strengthened through practice; the new learned responses, in turn, may lead to more fundamental changes in attitudes and emotions. The social learning perspective is another relatively simple theory to use, stressing the importance of effective role models, who by their example demonstrate exactly what behavior is expected.

Cognitive, social learning, psychodynamic, and humanistic theories remind us to consider internal factors—perceptions, thoughts, ways of processing information, feelings, and emotions. These factors cannot be ignored because, ultimately, it is the learner who controls and regulates learning: how information is perceived, interpreted, and remembered and whether the new knowledge is expressed or performed. In practice, learning theories should not be considered mutually exclusive but operate together to change attitudes and behavior. For example, patients undergoing painful procedures are first taught systematic desensitization (behaviorist) and while experiencing pain or discomfort encouraged to employ imagery, such as thinking about a favorite, beautiful place or imagining the healthy cells "gobbling up" the unhealthy cells (cognitive). Staff are highly respectful, upbeat, and emotionally supportive of each patient (humanistic) and create the time and opportunity to listen to patients discuss some of their deepest fears and concerns (psychodynamic). Waiting rooms and lounge areas for patients and their families are designed to be comfortable, friendly, and pleasant to facilitate conversation and interaction (social learning).

Another generalization from this discussion is that some learning theories are better suited to certain kinds of individuals than to others. While theoretical assumptions about the learner range from passive to highly active, passive individuals may learn more effectively from behaviorist techniques, whereas curious, highly active, and self-directed persons may do better with cognitive and humanistic approaches. Also, keep in mind that some learners require external reinforcement and incentives, whereas other learners do not seem to need—and may even resent—attempts to manipulate and reinforce them. Individuals who are well educated, verbal, and reflective may be better candidates for cognitive and psychodynamic approaches, whereas behaviorist approaches may be more suitable for persons who are uncomfortable dealing with abstractions or scrutinizing and communicating their thoughts and emotions or whose cognitive processes are impaired. In addition, each individual's preferred modes of learning may help determine the selection of suitable theoretical approaches. That is, while some individuals learn by acting and responding (behaviorist), the route to learning for others may be through perceptions and thoughts (cognitive) or through feelings and emotions (humanistic and psychodynamic). Most people appear to benefit from demonstration and example (social learning).

COMMON PRINCIPLES OF LEARNING

Taken together, the theories discussed in this chapter indicate that learning is a more complicated process than any one theory implies. Besides the distinct considerations for learning suggested by each theory, their similarities point to some core features of learning. The issues raised at the beginning of the chapter can be answered by synthesizing the learning theories and identifying their common principles.

How Does Learning Occur?

Learning takes place as individuals interact with their environment and incorporate new information or experiences with what they already know or have learned. Factors in the environment that affect learning include the structure or pattern of stimuli, the effectiveness of role models and reinforcements, feedback for correct and incorrect responses, and opportunities to process and apply learning to new situations. The individual exerts significant control over learning, often involving

TABLE 3–3. Summary of learning theories

Learning Procedures	Assumptions About Learner	Educator's Task	Sources of Motivation	Transfer of Learning
Behaviorist				
Environmental stimulus conditions and reinforcement promote changes in responses. To change behavior, change the environment.	Passive, reactive learner responds to environmental conditions (stimuli and reinforcement).	Active educator manipulates stimuli and reinforcement to direct learning and change.	Drive reduction	Practice; similarity in stimulus conditions and responses between learning and new situations
Cognitive				
Internal perception and thought processing within context of human development promote learning and change. To change behavior, change cognitions.	Active learner determines patterning of experiences; is strongly influenced by attributions.	Active educator structures experiences (through organization and meaningfulness) to encourage the reorganization of cognitions.	Goals Expectations Disequilibrium	Mental and physical activity Common patterns Understanding Learning to learn
Social Learning				
External role models and their perceived reinforcement along with learner's internal influences. To change behavior, change role models, perceived reinforcement, and the learner's self-regulating mechanisms.	Active learner observes others and regulates decision to reproduce behavior.	Active educator models behavior, encourages perception of reinforcement, carefully evaluates learning materials for social messages, and attempts to influence learner's self-regulation.	Socialization experiences, role models, and self-reactive influences (observe self, set goals, and reinforce performance)	Similarity of setting and role models' behavior

Psychodynamic				
Internal forces such as developmental stage, childhood experiences, emotional conflicts, and ego strength influence learning and change. To change behavior, change interpretations and make unconscious motivations conscious.	Active learner's lifestyle, past experiences, and current emotional conflicts influence what is learned and how it is remembered and performed.	Educator as a reflective interpreter makes sense of learner's personality and motivation by listening and posing questions to stimulate conscious awareness, insight, and ego strength.	Pleasure principle and reality principle Imbalance Conscious and unconscious influence of conflict, development and defense mechanisms.	Personality conflict, resistance, and transference associated with learning situations may act as barrier.
Humanistic				
Internal feelings about self, ability to make wise choices, and needs affect learning and change. To change behavior, change feelings, self-concept, and needs.	Active learner attempts to actualize potential for positive self-growth and confirm self-concept; is spontaneous, creative, and playful.	Facilitative educator encourages positive self-growth, listens empathetically, allows freedom of choice, and respects learner.	Needs, desire for positive self-growth, and confirmation of self-concept.	Positive or negative feelings about self and freedom to learn promote or inhibit transfer.

considerations of his or her developmental stage, past history (habits, cultural conditioning, socialization, childhood experiences and conflicts), cognitive style, dynamics of self-regulation, conscious and unconscious motivations, personality (stage, conflicts, self-concept), and emotions.

A critical influence on whether learning occurs or not is motivation. The learning theories reviewed here suggest that in order to learn, individuals must want to gain something (receive rewards and pleasure, meet goals and needs, confirm expectations, grow in positive ways, resolve conflicts), which in turn arouses the learner by creating tension (drives to be reduced, disequilibrium and imbalance) and the propensity to act or change behavior. The relative success or failure of the learner's performance may have an impact on subsequent learning experiences. In some cases, an inappropriate, maladaptive, or harmful previously learned behavior may need to be extinguished and then replaced with a more positive response.

What Kinds of Experiences Facilitate or Hinder the Learning Process?

This is where the educator's selection of learning theories and structuring of the learning experience become important. To be effective, educators must have knowledge (of the material to be learned, the learner, and educational psychology), and they must be competent (imaginative, flexible, able to employ teaching methods, display solid communication skills, and have the ability to motivate others). All the learning theories discussed in this chapter indicate the need to recognize and relate the new information to the learner's past experiences (old habits, familiar patterns, childhood memories, feelings about the self, and what is valued, normative, and perceived as successful or rewarded in society).

Ignoring these considerations, of course, may hinder learning. Other impediments to learning may involve a lack of clarity and meaningfulness in what is to be learned, neglect or harsh punishment, poor role models and rewards for unhealthy behavior, confusing reinforcement, and inappropriate materials for the individual's ability, readi-

ness to learn, or stage of life-cycle development. Moreover, learners with negative socialization experiences, deprived of stimulating environments, without goals and realistic expectations for themselves are unlikely to want to learn.

What Helps Ensure that Learning Becomes Relatively Permanent?

First, organizing the learning experience, making it meaningful, and pacing the presentation in keeping with the learner's ability to process information enhance the likelihood of learning. Second, learning is strengthened by practicing (mentally and physically) new knowledge or skills under varied conditions. The third issue concerns reinforcement. Although reinforcement may or may not be necessary, some theorists have argued that reinforcement may be helpful because it serves as a signal to the individual that learning has occurred (Hill, 1990). A fourth consideration involves whether learning transfers beyond the initial educational setting. Learning cannot be assumed to be relatively lasting or permanent; it must be assessed and evaluated soon after the learning experience as well as by follow-up measurements at later times. Research skills, knowledge of evaluation procedures, and the willingness and resources to engage in educational assessment are now considered essential aspects of the learning process. Evaluation feedback can then be used to revamp and revitalize learning experiences.

SUMMARY

This chapter demonstrates that learning is complex. Readers may feel overwhelmed by the diverse theories, sets of propositions, and cautions associated with employing the various approaches. Yet, like the blind men exploring the elephant, each theory gives focus to an important dimension that affects the overall learning process, and together the theories provide a wealth of complementary strategies. There is, of course, no single, best way to approach learning, although all the theories indicate the need to be sensitive to the unique characteristics and motivations of each learner. Educators cannot be expected to know everything about the learning process. More important, perhaps, is that they can determine what needs to be known, where to find the necessary information, and how to help others benefit directly from the learning experience.

References

Bandura, A. (1977). *Social learning theory*. Englewood Cliffs, NJ: Prentice-Hall.

Bandura, A. (1986). *Foundations of thought and action: A social-cognitive theory*. Englewood Cliffs, NJ: Prentice-Hall.

Bigge, M.L., & Shermis, S.S. (1992). *Learning theories for teachers,* 5th ed. New York: HarperCollins.

Bootzin, R.R. (1975). *Behavior modification and therapy*. Cambridge, MA: Winthrop.

Bruner, J.S. (1966). *Toward a theory of instruction*. Cambridge, MA: Harvard University Press.

Buscaglia, L. (1982). *Living, loving and learning*. New York: Fawcett Columbine.

Dunkel-Schetter, C., & Wortman, C.B. (1982). The interpersonal dynamics of career: Problems in social relationships and their impact on the patient. In H. Freeman (Ed.), *Interpersonal issues in health care* (pp. 69-100). New York: Academic Press.

Erikson, E. (1968). *Identity: Youth and crisis*. New York: Norton.

Farnham-Diggory, S. (1992). *Cognitive processes in education,* 2nd ed. New York: HarperCollins.

Field, K.A., Cohler, B.J., & Wool, G. (Eds.). (1989). *Learning and education: Psychoanalytic perspectives*. Madison, CT: International Universities Press.

Fiske, S.T., & Taylor, S.E. (1991). *Social cognition*. New York: McGraw-Hill.

Flavell, J.H. (1977). *Cognitive psychology*. Englewood Cliffs, NJ: Prentice-Hall.

Flavell, J.H., & Markman, E. (Eds.). (1983). *Handbook of child psychology*, Vol. 3. New York: Wiley.

Gage, N.L., & Berliner, D.C. (1988). *Educational psychology,* 4th ed. Boston: Houghton Mifflin.

Gage, N.L., & Berliner, D.C. (1992). *Educational psychology,* 5th ed. Boston: Houghton Mifflin.

Gagné, R.M. (1985). *The conditions of learning,* 4th ed. New York: Holt, Rinehart & Winston.

Gagné, R.M., Briggs, L.J., & Wagner, W.W. (1988). *Principles of instructional design*. New York: Holt, Rinehart & Winston.

Giaconia, R.M., & Hedges, L.V. (1982). Identifying features of effective open education. *Review of Educational Research, 52*, 579-602.

Henton, W.W., & Iverson, I.H. (1978). *Classical conditioning and operant conditioning*. New York: Springer-Verlag.

Hilgard, E.R., & Bower, G.H. (1966). *Theories of learning,* 3rd ed. New York: Appleton-Century-Crofts.

Hill, W.F. (1990). *Learning: A survey of psychological interpretations,* 5th ed. New York: Harper & Row.

Huyck, M.H., & Hoyer, W.J. (1982). *Adult development and aging*. Belmont, CA: Wadsworth.

Klein, S.B., & Mowrer, R.R. (Eds.). (1989). *Contemporary learning theories: Pavlovian conditioning and the status of traditional learning theory*. Hillsdale, NJ: Lawrence Erlbaum.

Kohler, W. (1947). *Gestalt psychology*. New York: Mentor Books.

Kohler, W. (1969). *The task of gestalt psychology*. Princeton, NJ: Princeton University Press.

Kramer, D.A. (1983). Post-formal operations? A need for further conceptualization. *Human Development, 26*, 91-105.

Kübler Ross, E. (1969). *On death and dying*. New York: Macmillan.

Maslow, A. (1954). *Motivation and personality*. New York: Harper & Row.

Miller, N.E., & Dollard, J. (1941). *Social learning and imitation*. New Haven, CT: Yale University Press.

Modgil, S., & Modgil, C. (Eds.). (1987). *B.F. Skinner, consensus and controversy*. New York: Falmer Press.

Notterman, J.M., & Drewry, H.N. (1993). *Psychology and education.* New York: Plenum.

Pattison, E.M. (1977). *The experience of dying*. Englewood Cliffs, NJ: Prentice-Hall.

Pfeffer, J. (1985). Organizations and organizational theory. In G. Lindzey & E. Aronson (Eds.), *Handbook of social psychology,* 3rd ed. Vol. 1, *Theory and method* (pp. 379-440). New York: Random House.

Piaget, J., & Inhelder, B. (1969). *The psychology of the child* (H. Weaver, Trans.). New York: Basic Books.

Pine, G.J. (1977). *Learner-centered teaching: A humanistic view*. Denver, CO: Love.

Puckett, J.M., & Reese, H.W. (Eds.). (1993). *Mechanisms of everyday cognition*. Hillsdale, NJ: Lawrence Erlbaum.

Redman, B.L. (1993). *The process of patient education,* 7th ed. St. Louis: Mosby.

Riegel, K.F. (1973). Dialectic operations: The final period of cognitive development. *Human Development, 16,* 346-370.

Rogers, C. (1961). *On becoming a person*. Boston: Houghton Mifflin.

Rogers, C. (1994). *Freedom to learn*. New York: Merrill.

Rosenthal, T.L., & Zimmerman, B.J. (1978). *Social learning and cognition*. New York: Academic Press.

Sherif, C.W. (1976). *Orientation in social psychology*. New York: Harper & Row.

Sherif, M., & Sherif, C.W. (1969). *Social psychology*. New York: Harper & Row.

Skinner, B.F. (1974). *About behaviorism*. New York: Vintage Books.

Skinner, B.F. (1989). *Recent issues in the analysis of behavior*. Columbus, OH: Merrill.

Sternberg, R.J. (1991). A triarchic model for teaching intellectual skills. In A. McKeough & J.L. Lupart (Eds.), *Toward the practice of theory-based instruction* (pp. 92-116). Hillsdale, NJ: Lawrence Erlbaum.

Taylor, S.E. (1986). *Health psychology*. New York: Random House.

Taylor, S.E., Peplau, L.A., & Sears, D.O. (1994). *Social psychology*, 8th ed. Englewood Cliffs, NJ: Prentice-Hall.

Wahba, M.A., & Bridwell, L.G. (1976). Maslow reconsidered: A review of research on the need hierarchy theory. *Organizational Behavior and Research, 15*, 212-240.

Wolpe, J. (1982). *The practice of behavior therapy,* 3rd ed. New York: Pergamon.

PART II

Characteristics of the Learner

CHAPTER 4

Determinants of Learning

Sharon Kitchie

CHAPTER HIGHLIGHTS

Educator's Role in Learning

Assessment of the Learner

Assessing Learning Needs

Methods to Assess Learning Needs
- Informal Conversations
- Structured Interviews
- Focus Groups
- Self-Administered Questionnaires
- Tests
- Observations
- Patient Charts
- Assessing Learning Needs of Nursing Staff

Readiness to Learn
- Physical Readiness
- Emotional Readiness
- Experiential Readiness
- Knowledge Readiness

Learning Styles
- Six Learning Style Principles

Learning Style Instruments
- Right-Brain/Left-Brain and Whole-Brain Thinking
- Field-Independent/Field-Dependent Embedded Figures Test
- Dunn and Dunn Learning Style Inventory
- Myers-Briggs Type Indicator
- Kolb Learning Style Inventory
- Gregorc Style Delineator
- 4MAT System
- Gardner's Seven Types of Intelligence
- Recent Discoveries About Learning Styles
- Interpretation of the Use of Style Instruments

KEY TERMS

determinants of learning   learning needs
readiness to learn   learning styles

OBJECTIVES

After completing this chapter, the reader will be able to

1. State the nurse educator's role in the learning process.
2. Identify the three components of what is known as "determinants of learning."
3. Describe the steps involved in the assessment of learning needs.
4. Explain methods that can be used to assess learner needs.
5. Discuss the factors that need to be assessed in each of the four types of readiness to learn.
6. Describe what is meant by learning styles.
7. Discriminate between the major learning styles identified.
8. Discuss ways to assess learning styles.

In a variety of settings, nurses are responsible for the education of patients, families, nursing staff, other health-care staff, and nursing students. Several factors have made using principles of learning particularly challenging for the nurse educator to meet learners' needs for information. For example, same-day surgery has compressed patient and family contact with the nurse. Often the teachable moment is gone because of shortened hospital stays. In the case of staff, many times the difficulty with meeting learners' needs is due to the various educational and experiential levels of staff and time constraints in the practice arena. To meet these challenges, the nurse educator must know what determines how well a person learns. This is done by assessing the needs of the learner, recognizing factors involved in the readiness to learn, and being able to correlate teaching interventions with learning styles to maximize opportunities for learning. This chapter will address the determinants of learning in relation to the patient teaching and staff education component of the practice of nursing.

EDUCATOR'S ROLE IN LEARNING

The role of educating can be one of the most challenging and essential interventions a nurse has to perform. To do it well, the nurse must identify the information learners need as well as consider their readiness to learn and their styles of learning. Nevertheless, the learner is the single most important person in the education process. Learning can actually occur without an educator, but learning is enhanced by the addition of an educator who can serve as a facilitator. Just providing information to the learner, however, does not mean that learning has occurred. There is no guarantee that the learner will learn the information given, but there is more of an opportunity to learn if the educator assesses the determinants of learning.

Assessment enables the nurse, as an educator, to facilitate the process of learning by arranging experiences within the environment to help the learner find meaning and purpose for learning. An assessment of the determinants of learning enables the educator to present information in a variety of ways, which a learner cannot do alone. The educator manipulates the environment so that the learner's experience is put into meaningful parts and wholes to reach the learner's unique potential. This enables the learner to incorporate the information into behavior. The educator plays a crucial role in the learning process by (1) assessing problems or deficits, (2) providing appropriate information and presenting it in unique ways, (3) identifying progress being made, (4) giving feedback and follow-up, (5) reinforcing learning in the acquisition of knowledge, the performance of a skill, or a change in attitude, and (6) evaluating learners' abilities.

The educator is vital in giving support, encouragement, and direction during the process of learning. Learners may make choices on their own, but these choices may be limited or inappropriate. The educator can help to identify optimal learning approaches and then provide assistance in choosing learning activities that can both support and challenge the learner based on individual learning needs, readiness to learn, and learning style.

ASSESSMENT OF THE LEARNER

The importance of assessment of the learner may seem self-evident, but often only lip service is given to the assessment phase of the educational process. It is not unusual to witness different patients with the same condition being taught with the same materials in the same way (Haggard, 1989). Frequently the nurse delves into teaching before addressing all the determinants of learning. Nursing assessment of needs, readiness, and styles of learning is the first and most important step in instructional design, but it is the one most often neglected. For years nurses have been taught that any nursing intervention should be preceded by an assessment, and few would deny that this is the correct approach, no matter whether planning for giving direct physical care, meeting the psychosocial needs of a patient, or teaching someone to be independent in self-care or the delivery of care. The effectiveness of nursing interventions is dependent on the scope, accuracy, and comprehensiveness of assessment prior to interventions. But why is assessment so significant and fundamental to the educational process, and why is it often overlooked or only partially carried out?

This initial step in the educational process helps validate the need for learning and the approach to be used in designing learning experiences. Persons who desire or require information to maintain optimal health or staff nurses who must have a greater scope or depth of knowledge to deliver quality care to patients deserve to have an assessment done by the educator so that the needs of the learner are appropriately addressed. There are many factors to consider with respect to the three determinants of learning, and assessments of all three should be based on theories, concepts, and principles. Assessments do more than identify and prioritize information for purposes of setting behavioral goals and objectives, planning instructional interventions, and being able to evaluate in the long run if the goals and objectives have been met by the learner. Good assessments ensure that optimal learning will occur with the least amount of stress and anxiety for the learner. Assessment prevents needless repetition of known material, saves time and energy on the part of both the learner and the educator, helps to establish rapport between the two parties (Haggard,

1989), and increases motivation to learn by addressing what the patient or staff member feels is most important to know or to be able to do. Lack of time, as a result of such factors as shortened hospital stays and limited contact in other settings with patients and families as well as tighter schedules of nursing staff as a result of increased practice demands, has led nurse educators to shortchange the assessment phase. In addition, many nurses, although expected and required to instruct others, are unfamiliar with the concepts and techniques of teaching. The nurse in the role of educator must become more familiar and comfortable with all the elements of instructional design, but particularly with the assessment phase because it provides the foundation for the rest of the educational process. Because of time constraints, which are a major concern when having to teach, nurses must become skilled in accurately carrying out assessments to have reserve time left for actual teaching.

Assessment of the learner includes attending to the three determinants (Haggard, 1989):

1. Learning needs (*what* the learner needs to learn).
2. Readiness to learn (*when* the learner is receptive to learning).
3. Learning style (*how* the learner best learns).

ASSESSING LEARNING NEEDS

Of the three determinants, learning needs must be examined first because there may be no reason to assess readiness to learn or learning styles if, by chance, learning needs are nonexistent. Assessment is essential to determine learning needs so that an instructional plan can be designed to address deficits in any of the cognitive, affective, or psychomotor domains (Gessner, 1989). The purpose of assessing learning needs is to discover what has to be taught and to determine the extent of instruction or if instruction is necessary at all. Not every individual perceives a need for education. An assessment is used to identify and prioritize the needs and interests of the learner. This information is used to set objectives and plan appropriate and effective teaching methodologies whereby education can begin at a point suitable to the learner rather than from an unknown or inappropriate place. Significant differences have been found between the perception of needs identified by patients versus the needs identified by nurses caring for them. In one study, there was only a 20% nurse-patient agreement score with respect to congruency on problems identified (Roberts, 1982).

Learning needs are defined as gaps in knowledge that exist between a desired level of performance and the actual level of performance (Healthcare Education Association, 1985). A learning need is the gap between what someone knows and what someone needs to know. These gaps exist because of a lack of knowledge, attitude, or skill.

Most learners, 90% to 95% of them according to the estimates of many educators in educational psychology (Bloom, 1968; Carroll, 1963; Bruner, 1966; Skinner, 1954), can master a subject with a high degree of success if given sufficient time and appropriate types of help. It is the task of the educator to determine exactly what needs to be learned and be able to identify an approach for presenting the material that will be best understood by the learner. That is to say, the teacher first must discover what the needs of the learner are and then find the most appropriate means of instruction that will enable the learner to master the subject under consideration.

The following are important steps in the assessment of learning needs:

1. *Identify the learner:* Who is the audience? If the audience is one individual, is there a single need or many needs that have to be fulfilled? Is there more than one learner, and if so, are their needs congruent or diverse? The development of formal and informal education programs for patients and their families, nursing staff, or students must be based on accurate identification of the learner. For example, an educator may believe that all postpartum mothers need a formal class on safety issues for the newborn. This may be based on the educator's interaction with one patient and may not be true of all postpartum mothers. The manager of a health-care agency might request an in-service workshop for all staff on documentation of infection control because of an isolated incident of one staff member's failing to report the time at which isolation techniques were begun. This break in protocol may or may not indicate that everyone needs to have an update.

2. *Choose the right setting:* Establishing a trusting environment will help learners feel a sense of security in confiding information, believe their concerns are taken seriously and thought of as important, and feel respected. Assuring privacy and confidentiality is essential to establishing a trusting relationship (Rankin & Stallings, 1990).

3. *Collect data on the learner:* Once the learner is identified, the educator can determine characteristic needs of the population by exploring typical health problems or issues of interest to that population. Subsequently, a literature search can assist in identifying the type and extent of content to be included in teaching sessions as well as the educational strategies for teaching a specific population based on the analysis of needs.

4. *Include the learner as a source of information:* Learners themselves are usually the most important source of needs assessment data. Allow the patient and/or family members to identify what is important to them, what types of social support systems are available or perceived to be available, and how their social support system can help. If the audience for teaching is staff members or students, solicit them for information as to what areas of practice they feel they need new or additional information. Actively engaging learners in defining their own problems and needs allows them to learn in the process and also motivates them to learn because they have an investment in planning for a program specifically tailored to their unique circumstances.

5. *Involve members of the health-care team:* Other health-care professionals may have insight into patient or family needs or the educational needs of the nursing staff or students as a result of their frequent contacts with consumers as well as caregivers. Nurses are not the sole teachers and they must remember to collaborate with other members of the health-care team for a richer assessment of learning needs. In addition, associations such as the American Heart Association, March of Dimes, American Diabetes Association and the Muscular Dystrophy Association are examples of organizations within the health-care field that are also excellent sources of information.

6. *Prioritize needs:* A list of needs can become endless and seemingly impossible to accomplish. Maslow's (1970) hierarchy of human needs helps the educator prioritize identified learning needs (Figure 4–1). The educator can then assist

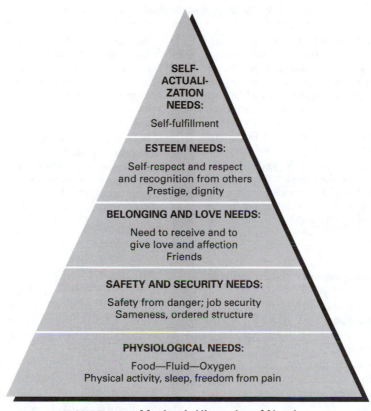

FIGURE 4–1.   Maslow's Hierarchy of Needs

SOURCE: Reprinted by permission from M. Lafleur-Brooks, *Health Unit Coordinating*, p. 48, Philadelphia: W.B. Saunders, 1979.

the learner to meet basic needs first. Learning of other needs will be delayed if basic needs are not attended to first and foremost. For example, learning about a low-sodium diet will not occur if a patient faces problems with basic physiological needs such as pain and discomfort. These needs must be addressed first before any other learning can occur.

Setting priorities for learning is often difficult when faced with many learning needs in several areas. An effort to prioritize the identified needs will help the patient or nursing staff to set realistic and achievable learning goals. Choosing what information to cover is imperative, and choices must be deliberate. Learning needs must be prioritized based on the criteria in Table 4–1 (Healthcare Education Association, 1985, p. 23) to foster maximum learning.

Not all learners need to know everything, and assessment can help to discriminate the "need to know" from the "nice to know" information. If pa-

tients want to know the pathophysiology of their disease, that's fine, but it is not fundamental to learning how to carry out self-care activities that are essential for discharge from the hospital. Often, highly technical information will serve only to confuse and distract patients from learning what they need to know to comply with their regimen (Ruzicki, 1989). There may be needs that are not amenable to education. It is important to sort out types of learning needs from nonlearning needs. This will help the educator know when action other than education would be more appropriate. Education in and of itself is not always the answer to a problem. Often, when something goes wrong, when something is not being done, when a patient is not following a prescribed regimen, or when a staff member does not adhere to protocol, it is believed that more education is necessary. Always look for other needs that are nonlearning. For example, the nurse discovers that the patient is not

TABLE 4–1.   Criteria for prioritizing learning needs

Mandatory: Needs that must be learned for survival or situations in which the learner's life or safety is threatened. Learning needs in this category must be met immediately. For example, a patient who has experienced a recent heart attack needs to know the signs and symptoms and when to get immediate help. The nurse who works in a hospital must learn how to do cardiopulmonary resuscitation or be able to carry out correct isolation techniques for self-protection.

Desirable: Needs that are not life-dependent but are related to well-being or the overall ability to provide quality care situations involving changes in institutional procedure. For example, it is important for patients who have cardiovascular disease to under-

stand the effects of a high-fat diet on their condition. It is desirable for nurses to update their knowledge by attending an in-service program when hospital management decides to focus more attention on the appropriateness of patient education materials in relation to the patient populations being served.

Possible: Needs for information that is "nice to know" but not essential or required or situations in which the learning need is not directly related to daily activities. The patient who is newly diagnosed as having diabetes mellitus most likely does not need to know about traveling across time zones or staying in a foreign country because this information does not relate to the patient's everyday activities.

---

taking his medication and may begin a teaching plan without adequate assessment. The patient may already understand the importance of taking a prescribed medication, know how to administer it, and be willing to follow regimen but may not have the finances necessary to purchase the medication. In this case, the patient does not have a learning need but requires help in exploring financing options or mechanisms to be able to obtain the medication.

7. *Determine availability of educational resources:* A need may be identified, but it may be useless to proceed with interventions if the proper educational resources are not available, are unrealistic to obtain, or do not match the learner's needs. In this case, it may be better to focus on the other identified needs at this point in time. For example, a patient who has asthma needs to learn how to use an inhaler and peak flow meter. The nurse educator determines that this patient learns best by the nurse's giving a demonstration on the use of the inhaler and peak flow meter and then allowing the patient the opportunity to do a return demonstration. If the proper equipment is not available for demonstration/return demonstration at that moment in time, it might be better for the nurse educator to concentrate on teaching the signs and symptoms the patient might experience when having poor air exchange than to cancel the encounter altogether. Thereafter, the educator would work immediately on obtaining the necessary equipment for future encounters.

8. *Assess demands of the organization:* This will yield information that reflects the climate of the organization. What is the organization's philosophy, mission, strategic plan, and goals? The educator should be familiar with standards of performance required in various employee categories along with job descriptions and hospital, professional, and agency regulations. If the organization is focused on health promotion versus trauma care, then there likely will be a different educational focus or emphasis that dictates learning needs of both consumers and employees.

9. *Take time-management issues into account:* Because time constraints are a major impediment to the assessment process, Rankin and Stallings (1990) suggest the educator should emphasize some important points with respect to time-management issues:

- Although close observation and active listening take time, it is much more efficient and effective to do a good initial assessment than to have to waste time going back to discover the obstacles to learning that prevented progress in the first place.
- Learners must be given time to offer their own perceptions of their learning needs if the educator expects them to take charge and become actively involved in the learning process.
- Assessment can be made anytime and anywhere the educator has formal or informal contact with learners. Data collection does not have to be restricted to a specific, prede-

termined schedule. With patients, there are many potential opportunities such as when giving a bath, serving a meal, making rounds, distributing medications, and so forth. For staff, assessments can be made when stopping to talk in the hallway or while enjoying lunch or break time together.

- Informing someone ahead of time that the educator wishes to spend time discussing problems or needs gives them advanced notice to sort out their thoughts and feelings.
- Minimizing interruptions and distractions during planned assessment interviews maximizes productivity such that the educator might accomplish in 15 minutes what otherwise might have taken the educator an hour in less directed, more frequently interrupted circumstances.

METHODS TO ASSESS LEARNING NEEDS

The nurse in the role of educator must obtain objective data about the learner as well as subjective data from the learner. The following are various methods that can be used to assess learner needs and should be used in conjunction with one another to yield the most reliable information (Haggard, 1989).

Informal Conversations

Often learning needs will be discovered during informal conversations that take place between the nurse and patient or family. The nurse educator must rely on active listening. Open-ended questions will encourage learners to reveal information about what they perceive their learning needs to be.

Structured Interviews

The structured interveiw is perhaps the most common form of needs assessment to solicit the learner's point of view. The nurse asks the learner direct and often predetermined questions to gather information about learning needs. As with the gathering of any information from a learner in the assessment phase, the nurse should strive to establish a trusting environment, use open-ended questions, choose a setting that is free of distractions, and allow the learner to state what is believed to be the learning needs. It is important to remain non-judgmental when collecting information about the learner's strengths, beliefs, and motivations. Notes should be taken with the learner's permission, so important information is not lost. The telephone is a good tool to use for an interview if it is impossible to ask questions in person. The major drawback of a telephone interview, however, is the inability on the part of the nurse educator to perceive nonverbal cues from the learner.

Interviews yield answers that may reveal uncertainties, conflicts, inconsistencies, unexpected problems, anxieties, fears, and present knowledge base. Examples of questions that could be asked of a patient as learner are as follows: What do you think caused your problem? How severe is your illness? What does your illness/health mean to you? What do you do to stay healthy? What results do you hope to obtain from treatments? What are your strengths and weaknesses? If the learner is a staff member or student, the following questions could be asked: What do you think you will have the most problem in learning? Is there any skill that you have doubts you can perform? What problems have you encountered in the past when you have had to deal with a patient who has had this illness? What do you see as your strengths and weaknesses? These types of questions help to determine the needs of the learner and serve as a foundation for beginning to plan for the education of the learner.

Focus Groups

Focus groups involve getting together a small number (4 to 12) of potential learners (Breitrose, 1988) to determine areas of educational need by using group discussion to identify points of view or knowledge about a certain topic. A facilitator leads the discussion by asking questions. The questions are open-ended, and detailed discussion of each question is encouraged by the facilitator. These groups of potential learners should be homogeneous with similar characteristics such as age, gender, and past experience with the topic under discussion. However, if the purpose of the focus group is to solicit attitudes about a particular subject or to discuss ethical issues, for example, it may not be necessary to have a homogeneous group.

Self-Administered Questionnaires

The learner's written responses to questions about learning needs can be obtained by self-administered questionnaires. Checklists are one of the most common forms of questionnaires. Checklists are easy to administer, provide more privacy than interviews, and are easy to tabulate. Learners seldom object to this method of obtaining information about their learning needs. Because checklists usually reflect what the nurse educator perceives as needs, there should also be a space for the learner to add any other items of interest or concern.

Tests

Written pretests given before teaching is planned can help identify the knowledge level of the potential learner regarding a particular subject and assist in identifying specific needs of the learner. This approach also prevents the educator from including in the teaching plan repetition of already known material. Furthermore, pretest results also are useful to the educator after the completion of teaching to determine if learning has taken place by comparing pretest scores to posttest scores.

Observations

Observations can provide useful data related to needs. Observing health behaviors in several different time periods can help to determine established patterns of behavior. It must be remembered that conclusions cannot be drawn from a single observation. Actually watching the learner perform a skill is an excellent way of assessing a psychomotor need. Are all steps performed correctly? Is there any difficulty with manipulating various equipment? Does the learner require prompting? Learners may believe they can accurately perform a skill or task (e.g., walking with crutches, changing a dressing, giving an injection), but the educator can best determine what additional learning may be needed by observing the skill performance.

Patient Charts

Often documentation in patient charts will provide patterns that reveal learning needs. Physi-cians' progress notes, nursing care plans, nurses' notes, and discharge planning forms can also provide further information on learning needs. Remember not to disregard the valuable insights other members of the health-care team can provide with respect to the needs of the learner.

Assessing Learning Needs of Nursing Staff

The following are additional methods that can be used specifically to determine the learning needs of nursing staff.

Written Job Descriptions

A written description of what is required to effectively carry out job responsibilities is a source to determine potential learning needs of staff. This can be the basis of establishing content in an orientation program for new staff or of designing continuing education opportunities for seasoned nurses.

Formal and Informal Requests

Many times staff will be asked for ideas for educational programs, which reflect what they perceive as needs. When doing a formalized educational program, the educator must verify that these requests are congruent with the needs of other staff members.

Quality Assurance Reports

Trends found in incident reports indicating safety violations or errors in procedures are a source for establishing learning needs of staff that education could adequately address.

Chart Audits

Audits of charts help identify trends in practice. Is there a learning need by staff in terms of the actual charting? Or is an intervention being newly implemented that was not done before and the record indicates some inconsistency with implementation?

Rules and Regulations

A thorough knowledge of hospital, professional, and health-care requirements helps to identify possible learning needs of staff. It is important for the educator to monitor new rules of practice that may arise from changes occurring within an institution or external to the organization but have implications for the delivery of care.

Knox Four-Step Appraisal

Panno (1992) describes a systematic approach, called the Knox Four-Step Appraisal, for assessing learning needs of caregivers and the organizations in which they practice. The four steps are (1) defining the target population, (2) analyzing learner and organizational needs, (3) analyzing the perceived needs of the learner and comparing these to the actual needs, and (4) using data to prioritize learning needs identified. This organizing framework can be used to assess multiple caregiver levels, the registered nurse to the nursing assistant, which are typically the target audiences for programs by nursing education departments within an institution. Panno points out that often plans for educational activities are based on personal preference, mandates from administration, intuition, or trends in the profession, which may meet the sponsor's needs but not the needs of the learner. The Knox needs assessment appraisal tool is useful because it benefits all involved and is a process that justifies the resources required for the assessment process.

READINESS TO LEARN

Once the learning needs have been identified, the next step is to determine the learner's readiness to receive information. *Readiness to learn* can be defined as the time when the learner demonstrates an interest in learning the type or degree of information necessary to maintain optimal health or to become more skillful in a job. Readiness to learn is when the learner is receptive to learning and is willing and able to participate in the learning process. The educator must never overuse the expression "the patient is not ready to learn." It is the responsibility of the educator to discover through assessment when exactly patients are *ready* to learn and what they *want* to learn. For example, the educator needs to adapt the content to be learned to fit with what the learner is ready to learn. In preparing to teach a patient, the educator must determine what needs to be known about the illness to assist the patient to move toward independence in self-care.

Assessing readiness to learn requires the educator to first understand what needs to be taught and to be competent in collecting and validating information. The same methods that were used to assess learning needs can also be used for assessing readiness to learn, such as making observtions, conducting interviews, gathering information from the learner as well as other health-care team members, and reviewing written data in charts.

An assessment of readiness to learn must be done prior to the time when actual learning is to occur. No matter how important the information is or how much the educator feels the recipient of teaching needs the information, if the learner is not ready, the information will not be absorbed. If educational objectives are set by the educator prior to assessing readiness to learn, then both the educator's and the learner's time could very well be wasted because the established objectives may be beyond the readiness of the learner. The educator must give thought as to what is required of the learner, that is, what needs to be learned, what the learning objectives should be, and in which domain and at what level of learning these objectives should be classified. The educator will then have an idea about what to focus on in the assessment of the learner's abilities.

Timing, that is, the point at which teaching should take place, is very important because anything that affects physical or psychological comfort can affect a learner's ability and willingness to learn. A learner who is unreceptive to information at one time may be more receptive to the same information at another time. Within the health-care system, the nurse often has limited contact with patients and family members. This contact may occur during a 2-day stay in the hospital or a 1-hour visit in the outpatient setting. The patient's readiness to learn is confined to that particular time and is based on learning being brief and basic. Timing is also an important factor with the nursing staff because readiness to learn is based on current demands of practice and needs to correspond to the ever constant changes in practice. Adults, whether they be the patient or family or the nursing staff or students, are eager to learn when the subject of teaching is relevant and applicable to their everyday concerns.

Before teaching can begin, the educator must take the time to first take a PEEK (Lichtenthal, 1990) at the four types of readiness to learn. Readiness to learn can be determined by the learner's characteristics as follows: *P*hysical readiness, *E*motional readiness, *E*xperiential readiness, and *K*nowledge readiness.

These four types of readiness to learn may or may not prove to be obstacles to learning, but the few minutes the educator spends assessing learning readiness can help overcome these possible obstacles. The following factors must be taken into consideration (Table 4–2).

Physical Readiness

There are several physical factors related to readiness that need to be considered by the educator because they may have an adverse impact on the degree to which learning will occur (Singer, 1972). There are five major components to physical readiness: measures of ability, complexity of task, environmental effects, health status, and gender.

TABLE 4–2.   Take time to take a PEEK at the four types of readiness to learn

P=Physical readiness
- Measures of ability
- Complexity of task
- Environmental effects
- Health status
- Gender

E=Emotional readiness
- Anxiety level
- Support system
- Motivation
- Risk-taking behavior
- Frame of mind
- Developmental stage

E=Experiential readiness
- Level of aspiration
- Past coping mechanisms
- Cultural background
- Locus of control
- Orientation

K=Knowledge readiness
- Present knowledge base
- Cognitive ability
- Learning disabilities
- Learning styles

SOURCE: From C. Lichtenthal, *A Self-Study Model on Readiness to Learn*, August 1990. Reprinted with permission from Cheryl Lichtenthal.

Measures of Ability

If the task requires gross movements using the large muscles of the body, then adequate strength, flexibility, and endurance must be present. Walking on crutches is a good example of a psychomotor skill for which a patient must have the physical ability to be ready to learn. If the educator is conducting an in-service workshop for staff on the subject of lifting and transfer activities of patients, the nurse as educator must be cognizant of the endurance level required of the staff for them to be able to return demonstrate this skill. In addition, for information to be accurately processed, sense organs and receptors must be adequately functioning. For example, if a person has a visual deficit, are eyeglasses available to allow the patient to see the lines on an insulin syringe? If not, the individual is not physically ready to learn. Measures involving visual and auditory acuity as well as the capacity to perform adequate movements affect the ability to learn. Creating a stimulating and accepting environment by using instructional tools to match learners' sensory abilities will help to pique their interest in learning.

Complexity of Task

In learning to perform a skill, the nurse educator must take into account the difficulty level of the subject or task to be mastered by the learner. Variations in the complexity of the task affect the extent to which behavioral changes are necessary in the cognitive, affective, and psychomotor domains. Psychomotor skills, in particular, require different degrees of manual dexterity and physical energy output. Once acquired, however, they are usually retained better and longer than learning in the other domains (Greer et al., 1972). Once ingrained, psychomotor skills become habitual and may be difficult to alter. For example, if the learner has been performing a psychomotor skill over a long period of time and then the procedural steps of the task change, the learner will need to unlearn those steps and relearn a new way. This may increase the complexity of the task and put additional physical demands on the learner as a result of lengthening the time needed to adjust to doing something in a new way. Older adults or those with low literacy skills will likely find the effort particularly difficult and time-consuming and may even refuse to make a change.

Environmental Effects

An environment conducive to learning will help to keep the learner's attention and stimulate interest in learning. For example, extremely high levels of noise can interfere with the accuracy and precision in performing manual dexterity tasks. Noise induces vibration of body parts and negatively affects concentration levels. Intermittent noise tends to have greater disruptive effects than the more rapidly habituated steady-state noise. Intermittent use of a jackhammer in the street outside the patient's room, for instance, is more disruptive to a nurse's ability to perform skills than a constant roar of traffic coming from the same street.

The older adult, in particular, needs more time to react and respond to stimuli. The increased inability to receive and transmit information is a symptom of older age. Thus, tasks requiring large amounts of strength, endurance, speed, or flexibility can be difficult for the older person. Complex motor tasks, with too much information given during demonstration by the educator, may result in the older learner becoming overwhelmed and can contribute to a tendency for an older person to focus on irrelevant information rather than on cues relevant to accomplishing the task at hand. When an activity is self-paced, the older learner will respond more favorably. Breaking down complex learning material into more simplified steps is helpful for all learners in improving their retention of information, reducing inattention and confusion, and decreasing energy demands, thereby increasing physical readiness to learn.

Health Status

Assessment of the learner's health status is important to determine the amount of energy available as well as present comfort level because both of these factors impact heavily on readiness to learn. Energy-reducing demands caused by the body's response to illness require the learner to expend large amounts of physical and psychic energy, with little reserve left for actual learning. A person's health status, which can be classified as well, acutely ill, or chronically ill, must be taken into serious consideration when assessing for readiness.

Learners who are healthy have energy available for learning. Readiness to learn about health-promoting behaviors is based on their perception of self-responsibility. The extent to which an illness is perceived to potentially affect future well-being influences someone's desire to learn preventive and promotion measures. If learners feel a threat to their quality of life, more information will be sought in an attempt to control the negative impact of an illness (Bubela & Galloway, 1990). This type of response behavior can be best understood by examining the Health Belief Model and the Health Promotion Model described in Chapter 6.

Learners who are acutely ill focus their energies on the physiological and psychological demands of their illness. Learning is at a minimum because most of their energy is needed for the demands of the illness and gaining immediate relief. Any learning that may occur is related to treatments, tests, and minimizing pain or other discomforts. As these patients improve and the acute phase of illness diminishes, they can then focus on learning follow-up management and the avoidance of complications. The educator must assess an acutely ill person's readiness to learn by observing energy levels and comfort status. One observation that can signify increased energy and comfort levels is the ability to move more readily without becoming easily fatigued. Improvement in physical status usually results in more receptivity to learning. However, medications that can induce side effects, such as drowsiness, mental depression, impaired depth perception, decreased ability to concentrate, and learner fatigue, will also reduce task-handling capacity. Giving a patient a sedative prior to a learning experience will result in less apprehension, but cognitive and psychomotor abilities will be impaired, thus requiring a longer time, more physical output, and more frustration for the learner to master a skill (Greer et al., 1972).

Chronic illness, on the other hand, has no time limits and is of long-term duration. A patient with a chronic condition, however, may experience acute episodes either as an exacerbation of the chronic disease or as a separate event, such as a motor vehicle accident. The physiological and psychological demands vary in chronic illness and are not always predictable. Patients go through different stages in adjusting to their illness. If the learner is in the avoidance stage, readiness to learn will be limited to simple explanations because the patient's energy is being spent on the stress involved in emotionally attempting to deny the illness. Energy levels become more stable when the patient becomes aware of the realities of the situation or symptoms become too obvious to avoid. Readiness to learn will be indicated by the questions the patient may ask. Readiness to learn must never be assumed but should always be assessed during each encounter with the chronically ill patient.

Gender

Research has indicated that women overall are more receptive to medical care and take less risks to their health than men. This may be because women traditionally have been in the role of caregiver and therefore are more open to health promotion teaching. In addition, they have more frequent contacts with health providers while bearing and raising children. Men, on the other hand, tend to be less receptive to health-care interventions and are more likely to be risk takers. Since a good deal of this behavior is thought to be socially induced, changes are beginning to be seen in the health-seeking behavior of men and women as increased attention is being paid to healthier lifestyles and because of the blending of gender roles in the home and workplace.

Emotional Readiness

The learner must be emotionally ready to learn. As with physical readiness, emotional readiness also includes several factors that need to be assessed.

Anxiety Level

Anxiety is a factor that influences the ability to perform at a cognitive, affective, and psychomotor level. Depending on the level of anxiety, it may or may not be a hindrance to the learning of new skills. Fear is a major contributor to anxiety and thus negatively impacts on readiness to learn in any of the learning domains. The performance of a task in and of itself may be fear inducing to a patient because of its very nature or meaning. For example, having to learn self-administration of a medication by injection may produce fear for the patient because of the necessity of inflicting pain on oneself and the perceived danger of the needle breaking off into the skin. A staff member or nursing student may have real difficulty mastering a skill because of the fear of harming a patient or of failing to do a procedure correctly.

Fear may also lead patients to deny their illness, which interferes with their ability to learn. If a situation is life-threatening or overwhelming, anxiety will be high, and readiness to learn will be diminished. While teaching may be imperative for survival, learning usually can take place only if instructions are repeated over and over again. In such circumstances, families and support persons should be educated instead. In later stages of adaptation, acceptance of illness will allow the individual to be more receptive to learning because anxiety levels will be less acute.

Some degree of anxiety is a motivator to learn, but low or high anxiety will interfere with readiness to learn. On either end of the continuum, mild or severe anxiety leads to inaction on the part of the learner, whereas moderate anxiety will drive someone to take action. As the level of anxiety begins to increase, emotional readiness peaks and then begins to decrease (Figure 4–2). Discovering what stressful events or major life changes the learner is experiencing will give the educator clues as to that person's emotional readiness to learn.

Support System

The availability and strength of a support system also influence emotional readiness and are closely tied to how anxious someone might feel. If there are persons in the patient's support system to assist with self-care activities at home, then they should be present during at least some of the teaching sessions to learn how to help the patient if the need arises. A strong support system decreases anxiety, while the lack of one increases anxiety levels.

Motivation

The motivation and interest on the part of the learner to achieve a task also lead to more meaningful teaching-learning experiences. Emotional readiness is strongly associated with motivation. Knowing the motivational level of the learner assists the educator in determining when someone is ready to learn. The learner must have intentions of improving performance. Otherwise, merely going through the motions in a haphazard or mechanical manner, disregarding important learning cues, and demonstrating purposeless activity will not result in task mastery. Assessment of emotional readiness involves ascertaining the level of motivation, not necessarily the reasons for the motiva-

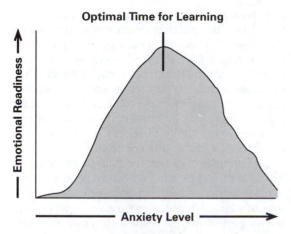

Optimal Time for Learning

Emotional Readiness →

Anxiety Level →

FIGURE 4–2.   Effect of Anxiety on Emotional Readiness to Learn

tion. There are many reasons why a learner may be motivated to learn, and almost any reason to learn is valid. The level of motivation is related to what learners perceive as an expectation of themselves or others. Interest in informal or formal educator-learner interactions is a cue to motivation. The learner who is ready to learn shows an interest in what the nurse educator is doing by demonstrating a willingness to participate or to ask questions. Prior learning experiences, whether they be past accomplishments or failures, will be reflected in the current level of motivation demonstrated by the learner for accomplishing the task at hand (see Chapter 6).

Risk-Taking Behavior
Taking risks is intrinsic in the activities people perform daily. Many activities are done without thinking about the outcome. According to Joseph (1993), some patients, by the very nature of their personality, will take more risks than others. The educator can help patients develop strategies to help reduce the risk of their choices. If patients prefer to participate in activities that may shorten their life spans, then instead of repeating over and over a rigid treatment plan, the educator must be willing to teach these patients how to recognize certain body symptoms and then what to do. Health-care providers also have risk-taking behavior. Understanding how much individual risk taking nurses have or do not have helps the educator

understand why some learners may be hesitant to try new approaches to delivering care. Wolfe (1994) states that taking risks can be threatening when the outcomes are not guaranteed. Educators can help nurses and other health-care providers learn how to take risks. First, the decision has to be made to take the risk. The next step is to develop strategies to minimize the risk. The learner then needs to develop a worst, best, and most probable case scenario. Lastly, the learner can decide if the worst-case scenario developed can be lived with.

Frame of Mind
Frame of mind involves concern about the here and now. If survival is of primary concern, then readiness to learn will be focused on meeting basic human needs. Physical needs such as food, warmth, comfort, and safety as well as psychosocial needs of feeling accepted and secure must be met before someone can focus on higher learning. People from lower socioeconomic levels tend to have an immediate orientation to present-day concerns because they are trying to satisfy everyday needs. Children and teenagers also regard life in the here and now because they are developmentally focused on what makes them happy and satisfied and are more into concrete than abstract thought. Adults who have reached self-actualization and whose basic needs are met are more ready to learn health promotion tasks and are said to have a more futuristic orientation.

Developmental Stage
Each task associated with human development produces a peak time for readiness to learn, known as a "teachable moment" (Tanner, 1989). Unlike children, adults can build on past experiences and are strongly driven to learn information that will help them to cope better with real-life tasks. They see learning as relevant when they can apply new knowledge to help them solve immediate problems. Children, on the other hand, desire to learn for learning sake and actively seek out experiences that give them pleasure and comfort (see Chapter 5).

Experiential Readiness

Experiential readiness refers to the learner's past experiences with learning. Before starting to teach, the educator should assess whether previous learning experiences have been positive or negative in overcoming problems or accomplishing a new task. Someone who has had negative experiences with learning is not likely to be motivated or willing to take a risk in trying to change behavior or acquire new behaviors.

Level of Aspiration

The extent to which someone is driven to achieve is related to the type of short- and long-term goals established, not by the educator, but by the learner. Previous failures and past successes influence what goals learners set for themselves. Early successes are important motivators in learning subsequent skills. Satisfaction, once achieved, elevates the level of aspiration, and this in turn increases the probability of continued performance output in undertaking future endeavors to change behavior.

Past Coping Mechanisms

The coping mechanisms someone has been using must be explored to understand how the learner has dealt with previous problems. Once these mechanisms are identified, the educator must determine if past coping strategies have been effective and, if so, whether these will work well under the present learning situation.

Cultural Background

Knowledge on the part of the educator about other cultures and being sensitive to behavioral differences between cultures are important to avoid teaching in opposition to cultural beliefs (see Chapter 8). Assessment of what an illness means to the patient from the patient's cultural perspective is imperative in determining readiness to learn. Remaining sensitive to cultural influences allows the teacher to bridge the gap when necessary between the medical health-care culture and the patient's culture. Building on the learner's knowledge base or belief system (unless it is dangerous to well-being), rather than attempting to change it or claim it is wrong, will encourage rather than dampen readiness to learn. Language is also a part of culture and may prove to be a significant obstacle to learning if the educator and the learner do not fluently speak the same language. Assessing whether the learner understands English

well enough is the first step. Often a relative, a friend, or a designated person within the health-care system can be called on, if necessary, to act as an interpreter. Enlisting the help of someone else to bridge cultural differences may at times, however, have a negative impact on learning, depending on the sensitivity of the topic and the need for privacy. There may be instances when the patient does not want family members or associates to know about a health concern or illness.

Remember, also, that medical terminology in and of itself may be a foreign language to many patients whether or not they are from another culture. In addition, sometimes a native language does not have an equivalent word to describe the terms that are being used in the teaching situation. Differences in language compound the cultural barrier. Teaching should not be started unless you have determined that the learner understands you and that you have an understanding of the learner's culture (see Chapter 8).

Locus of Control

Whether readiness to learn comes from internal or external stimuli can be determined by ascertaining the learner's previous life patterns of responsibility and assertiveness. When patients are internally motivated to learn, they have what is known as an internal locus of control. They are ready when they feel a need to know about something. The drive to learn comes from within themselves. Usually this type of learner will indicate a need by asking questions. When someone asks a question, the time is prime for learning. If patients have an external locus of control, that is, they are externally motivated, then someone other than themselves has to encourage a feeling of wanting to know something. The responsibility often falls on the educator's shoulders to motivate them to want to learn.

Orientation

The tendency to adhere to a parochial or cosmopolitan point of view is known as orientation. Patients with a parochial orientation tend to be more close-minded in their thinking, are more conservative in their approach to situations, are less willing to learn new material, and place the most trust in traditional authority figures like the physician. This type of orientation is seen most often in people who have been raised in a small-town atmosphere or who come from cohesive neighborhoods or protective family environments. Conversely, people who exhibit a cosmopolitan orientation most likely have a more worldly perspective on life due to broader experiences outside their immediate spheres of influence. These individuals are more likely to be receptive to new ideas and to opportunities to learn new ways of doing things. One must be careful not to unfairly stereotype individuals, but learners usually possess representative characteristics of one or the other of these two opposing types of orientation.

Knowledge Readiness

Knowledge readiness refers to the learner's present knowledge base, the level of learning capability, and the preferred style of learning. These components must be assessed to determine readiness to learn, and teaching should be planned accordingly.

Present Knowledge Base

How much someone already knows about a particular subject or how proficient they are at performing a task is an important factor to determine before designing and implementing instruction. If the educator makes the mistake of teaching subject material that has already been learned, then the educator risks, at the very least, creating boredom and disinterest in the learner, or, at the extreme, causing insult to the learner, which could result in resistance to further learning. Always find out what the patient already knows prior to teaching, and build on this knowledge base to encourage readiness to learn.

Cognitive Ability

The extent to which information can be processed is indicative of the level at which the learner is capable of learning. The educator must match behavioral objectives to the cognitive ability of the learner, or failure to achieve will result. The learner who is capable of understanding, memorizing, recalling, or recognizing subject material is functioning at a lower level than the learner who demonstrates problem solving, concept formation, or application of information. For example, the educator can assume that nursing staff or students who are able to answer questions about cardiopulmonary resuscitation (CPR) on a written test understand the subject. This does not mean, however, that the staff member or student can perform CPR in the clinical setting. Patients who can identify the risk factors of hypertension are functioning at the lower level in the cognitive domain and may have difficulty generalizing the information to find ways of incorporating a low-salt diet into their lifestyle. The level at which the learner is able to learn is of major importance when designing instruction.

Individuals with cognitive impairment due to mental retardation present a special challenge to the educator and will require simple explanations and step-by-step progression of instruction with frequent repetition. Be sure to make information meaningful to those with cognitive impairments by teaching at their level and communicating in ways that the learner will be able to understand. Enlisting the help of members of the patient's support system by teaching them requisite skills will allow them to positively contribute to the reinforcement of self-care activities.

Learning Disabilities

Other than those caused by mental retardation, learning disabilities and low-level reading skills are not necessarily indicative of an individual's intellectual abilities but will require special or innovative approaches to instruction to sustain or bolster readiness to learn. It is easy for low-literacy and learning-disabled persons to become easily discouraged unless the teacher recognizes their special needs and seeks ways to help them accommodate or overcome their problems with processing information (see Chapter 9).

Learning Styles

There are various preferred styles of learning, and assessing how someone learns best will help the educator to vary teaching approaches accordingly. Knowing what teaching methods and materials a learner is most comfortable with or, conversely, does not tolerate well will help the educator to tailor teaching to meet the needs of individuals with different styles of learning, thereby increasing their readiness to learn. For more information see the following discussion on learning styles.

LEARNING STYLES

Learning styles refers to the way individuals process information (Guild & Garger, 1985). Each learner is unique and complex, with a distinct learning style preference, which distinguishes one learner from another. The learning style models are based on the premise that certain characteristics of style are biological in origin, whereas others are sociologically developed as a result of environmental influences. Recognizing that people have different approaches to learning helps the nurse educator to understand the various educational interests and needs of diverse populations. Accepting diversity of style can help educators create the atmosphere for learning that offers experiences that encourage each individual to reach his or her full potential. Understanding learning style also helps educators to make deliberate decisions about program development and instructional design (Arndt & Underwood, 1990).

No learning style is either better or worse than another. Given the same content, most learners can assimilate information with equal success, but how they go about mastering the content is determined by their individual style. The more flexible the educator is in using teaching methodologies related to individual learning styles, the greater the likelihood that learning will occur.

Six Learning Style Principles

Six principles have emerged from research about learning styles (Friedman & Alley, 1984). To develop these six principles, Friedman and Alley reviewed an enormous volume of literature, which included more than 30 different learning style instruments. The six principles are as follows (the reference to "student" can be interpreted as any learner who is the recipient of teaching):

1. *Both the style by which the teacher prefers to teach and the style by which the student prefers to learn can be identified.* Identification of different styles offers specific clues as to the way a person learns. By understanding one's own learning style, the educator can appreciate why it may be easier to help one style of learner to master information while it may be more difficult to work with

another learner who needs an entirely different approach to learning.

2. *Teachers need to guard against over-teaching by their own preferred learning styles.* Nurse educators need to realize that just because they gravitate to learning a certain way does not mean that everyone else can or wants to learn this way. It is much easier for the educator to change the teaching approach than for the learner to adapt to the teacher's style.

3. *Teachers are most helpful when they assist students in identifying and learning through their own style preferences.* Making learners aware of their individual style preferences will lead to an understanding of which teaching-learning approaches work best for them. Also, an awareness of their preference for a particular learning style sensitizes learners to the fact that whatever style is most comfortable for them may not be the best approach for others.

4. *Students should have the opportunity to learn through their preferred style.* The nurse educator can provide the means by which each learner can experience successful learning. Visual learners, for example, should be given movies, computer simulations, and videos from which to learn rather than insisting that they read. Concrete and abstract thinkers need to capitalize on their strengths; concrete thinkers need facts, and abstract thinkers need theories.

5. *Students should be encouraged to diversify their style preferences.* Today learners are constantly faced with learning situations where one approach to learning will not suffice if they are to reach their fullest potential. However, without encouragement, learners will automatically gravitate to using their preferred style of learning. The more frequently learners are exposed to different methods of learning, the less stressful those methods will be in future learning situations.

6. *Teachers can develop specific learning activities that reinforce each modality or style.* Nurse educators must become aware of various methods and materials available to address and augment the different learning styles. To be effective, educational strategies should be geared to different learning styles because using only a limited number of approaches will selectively exclude many learners.

Three mechanisms to determine learning style are observation, interviews, and administration of learning style instruments. By observing the learner in action, the educator can determine how the learner problem solves. When doing a math calculation, does the learner write every step down or only the answer? Learning style can also be determined by interview. The educator can ask the learner about preferred ways of learning as well as the environment most comfortable for learning. Is a warm or cold room more conducive to concentration? Is group discussion or self-instruction more preferable? The last mechanism to determine learning style is by administration of learning style instruments.

All of these three techniques should be used to determine learning style. This can be looked at as parallel to the nursing process. Once data are gathered through interview, observation, and instrument administration, then learning style can be validated by the educator, and methods and materials for instruction can be chosen to match the preferred style of the learner. Nurse educators can also use the learning style approach in directing patients, nursing students, or the nursing staff toward ways they best can learn. Implications for using the learning style approach to instruction are enormous and exciting. If learning styles of the nurses participating in the clinical or academic setting have been assessed and identified, then educational experiences to complement those styles can be designed. Adapting educational experiences to coincide with learning styles thus increases the likelihood that learning will take place. Understanding and recognizing various styles are useful when making decisions about planning, implementing, and evaluating educational programs.

LEARNING STYLE INSTRUMENTS

A word of caution: Before using any learning style instrument, it is important to determine its reliability and validity. Another factor to consider is that an all-inclusive instrument does not exist that can measure all domains of learning—cognitive, affective, and psychomotor—and therefore, it is best to use more than one measurement for assessment. Also, the educator should not rely heavily on these instruments because they are not for diagnosis but to validate what the learner perceives in comparison to what the educator perceives. These instruments will help the nurse in developing a more personalized form of instruction. It is not the intent of this chapter to review all the instruments that are available, but rather to highlight those instruments that are the most useful to nurse educators for assessment purposes.

The identification and application of learning styles is still an emerging movement and is just beginning to be applied to the health education field. Researchers to date have defined learning styles differently, but often the concepts are overlapping. The remainder of this chapter will look at some of the different, better-known theories on learning styles. These do not offer any single framework for instructional design but do provide the educator with a more profound view of the learner than known previously (Villejo & Meyers, 1991).

Right-Brain/Left-Brain and Whole-Brain Thinking

Twenty-five years ago Dr. Roger Sperry and his research team established that the brain functions in many ways as two brains (Sperry, 1977; Herrman, 1988). The brain is composed of two hemispheres that have separate and complementary functions. Studies were conducted on people whose hemispheres were separated to observe how each hemisphere functions. The left hemisphere of the brain was found to be the vocal and analytical side, which is used for verbalization and for reality-based and logical thinking. The right hemisphere was found to be the emotional, visual-spatial, nonverbal hemisphere. Thinking processes using the right brain are intuitive, subjective, relational, holistic, and time free. Sperry and his colleagues discovered that learners are able to use both sides of the brain because of a connector between the two hemispheres called the corpus callosum.

There is no correct or wrong side of the brain. Each hemisphere gathers in the same sensory information but handles the information in different ways. One hemisphere may take over and inhibit the other in processing information, or the task may be divided between the two sides with each handling the part best suited to its way of processing information. Educators need to know which side of the brain is better equipped for certain kinds of tasks and, thus, which is the most effective way to present information to learners who may have a dominant brain hemisphere (Table 4–3). These findings are important for instructional design because educators have limited time and contact with the learner and need to meaningfully present the material to be learned. Brain hemisphericity is linked to cognitive learning style or the way individuals perceive and gather information to problem solve, complete assigned tasks, relate to others, and meet the daily challenges of life.

Knowledge of one's own brain hemispherical performance can aid educators in identifying strengths and weaknesses in their teaching methods. The Brain Preference Indicator (BPI) is a set of questions used to determine hemispheric dominance. The BPI instrument can reveal a general style of thought that results in a consistent pattern of behavior in all areas of the individual's life. More information about the BPI can be found in *Whole-Brain Thinking* by Wonder and Donovan (1984). Statistics show that most learners have left-brain dominance and that only approximately 30% have right-brain dominance (Gondringer, 1989). This may be because the Western world is geared toward rewarding left-brain skills to the extent that

right-brain skills go undeveloped. Teaching methods need to be used that enable the learner to use both sides of the brain. For example, to stimulate the development of left-brain thinking, the nurse educator would choose to use objectives and a course outline, and to stimulate the development of the right brain, the nurse educator might choose to use soft music in the background at a slow even rhythm. By employing teaching strategies aimed at helping the learner use both brain hemispheres, the educator will facilitate more effective and efficient learning. Whole-brain thinking allows the learner to get the best of both worlds, in terms of thought processes. Duality of thinking is what educators should strive to teach to encourage learners to reach their full learning potential.

Field-Independent/ Field-Dependent Embedded Figures Test

An extensive series of studies by H. Witkin and associates (1971a) identified two styles of learning in the cognitive domain. These two cognitive styles are based on the bipolar distribution of characteristics of learners affecting the manner in which learners process and structure information in the environment. Learners have preference styles for certain environmental cues: a field-dependent person's perception is influenced by or immersed in the surrounding field; a field-independent person

TABLE 4–3. Examples of hemisphere functions

Left-Hemisphere Functions	*Right-Hemisphere Functions*
Thinking is critical, logical, convergent, focal	Thinking is creative, intuitive, divergent, diffuse
Analytical	Synthesizing
Prefers talking and writing	Prefers drawing and manipulating objects
Responds to verbal instructions and explanations	Responds to written instructions and explanations
Recognizes/remembers names	Recognizes/remembers faces
Relies on language in thinking and remembering	Relies on images in thinking and remembering
Solves problems by breaking them into parts, then approaches the problem sequentially, using logic	Solves problems by looking at the whole, the configurations, then approaches the problem through patterns, using hunches
Good organizational skills, neat	Loose organizational skills, sloppy
Likes stability, willing to adhere to rules	Likes change, uncertainty
Conscious of time and schedules	Frequently loses contact with time and schedules
Algebra is the preferred math	Geometry is the preferred math
Not as good at interpreting body language	Good at interpreting body language
Controls emotions	Free with emotions

perceives items as separate or differentiated from the surrounding field.

Witkin and associates (1971b) devised a tool called the Embedded Figures Test (EFT) to measure field independence/dependence. The tool measures how a person's perception of an item is influenced by the context in which it appears. Bonham (1988) noted that the EFT is designed to measure a person's ability to find simple geometric figures within complex drawings. This tool takes approximately 30 minutes to complete. Witkin's work is based on 35 years of psychological research on over 2000 subjects. Educators must keep in mind that the tool is based on psychological research when they attempt to broadly apply findings to the educational setting (Witkin et al., 1977).

Field-dependent individuals are more socially oriented, more aware of social cues, and able to reveal their feelings. They are more dependent on others for reinforcement. They have a need for extrinsic motivation and externally defined objectives. Field-dependent individuals learn better if the material to be learned has a social context. They are more easily affected by criticism, take a passive, spectator role, and change their opinions in the face of peer pressure.

Field-independent individuals have internalized frames of reference and experience themselves as separate or differentiated from others and the environment. They are less sensitive to social cues, are not affected by criticism, favor an active participant role, and are eager to test out their ideas or opinions in a group.

Garity (1985) states that these individual differences in characteristics and interpersonal behavior can be used as a basis for looking at different learning styles. Understanding these differences can facilitate the way educators work with learners and structure the learning task and environment (Table 4-4).

Bonham (1988) points out in her analysis of learning style instruments that the ability to do something is being measured by the EFT, not the manner (style) in which it is done. There is no way to tell whether a person is good at both approaches and could choose which style is most effective in a given situation (Shipman & Shipman, 1985; Witkin & Goodenough, 1981). Adults generally do not do well on tests in which speed is important (Botwinick, 1978), but speed is important in this assessment tool. Field independence/dependence might be related to hemispheric brain processes (Chall & Mirsky, 1978). The studies in *Sex and the Brain* (Durden-Smith & deSimone, 1983) show that the males' right hemisphere is stronger than their left, and in females the opposite is true. Males have better visual-spatial abilities, and females have better linguistic skills. Thus females generally do not do as well as males on tests of spatial ability.

The best time to use the EFT seems to be when the educator wants to measure field independence, not field dependence, in a context in which the educator wants to test the extent to which learners are able to ignore distractions from other persons who may offer incorrect information or ideas. Men should be measured only against other men, and women against women, to reduce

TABLE 4–4. Characteristics of field-dependent and field-independent learners

Field-Dependent	**Field-Independent**
Are easily affected by criticism	Are not affected by criticism
Will conform to peer pressure	Will not conform to peer pressure
Are influenced by feedback (grades and evaluations)	Are less influenced by external feedback
Learn best when material is organized	Learn best by organizing their own material
Have a social orientation to the world	Have an impersonal orientation to the world
Place emphasis on facts	Place emphasis on applying principles
Prefer learning to be relevant to own experience	Are interested in new ideas or concepts for own sake
Need external goals, objectives, and reinforcements	Provide self-directed goals, objectives, and reinforcement
Prefer discussion method	Prefer lecture method

the differential effect of the task on the sexes. The results should be used in helping individuals know why they may have trouble with a particular learning experience (Bonham, 1988).

The educator can also use this instrument to determine if a learner sees the whole first (global, field-independent) and then the individual parts (specific, field-dependent) or vice versa. This is important in the approach the educator uses to facilitate learning. The field-independent person will want to know the end result of teaching and learning prior to concentrating on the individual parts of the process, whereas the field-dependent person will want to know the individual parts in sequence prior to looking at the expected overall outcome of teaching-learning efforts.

Dunn and Dunn Learning Style Inventory

In 1967, Rita and Kenneth Dunn set out to develop an instrument that would assist educators in identifying those characteristics that allow individuals to learn in different ways. What has evolved since then is a highly tested and continuously revised instrument that has proved to be both valid and reliable. The Dunn and Dunn Learning Style Inventory is a self-reporting instrument that is widely used in the identification of how individuals prefer to function, learn, concentrate, and perform in their educational activities. It is available in three different forms: for grades 3–5; for grades 6–12; and in the adult version, called the Productivity Environmental Preference Survey (PEPS). Dunn and Dunn (1978) identified four basic stimuli (Figure 4-3) that affect a person's ability to learn:

1. Environmental elements (such as sound, light, temperature, design), which are biological in nature.
2. Emotional elements (such as motivation, persistence, responsibility, and structure), which are developmental and emerge over time as an outgrowth of experiences that have happened at home, school, and play or work.
3. Sociological patterns, which are indicative of the desire to work alone or in groups or a combination of these two approaches.

4. Physical elements (such as perceptual strength, intake, time of day, and mobility), which are also biological in nature and relate to the way learners function physically.

The Environmental Elements

Sound Individuals react to sound in different ways. Some need complete silence, others are able to block out sounds around them, while others require sound in their environment for learning. Cognizant of the effect of sound on learning, the educator should permit learners to study either in silent areas for those who need quiet or, for those who need noise, with music from headsets to prevent interfering with those who need quiet.

Light Some learners work best under bright lights, and others need dim or low lighting. The educator should provide lighting conducive to learning by moving furniture around to establish both well- and dimly lit areas to permit learners to sit where they are most comfortable.

Temperature Some learners have difficulty thinking or concentrating if a room is too hot or, conversely, if it is too cold. The educator needs to make learners aware of the temperature of the environment and encourage them to wear lighter or heavier clothing. If windows are available, they should be opened to permit variable degrees of temperature in the room to accommodate different comfort levels.

Design Dunn and Dunn established that when learners are seated on wooden, steel, or plastic chairs, 75% of the total body weight is supported on only 4 square inches of bone. This results in stress on the tissues of the buttocks, which causes fatigue, discomfort, and the need for frequent body changes. Hard surfaces are especially disturbing for those learners who are not well padded (Dunn & Dunn, 1987). Also, some learners are more relaxed and can learn better in an informal environment by being able to position themselves in a lounge chair, on the floor, on pillows, or on carpeting. Others cannot learn in an informal environment because it makes them drowsy and unable to achieve. If possible, the educator should vary the

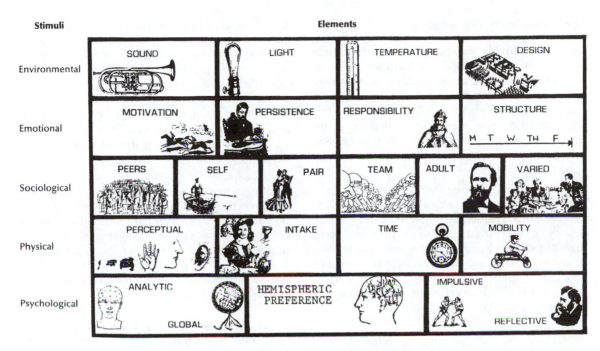

FIGURE 4–3.   Dunn and Dunn's Learning Style Elements

SOURCE: R. Dunn, "Can Students Identify Their Own Learning Styles." *Educational Leadership, 40*, 5:61. Reprinted by permission of the Association for Supervision and Curriculum Development. Copyright © 1983 by ASCD. All rights reserved.

furniture in the classroom to allow some to sit more informally while learning.

The Emotional Elements

Motivation   Motivation, or the desire to achieve, increases when learning success increases. Unmotivated learners need short learning assignments that enhance their strengths. Motivated learners, on the other hand, are eager to learn and should be told exactly what they are required to do, with resources available so they can self-pace their learning.

Persistence   Learners differ in their preference to want either to complete tasks that are begun in one sitting or to take periodic breaks and return to the task at a later time. By giving learners objectives and a time interval for completion of a task ahead of time, those with long attention spans can get the job done in a block of time, while those whose attention span is short can take the opportunity for breaks without feeling guilty or rushed.

Responsibility   Responsibility involves the desire to do what the learner thinks is expected. It is related to the concept of conformity or following through on what an educator asks or tells the learner to do. Learners with low responsibility scores usually are nonconforming. They do not like to do something because someone asks them to do it. Knowing this, the educator should give choices and allow learners to select different ways to complete the assignment. When given appropriate choices, the nonconformist will likely be more willing to meet expectations set forth.

Structure   Structure refers to either the preference for specific directions, guidance, or rules prior to carrying out an assignment or the preference for doing an assignment without structure in the learner's own way. Structure should vary in the amount and kind that is provided, depending on the learner's ability to make responsible decisions.

The Sociological Elements

Learning alone   Some learners prefer to study by themselves, others prefer to learn with a friend or colleague. When learners prefer to be with others, group discussion and role playing facilitate learning. For learners who do not do well learning with others because they tend to socialize or are unable to concentrate, self-instruction, one-to-one interaction, or lecture-type methods are the best approaches.

Presence of an authority figure   Some learners feel more comfortable when someone with authority or recognized expertise is present during learning. Others become fearful, are embarrassed to show inability, and often become too tense to concentrate. Depending on the style of the learner, either one-to-one interaction or self-study may be the appropriate approach.

Variety of ways   Some learners can learn as well alone as they can with authority figures and with peer groups; that is, these learners are versatile in their style of learning and would benefit from variety as opposed to routine approaches.

The Physical Elements

Perceptual strengths   Four types of learners constitute this category: those with auditory preferences, who learn best while listening to verbal instruction; those with visual preferences, who learn best from reading or observation; those with tactile preferences, who learn best when they can underline as they read, take notes when they listen, and otherwise keep their hands busy; and those with kinesthetic preferences, who absorb and retain information best when allowed to perform whole-body movement or participate in simulated or real-life experiences.

Auditory learners learn best by listening and should be introduced to new information first by hearing about it, followed by verbal feedback for reinforcement of the information. Lecture and group discussion are instructional methods best suited to their style. Visual learners learn more easily by viewing, watching, and observing, and therefore, simulation and demonstration methods of

instruction are most beneficial to their learning. Tactile learners learn through touching, manipulating, and handling objects. They remember more when they write, doodle, draw, or move their fingers. The use of models and computer-assisted instruction is most suitable for their learning style. Kinesthetic learners learn more easily by doing and experiencing and profit from opportunities for field trips, role playing, interviewing, and participating in return demonstration.

Intake   Some learners need to eat, drink, chew, or bite objects while concentrating, and others prefer no intake until after they have finished studying. A list of rules needs to be established to satisfy the oral needs of those who prefer intake while learning as long as it is not offensive to others or does not interfere with building rules and regulations of the agency.

Time of day   Some learners perform better at one time of day than another. The four time-of-day preferences are on a continuum, and the educator needs to identify these preferences with an effort toward structuring teaching and learning to occur during the times that are most suitable for the learner:

> *Early-morning learners*—The ability to concentrate and focus energies on learning are oriented to this time of day.
>
> *Late-morning learners*—The energy curve peaks before noontime, when their ability to perform is at its height.
>
> *Afternoon learners*—The energy curve is highest in the mid to late afternoon, and they perform best during this time of day.
>
> *Evening learners*—The ability to concentrate and focus energies on learning is oriented to this time of day.

Mobility   Mobility refers to how still the learner can sit and for how long a period of time. Some learners need to move about, while others can sit for hours engaged in learning. For those who require mobility, provide opportunity for movement by assigning them to less restrictive sections of the room.

Dunn and Dunn stress that the PEPS is not intended to be used as an indicator of underlying psychological factors, value systems, or the quality of attitudes. This instrument yields information concerned with the patterns through which learning occurs but does not assess the finer aspects of an individual's skills, such as the ability to outline procedures, and organize, classify, or analyze new material. It indicates how people prefer to learn, not the abilities they possess.

Myers-Briggs Type Indicator

The Myers-Briggs Type Indicator (MBTI) is a forced choice, self-report inventory based on the Jungian theory of type. Since its development in the 1920s, this instrument has undergone several revisions, and its reliability and validity are well established. C. G. Jung, a Swiss psychiatrist, developed a theory that explains personality similarities and differences by identifying the ways people prefer to take in and make use of data from the world around them. Jung proposed that people have to operate in a variety of different ways depending on the circumstances. Despite these situational adaptations, each individual will tend to develop comfortable patterns, which dictate behavior in certain predictable ways. Jung used the word "types" to identify these styles of personality.

Katherine Briggs and her daughter Isabel Briggs Myers became convinced that Jung's theories had an application for increasing human understanding (Myers, 1980). They developed an instrument based on Jung's theories that would permit people to learn about their own type of behavior and thus understand themselves better with respect to the way in which they interact with others. The instrument uses forced-choice questions and word pairs to measure four dimensions of behavior as indicated by the following dichotomous preferences (Figure 4–4):

1. *Extraversion-Introversion* (EI) reflects an orientation to either the outside world of people and things or to the inner world of concepts and ideas. This dimension describes the extent to which our behavior is determined by our attitudes toward the world. Jung invented the terms from Latin words meaning outward turning (extraversion) or inward turning (introversion). Jung said extraverts operate comfortably and successfully by

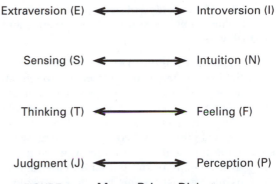

FIGURE 4–4. Myers-Briggs Dichotomous Dimensions or Preferences

interacting with things external to themselves, such as other people, experiences, and situations. Extraverts like to clarify thoughts and ideas through talking and doing. Those who operate more comfortably in an extraverted way think aloud. Introverts, on the other hand, are more interested in the internal world of their minds, hearts, and souls. Introverts like to brew over thoughts and actions, reflecting on them until they become more personally meaningful. Those who operate more comfortably in an introverted way are often thoughtful, reflective, and slow to act because they need time to translate internal thoughts to the external world. Introverts have their thoughts well formulated before they are willing to share them with others.

2. *Sensing-Intuition* (SN) describes perception as coming directly through the five senses or indirectly by way of the unconscious. This dimension explains how people understand what is experienced. People who fall into the sensing category view the world through their senses—vision, hearing, touch, taste, and smell. They observe what is real, what is factual, and what is actually happening. Seeing (or other sense experiences) is believing. These sensory functions allow the individual to observe carefully, gather facts, and focus on practical actions. Conversely, those people who are associated with the intuition category tend to read between the lines, focus on meaning, and attend to what is and what might be. Intuitives view the world through possibilities and relationships and are tuned into subtleties of body language and tones of voice. This kind of perception leads them to examine problems and issues in creative and original ways.

3. *Thinking-Feeling* (TF) is the approach used by individuals to arrive at judgments through impersonal, logical, or subjective processes. Thinkers analyze information, data, situations, and people and make decisions based on logic. They are careful and slow in the analysis of the data because accuracy and thoroughness are important to them. They trust objectivity and put faith in logical predictions and rational arguments. Thinkers explore and weigh all alternatives, and the final decision is reached unemotionally and carefully. In the feeling dimension, on the other hand, the approach to decision making is through a subjective, perceptive, empathetic, and emotional perspective. The feeling person searches for the effect of a decision on themselves and others. They consider alternatives and examine evidence to develop a personal reaction and commitment. They believe the decision-making process is complex and not totally objective. Circumstantial evidence is extremely important, and they see the world as gray rather than black and white.

Jung said that everyone uses these opposing perceptions to some degree in each of the three dimensions (EI, SN, TF) when dealing with people and situations, but they tend to have a preference for one way of looking at the world. They become more skilled in arriving at a decision in either a thinking or feeling way and can function as an extravert at one time and as an introvert at another time, but they tend to develop patterns that are most typical and comfortable.

In addition to Jung's dimensions, Myers and Briggs discovered another dimension they labeled *Judgment-Perception* (JP), whereby an individual comes to a conclusion about something or becomes aware of something. Each individual has a preference for either the judging function or the perceptive function. The desire to regulate and bring closure to circumstances in life is called judgment, and the desire to be open-minded and understanding is known as perception.

By combining the different dimensions, Myers and Briggs identified 16 different personality

ISTJ	ISFJ	INFJ	INTJ
ISTP	ISFP	INFP	INTP
ESTP	ESFP	ENFP	ENTP
ESTJ	ESFJ	ENFJ	ENTJ

FIGURE 4–5. Myers-Briggs Types

SOURCE: Modified and reproduced by special permission of the publisher, Consulting Psychologists Press, Inc., Palo Alto, CA 94303 from *Introduction to Type* by Isabel Briggs Myers. Copyright 1987 by Consulting Psychologists Press, Inc. All rights reserved. Further reproduction is prohibited without the publisher's written consent.

types, each with its own strengths and interests (Figure 4–5). The Myers-Briggs Type Indicator can be useful for the educator to understand the many different ways in which learners perceive and judge information when learning (Table 4–5). These preferences can be reflected in how the educator teaches based on how the learner learns. The logical, detailed educator (sensing-thinking) may have difficulty communicating with a learner who is more holistically oriented (intuitive-feeling). What each values and believes to be most important to be learned or discussed may be different and can lead to misunderstanding and conflicts (Bargar & Hoover, 1984) unless the educator realizes this and adapts teaching to meet the style of the learner. The sensing-thinking learner's preferred learning style emphasizes hands-on experience, demonstration, and application of concepts, whereas intuitive-thinking learners prefer emphasis on the theoretical concerns before they can concentrate on the practical applications.

Kolb Learning Style Inventory

David Kolb (1984), a management expert from Case Western Reserve University, developed an experiential learning model in the early 1970s. Kolb believes knowledge is a transformational process

TABLE 4–5.   Myers-Briggs types: Examples of learning

Extravert	*Introvert*
Likes group work	Likes quiet space
Dislikes slow-paced learning	Dislikes interruptions
Likes action and to experience things in order to learn	Likes learning that deals with thoughts, ideas
Offers opinions without being asked	Offers opinions only when asked
Asks questions to check on the expectations of educator	Asks questions to allow understanding of learning activity
Sensing	*Intuition*
Practical	Always likes something new
Realistic	Imaginative
Observant	Sees possibilities
Learns from orderly sequence of details	Prefers the whole concept versus details
Thinking	*Feeling*
Low need for harmony	Values harmony
Finds ideas and things more interesting than people	More interested in people than things or ideas
Analytical	Sympathetic
Fair	Accepting
Judgment	*Perception*
Organized	Open-ended
Methodical	Flexible
Work oriented	Play oriented
Controls the environment	Adapts to the environment

that is continuously created and recreated. Learning is a continuous process grounded in the reality that the learner is not a blank slate. Every learner approaches a topic to be learned with preconceived ideas. Kolb's theory on learning style is that learning is a cumulative result of past experiences, heredity, and the demands of the present environment. These factors combine to produce different individual orientations to learning. By knowing each learner's preferred style, the nurse educator is better equipped to assist learners in refining or modifying these preconceived ideas so real learning can occur.

Kolb's model, known as the Cycle of Learning, includes four modes of learning, which reflect two major dimensions of perception and processing. He hypothesized that learning results from the way learners perceive as well as how they process what they perceive. The dimension of perception involves two opposite perceptual viewpoints. Some learners perceive through *concrete experience* (CE mode), while others perceive through *abstract conceptual-*

ization (AC mode). At the CE stage of the learning cycle, learners tend to rely more on feelings than on a systematic approach to problems and situations. Learners who fall into this category like relating with people, benefit from specific experiences, and are sensitive to others. They learn from feeling. At the AC stage, on the other hand, learners rely on logic and ideas rather than on feelings to deal with problems or situations. People who fall into this category use systematic planning and logical analysis to solve problems. They learn by thinking.

The process dimension also has two opposing orientations. Some learners process information through *active experimentation* (AE mode), while others process information through *reflective observation* (RO mode). At the AE stage of the learning cycle, learning is active, and learners like to experiment to get things done. They like to influence or change situations and see the results of their actions. They like involvement and are risk takers. They learn by doing. At the RO stage of the learning cycle, learners rely on objectivity, careful

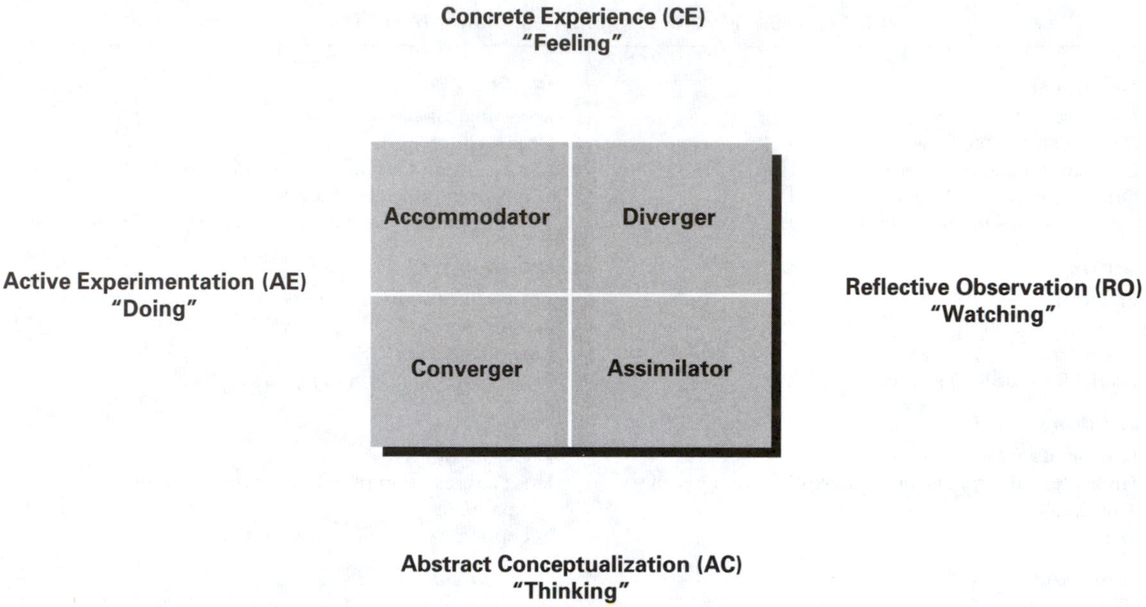

Concrete Experience (CE)
"Feeling"

Active Experimentation (AE)
"Doing"

Accommodator	Diverger
Converger	Assimilator

Reflective Observation (RO)
"Watching"

Abstract Conceptualization (AC)
"Thinking"

FIGURE 4–6.   Kolb's Learning Style Inventory

SOURCE: Kolb, D. *Experiential Learning: Experience as a Source of*
Learning and Development © 1984, Figures 3.1, 4.2. Reprinted by
permission of Prentice-Hall, Inc., Upper Saddle River, NJ.

judgment, personal thoughts, and feelings to form opinions. People who fall into this category look for meaning of things by viewing them from different perspectives. They learn by watching and listening.

Kolb described learning style as a combination of the above basic learning modes (CE, AC, AE, and RO) and labeled styles into separate learning style types that best define the strengths and weaknesses of a learner. The learner predominantly demonstrates characteristics of one of the following style types: (1) diverger, (2) assimilator, (3) converger, (4) accommodator (Figure 4-6).

The *diverger* combines the learning modes of CE and RO. People with this learning style are good at viewing concrete situations from many points of view. They like to observe, gather information, and gain insights rather than take action. Working in groups to generate ideas appeals to them. They place a high value on understanding for knowledge's sake and like to personalize learning by connecting information with something familiar in their experiences. They have active imaginations, enjoy being involved, and are sensi-

tive to feelings. Divergent thinkers learn best, for example, through group discussions and participating in brainstorming sessions.

The *assimilator* combines the learning modes of AC and RO. People with this learning style demonstrate the ability to understand large amounts of information by putting it into concise and logical form. They are less interested in people and more focused on abstract ideas and concepts. They are good at inductive reasoning, value theory over practical application of ideas, and need time to reflect on what has been learned and how information can be integrated into their past experiences. They rely on knowledge from experts. Assimilative thinkers learn best, for example, through lecture, one-to-one instruction, and self-instruction methods with ample reading materials to support their learning.

The *converger* combines the learning modes of AC and AE. People with this learning style type find practical application for ideas and theories and have the ability to use deductive reasoning to solve problems. They like structure and factual information, and they look for specific solutions to problems. Learners with this style prefer technical tasks rather than dealing with social and interpersonal issues. Kolb postulates that individuals with this learning style have skills that are important for specialist and technology careers. The convergent thinker learns best, for example, through demonstration–return demonstration methods of teaching accompanied by handouts and diagrams.

The *accommodator* combines the learning modes of CE and AE. People with this learning style learn best by hands-on experience and enjoy new and challenging situations. They act on intuitive and gut feelings rather than on logic. They are risk takers who like to explore all possibilities and learn by experimenting with materials and objects. Accommodative thinkers are perhaps the most challenging to educators because they demand new and exciting experiences and are willing to take risks that might endanger their safety. Role playing, gaming, and computer simulations, for example, are methods of teaching most preferred by this style of learner.

Kolb's Learning Style Inventory is a self-report instrument that measures learning style types and is based on Piaget's and Guilford's theories of thinking, creativity, and intellect. The instrument rank orders four word phrases in a list of sets. Each word phrase represents one of the four learning modes. A scoring process reduces the ranking evidence to four mode scores (CE, RO, AC, and AE) and then further reduces these down into two dimension scores (concrete-abstract and reflective-active). The predominant score indicates the learner's style (diverger, assimilator, accommodator, or converger).

Knowledge of learning style differences enables the educator to enhance individuals' strengths and to assist learners in developing additional ways of learning. Kolb believes that understanding a person's learning style, its strengths and weaknesses, is a major step toward increasing learning power and helping learners to get the most from their learning experiences. By using different teaching strategies to address these four learning styles, particular modes of learning can be matched, at least some of the time, with the educator's methods of teaching. For every group of learners, about 25% will fall into each of the four categories. If the educator predominantly uses only one method of teaching, such as the lecture to promote learning, then 75% of all learners will be selectively excluded. When teaching groups of learners, instruction should begin with activities best suited to the divergent thinker and progress sequentially to include activities for the assimilator, converger, and accommodator, respectively (Arndt & Underwood, 1990). This is because learners must first have foundational knowledge of a subject before they can test out information. Otherwise, they will be operating from a level of ignorance. They must first have familiarity with facts and ideas before they can explore and test concepts.

Gregorc Style Delineator

Anthony Gregorc's extensive research on learning style (1982) identifies four sets of dualities. These are perception, ordering, processing, and relating, thus bringing more depth to his model than other theories. Based on his research, Gregorc developed an instrument called the Gregorc Style Delineator. This is a self-analysis instrument designed to assess a person's learning style. Sets of words are ranked, a numerical score is derived from each of the four patterns, and the scores are then plotted on a grid (Figure 4–7).

Gregorc states that learning style consists of distinctive and observable behavior that provides cues about the mediation abilities of individuals. He states that the human mind has channels through which it receives and expresses information most efficiently and effectively. The power, capacity, and dexterity to utilize these channels are collectively termed mediation abilities. Two mediation abilities of the mind are how people perceive and how they order knowledge. Perception is seen as a continuum with two opposite tendencies—concrete and abstract. Ordering is also on a continuum, with sequential and random tendencies. The other two mediation abilities of processing and relating are still being refined.

Learners vary in the balance of these four qualities of perception and ordering and create four learning patterns known as concrete sequential (CS), abstract sequential (AS), abstract random (AR), and concrete random (CR). In each of these patterns, learners demonstrate perceived attitudes, motivations, and reasoned thought toward the learning environment.

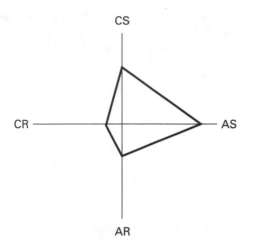

FIGURE 4–7.   Gregorc Style Delineator

SOURCE: Adapted from Gregorc, A. *An Adult's Guide to Style*. Columbia, CT: Gregorc Associates, Inc., 1982.

Concrete sequential (CS) learners tend to operate in a highly structured, conservative manner in which specific details and time schedules are critical. Objectives are important to CS learners as well as a clear beginning and a clear end to the task. These learners do not tolerate being interrupted during the performance of a skill because questioning throws the learning sequence off and causes the CS learner to have difficulty completing the skill. External distractions should be eliminated because the CS individual learns better in a quiet environment as opposed to a noisy environment. It is important that if more than one educator is involved in an interaction with the learner that they all provide the same information in the same sequence. Consistency is important because CS learners can detect a minute flaw or variance in details. A CS learner likes recognition or a compliment on a job well done in learning. "Thank-you" and "good" are terms the CS learner likes to hear. Standards that CS individuals set for themselves are extremely high. The educator must be aware that words used should be concise and that the CS learner will interpret words and labels literally. Learning can be enhanced by using handouts, demonstration teaching, hands-on opportunities with guided practice, lectures with visual aids, and computer-aided instruction.

Abstract sequential (AS) learners are global thinkers and surround themselves with language and other symbols of knowledge. They also like to deal with abstract ideas, and their style of learning continually leads to further understanding. These types of learners also do not learn well when sequence is interrupted. The AS learner needs facts and written documentation to refer to, such as statistics and resource references. Usually when learning, the AS individual does not display emotion and has difficulty picking up subtle verbal and nonverbal cues. The AS learner also needs a quiet environment in order to concentrate and learn. Learning can be enhanced by audiotapes, lectures, and supplemental reading.

Abstract random (AR) learners value relationships over time-bound structures. They think in global terms, and their thinking processes are anchored in feelings. Often AR learners will direct attention to information that has personal meaning to them. Learning can be enhanced with color, music, pictures, drawings, symbols, poetry, and humor. Educators need to know that the AR learner will ask questions randomly during teaching episodes and likes a busy environment for learning. Learning is best achieved in groups, with the opportunity for discussion and question-and-answer sessions.

Finally, *concrete random* (CR) learners tend to seek alternatives and create choices where none existed before. The CR learner is very inquisitive and will question motives. Attention is focused on the process, and the CR individual will make intuitive leaps or insights. The "why" is more important than the "how." The CR learner does not like detail and has difficulty with step-by-step learning. Learning for the CR individual is enhanced with simulations, computer and board games, case studies, and brainstorming sessions.

Gregorc believes that most people have the ability to operate to some extent in all four styles, although 90% of learners are better able to operate in only one or possibly two learning styles. In a new or stressful learning situation, the learner will exhibit stronger characteristics of one particular style. The Gregorc Style Delineator instrument is designed to measure the extent to which a learner's pattern of thinking reflects the four modes. A higher score in a mode indicates a stronger orientation to that mode. With an understanding of these modes, the educator can design teaching methods based on the individual styles of learners.

4MAT System

McCarthy (1981) developed a model based on previous research on learning styles and brain functioning. In particular, she used Kolb's model combined with right/left-brain research findings to create the 4MAT System (Figure 4–8). McCarthy's model describes four types of learners and also defines the learning process as a natural sequence from type one to type four. Educators can address all four learning styles by teaching sequentially, thus attending to all types of learners. Learners are then able to work with their own strongest learning style while at the same time developing the ability through exposure to work in the other quadrants. To use this sequence, learners begin in the first quadrant, known as type one, and engage the right brain by sensing and feeling their way through an experience and eventually moving to the left brain to analyze what they experienced. They ask, "Why is this important? Why should I try to learn this?" The next quadrant is type two, in which learning also begins with the right brain to make observations and integrate data with present knowledge. Learners then engage the left brain to think about new theories and concepts relative to these observations. They ask, "What is it I am supposed to be learning? What is the relationship?" Type three learners in the third quadrant begin with the left brain by working with defined concepts, then shifting to the right brain to experiment with what has to be learned. They ask, "How does this work? How can I figure this out?" Finally, type four learners will also begin with the left brain by analyzing the practicality of what has been learned but then move to the right brain to show mastery through application and the sharing of findings with others. They ask, "If I learn this, what can I do with it? Can I apply it?"

The learning sequence is circular and cyclic, beginning at type one and moving to type four, which is characteristic of a higher level and greater complexity of learning. Based on this model, it is important for the educator to begin type one learning by including personal meaning for the learner to make the learning experience relevant and to answer the "why" question. Next, it is essential to introduce new knowledge based on accurate information to answer the "what" question. The third step in sequential learning is to deal with reality in a practical manner through application of knowledge to enable learners to answer the "how" question. Finally, in the fourth step, the learning experience must allow the learner to be innovative and inspiring and create new possibilities so the "if" question is answered. The educator needs to determine cognitive skill and attitude changes to be attained by all learners to be certain teaching matches expected outcomes. By using this sequential approach to learning, the educator can instill personal meaning and motivation for what is to be learned (type one), assist the learner in the acquisition of the new knowledge and concepts (type two), allow for active experimentation (type three), and finally provide the opportunity for more complex synthesis and extension through practical application (type four). Through use of the 4MAT System, each learning style will then have an opportunity to exert itself at least part of the time.

Gardner's Seven Types of Intelligence

Most theories and measurement instruments on learning style focus on the adult as learner. However, children also have their own way of learning. Learning styles of children can be assessed from the standpoint of growth and each individual's unique pattern of neurological functioning. Psychologist Howard Gardner (1983) developed the theory of seven different kinds of intelligence, and this theory is useful in looking at styles of learning in children. Gardner based his theory on findings from brain research, developmental work with children, and psychological testing. He identified seven kinds of intelligence located in different parts of the brain: linguistic, logical-mathematical, spatial, musical, bodily-kinesthetic, interpersonal, and intrapersonal. All learners have all the seven kinds of intelligence but in different proportions.

Linguistic intelligence seems to be in the Broca's area of the left side of the brain for most people. Children who have a preference for this type of intelligence have highly developed auditory skills and think in words. They like to write, tell stories, spell words accurately, enjoy reading, and can recall

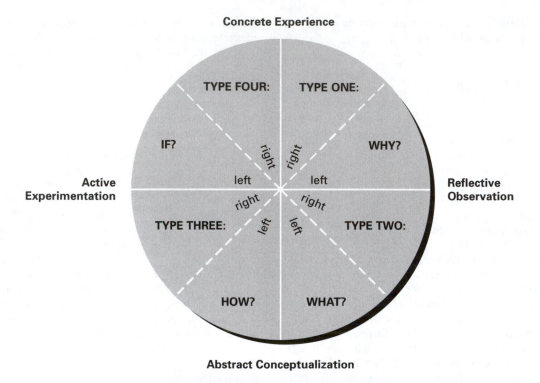

FIGURE 4–8. McCarthy's 4MAT System

SOURCE: From P. B. Guild and S. Garger, *Marching to Different Drummers*. Alexandria, VA: Association for Supervision and Curriculum Development, 1985.

names, places, and dates. These children learn best by verbalizing, hearing, or seeing words. Word games or crossword puzzles are an excellent method for helping these children learn new material.

Logical-mathematical intelligence involves both sides of the brain. The right side deals with concepts, and the left remembers the symbols. The children who are strong in this intelligence explore patterns, categories, and relationships. In the adolescent years, they have the ability of logical thinking with a high degree of abstraction. As learners, they question a lot of things and ask where, what, and when. A question this learner could ask is, "If people are always supposed to be good to each other, then why do people always say they are sorry?" They can do arithmetic problems quickly in their heads, like to learn by computers, and do experiments to test concepts they do not understand. They enjoy strategy board games such as chess or checkers.

Spatial intelligence is related to the right side of the brain. These children learn by images and pictures. They enjoy such things as building blocks, jigsaw puzzles, and daydreaming. They like to draw or do other art activities, can read charts and diagrams, and learn with visual methods such as videos or photographs.

Musical intelligence is also related to the right side of the brain. These children can be found singing a tune, telling you when a note is off-key, playing musical instruments with ease, dancing to music, and keeping time rhythmically. They are also sensitive to sounds in the environment such as the sound of walking on snow on a cold winter morning. Often musical intelligence children learn best with music playing in the background.

Bodily kinesthetic intelligence includes the basal ganglia and cerebellum of the brain in addition to other brain structures. These children learn by processing knowledge through bodily sensations. They need to learn by moving or acting things out. It is difficult for these learners to sit still for long periods of time. They are good at athletic sports and have highly developed fine-motor coordination. Use of body language to communicate and copying people's behaviors or movements come easily for this group of learners.

Interpersonal intelligence involves the prefrontal lobes of the brain. These children understand people, are able to pick up on other's feelings, tend to have a lot of friends, and are gifted in the social skills. They learn best in groups and gravitate toward activities that involve others.

Intrapersonal intelligence, like interpersonal intelligence, involves the prefrontal lobes of the brain. These children have strong personalities and prefer the inner world of feeling and ideas and like being alone. They are very private individuals, like a quiet area to learn, and many times need to be by themselves in order to learn. They tend to be self-directed and self-confident. They learn well with independent, self-paced instruction.

Educators should always approach a child's learning using concepts from the seven intelligences (Armstrong, 1987). Often it can be difficult to assess the preferred learning style of a child when the child is facing an illness or surgery. Asking some key questions of the child or parents may give the educator some clues as to the preferred style of learning. What does the child already know how to do? What subjects does the child excel in or like best? What kinds of hobbies does the child have? What excites this child? What kinds of toys does the child play with? What inner qualities does the child possess, such as courage, playfulness, curiosity, friendliness, or creativity? What talents does the child have? Does the child like to take things apart and put them back together?

By using the theory of the seven intelligences, the educator can assess each child's style of learning and tailor teaching accordingly. For example, if the educator wants to assist a child in learning about a kidney disorder, then one of seven different approaches can be used, depending on the child's style of learning:

Linguistic—Practice quizzing the child orally on the different parts of the kidney, the disease itself, and how to take care of oneself.

Spatial—Have a diagram or chart that allows the child to associate different colors or shapes with concepts. Storytelling can be used illustrating a child with the same chronic illness.

Kinesthetic—Have a kidney model available that can be felt, taken apart, and manipulated. Have the child identify tactile features of the kidney or "act out" appropriate behavior.

Logical-mathematical—Group concepts into categories, starting with simple generalizations or health behaviors. Reasoning works well in showing the child the consequences of actions.

Musical—Teach self-care or the material to be learned by putting information into a song. Soft music also serves as a relaxing influence on the child.

Interpersonal—Have a group of children play a card game such as a version of Old Maid that matches information with medical pictures or pictures of health-care activities and procedures. Use group work for problem-solving activities.

Intrapersonal—Suggest that the child get active in writing to friends, family, or local and state government officials to advocate for kidney disease. They need to research the facts and then convey these findings to others. These children learn best by one-to-one teaching and through use of self-learning modules.

Recent Discoveries About Learning Styles

Recent theories on learning style have addressed the novice-to-expert concept. These theories are particularly applicable when assessing learning of professional nursing staff and students. How one proceeds from a novice to an expert learner in each learning domain is illustrated in an article entitled "The Mind's Journey from Novice to Expert," by John Bruer (1993). Bruer discusses how progress made by cognitive scientists in understanding the learning process can help educators promote subjects' optimal learning. Cognitive scientists have determined how expertise in a particular subject matter requires mastery of a distinct knowledge base in a specific domain. In the same article, Newell and Simon (1972) argue that to understand learning in a particular domain, the educator must begin with a detailed analysis of how people solve problems in that domain. By analyzing chess players, Chase and Simon (1973) found that experts see chunks and that novices, in contrast, see individual pieces. The experts envision potential moves, and this approach permits them to choose the best strategies because they operate using information-rich chunks. Chunking, rather than concentrating on each move, accounts for the experts' superiority.

In this classic example of chess players, Bruer (1993) acknowledges that novices see the chessboard in terms of individual pieces. They can store the positions of only five or six pieces in their short-term memory. This number saturation is consistent with what research has shown to be our working memory span capacity. Therefore, if each chunk contains four or five pieces and experts are able to hold five such chunks in their working memory, then the experts can reproduce accurately the positions of 20 to 25 individual pieces. In addition, Simon and Chase (1973) found that when experts reproduce the positions of chess pieces on the board, they did so in chunks. Thus, if an educator knows how a novice solves a particular problem in a domain, compared with the way an expert thinks, then learning can be traced to changes that occur in mental processes in moving from novice to expert. Learning is the process by which novices become experts.

Interpretation of the Use of Style Instruments

Learning style is an important consideration in the teaching-learning process. However, caution must be exercised in assessing styles in order not to ignore other factors that are equally important in learning such as readiness and capabilities to learn, educational background, and rates of learning. Styles, which vary from person to person, also differ from capabilities in that the style by which someone learns describes how that individual processes stimuli as opposed to defining how much and how well the information is processed (Thompson & Crutchlow, 1993). Many learning

theorists advocate that learning style be matched with a similar teaching style for learners to attain an optimum level of achievement. However, research in this area is clouded by inconsistent findings. Some studies have found that learning styles have no significant effect on achievement of learning. It may be that learning occurs not so much as a result of matching teacher and learner styles but that when the educator uses a variety of different teaching approaches rather then relying on just one, learners feel less stressed. Therefore, learners will be more satisfied overall with the learning experience and thus will be more motivated to learn. Nevertheless, using teaching methods that coincide with the dominant learning style of individuals is usually considered the best way to effect the greatest learning achievement (deTornay & Thompson, 1987). Application of learning style theory to facilitate education allows the teacher to approach each learner holistically by recognizing that not all learners process information in the same way (Arndt & Underwood, 1990).

Much of the research implies that individuals have a certain learning style that prevails over time; however, the use of certain styles also may depend on the context in which learners are operating at any given moment. The concept of matching styles implies that individuals are static, which contradicts the purpose of education. Learners need to experience some discomfort in order to grow. Educators need to generate "dynamic disequilibrium" rather than creating an environment that is too harmonious (Joyce, 1984).

When selecting a learning style instrument, the educator must first evaluate the instrument for validity, reliability, and the population for which it is to be used. In addition, the ease of administering the instrument as well as the ease of analyzing the results needs to be taken into consideration. Also, copyright laws must be adhered to, which means that the instrument must be bought or the author's permission must be obtained before the tool is used.

When considering using a learning style instrument for purposes of assessment, the nurse educator is encouraged to use more than one learning style instrument. If the educator focuses on only one model, then the possibility arises of trying to make the learner fit. By using more than one model, given the learning situation, the educator may find that one learning style is more appropriate than another. The educator will also have more strategies for dealing with problems or unique situations.

Because it may not always be practical to use learning style instruments because of cost, time, or appropriateness of the instrument fit for a specific population, there are some general guidelines educators should follow when assessing individual learning styles:

- Become familiar with the different instruments available and the ways in which styles are classified so that it becomes easier to recognize various learning styles.
- Identify key elements of an individual's learning style by observing and asking questions to verify observations and then matching instructional methods and materials to those unique qualities. For example, such questions could include the following: Do you prefer to attend lectures or group discussions? Which do you like to do better, read or view a film? Would you like me to demonstrate this skill first, or would you rather learn by doing while I talk you through the procedure?
- Always allow learners the opportunity to say when the teaching method is not working for them.
- Place emphasis on assessing learning styles as a way to increase understanding both from the educator's and the learners' perspectives. No one style is better than another, and everyone should realize that there are a variety of learning modalities.
- Be cautious about saying that certain instructional methods are always more effective for certain styles. Remember that everyone is unique, and there are many different ways to impact on learning.
- Encourage learners to expand their style ranges rather than to seek only comfortable experiences.

Caution must be exercised when using any of these instruments to assess learning style. The educator must remember not to place too much emphasis or reliance on these tools to categorize learners. It should not be the intent of educators to stereotype learners as to style but to ensure that each individual learner is given an equal opportunity to learn the best or most comfortable way. These instruments may help the educator to understand how someone prefers to learn so that a diversity of appropriate teaching methods and materials can be chosen to meet the needs of all learners.

SUMMARY

In this chapter, the importance of the assessment phase of learning has been stressed because the educator must be aware of as well as know how to determine learning needs, the learner's readiness to learn, and the learner's individual learning style prior to planning for any educational encounter.

Learning is a complex concept that is not directly seen but can be inferred from permanent changes that occur in the learner's behavior. Learning takes place in all three of the cognitive, psychomotor, and affective domains. Behavioral objectives for these three domains should not be set until the educator establishes *what* the needs of the learner are, *when* the learner is ready to learn, and *how* the learner best learns. Learning by the patient, family member, or nurses and other health-care professionals requires that the educator identify learning approaches and activities based on the individuals' determinants of learning.

Identifying and prioritizing the learning needs mean finding out what the learner feels is important. Once these needs are established, the educator must assess the learner's readiness to learn based on the physical, emotional, experiential, and knowledge components particular to each learner so that teaching interventions can be adjusted to facilitate the learning process. The last determinant of learning is assessing the learner's learning style. Assessment of learning style by way of interviewing, observing, and instrument measurement can reveal how individuals best learn as well as how they prefer to learn. By accepting the diversity of style among learners, the educator can create a versatile atmosphere and provide optimal experiences that encourage all learners to reach their full potential. Whoever the audience may be, the nurse educator should be able to identify and select approaches and activities most beneficial for the learner based on the three determinants of learning.

References

Armstrong, T. (1987). *In their own way*. New York: St. Martin's Press.

Arndt, M.J., & Underwood, B. (1990). Learning style theory and patient understanding. *Journal of Continuing Education in Nursing, 21*(1), 28-31.

Bargar, R., & Hoover, R. (Winter 1984). Psychological type and the matching of cognitive styles. *Theory into Practice, 23*(1), 56-63.

Bloom, B. (1968). Learning for mastery. *Instruction and Curriculum, Topical Papers and Reprints No. 1* (Durham, NC: National Laboratory for Higher Education.)

Bonham, L. A. (1988). Learning style instruments: Let the buyer beware. *Lifelong Learning: 11*(6),14-17.

Botwinick, J. (1978). *Aging and behavior*, 2nd ed. New York: Springer.

Breitrose, P. (1988). *Focus groups—When and how to use them: A practical guide*. Stanford University, Palo Alto, CA: Health Promotion Resource.

Bruer, J. (Summer 1993). The mind's journey from novice to expert. *American Educator, 17*(2), 6-15, 38-46.

Bruner, J. (1966). *Toward a theory of instruction*. Cambridge, MA: Harvard University Press.

Bubela, N., & Galloway, S. (1990). Factors influencing patients' informational needs at time of hospital discharge. *Patient Education and Counseling, 16*, 21-28.

Carroll, I. (1963). A model of school learning. *Teachers College Record, 64*, 723-733.

Chall, J., & Mirsky, A. (Eds.). (1978). Education and the brain. *Seventy-seventh yearbook of the National Society for the Study of Education*, Part 2. Chicago: University of Chicago Press.

Chase, W.G., & Simon, H.A. (1973). Perception in chess. *Cognitive Psychology, 4*, 55-81.

deTornay, R., & Thompson, M.A. (1987). *Strategies for teaching nursing*, 3rd ed. Albany, NY: Delmar.

Dunn, K., & Dunn, R. (March 1987). Dispelling outmodeled beliefs about student learning. *Educational Leadership, 44*(6), 55-62.

Dunn, R., & Dunn, K. (1978). *Teaching students through their individual learning styles: A practical approach*. Reston, VA: National Association of Secondary School Prinicpals.

Durden-Smith, J., & deSimone, D. (1983). *Sex and the brain*. New York: Arbor House.

Friedman, P., & Alley, R. (Winter 1984). Learning/teaching styles: Applying the principles. *Theory into Practice 23*(1), 77-81.

Gardner, H. (1983). *Frames of mind*. New York: Basic Books.

Garity, J. (1985). Learning styles: Basis for creative teaching and learning. *Nurse Educator, 10*(2), 12-16.

Gessner, B. (Sept. 1989). Adult education: The cornerstone of patient education. *Nursing Clinics of North America, 24*(3), 589-595.

Gondringer, N. (1989). Whole brain thinking: A potential link to successful learning. *Journal of the American Association of Nurse Anesthetists, 57*(3), 217-219.

Greer, G., Hitt, J. D, Sitterly, T.E., & Slebodnick, E. B. (1972). An examination of four factors impacting on psychomotor performance effectiveness. In D.P. Ely (Ed.), *Psychomotor domain: A resource book for media specialists*. Washington, DC: Gryphon House.

Gregorc, A.F. (1982). *An adult's guide to style*. Maynard, MA: Gabriel Systems.

Guild, P.B., & Garger, S. (1985). *Marching to different drummers*. Alexandria, VA: Association for Supervision and Curriculum Development.

Haggard, A. (1989). *Handbook of patient education*. Rockland, MD: Aspen.

Healthcare Education Association. (1985). *Managing hospital education*. Laquana Niquel, CA: Healthcare Education Associates.

Herrman, N. (1988). *The creative brain*. Lake Lure, NC: Brain Books.

Joseph, D.H. (1993). Risk: A concept worthy of attention. *Nursing Forum, 28*(1), 12-16.

Joyce, B. (1984). Dynamic Disequilibrium: The intelligence of growth. *Theory into Practice, 23*(1), 26-34.

Kolb, D.A. (1984). *Experiential learning: Experience as the source of learning and development*. Englewood Cliffs, NJ: Prentice-Hall.

Lichtenthal, C. (1990). *A self-study model on readiness to learn*. Unpublished.

Maslow, A. (1970). *Motivation and personality*. New York: Harper & Row.

McCarthy, B. (1981). *The 4Mat system: Teaching to learning styles with right/left mode techniques*. Barrington, IL: Excel.

Myers, I.B. (1980). *Gifts differing*. Palo Alto, CA: Consulting Psychologists Press.

Newell, A., & Simon, H.A. (1972). *Human problem solving*. Englewood Cliffs, NJ: Prentice-Hall.

Panno, J.M. (Nov./Dec.1992). A systematic approach for assessing learning needs. *Journal of Nursing Staff Development, 8*(6), 267-273.

Rankin, S.H., & Stallings, L.D. (1990). *Patient education: Issues, principles and practices*, 2nd ed. Philadelphia: Lippincott.

Roberts, C. (Sept. 1982). Identifying the real patient problems. *Nursing Clinics of North America, 17*(3), 484-485.

Ruzicki, D.A. (Sept. 1989). Realistically meeting the educational needs of hospitalized acute and short-stay patients. *Nursing Clinics of North America, 24*(3), 629-636.

Shipman, S., & Shipman, V.C. (1985). Cognitive styles: Some conceptual, methodological, and applied issues. In E.W. Gordon (Ed.), *Review of research in education,* Vol. 12. Washington, DC: American Educational Research Associates.

Simon, H.A., & Chase, W.G. (1973). Skill in chess. *American Scientist, 61,* 394-403.

Singer, R. N. (1972). The psychomotor domain: General considerations. In D.P. Ely (Ed.), *Psychomotor domain: A resource book for media specialists.* Washington, DC: Gryphon House.

Skinner, B.F. (1954). The science of learning and the art of teaching. *Harvard Educational Review, 24,* 86-97.

Sperry, R.W. (1977). Bridging science and values: A unifying view of mind and brain. *American Psychologist 32*(4), 237-245.

Tanner, G. (Aug. 1989). A need to know. *Nursing Times, 85*(31), 54-56.

Thompson, C. & Crutchlow, E. (Jan.-Feb. 1993). Learning style research: A critical review of the literature and implications for nursing education. *Journal of Professional Nursing, 9*(1), 34-40.

Villejo, L., and Myers, C. (May 1991). Brain function, learning styles, and cancer patient education. *Seminars in Oncology Nursing, 7*(2), 97-104.

Witkin, H., & Goodenough, D.R. (1981). *Cognitive styles: Essence and origins.* New York: International Universities Press.

Witkin, H., Moore, C.A., & Oltman, P.K. (1977). Cognitive styles and their educational implications. *Review of Educational Research, 47,* 1-64.

Witkin, H., Oltman, P.K., Raskin, E., & Karp, S. (1971a). *A manual for the Embedded Figures Tests.* Palo Alto, CA: Consulting Psychologists Press.

Witkin, H., Otlman, P.K., Raskin, E., & Karp, S. (1971b). *Group Embedded Figures Test.* Palo Alto, CA: Consulting Psychologists Press.

Wolfe, P. (Jan. 1994). Risk taking: Nursing's comfort zone. *Holistic Nurse Practice, 8*(2), 43-52.

Wonder, J. & Donovan, M. (1984). *Whole-brain thinking.* New York: Ballantine.

CHAPTER 5

Teaching Strategies Specific to Developmental Stages of Life

Susan B. Bastable

CHAPTER HIGHLIGHTS

Developmental Characteristics

The Developmental Stages of Childhood
    Infancy and Toddlerhood
    Preschooler
    School-Aged Childhood
    Adolescence

The Developmental Stages of Adulthood
    Young Adulthood
    Middle-Aged Adulthood
    Older Adulthood

The Role of the Family in Patient Education

KEY TERMS

physical maturation	cognitive development
psychosocial development	pedagogy
andragogy	gerogogy
crystallized intelligence	fluid intelligence

OBJECTIVES

After completing this chapter, the reader will be able to

1. Identify the physical, cognitive, and psychosocial characteristics of learners that influence learning at various stages of growth and development.
2. Recognize the role of the nurse as educator in assessing stage-specific learner needs according to maturational levels.
3. Determine the role of the family in patient education.
4. Discuss appropriate teaching strategies effective for learners at different developmental stages.

When planning, designing, and implementing an educational program, the nurse as educator must carefully consider the characteristics of learners with respect to their developmental stage in life. The more heterogeneous the target audience, the more complex the development of an educational program to meet the diverse needs of the population. Conversely, the more homogeneous the population of learners, the more straightforward the approach to teaching. An individual's developmental stage significantly influences the ability to learn. To meet the health-related educational needs of learners, a developmental approach must be used. There are three major stage-range factors associated with learner readiness—physical, cognitive, and psychosocial maturation—which must be taken into account at each developmental period throughout the life cycle. Developmental psychologists have for years explored the various patterns of behavior particular to stages of development. Educators, more than ever before, acknowledge the impact of growth and development on an individual's willingness and ability to make use of instruction.

This chapter has specific implications for staff nurses and staff development and in-service nurse educators because of the recent mandates by the Joint Commission on Accreditation of Healthcare Organizations (JCAHO). For healthcare agencies to meet JCAHO accreditation requirements, teaching plans must address stage-specific competencies of the learner. In this chapter, the distinct life stages of learners are examined from the perspective of physical, cognitive, and psychosocial development; the role of the nurse in assessment of stage-specific learner needs; the role of the family in the teaching-learning process; and the teaching strategies specific to meeting the needs of learners at various developmental stages of life.

A deliberate attempt has been made to minimize reference to age as the criterion for categorization of learners. Research shows that chronological age per se is not a good predictor of learning ability. At any given age, there can be a wide variation in the acquisition of abilities related to physical, cognitive, and psychosocial maturation. Thus, the term *developmental stage* will be used based on the confirmation by psychologists that human growth and development are sequential but not always specifically age-related.

Although this chapter focuses on the patient as the learner throughout the life span, the stage-specific characteristics of adulthood and the associated teaching principles of adult learning presented can be applied to any audience of older learners, whether the nurse is instructing the general public in the community or teaching continuing education to staff nurses. Emphasis is placed on the learning needs of the adult learner because the middle-aged and older adult constitute the largest percentage of the patient population. Furthermore, all nurses have had courses in developmental psychology and pediatrics in their basic nursing education programs, which thoroughly cover the content of childhood development.

DEVELOPMENTAL CHARACTERISTICS

Actual chronological age is only a relative indicator of someone's physical, cognitive, and psychosocial stage of development. Unique as each individual is, however, there are typical developmental trends that have been identified as milestones of normal progression through the life cycle. When dealing with the teaching-learning process, it is imperative to examine the developmental phases as an individual progresses from infancy to senescence to appreciate the behavioral changes that occur in the cognitive, affective, and psychomotor domains. As influential as age can be to learning readiness, it should never be examined in isolation. Growth and development interact with experiential background, physical and emotional health status, and personal motivation, as well as numerous environmental factors such as stress, the surrounding conditions, and the available support systems, to affect a person's ability and readiness to learn.

If the nurse as educator is to encourage learners to be responsible for their own health, then learners must be recognized as an important source of data regarding their health status. Before any learning can occur, the nurse must assess how much knowledge the learner already possesses with respect to the topic to be taught. With the child as client, for example, new content should be introduced at appropriate stages of development and built on the child's previous knowledge base and experiences.

The major question underlying the planning for educational experiences is, when is the most appropriate or best time to teach the learner? The answer is when the learner is ready—the "teachable moment" as defined by Havighurst (1976)—that point in time when the learner is most receptive to a teaching situation. It is important to remember that the nurse as educator does not always have to wait for teachable moments to occur; it is quite possible for the teacher to create these teachable moments by taking an interest in and attending to the needs of the learner. When assessing readiness to learn, the nurse educator must determine not only if an interpersonal relationship has been established, if prerequisite knowledge and skills have been mastered, and if the learner ex-

hibits motivation, but also if the plan for teaching matches the developmental level of the learner (Hussey & Hirsh, 1983).

THE DEVELOPMENTAL STAGES OF CHILDHOOD

Pedagogy is the art and science of helping children to learn. The different stages of childhood are divided according to what developmental theorists and educational psychologists define as specific patterns of behavior seen in particular phases of growth and development. The following is a review of the teaching strategies to be used in the four stages of childhood in relation to the physical, cognitive, and psychosocial maturational levels indicative of learner readiness (Table 5-1).

Infancy and Toddlerhood

The field of growth and development is highly complex, and at no other time is physical, cognitive, and psychosocial maturation so changeable as during the very early years of childhood. Because of the dependency of this age group, the main focus of instruction is geared toward the parents, who are considered to be the primary learners rather than the very young child. However, the older toddler should not be excluded from health-care teaching and can participate to some extent in the education process (Hussey & Hirsh, 1983).

Physical, Cognitive, and Psychosocial Development

At no other time in life is physical maturation so rapid as during the period of development from infancy to toddlerhood. Exploration of self and the environment becomes paramount and a stimulant for further physical development. Patient education must focus on teaching the parents of very young children the importance of stimulation and the practice of safety measures.

Piaget (1951, 1952, 1976), the noted expert in defining the key milestones in the cognitive development of children, labeled the stage of infancy to toddlerhood as the *sensorimotor* period. As children mature from infancy to toddlerhood, learning is enhanced through sensory experiences and through movement and manipulation of objects in the environment. Motor activities promote their understanding of the world and an awareness of themselves as well as others' reactions in response to their own actions. The toddler has the rudimentary capacity for basic reasoning, understands object permanence, has the beginnings of memory, and begins to develop an elementary concept of causality. With limited ability to recall past happenings or anticipate future events, the toddler is oriented primarily to the "here and now" and has little tolerance for delayed gratification. The child who has lived with strict routines and plenty of structure will have more of a grasp of time than those who live in an unstructured environment. Children at this stage have short attention spans, are easily distracted, are egocentric in their thinking, and are not amenable to correction of their own ideas. Unquestionably, they believe their own perceptions to be reality. Asking questions is the hallmark of this age group, and curiosity abounds as they explore places and things. They can respond to simple, step-by-step commands and obey such directives as "kiss Daddy goodnight" or "put your hat on" (Petrillo & Sanger, 1980; Levine, 1983). Language skills are acquired rapidly during this period, and parents should be encouraged to foster this aspect of development by talking with and listening to their child. As they progress through this phase, children begin to engage in fantasizing and "make-believe" play. Because they are unable to distinguish fact from fiction and have limited cognitive capacity for understanding cause and effect, a child may feel that illness and hospitalization are a punishment for something done wrong.

According to Erikson (1963), the noted authority on psychosocial development, the period of infancy is one of *trust versus mistrust*. This is the time when children must work through their first major dilemma of developing a sense of trust with their primary caretaker. As the infant matures into toddlerhood, *autonomy versus shame and doubt* emerges as the central issue. During this period of psychosocial growth, toddlers must learn to balance feelings of love and hate and learn to cooperate and control willful desires. Children progress sequentially through accomplishing the tasks of developing basic trust in their environment to reaching increasing levels

of independence and self-assertion. Their newly discovered sense of independence often is expressed by demonstrations of negativism. Children may have difficulty in making up their minds, and, aggravated by personal and external limits, their level of frustration and feelings of ambivalence are often expressed in words and behaviors, such as in exhibiting temper tantrums to release tensions (Falvo, 1994). With peers, play is a parallel activity, and it is not unusual for them to end up in tears because they have not yet learned about tact, fairness, or rules of sharing (Babcock & Miller, 1994). Toddlers like routines because it gives them a sense of security, and they gravitate toward ritualistic ceremonial-like exercises when carrying out activities of daily living. Separation anxiety also is characteristic of this stage of development and is particularly apparent when children are hospitalized and feel insecure in an unfamiliar environment. This anxiety is often compounded when they are subjected to medical procedures and other health-care interventions performed by people who are strangers to them.

Teaching Strategies

Patient education for infancy through toddlerhood need not be illness related. Usually less time is devoted to teaching parents about illness care, and considerably more time is spent teaching aspects of normal development, safety, health promotion, and disease prevention. When the child is ill, the first priority for teaching interventions would be to assess the parent's and child's anxiety levels and help them cope with their feelings of stress related to uncertainty and guilt. Anxiety on the part of the child and parent can adversely affect their readiness to learn.

Although teaching activities primarily are directed to the main caregiver(s), children at this developmental stage in life have a great capacity for learning. Toddlers are capable of some degree of understanding procedures they may experience. Because of the natural tendency for a child to be intimidated by unfamiliar people, it is imperative that a primary nurse be assigned to establish a relationship with the child and parents. This approach will not only provide consistency in the teaching-learning process but also help to reduce the child's fear of strangers. Parents should be

TABLE 5–1. Stage-appropriate teaching strategies

Learner	General Characteristics	Teaching Strategies	Nursing Interventions
INFANCY-TODDLERHOOD			
Approximate age: Birth–3 yr Cognitive stage: Sensorimotor (Birth–12 mo) Psychosocial stage: Trust vs. mistrust Autonomy vs. shame and doubt (1–3 yr)	Dependent on environment Needs security Explores self and environment Natural curiosity	Orient teaching to caregiver Use repetition and imitation of information Stimulate all senses Provide physical safety and emotional security Allow play and manipulation of objects	Welcome active involvement Forge alliances Encourage physical closeness Provide detailed information Answer questions and concerns Ask for information on child's strengths/limitations and likes/dislikes
PRESCHOOLER			
Approximate age: 3–6 yr Cognitive stage: Preoperational Psychosocial stage: Initiative vs. guilt	Egocentric Thinking precausal, concrete, literal Believes illness self-caused and punitive Limited sense of time Fears bodily injury Cannot generalize Animistic thinking (objects possess life or human characteristics) Centration (focus is on one characteristic of an object) Separation anxiety Motivated by curiosity Active imagination, prone to fears Play is his/her work	Use warm, calm approach Build trust Use repetition of information Allow manipulation of objects and equipment Give care with explanation Reassure not to blame self Explain procedures simply and briefly Provide safe, secure environment Use positive reinforcement Encourage questions to reveal perceptions/feelings Use simple drawings and stories Use play therapy, with dolls and puppets Stimulate senses: visual, auditory, tactile, motor	Welcome active involvement Forge alliances Encourage physical closeness Provide detailed information Answer questions and concerns Ask for information on child's strengths/limitations and likes/dislikes

SCHOOL-AGED CHILDHOOD

Approximate age: 7–11 yr
Cognitive stage: Concrete operations
Psychosocial stage: Industry vs. inferiority

More realistic and objective
Understands cause and effect
Deductive/inductive reasoning
Wants concrete information
Able to compare objects and events
Variable rates of physical growth
Reasons syllogistically
Understands seriousness and consequences of actions
Subject-centered focus
Immediate orientation

Encourage independence and active participation
Be honest, allay fears
Use logical explanation
Allow time to ask questions
Use analogies to make invisible processes real
Establish role models
Relate care to other children's experiences; compare procedures
Use subject-centered focus
Use play therapy
Provide group activities
Use drawings, models, dolls, painting, audio- and video-tapes

Welcome active involvement
Forge alliances
Encourage physical closeness
Provide detailed information
Answer questions and concerns
Ask for information on child's strengths/limitations and likes/dislikes

ADOLESCENCE

Approximate age: 12–18 yr
Cognitive stage: Formal operations
Psychosocial stage: Identity vs. role confusion

Abstract, hypothetical thinking
Can build on past learning
Reasons by logic and understands scientific principles
Future orientation
Motivated by desire for social acceptance
Peer group important
Intense personal preoccupation, appearance extremely important (imaginary audience)
Feels invulnerable, invincible/immune to natural laws (personal fable)

Establish trust, authenticity
Know their agenda
Address fears/concerns about outcomes of illness
Identify control focus
Include in plan of care
Use peers for support and influence
Negotiate changes
Focus on details
Make information meaningful to life
Ensure confidentiality and privacy
Arrange group sessions
Use audiovisuals, role play, contracts, reading materials
Provide for experimentation and flexibility

Explore emotional and financial support
Determine goals and expectations
Assess stress levels
Respect values and norms
Determine role responsibilities and relationships
Allow for 1:1 teaching without parents present, but with adolescent's permission; inform family of content covered

TABLE 5–1. Stage-appropriate teaching strategies (Continued)

	Learner	General Characteristics	Teaching Strategies	Nursing Interventions
YOUNG ADULTHOOD				
Approximate age:	18–40 yr	Autonomous	Use problem-centered focus	Explore emotional, financial,
Cognitive stage:	Formal operations	Self-directed	Draw on meaningful	and physical support system
Psychosocial stage:	Intimacy *vs.* isolation	Uses personal experiences to	experiences	Assess motivational level for
		enhance or interfere with	Focus on immediacy of	involvement
		learning	application	Identify potential obstacles and
		Intrinsic motivation	Encourage active participation	stressors
		Able to analyze critically	Allow to set own pace, be	
		Makes decisions about per-	self-directed	
		sonal, occupational, and	Organize material	
		social roles	Recognize social role	
		Competency-based learner	Apply new knowledge through	
			role play and hands-on	
			practice	
MIDDLE-AGED ADULTHOOD				
Approximate age:	40–65 yr	Sense of self well-developed	Focus on maintaining indepen-	Explore emotional, financial,
Cognitive stage:	Formal operations	Concerned with physical	dence and reestablishing	and physical support system
Psychosocial stage:	Generativity *vs.*	changes	normal life patterns	Assess motivational level for
	self-absorption and	At peak in career	Assess positive and negative	involvement
	stagnation	Explores alternative lifestyles	past experiences with	Identify potential obstacles and
		Reflects on contributions to	learning	stressors
		family and society	Assess potential sources of	
		Reexamines goals and values	stress due to mid-life crisis	
		Questions achievements and	issues	
		successes	Provide information to coincide	
		Has confidence in abilities	with life concerns and	
		Desires to modify unsatisfactory	problems	
		aspects of life		

Approximate age: 65 yr and over
Cognitive stage: Formal operations
Psychosocial stage: Ego integrity vs. despair

Cognitive changes
Decreased ability to think abstractly, process information
Decreased short-term memory
Increased reaction time
Increased test anxiety
Stimulus persistence (afterimage)
Focuses on past life experiences

Use concrete examples
Build on past life experiences
Make information relevant and meaningful
Present one concept at a time
Allow time for processing/ response (slow pace)
Use repetition and reinforcement of information
Avoid written exams
Use verbal exchange and coaching
Establish retrieval plan (use one or several clues)
Encourage active involvement
Keep explanations brief
Use analogies to illustrate abstract information

Sensory/motor deficits
Auditory changes
Hearing loss, especially high-pitched tones, consonants (S, Z, T, F, & G), and rapid speech
Visual changes
Farsighted (needs glasses to read)
Lenses become opaque (glare problem)
Smaller pupil size (decreased visual adaptation to darkness)
Decreased peripheral perception

Speak slowly, distinctly
Use low-pitched tones
Face client when speaking
Minimize distractions
Avoid shouting
Use visual aids to supplement verbal instruction
Avoid glares, use soft white light
Provide sufficient light
Use white backgrounds and black print
Use large letters and well-spaced print
Avoid color coding with blues, greens, purples, and yellows
Increase safety precautions/provide safe environment

Involve principal caregivers
Encourage participation
Provide resources for support (respite care)
Assess coping mechanisms
Provide written instructions for reinforcement
Provide anticipatory problem solving (what happens if . . .)

TABLE 5–1. Stage-appropriate teaching strategies (Continued)

Learner	General Characteristics	Teaching Strategies	Nursing Interventions
OLDER ADULTHOOD (*continued*)	Yellowing of lenses (distorts low-tone colors: blue, green, violet) Distorted depth perception Fatigue/decreased energy levels Pathophysiology (chronic illness)	Ensure accessibility and fit of prostheses (i.e., glasses, hearing aid) Keep sessions short Provide for frequent rest periods Allow for extra time to perform Establish realistic short-term goals	
	Psychosocial changes Decreased risk taking Selective learning Intimidated by formal learning	Give time to reminisce Identify and present pertinent material Use informal teaching sessions Demonstrate relevance of information to daily life Assess resources Make learning positive Identify past positive experiences Integrate new behaviors with formerly established ones	

present whenever possible during learning activities to allay stress, which could be compounded by separation anxiety.

Ideally, health teaching should take place in an environment familiar to the child, such as the home or day-care center. When the child is hospitalized, the environment selected for teaching and learning sessions should be as safe and secure as possible, such as the child's bed or the playroom, to increase the child's sense of feeling protected. Movement is an important mechanism by which toddlers communicate. Immobility due to illness or hospital confinement increases children's anxiety by restricting activity. Nursing interventions should be chosen that promote children's use of gross motor abilities and that stimulate their visual, auditory, and tactile senses. Developing a rapport with children through simple teaching will help to elicit their cooperation and active involvement. The approach to children should be warm, honest, calm, accepting, and matter-of-fact. A smile, a warm tone of voice, a gesture of encouragement, or a word of praise goes a long way in attracting their attention and helping children adjust to new circumstances. Fundamental to the child's response is how the parents respond to health-care personnel and medical interventions.

The following teaching strategies are suggested to convey information to this age group. These strategies feed into children's natural tendency for play and their need for active participation and sensory experiences:

FOR SHORT-TERM LEARNING

- Read simple stories from books with lots of pictures.
- Use dolls and puppets to act out feelings and behaviors.
- Use simple audiotapes with music and videotapes with cartoon characters.
- Role-play to bring the child's imagination closer to reality.
- Give simple, concrete, nonthreatening explanations to accompany visual and tactile experiences.
- Perform procedures on a teddy bear first to help the child comprehend what an experience will be like.
- Allow the child something to do—squeeze your hand, hold a Band-Aid, cry if it hurts—to

channel their responses to an unpleasant experience.
- Keep teaching sessions brief (no longer than about 5 minutes each) because of the child's short attention span.
- Cluster teaching sessions close together so that children can remember what they learned from one instructional encounter to another.
- Avoid analogies and explain things in straightforward and simple terms because children take their world literally and concretely.
- Individualize the pace of teaching according to the child's responses and level of attention.

FOR LONG-TERM LEARNING

- Focus on rituals, imitation, and repetition of information in the form of words and actions to hold the child's attention.
- Use reinforcement as an opportunity for children to achieve permanence of learning through practice.
- Employ the teaching methods of gaming and modeling as a means by which children can learn about the world and test their ideas over time.
- Encourage parents to act as role models because their values and beliefs serve as a reinforcement of healthy behaviors and impact significantly on the child's development of attitudes and behaviors.

Preschooler

Preschool children continue with development of skills learned in the earlier years of growth. Their sense of identity becomes clearer, and their world expands to encompass involvement with others external to the family unit. Children in this developmental category acquire new behaviors that give them more independence from their parents and allow them to care for themselves more autonomously. Learning during this time period occurs through interactions with others and through mimicking or modeling the behaviors of playmates and adults.

Physical, Cognitive, and Psychosocial Development

The physical maturation of preschoolers is an extension of their prior growth. Fine and gross motor skills become increasingly more refined and coordinated so that they now are able to carry out activities of daily living with greater independence. Although their efforts are more coordinated, supervision of activities is still required because they lack judgment in carrying out the skills they have developed.

The preschooler's stage of cognitive development is labeled by Piaget (1951, 1952,1976) as the *preoperational* period. The young child continues to be egocentric and is essentially unaware of others' thoughts or the existence of others' points of view. Preschoolers can recall past experiences and anticipate future events. They can classify objects into groups and categories but with only a vague understanding of their relationships. Thinking remains literal and concrete—they believe what is seen and heard. Reasoning is transductive, that is, from the particular to the particular, rather than inductive or deductive. Precausal thinking allows preschoolers to understand that people can make things happen, but they are unaware of causation as the result of invisible physical and mechanical forces. They often believe that they can influence natural phenomena, and their beliefs reflect animistic thinking—the tendency to endow inanimate objects with life and consciousness (Pidgeon, 1977).

Preschoolers are very curious, can think intuitively, and pose questions about almost anything. They want to know the reasons, cause, and purpose for everything (the whys) but are unconcerned at this point with the process (the hows). Fantasy and reality are not well differentiated. Children in this cognitive stage mix fact and fiction, tend to generalize, think magically, develop imaginary playmates, and believe they can control events with their thoughts. However, they do possess self-awareness and realize that they are vulnerable to outside influences. The preschooler also continues to have a limited sense of time. For children of this age, being made to wait 15 minutes before they can do something can feel like an eternity. They do, though, understand the timing of familiar events in their daily lives, such as when breakfast or dinner is eaten and when they can play or watch their favorite television program. Their attention span begins to lengthen such that they can usually remain quiet long enough to listen to a song or hear a short story read.

In the preschool stage, children begin to develop sexual identity and curiosity, an interest that may cause parents considerable discomfort. Cognitive understanding of their bodies related to structure, function, health, and illness becomes more specific and differentiated. They can name external body parts but have only an ill-defined concept of the size and shape of internal organs and the function of body parts (Kotchabhakdi, 1985). Explanations of the purpose of and reasons for a procedure are still beyond their level of reasoning, and therefore, explanations have to be kept very simple and matter-of-fact (Pidgeon, 1985). They have a fear of body mutilation and pain, which not only stems from their lack of understanding of the body but also is compounded by their active imagination. Their ideas regarding illness also are primitive with respect to cause and effect; illness is a punishment for something they did wrong, either through omission or commission. Health, on the other hand, may be identified with doing things right. Health allows them to play with friends and participate in desired activities; illness prevents them from doing so (Hussey & Hirsh, 1983).

Erikson (1963) has labeled the preschooler's psychosocial maturation level as the period of *initiative versus guilt*. Children take on tasks for the sake of being involved and on the move. Excess energy and a desire to dominate may lead to frustration and anger on their part. They show evidence of expanding imagination and creativity, are impulsive in their actions, and are curious about almost everything they see and do. Their growing imagination can lead to many fears—of separation, disapproval, pain, punishment, and aggression from others. Loss of body integrity is the preschooler's greatest threat, which significantly affects his willingness to interact with health-care personnel (Poster, 1983; Vulcan, 1984). In this phase of development, children begin interacting with playmates rather than just playing alongside one another. Appropriate social behaviors demand that they learn to wait for others, give others a turn, and recognize the needs of others. Play in the mind of a child is equivalent to the work performed by adults. Play can be as equally productive as adult work and is a means for self-education of the physical and social world. Play helps the child act out feelings and experiences to master fears, develop role skills, and express joys, sorrows, and hostilities. Through play, the preschooler also begins to share ideas and imitate parents of the same sex. Role-playing is typical of this age as the child attempts to learn the responsibilities of family members and others in society.

Teaching Strategies

The nurse's interactions with preschool children and their parents are often sporadic, usually occurring during occasional well-child visits to the pediatrician's office or when minor medical problems arise. During these interactions, the nurse should take every opportunity to teach parents about health promotion and disease prevention measures, to provide guidance regarding normal growth and development, and to instruct about medical recommendations when illnesses do arise. Parents can be a great asset to the nurse in working with children in this developmental phase, and they should be included in all aspects of the educational plan and the actual teaching experience (Ryberg & Merrifield, 1984). Parents can serve as the primary resource to answer questions about their child's disabilities, their idiosyncrasies, their favorite toys—all of which may affect their ability to learn (Hussey & Hirsh, 1983).

Children's fear of pain and bodily harm is uppermost in their minds, whether they are well or ill. Because of preschoolers' fantasies and active imaginations, it is most important for the nurse to reassure them and allow them to express themselves openly about their fears (Heiney, 1991). Choose your words carefully when describing procedures. Preschoolers are familiar with many words, but using terms like "cut" or "knife" is frightening to them. Instead, use less threatening words like "fix," "sew," or "cover up the hole." "Band-Aids" rather than "dressings" is a much more understandable term, and bandages are thought by children to have magical healing powers (Babcock & Miller, 1994).

Although still dependent on family, the preschooler has begun to have increasing contact with the outside world and is usually able to interact more comfortably with others. However, significant adults in a child's life should be invited as participants during teaching sessions. They can provide support to the child, substitute as the teacher if the child is reluctant to interact with the nurse, and can reinforce teaching at a later point in time. The primary caretakers, usually the mother and father, are the recipients of the majority of the nurse's teaching efforts. They will be the learners to assist the child in achieving desired health outcomes (Hussey & Hirsh, 1983; Kennedy & Riddle, 1989). The following specific teaching strategies are recommended:

FOR SHORT-TERM LEARNING

- Provide physical and visual stimuli because language ability is still limited, both for purposes of expressing ideas as well as comprehending verbal instructions.
- Keep teaching sessions short (no more than 15 minutes) and scheduled sequentially at close intervals so that information is not forgotten.
- Relate information needs to activities and experiences familiar to the child.
- Encourage the child to participate in selecting between a limited number of teaching-learning options, such as playing with dolls or reading a story, which promotes active involvement and helps to establish a nurse-client rapport.
- Arrange small group sessions with peers as a way to make teaching less threatening and more fun.
- Give praise and approval, through both verbal expressions and nonverbal gestures, which are real motivators for learning.
- Give tangible rewards, such as badges or small toys, immediately following a successful learning experience as reinforcers in the mastery of cognitive and psychomotor skills.
- Allow the child to manipulate equipment and play with replicas or dolls to learn about body parts. Special kidney dolls, ostomy dolls with stomas, or orthopedic dolls with splints and tractions provide opportunity for hands-on experience.
- Use storybooks to emphasize the humanity of health-care personnel, to depict relationships between child, parents, and others, and to assist with helping the child identify with particular situations.

FOR LONG-TERM LEARNING

- Enlist the help of parents, who can play a vital role in modeling a variety of healthy habits, such as practicing safety measures and eating a balanced diet.

- Reinforce positive health behaviors and the acquisition of specific skills.

School-Aged Childhood

School-aged children have progressed in their physical, cognitive, and psychosocial skills to the point where most begin formal training in structured school systems. They approach learning with enthusiastic anticipation, and their minds are open to new and varied ideas. Children at this developmental level are motivated to learn because of their natural curiosity and their desire to understand more about themselves, their bodies, their world, and the influence that different things in the world have on them (Hussey & Hirsh, 1983). This is a period of great change for them, when attitudes, values, and perceptions of themselves, their society, and the world are shaped and expanded. Visions of their own environment and the cultures of others take on more depth and breadth.

Physical, Cognitive, and Psychosocial Development

The gross- and fine-motor abilities of school-aged children are increasingly more coordinated so that they are able to control their movements with much greater dexterity than ever before. Involvement in all kinds of curricular and extracurricular activities helps them to fine-tune their psychomotor skills. Physical growth during this phase is highly variable, with the rate of development differing from child to child. Toward the end of this developmental period, girls more so than boys on the average begin to experience prepubescent bodily changes and tend to exceed the boys in physical maturation. Growth charts, which monitor the rate of growth, are a more sensitive indicator of health or disability than actual size (Burkett, 1989).

Piaget (1951, 1952, 1976) has labeled the cognitive development in the school-aged child as the period of *concrete operations*. This is the time when logical thought processes and the ability to reason develop. School-aged children are able to think more objectively, are willing to listen to others, and will selectively use questioning to find answers to the unknown. At this stage, they begin to reason syllogistically, that is, they can consider two premises and draw a logical conclusion from

them (Elkind, 1984). They are intellectually able to understand cause and effect in a concrete way. Concepts are beginning to be mastered (Babcock & Miller, 1994), such as conservation (a piece of clay weighs the same no matter whether it changes shape), reversibility (liquid is the same amount whether it is poured into a tall glass or into a short wide cup), and inferred reality (an object remains its original color even when a black filter is put in front of it). Fiction and fantasy are separate from fact and reality. The skills of memory, decision making, insight, and problem solving are all more fully developed. Children in this phase of development are capable of engaging in systematic thought through inductive reasoning. They are able to classify objects and systems, express concrete ideas about relationships and people, and can carry out mathematical operations (Lambert, 1984). Also, they begin to understand and use sarcasm as well as to employ well-developed language skills for telling jokes, conveying complex stories, and communicating increasingly sophisticated thoughts. However, thinking is still quite literal, with only a vague understanding of abstractions. Early on in this phase, children are reluctant to do away with magical thinking in exchange for reality thinking. Cherished beliefs, such as the existence of Santa Claus or the tooth fairy, are clung to for the fun and excitement that the fantasy provides them, even when they have information that proves contrary to their beliefs.

School-aged children have developed the ability to concentrate for extended periods, can tolerate delayed gratification, are responsible for independently carrying out activities of daily living, have a good understanding of the environment as a whole, and can generalize from experience. They understand time, can predict time intervals, are oriented to the past and present, have some grasp and interest in the future, and have a vague appreciation for how immediate actions can have implications over the course of time. Special interests in topics of their choice begin to emerge, and they can pursue subjects and activities with devotion to increase their talents in particular areas.

Children at this cognitive stage can make decisions and act in accordance with how events are interpreted, but they understand only to some extent the seriousness or consequences of their choices. Children in the early period of this developmental phase know the functions and names of many common body parts, whereas older children have a more specific knowledge of anatomy and can differentiate between external and internal organs with a beginning understanding of their complex functions (Kotchabhakdi, 1985).

In the shift from precausal to causal thinking, the child begins to incorporate the idea that illness is related to cause and effect and can recognize that germs create disease. Illness is thought of in terms of social consequences and role alterations, such as the realization that they will miss school and outside activities, people will feel sorry for them, and they will be unable to maintain their usual routine (Banks, 1990). Research indicates that there are, however, systematic differences in children's reasoning skills with respect to understanding body functioning and the cause of illness as a result of their experiences with illness. Children suffering from chronic diseases have been found to have more sophisticated conceptualization of illness causality and body functioning than do their healthy peers. Piaget (1976) postulated that experience with a phenomenon catalyzes a better understanding of it. On the other hand, the stress and anxiety resulting from having to live with a chronic illness have been shown to interfere with a child's general cognitive performance. Chronically ill children have a less refined understanding of the physical world than healthy children and often are unable to generalize what they learned about a specific illness to a broader understanding of illness causality (Perrin et al., 1991). Thus, illness may act as an intrusive factor in overall cognitive development.

Erikson (1963) characterizes school-aged children's psychosocial stage of life as *industry versus inferiority*. During this period, children begin to gain an awareness of their unique talents and special qualities that distinguish them from one another. They begin to establish their self-concept as members of a social group larger than their own nuclear family and start to compare family values with those of the outside world. The school environment, in particular, facilitates their gaining a sense of responsibility and reliability. With less dependency on family, they extend their intimacy to include special friends and social groups. Relationships with peers and adults external to the home environment become important influences in their development of self-esteem and their suscep-

tibility to social forces outside the family unit. School-aged children fear failure and being left out of groups. They worry about their inabilities and become self-critical as they compare their own accomplishments to those of their peers. They also fear illness and disability that could significantly disrupt their academic progress, interfere with social contacts, decrease their independence, and result in loss of control over body functioning.

Teaching Strategies

With their increased ability to comprehend information and their desire for active involvement and control of their lives, it is very important to include school-aged children in patient education efforts. The nurse in the role of educator should explain illness, treatment plans, and procedures in simple, logical terms in accordance with the child's level of understanding and reasoning. Although school-aged children are able to think logically, the ability for abstract thought is limited. Therefore, teaching should be presented in concrete terms with step-by-step instructions (Pidgeon, 1985). It is imperative that you observe children's reactions and listen to their verbal feedback to be certain that information shared has not been misinterpreted or confused.

To the extent feasible, parents should be informed of what their child is being taught. Teaching parents directly is encouraged so they may be involved in fostering their child's independence, providing emotional support and physical assistance, and giving guidance regarding the correct techniques or regimens in self-care management. Siblings and peers also should be considered as sources of support (Hussey & Hirsh, 1983). In attempting to master self-care skills, children thrive on praise from others important in their lives as rewards for their accomplishments and successes.

Education for health promotion and health maintenance most likely occurs in the school system by the school nurse, but the parents as well as the nurse outside the school setting should be told what content is being addressed. Information then can be reinforced and expanded on when in contact with the child in other care settings. Numerous opportunities for nurses to teach the individual child or groups of school-aged children about health promotion and disease and injury prevention are available in schools, physicians' offices, community centers, outpatient clinics, or hospitals. Health education for children of this age can be very fragmented because of the many encounters they have with nurses in a variety of settings. The school nurse, in particular, is in an opportune position to coordinate the efforts of all other providers to avoid duplication of teaching content or the giving of conflicting information as well as to provide reinforcement of learning.

The specific conditions that may come to the attention of the nurse in caring for children at this phase of development are problems such as behavioral disorders, hyperactivity, learning disorders, diabetes, asthma, and enuresis. Extensive teaching may be needed to help children and parents understand a particular condition and how to overcome or deal with it. The need to sustain or bolster their self-image and self-esteem requires that children be invited to participate, to the extent possible, in planning for and carrying out learning activities. Because of children's fears of falling behind in school, being separated from peer groups, and being left out of social activities, teaching must be geared to fostering normal development despite the limitations that may be imposed by illness (Falvo, 1994).

Because school-aged children are used to the structured, direct, and formal learning in the school environment, they are receptive to a similar teaching-learning approach when hospitalized or confined at home. The following teaching strategies are suggested when caring for children in this developmental stage of life:

FOR SHORT-TERM LEARNING

- Allow school-aged children to take responsibility for their own health care because they are not only willing but also capable of manipulating equipment with accuracy. Because of their adeptness in relation to manual dexterity, mathematical operations, and logical thought processes, they can be taught, for example, to calculate and administer their own insulin or use an asthma inhaler as prescribed.
- Teaching sessions can be extended to last up to 30 minutes each because the increased cognitive abilities of school-aged children aids in the retention of information. However, lessons should be spread apart to allow for comprehension of large amounts of content and to provide opportunity for the practice of newly acquired skills between sessions.
- Use diagrams, models, pictures, videotapes, and printed materials as adjuncts to various teaching methods because an increased facility with language (both spoken and written) as well as with mathematical concepts allows for them to work with more complex instructional tools.
- Choose audiovisuals and printed materials that show peers undergoing similar procedures or facing similar situations.
- Clarify any scientific terminology and medical jargon used.
- Use analogies as an effective means of providing information in meaningful terms, such as "A chest x-ray is like having your picture taken" or "White blood cells are like police cells that can attack and destroy infection."
- Use one-to-one teaching sessions as a method to individualize learning relevant to the child's own experiences and as a means to interpret the results of nursing interventions particular to the child's own condition.
- Provide time for clarification, validation, and reinforcement of what is being learned.
- Select individual instructional techniques that provide opportunity for privacy, an increasingly important concern for this group of learners, who often feel quite self-conscious and modest when learning about bodily functions.
- Employ group teaching sessions with others of similar age and with similar problems or needs to help children avoid feelings of isolation and to assist them in identifying with their own peers.
- Prepare children for a procedure well in advance to allow them time to cope with their feelings and fears, to anticipate events, and to understand the purpose of a procedure, how it relates to their condition, and how much time it will take.
- Encourage participation in planning for procedures and events because active involvement will help the child to assimilate information more readily.
- Provide much needed nurturance and support, for it must be kept in mind that young children are not just small adults.

FOR LONG-TERM LEARNING

- Help school-aged children acquire skills that they can use to assume self-care responsibility for carrying out therapeutic treatment regimens on an ongoing basis with minimal assistance.
- Assist them in learning to maintain their own well-being and prevent illnesses from occurring.

Research suggests that lifelong health attitudes and behaviors begin in the early childhood phase of development and are intrapersonally consistent throughout the stage of middle childhood. The development of cognitive understanding of health and illness has been shown to follow a systematic progression parallel to the stage of general cognitive development. As the child matures, beliefs about health and illness become less concrete and more abstract, less egocentric, and increasingly differentiated and consistent. Motivation, self-esteem, and positive self-perception are personal characteristics that influence health behavior. It has been found that the higher the grade level of the child, the greater the understanding of illness and an awareness of body cues. Thus, children become more actively involved in their own health care as they progress developmentally (Farrand & Cox, 1993). Teaching should be directed at assisting them to incorporate positive health actions into their daily lives. Because of the importance of peer influence, group activities are an effective method of teaching health behaviors, attitudes, and values.

Adolescence

The stage of adolescence marks the transition from childhood to adulthood. During this prolonged and very changeable period of time, many adolescents and their families experience much turmoil. How adolescents think about themselves and the world significantly influences many health-care issues facing them, from anorexia to diabetes. Teenage thought and behavior give insight into the etiology of some of the major health problems of this group of learners (Elkind, 1984). Adolescents are known to be among the nation's most at-risk populations (American Association of Colleges of Nursing, 1994). For patient education to be effective, an understanding of the characteristics of the adolescent phase of development is crucial.

Physical, Cognitive, and Psychosocial Development

Adolescents vary greatly in their biological, psychological, social, and cognitive development. From a physical maturation standpoint, they are faced with adapting to rapid and significant bodily changes, which can temporarily result in clumsiness and poorly coordinated movement. Alterations in physical size, shape, and function of their bodies, along with the appearance and development of secondary sex characteristics, bring about a significant preoccupation with their appearance and a strong desire to express sexual urges (Falvo, 1994).

Piaget (1951, 1952, 1976) termed this stage of cognitive development as the period of *formal operations*. Adolescents have attained a new, higher-order level of reasoning superior to earlier childhood thoughts. They are capable of abstract thought and complex logical reasoning described as propositional as opposed to syllogistic. Their reasoning is both inductive and deductive, and they are able to hypothesize and apply the principles of logic to situations never encountered before. Adolescents can conceptualize and internalize ideas, debate various points of view, understand cause and effect, comprehend complex explanations, and respond appropriately to multiple-step directions (Heiney, 1991; Day, 1981).

Formal operational thought enables adolescents to conceptualize invisible processes and make determinations about what others say and how they behave. With this capacity, teenagers can become obsessed with what others are thinking and begin to believe that everyone is concerned about the same things they are—namely, themselves and their activities. Elkind (1984) labeled this belief as the "imaginary audience," which has considerable influence over an adolescent's behavior. This imaginary audience explains the pervasive self-consciousness of adolescents, who, on the one hand, may feel embarrassed because they believe everyone is looking at them and, on the other hand, desire to be looked at and thought about because this confirms their sense of specialness and uniqueness.

Adolescents are able to understand the concept of health and illness, the multiple causes of diseases, the influence of variables on health status, and the ideas associated with health promotion and disease prevention. They understand illness as a process resulting from a dysfunction or nonfunction of a part or parts of the body and can comprehend the outcomes or prognosis of an illness. They also are able to identify health behaviors but may reject practicing them or begin to engage in risk-taking behaviors because of the social pressures they receive from peers as well as their feelings of invincibility. Elkind (1984) has called this belief of invulnerability the "personal fable." The personal fable leads the adolescent to believe that *other* people grow old and die, but not *them; other* people may not realize their personal ambitions, but *they* will. The fable has value in that it allows individuals to carry on with their lives even in the face of all kinds of dangers. But this fable also leads teenagers to believe they are cloaked in an invisible shield that will protect them from bodily harm despite any risks to which they may subject themselves. They can understand implications of future outcomes, but their immediate concern is with the present.

Erikson (1968) has labeled the psychosocial dilemma adolescents face as one of *identity versus role confusion*. They indulge in comparing their self-image with an ideal image. Adolescents find themselves in a struggle to establish their own identity, match their skills with career choices, and determine their "self." They work to emancipate themselves from their parents, seeking independence and autonomy so they can emerge as more distinct individual personalities. Teenagers have a strong need for group belongingness, friendship, peer acceptance, and peer support. They tend to rebel against any actions or recommendations by adults whom they consider authoritarian. Their concern over personal appearance and their need to look and act like their peers drive them to conform to the dress and behavior of this age group, which is usually contradictory and nonconformist in relation to the models, codes, and values of their parents' generation. Conflict, toleration, or alienation characterizes the relationship between adolescents and their parents and other authority figures. Adolescents seek to develop new and trusting relationships outside the home but are vulnerable to the opinions of those they emulate. Adolescents demand personal space, control, privacy, and confidentiality. Illness, injury, and hospitalization to them means dependency, loss of identity, a change in body image and functioning,

bodily embarrassment, confinement, separation from peers, and possible death.

Teaching Strategies

Although the majority of individuals at this phase of development remain relatively healthy, an estimated 20% of the United States's 31 million teenagers have at least one serious health problem such as asthma, diabetes, a range of disabilities as a result of injury, or psychological problems as a result of depression or physical and/or emotional maltreatment. In addition, adolescents are considered at high risk for teen pregnancy, the effects of poverty, drug or alcohol abuse, suicide, and sexually transmitted diseases such as venereal disease and AIDS. Greater than 30% of all adolescent deaths are a result of motor vehicle accidents. In spite of all these possible threats to their well-being, adolescents use medical services the least frequently of all age groups. Compounding this fact is the realization that adolescent health has not been a national priority and their health problems have been largely ignored by the health-care system (American Association of Colleges of Nursing, 1994). Thus, the educational needs of adolescents are broad and varied. The potential topics for teaching are numerous, ranging from sexual adjustment, contraception, and venereal disease to accident prevention, nutrition, and substance abuse.

Healthy teens have difficulty imagining themselves as sick or injured. Those with an illness or disability often comply poorly with medical regimens and continue to indulge in risk-taking behaviors. Because of their preoccupation with body image and functioning and the importance of peer acceptance and support, they view health recommendations as a threat to their autonomy and sense of control. Probably the greatest challenge to the nurse responsible for teaching the adolescent, whether healthy or ill, is to be able to develop a mutually respectful, trusting relationship. Adolescents, because of their well-developed cognitive and language abilities, are able to participate fully in all aspects of learning, but they need privacy, understanding, an honest and straightforward approach, and unqualified acceptance in the face of their fears of losing independence, identity, and self-control.

The existence of an imaginary audience and personal fable can contribute to the exacerbation of existing problems or cause new ones. Adolescents with disfiguring handicaps, who as young children exhibited a lot of spirit and strength, may now show signs of depression and lack of will. For the first time, they look at themselves from the standpoint of others and reinterpret behavior once seen as friendly as actually condescending. Teenagers may fail to use contraceptives because the fable tells them that *other* people will get pregnant or get venereal disease, but not *them*. Teenagers with chronic illnesses may stop taking prescribed medications because they feel they can manage without them to prove to others that they are well and free of medical constraints; *other* people with similar diseases need to follow therapeutic regimens, but not *them*.

Their language skills and ability to conceptualize and think abstractly give the nurse as educator a wide range of teaching methods and instructional tools from which to choose. The following teaching strategies are suggested when caring for adolescents:

FOR SHORT-TERM LEARNING

- Use one-to-one instruction to ensure confidentiality of sensitive information.
- Choose peer group discussion sessions as an effective approach to deal with many health problems on such topics as smoking, alcohol and drug use, safety measures, and teenage sexuality. Adolescents benefit from being exposed to others who have the same concerns or who have successfully dealt with problems similar to theirs.
- Use group discussion, role-playing and gaming as methods to clarify values and problem-solve, which feed into the teenager's need to belong and to be actively involved. Getting groups of peers together can be very effective in helping teens confront health challenges and to learn how to significantly change behavior (Fey & Deyes, 1989).
- Employ adjunct instructional tools, such as complex models, diagrams, and specific, detailed written materials, which can be used competently by many adolescents. Audiovisuals in the form of audiotapes, videotapes, simulated games, and interactive discs using the hardware of TV, audiocassette players, and computers usually are a comfortable approach to learning by adolescents, who have facility with technological equipment after years of academic and personal experience with telecommunications in the home and at school.
- Clarify any scientific terminology and medical jargon used.
- Share decision making whenever possible because control is an important issue for adolescents.
- Include them in formulating teaching plans related to teaching strategies, expected outcomes, and determining what needs to be learned and how it can best be achieved to meet their needs for autonomy.
- Suggest options so that they feel they have a choice about courses of action.
- Give a rationale for all that is said and done to help them feel a sense of control.
- Approach them with respect, tact, openness, and flexibility to elicit their attention and encourage their responsiveness to teaching-learning situations.
- Expect negative responses, which are common when their self-image and self-integrity are threatened.
- Avoid confrontation and acting like an authority figure. Instead of directly contradicting their opinions and beliefs, acknowledge their thoughts and then casually suggest an alternative viewpoint, such as "Yes, I can see your point, but what about the possibility of . . . ?"

FOR LONG-TERM LEARNING

- Accept adolescents' personal fable and imaginary audience as valid, rather than challenging their feelings of uniqueness and invincibility.
- Acknowledge that their feelings are very real because denying them their opinions simply will not work.
- Allow them the opportunity to test their own convictions. Let them know, for example, that while some other special people may get away without taking medication, others cannot. Suggest, if medically feasible, setting up a trial period with medications scheduled further apart or in lowered dosages to determine how they can manage.

Although much of patient education should be done directly with adolescents to respect their right to individuality, privacy and confidentiality, teaching effectiveness may be enhanced by including their families to some extent as well. The nurse as educator can give guidance and support to families so they can better understand adolescent behavior. Parents should be taught how to set realistic limits while at the same time fostering the adolescent's sense of independence. Through prior assessment of potential sources of stress, teaching both the parents and the adolescent as well as siblings can be enhanced. Because of the ambivalence the adolescent feels while in this transition stage from childhood to adulthood, health-care teaching, to be effective, must consider the learning needs of the adolescent as well as the parents (Falvo, 1994).

THE DEVELOPMENTAL STAGES OF ADULTHOOD

Andragogy, the term coined by Knowles (1990) to describe his theory of adult learning, is the art and science of helping adults learn. The concept of andragogy has served for years as a useful framework in guiding instruction for patient teaching and for continuing education of staff. The following are basic assumptions about Knowles's framework that have major implications for planning, implementing, and evaluating teaching programs for adults.

As the individual matures,

1. His or her self-concept moves from one of being a dependent personality to being an independent, self-directed human being.
2. He or she accumulates a growing reservoir of previous experience that serves as a rich resource for learning.
3. Readiness to learn becomes increasingly oriented to the developmental tasks of social roles.
4. The perspective of time changes from one of postponed application of knowledge to one of immediate application; there is a shift in orientation of learning from being subject centered to problem centered.

A limitation of Knowles's assumptions about child versus adult learners is that it is derived from studies done on healthy people. It is important to keep in mind, however, that illness and injury have the potential for significantly changing cognitive and psychological processes used for learning (Bille, 1980).

The period of adulthood constitutes three major developmental stages—that of the young adult, the middle-aged adult, and the older adult (see Table 5-1). Although adulthood, like childhood, can be divided into various developmental phases, the focus for learning is quite different. Whereas readiness to learn in the child is dependent on physical, cognitive, and psychosocial development, adults have essentially reached the peak of their physical and cognitive capacities. Instead, the emphasis for adult learning revolves around differentiation of life tasks and social roles with respect to employment, family, and other activities beyond the responsibilities of home and career (Whitman et al., 1992). In contrast to childhood learning, which is subject centered, adult learning is problem centered. The prime motivator to learn in adulthood is to be able to apply knowledge and skills for the solution of immediate problems. Unlike children, who like to learn for the sake of gaining an understanding of themselves and the world, adults must clearly perceive the relevancy in acquiring new behaviors or changing old ones for them to be willing and eager to learn. In the beginning of any teaching-learning encounter, adults want to know the benefit they will derive from their efforts at learning.

Unlike the child learner, who is dependent on authority figures for learning, the adult is much more self-directed and independent in seeking information. For adults, past experiences are internalized and form the basis for further learning. Adults already have a rich resource of stored information on which to build a further understanding of relationships between ideas and concepts. They are quicker than children at grasping relationships, and they do not tolerate learning isolated facts as well as children do (Table 5-2). Because they already have established ideas, values, and attitudes, they tend to be more resistant to change. In addition, adults must face barriers to learning, the extent to which children are not subjected. They have the burden of family, work, and social respon-

TABLE 5-2. Summary of adult learning principles

Adults learn best when:

Principle #1	Learning is related to an immediate need, problem, or deficit
Principle #2	Learning is voluntary and self-initiated.
Principle #3	Learning is person centered and problem centered.
Principle #4	Learning is self-controlled and self-directed.
Principle #5	The role of the teacher is one of facilitator.
Principle #6	Information and assignments are pertinent.
Principle #7	New material draws on past experiences and is related to something the learner already knows.
Principle #8	The threat to self is reduced to a minimum in the educational situation.
Principle #9	The learner is able to participate actively in the learning process.
Principle #10	The learner is able to learn in a group.
Principle #11	The nature of the learning activity changes frequently.
Principle #12	Learning is reinforced by application and prompt feedback.

SOURCE: Adapted from Burgireno (1985).

sibilities, which impact on their time, energy, and concentration for learning. Their need for self-direction also may present problems because various stages of illness as well as the health-care setting in which they may find themselves can force dependency. Anxiety, too, may impact negatively on their motivation to learn. They may feel too old or too out of touch with the formal learning of the school years, and if past experiences with learning were not positive, they may shy away from assuming the role of learner for fear of the risk of failure (Whitman et al., 1992).

There are a variety of reasons why adults pursue learning throughout their lives. Basically, three categories describe the general orientation of adults toward continuing education (Babcock & Miller, 1994):

1. *Goal-oriented learners* engage in educational endeavors to accomplish clear and identifiable objectives. Continuing education for them is episodic and occurs as a recurring pattern throughout their lives as they realize the need for or identify an interest in expanding their knowledge and skills. Adults who attend night courses or professional workshops do so to build their expertise in a particular subject or for advancement in their professional or personal lives.

2. *Activity-oriented learners* select educational activities primarily to meet social needs. The learning of content is secondary to their need for human contact. While they may choose to attend support groups, special interest groups, self-help groups, or academic classes because of an interest in a particular topic being offered, they join essentially out of their desire to be with and talk to other people in similar circumstances—retirement, parenting, divorce, or widowhood. Their drive is to alleviate social isolation or loneliness.

3. *Learning-oriented learners* view themselves as perpetual students who seek knowledge for knowledge sake. They are active learners all of their lives and tend to join groups, classes, or organizations with the anticipation that the experience will be educational and personally rewarding.

In most cases, all three types of learners initiate the learning experience for themselves. In planning educational activities for adults, it is important to know their motives for wanting to be involved. In caring for clients with various needs and problems, it is advantageous for the nurse as educator to understand the purpose and expectations of different continuing education groups to best serve as a referral or resource person for the learners.

Only recently has it been recognized that learning is a lifelong process that begins at birth and does not cease until the end of life. Growth and development are a process of becoming, and learning is inextricably a part of that process. As a person matures, learning is a significant and continuous task to maintain and enhance oneself.

Obviously, there are many differences between child and adult learners (Table 5–1). As the following discussion will clearly reveal, there also are differences in the characteristics of adult learners within the three developmental stages of adulthood.

Young Adulthood

Early adulthood is a time for establishing long-term, intimate relationships with other people, choosing a lifestyle and adjusting to it, deciding on an occupation, and managing a home and family. All of these decisions lead to changes in the lives of young adults that can be a potential source of stress for them. It is a time when intimacy and courtship are pursued and spousal and/or parental roles are developed.

Physical, Cognitive, and Psychosocial Development

During this period, physical abilities for most young adults are at their peak, and the body is at its optimal functioning capacity. The vast majority of individuals at this stage can master, if they so desire, almost any psychomotor skill they undertake to accomplish.

The cognitive capacity of young adults is fully developed, but with maturation, they continue to accumulate new knowledge and skills from an expanding reservoir of formal and informal experiences. These experiences add to their perceptions, allow them to generalize to new situations, and improve their abilities to critically analyze, problem solve, and make decisions about their personal, occupational, and social roles. Their interests for learning are oriented toward those experiences that are relevant for immediate application to problems and tasks in their daily lives. Young adults are motivated to learn about the possible implications of various lifestyle choices.

Erikson (1963) describes the young adult's stage of psychosocial development as the period of *intimacy versus isolation*. This is the time when individuals work to establish a trusting, satisfying, and permanent relationship with others. They strive to establish commitment to others in their personal, occupational, and social lives. The independence and self-sufficiency they worked to obtain in adolescence they are now working to maintain.

Young adults face many challenges as they take steps to control their lives. Many of the events they experience are happy and growth promoting from an emotional and social perspective, but they also can be disappointing and psychologically draining. The new experiences and multiple decisions they must make regarding choices for a career, marriage, parenthood, and higher education can be quite stressful. Young adults realize that the avenues they choose will impact on their lives for years to come.

Teaching Strategies

At this developmental stage, prior to the chronic diseases of the mid and older years, young adults are generally very healthy and tend to have limited exposure to health professionals. Their contact with the health-care system is usually for pre-employment, college, or pre-sport physicals, for a minor episodic complaint, or for pregnancy and contraceptive care. However, young adulthood is a crucial time for the establishment of behaviors that help individuals to lead healthy lives, both physically and emotionally. This is the time when many of the choices they make, if not positive ones, will be difficult to modify later. As Havighurst pointed out, this stage is full of "teachable moment" opportunities, but it is the most devoid of efforts by health providers to teach (Johnson-Saylor, 1980).

Health promotion is the most neglected aspect of health-care teaching at this stage of life. Yet, many of the health issues related to risk factors and stress management are important to deal with to help young adults establish positive health practices for preventing problems with illness in the future. The major factors associated with increased risk of death in later life, such as high blood pressure, elevated cholesterol, obesity, smoking, overuse of alcohol and drugs, and pertinent family history of major illnesses such as cancer and heart disease, all need to be addressed.

The nurse as educator must find a way of reaching and communicating with this audience about health promotion and disease prevention measures. Readiness to learn does not always require the nurse educator to wait for it to develop. Readiness can be fostered through experiences the nurse creates. Knowledge of the individual's lifestyle can be cues to concentrate on when determining specific aspects of education for the young adult. For example, if the individual is planning marriage, then teaching about family planning, contraception, and parenthood are potential topics to address. The motivation for adults to learn is in response to internal drives, such as need for self-esteem, a better quality of life, or job satisfaction, or in response to external motivators, such as job promotion, more money, or more time to pursue outside activities (Babcock & Miller, 1994).

When young adults are faced with acute or chronic illnesses, many of which may impact significantly on their lifestyle, they are stimulated to learn in order to maintain their independence and return to normal life patterns. It is likely they will view an illness or disability as a serious setback to achieving their immediate or future life goals. Since adults desire active participation in the educational process, it is important for the nurse as educator to allow them the opportunity for mutual collaboration in health education decision making. They should be encouraged to select what to learn (objectives), how they want material to be presented (instructional methods and tools), and what indicators will be used to determine the achievement of learning goals (evaluation) (Gessner, 1989). Also, it must be remembered that adults bring with them to the teaching-learning situation a variety of experiences that can serve as a foundation on which to build new learning. It is important to draw on their experiences to make learning relevant, useful, and motivating. Young adults are reluctant to expend the resources of time, money, and energy to learn new information, skills, and attitudes if they do not see the content of instruction as relevant to their current lives or anticipated problems (Babcock & Miller, 1994).

Teaching strategies must be directed at encouraging young adults to seek information that expands their knowledge base, helps them control their lives, and bolsters their self-esteem. Whether they be well or ill, young adults need to know about the opportunities available for learning. Making them aware of health issues and learning opportunities can occur in various settings such as physicians' offices, community clinics, outpatient departments, or hospitals, but these educational opportunities must be convenient and accessible to them in terms of their lifestyle with respect to

work and family responsibilities. Because they tend to be very self-directed in their approach to learning, young adults do well with written patient education materials and audiovisual tools that allow them to independently self-pace their learning. Group discussion is an attractive method for teaching and learning because it provides young adults opportunity to interact with others of similar age and situation, such as parenting groups, prenatal classes, or marital adjustment sessions. Although assessment prior to teaching will help to determine the level at which to begin teaching, no matter what the content, the enduring axiom to make learning easier and more relevant is to present concepts logically from simple to complex and establish conceptual relationships through specific application of information.

Middle-Aged Adulthood

Just as adolescence is the link between childhood and adulthood, midlife is the transition period between young adulthood and older adulthood. During middle age, many individuals have reached the peak in their careers, their sense of who they are is well-developed, their children are grown, and they have time to pursue other interests. It is a time for them to reflect on the contributions they have made to family and society and to reexamine their goals and values.

Physical, Cognitive, and Psychosocial Development

At this stage of maturation, a number of physiological changes begin to take place. Skin and muscle tone decreases, metabolism slows down, body weight tends to increase, endurance and energy levels lessen, hormonal changes bring about a variety of symptoms, and hearing and visual acuity begin to diminish. All these physical changes and others affect middle-aged adults' self-image and impact on their ability to learn as well as influence their motivation for learning about health promotion, disease prevention, and maintenance of health.

The ability to learn from a cognitive standpoint remains at a steady state throughout middle age. For many adults, the accumulation of life experiences and their proven record of accomplishments often allow them to come to the teaching-learning situation with confidence in their abilities as a learner. However, if their past experiences with learning were minimal or not positive, it is likely that their motivation will not be at a high level to facilitate learning. Physical changes, especially with respect to hearing and vision, may impede learning as well.

Erikson (1963) labeled this psychosocial stage of adulthood as *generativity versus self-absorption and stagnation*. Midlife marks a point at which adults realize that half of their life has been spent. This realization may cause them to question their level of achievement and success. Middle-aged adults, in fact, may choose to modify aspects of their lives that they perceive as unsatisfactory or adopt a new lifestyle as a solution to dissatisfaction. Concern for the lives of their grown children, recognizing the physical changes in themselves, and dealing with new roles of being a grandparent, as well as taking responsibility for their own parents whose health may be failing, are factors that may cause them to become aware of their own mortality. At this time, they may either feel greater motivation to follow health recommendations more closely, or just the opposite, they may deny illnesses or abandon healthy practices altogether (Falvo, 1994).

The later years of middle adulthood are the phase in which productivity and contributions to society are valued. It is an opportunity in life to feel a real sense of accomplishment from having cared for others—children, spouse, friends, their own parents, and colleagues for whom they have served as mentor. It is a time when individuals become oriented away from self and family to the larger community. New social interests and leisure activities are pursued as they find more free time from family responsibilities and demands of career. As they move toward retirement years, they begin to plan for what they want to do after culminating their career. This sparks their interest in learning about financial planning, alternative lifestyles, and how to remain healthy as they approach the later years.

Teaching Strategies

Depending on individual situations, middle-aged adults may be facing either a more relaxed lifestyle or an increase in stress level due to midlife crisis issues such as menopause, obvious physical changes in their bodies, responsibility for their own parents' declining health status, or concern about how finite their life really is. They may have regrets and feel they did not achieve the goals or live up to the values they had set for themselves in young adulthood or the expectations others had of them as young adults. The nurse in teaching this age group must be aware of their potential sources of stress, the health risk factors associated with this stage of life, and the concerns typical of midlife. Many misconceptions regarding physical changes such as menopause are common. Stress may interfere with their ability to learn or may be the stimulant for them to seek the help of health-care providers. Those who have lived healthy and productive lives are often motivated to make contact with health professionals to ensure maintenance of their healthy status. It is an opportune time on the part of the nurse educator to reach out to assist these middle-aged adults to cope with stress and to maintain optimal health status. Many need and want information related to chronic illnesses that can arise at this phase of life.

Adult learners need to be reassured or complimented on their learning competencies. Reinforcement for learning is internalized and serves to reward them for their efforts. Teaching strategies for learning are similar to those instructional methods and tools used for the young adult learner, but the content is different to coincide with the concerns and problems specific to this group of learners.

Older Adulthood

Older persons constitute approximately 12% of the U.S. population and make up the fastest growing segment of the population in our country today. By 2030, this number is expected to increase to 21%. Of the total amount of health-care expenditures, 36% are incurred by those over 65 years of age. Most older persons suffer from at least one chronic condition, and many have multiple conditions. On the average, they are hospitalized longer than persons in other age categories and require more teaching overall to broaden their knowledge of self-care. Because many older persons did not have the educational opportunities that are available to the young today, one-third of them have completed only 8 years or less of formal schooling. Low educational levels in the older adult contribute to their decreased ability to read and comprehend written materials (Jackson et al., 1994). Therefore, generally their educational needs are greater and more complex than for those persons in any of the other developmental stages. Numerous studies have documented that the older adult can benefit from health education programs. Their compliance, if they are given specific health directions, can be quite high. In light of considerable health-care cost expenditures for older people, education programs to improve their health status would be a cost-effective measure (Weinrich et al., 1989).

The teaching of older persons, known as *gerogogy,* is different from teaching adults (andragogy) and children (pedagogy). For teaching to be effective, gerogogy must accommodate the normal physical, cognitive, and psychosocial aging changes that occur at this phase of growth and development (Weinrich & Boyd, 1992). Until recently, little has been written about the special learning needs of older adults to take into account the physiological and psychological aging changes that affect their ability to learn. Age changes, which begin in the second decade of life, can create barriers to learning unless nurses understand these changes and adapt appropriate teaching interventions to meet the older person's needs (Weinrich et al., 1989). The following discussion of physical, cognitive, and psychosocial maturation is based on findings reported by numerous authors (Ellison, 1985; Weinrich et al., 1989; Culbert & Kos, 1971; Alford, 1982; Weinrich & Boyd, 1992; Palmore, 1977).

Physical, Cognitive, and Psychosocial Development

With advancing age, so many physical changes occur that it becomes difficult to establish normal boundaries. As a person grows older, normal physiological changes in all systems of the body are universal, progressive, decremental and intrinsic. The senses of sight, hearing, touch, taste, and smell are usually the first areas of decreased functioning noticed by older persons. Alterations in physiological functioning can lead secondarily to changes in learning ability. The sensory perceptive abilities

that relate most closely to learning capacity are visual and auditory changes. Hearing loss, which is very common beginning in the late 40s and 50s, includes diminished ability to discriminate high-pitched sounds. Visual changes such as cataracts, reduced pupil size, and presbyopia prevent older persons from being able to read small print, read words printed on glossy paper, or drive a car. Yellowing of the ocular lens produces color distortions and diminished color perceptions. In addition, other physiological changes affect organ functioning, which result in decreased cardiac output, lung performance, and metabolic rate, thereby reducing energy levels and lessening the ability to cope with stress. Nerve conduction velocity also is thought to decline by up to 15%, influencing reflex times and muscle response rates. The interrelatedness of each body system has a total negative cumulative effect on individuals as they grow older.

Aging affects the mind as well as the body. *Cognitive ability* changes with age as permanent cellular alterations invariably occur in the brain itself, resulting in an actual loss of neurons, which have no regenerative powers. Physiological research has demonstrated that people have two kinds of intellectual ability—fluid and crystallized intelligence. *Fluid intelligence* is the capacity to perceive relationships, to reason, and to perform abstract thinking. This kind of intelligence declines as degenerative changes occur. *Crystallized intelligence* is the intelligence absorbed over a lifetime such as vocabulary, general information, understanding social interactions, arithmetic reasoning, and ability to evaluate experiences. This kind of intelligence actually increases with experience as people age (Theis & Merritt, 1994). The decline in fluid intelligence results in the following specific changes:

1. *Slower processing time*: Older persons need more time to actually process and react to information, especially in terms of relationships between actions and results. However, if the factor of speed is removed from IQ tests, for example, older people can perform as well as younger ones.

2. *Persistence of stimulus (afterimage):* Older people can confuse a previous symbol or word with a new word or symbol just introduced.

3. *Decreased short-term memory:* Older people sometimes have difficulty remembering

events or conversations that occurred just hours or days before.

4. *Increased test anxiety*: Older people are especially anxious about making mistakes when performing, and when they do make an error, they become easily frustrated. Because of their anxiety, they may take an inordinate amount of time to respond to questions, particularly on tests that are written rather than verbal.

5. *Altered time perception*: For older persons, life becomes more finite, issues of the here and now are more important, and many adhere to the philosophy of Scarlett O'Hara, "I'll worry about that tomorrow." This philosophy can be detrimental when applied to health issues because it serves as a vehicle for denial.

Despite the changes in cognition as a result of aging, most research supports the premise that the ability of older adults to learn and remember is virtually as good as ever if special care is taken to slow the pace of presenting information, to ensure relevance of material, and to give appropriate feedback when teaching (Figure 5–1).

Erikson (1963) labeled the major psychosocial developmental task at this stage in life as *ego integrity versus despair*. This phase of older adulthood includes dealing with the reality of aging, the acceptance of the inevitability that we all will die, the reconciling of past failures with present and future concerns, and developing a sense of growth and purpose for those years remaining. The most common psychosocial tasks of aging involve changes in lifestyle and social status as a result of

- Retirement (mandatory at 70 years in this country)
- Illness or death of spouse, relatives, and friends
- The moving away of children, grandchildren, and friends
- Relocation to an unfamiliar environment such as a nursing home or senior citizens center

Depression, grief, and loneliness are common among older persons and are often related to the aforementioned developmental tasks. Many individuals experience multiple losses over a short period of time with respect to a previous support network of home, friends, family, and job. These

losses, which signify a threat to their own autonomy, independence, and decision making, result in isolation, financial insecurity, diminished coping mechanisms, and a decreased sense of identity, personal value, and societal worth. With aging, individuals begin to question their perception of a "meaningful life," that is, the potential for further enjoyment, pleasure, and satisfaction.

Although separate from biological aging but closely related are the many sociocultural factors that affect how older adults see themselves as competent individuals. The following traits regarding personal goals in life and the values associated with them are significantly related to motivation and learning (Ellison, 1985; Gessner, 1989; Culbert & Kos, 1971):

1. *Independence:* The ability to provide for one's needs is the most important aim of the majority of older persons, regardless of their state of health. Independence gives them a sense of self-respect, pride, and self-functioning so as not to be a burden to others. Health teaching is the tool to help them maintain or regain independence.

2. *Social acceptability:* The approval from others is a common goal of most older adults. It is derived from health, a sense of vigor, and feeling and thinking "young." In spite of declining physical attributes, the older adult often has residual fitness and functioning potentials. Health teaching can help to channel these potentials.

3. *Adequacy of personal resources:* Resources, both external and internal, are important considerations when assessing the older adult's current status. Life patterns, which include habits, physical and mental strengths, and economic situation, should be assessed to determine how to incorporate teaching to complement existing regimens with new required behaviors.

4. *Coping mechanisms:* The ability to cope with change during the aging process is indicative of the person's readiness for health teaching. Positive coping mechanisms allow for self-change as older persons draw on life experiences and knowledge gained over the years. Negative coping mechanisms indicate their focus on losses and that their thinking is immersed in the past. Emphasis on teaching is to explore alternatives, determine realistic goals, and support large and small accomplishments.

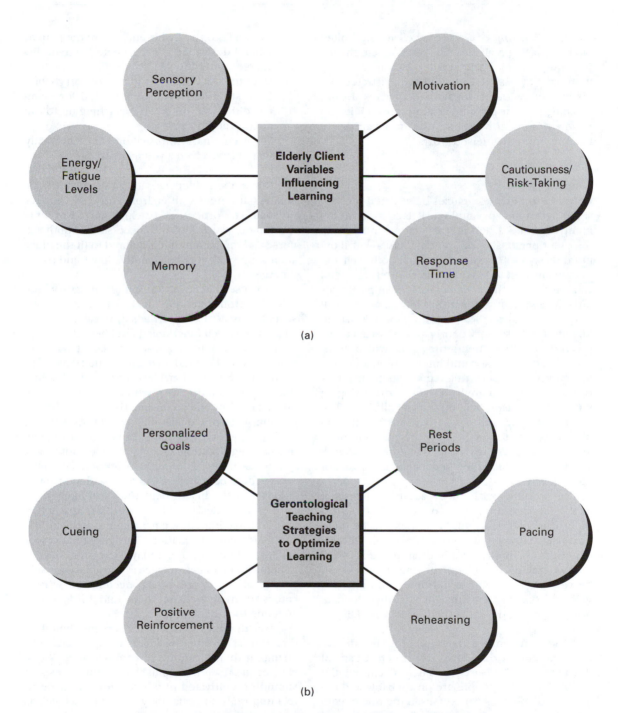

FIGURE 5–1.   (a) Elderly Client Variables Influencing Learning
(b) Gerontological Teaching Strategies to Optimize Learning.

SOURCE: Reprinted with permission from Rendon, D.C., Davis, D.K., Gioiella, E.C., & Tranzillo, M.J. (1986). The right to know, the right to be taught. *Journal of Gerontological Nursing, 12*(12), 34.

5. *Meaning of life:* For well-adapted older persons, having realistic goals allows them the opportunity to enjoy the smaller pleasures in life, whereas the less well-adapted are frustrated and dissatisfied with personal inadequacies. Health teaching must be directed at ways older adults can maintain optimal health so that they can derive pleasure from their leisure years.

Teaching Strategies

Learning in older adults can be affected by such sociological and psychological factors as retirement, economics, and mental status. Understanding older persons' developmental tasks will allow nurses to alter how they approach both well and ill individuals in terms of counseling, teaching, and establishing a therapeutic relationship. Nurses must be aware of the fact that older patients will frequently delay medical attention. Social isolation, loneliness, and sensory deprivation may lead to decreased cognitive functioning and will prevent early disease detection and intervention. A decline in psychomotor performance affects their reflex responses and their ability to handle stress. Coping with simple tasks becomes more difficult. The inability of older persons to handle stress has implications with respect to how they care for themselves (food, dress, taking medications) as well as the extent to which they understand the nature of their illnesses.

In working with older adults, reminiscing is a beneficial approach to use to establish a therapeutic relationship. Memories can be quite powerful. Talking with older persons about their experiences—marriage, children, grandchildren, jobs, community involvement, and the like—can be very stimulating. Furthermore, their answers will give the nurse an insight into their humanness, their abilities, and their concerns (Ellison, 1985).

Too many times nurses and other health professionals believe the adage "You can't teach an old dog new tricks." It is easy to fall into believing the myths that older people are unteachable and unmotivated (Kick, 1989). Nurses in the role of educator may not even be aware of their stereotypical attitudes toward older adults. To check yourself, think about the last time you gave instruction to an older patient, and ask yourself:

- Did I talk to the family and ignore the patient when I described some aspect of care or discharge planning?
- Did I tell the older person not to worry when he or she asked a question? Instead, for example, did I say, "Just leave everything up to the doctors and nurses."?
- Did I eliminate information that I normally would have given a younger patient?

Remember, older people can learn, but their abilities and needs differ from those of younger persons. The process of teaching and learning is much more rewarding and successful for both the nurse and the patient if it is tailored to fit the older adult's physical, cognitive, motivational, and social differences.

Because changes as a result of aging vary considerably from one individual to another, it is essential to assess each learner's physical, cognitive, and psychosocial functioning level before developing and implementing a teaching plan. It is important to keep in mind that older adults have an overall lower educational level of formal schooling than the population as a whole. Also, they were raised in an era when consumerism and health education were practically nonexistent. As a result, older people may feel uncomfortable in the teaching-learning situation and may be reluctant to ask questions. In the future, as the older population becomes more educated and in tune with consumer activism in the health field, they will likely have an increased desire to be more participatory in decision making and demand more detailed and sophisticated information. The proliferation of self-help literature and today's expectations for patients and families to take responsibility for self-care result in the present-day need for nurse educators to involve clients more fully in decisions affecting their health (Morra, 1991).

Health education for older persons should be directed at promoting their involvement and changing their attitiudes toward learning (Weinrich et al., 1989). A climate of mutual respect should be cultivated in which they are made to feel important for what they once were as well as for what they are today. Interaction needs to be supportive, not judgmental. Interventions work best when they take place in a casual, informal atmosphere. Individual and situational variables such as motivation, life experiences, educational background, socioeconomic status, health-illness status, and motor, cognitive, and language skills influence the ability of the older adult to learn.

Some of the more common aging changes that affect learning and the teaching strategies specific to meeting the needs of the older adult are summarized in Table 5-1. The following are specific tips to abide by when teaching older persons to create an environment for learning that takes into account major changes in their physical, cognitive, and psychosocial functioning (Picariello, 1986; Hallburg, 1976; Alford, 1982):

PHYSICAL NEEDS

1. To compensate for visual changes, teaching should be done in an environment that is brightly lit but without glare. Visual aids should include large print, well-spaced letters, and the use of primary colors. Bright colors and a visible name tag should be worn by the educator. Because of older persons' difficulty in discriminating certain shades of color, avoid blue, blue-green, and violet hues. Use white or off-white, flat mat paper and black print for posters, diagrams, and other written materials. Keep in mind that tasks that require discrimination of shades of color, such as test strips measuring the presence of sugar in the urine, may present learning difficulties for older patients. Color distortions can have an especially devastating effect on learning regarding medications. Avoid referring to pills by color in guiding patients to take medications as prescribed. Green, blue, and yellow pills may all appear gray to older persons. Additional accommodations should be made to meet physical needs, such as arranging seats so that the learner is reasonably close to the instructor and any visual aids that may be used. For patients who wear glasses, be sure they are readily accessible, lenses are clean, and frames are properly fitted.

2. To compensate for hearing losses, eliminate extraneous noise, avoid covering the mouth when speaking, directly face the learner, and speak slowly. Female instructors should wear bright lipstick, and male teachers can wear lip gloss. These techniques will assist the learner who may be seeking visual confirmation of what is being said. Low-pitched voices are heard best, but be careful not to drop your voice at the end of words or phrases. Do not shout because the decibel level is usually not a problem for the hearing impaired. The intensity of sound seems to be less important than the pitch and rate of auditory stimuli. Word speed should not exceed 140 words spoken per minute. Ask for feedback from the learner to determine if you are speaking too softly, too fast, or not distinctly enough. When addressing a group, microphones are useful aids. Be alert to nonverbal cues from the audience. Participants who are having difficulty with hearing your message may try to compensate by leaning forward, turning the "good" ear to the speaker, or cupping their hands to their ears. Ask older persons to repeat verbal instructions to be sure the entire message was heard and interpreted correctly.

3. To compensate for musculoskeletal problems, decreased efficiency of the cardiovascular system, and reduced kidney function, keep sessions short, schedule frequent breaks to allow for use of bathroom facilities, and allow time for stretching to relieve painful, stiff joints and to stimulate circulation.

4. To compensate for decline in central nervous system functioning and decreased metabolic rates, set aside more time for the giving and receiving of information and for the practice of psychomotor skills. Also, do not assume that older persons have the psychomotor skills to handle technological equipment for self-paced learning, such as tape recorders, videocassettes, and television. In addition, they may have difficulty with independently applying prostheses or doing dressing changes because of decreased strength and coordination. Be careful not to misinterpret the loss of energy and motor skills as a lack of motivation.

COGNITIVE NEEDS

1. To compensate for a decrease in fluid intelligence, provide older persons with more opportunity to process and react to information and to see relationships between concepts. Research has shown that older adults can learn anything if new information is tied to familiar concepts drawn from relevant past experiences. When teaching, avoid presenting long lists by dividing a series of directions for action into short, discrete, step-by-step messages and then waiting for a response after each one. For instance, if you want to give directions about following different menus depending on exercise levels, instead of saying, "Use menu A if you are not active; use menu B if you are fairly active; use menu C if you are very active," you should say, "You should use menu A if you are not active." Then wait for the learner's response, "That's what I should eat if I'm not very active?" and then follow up with the response, "That's right. And if you are fairly active, you should. . . ."

Older persons also tend to confuse previous words and symbols with a new word or symbol being introduced. Again, wait for a response before introducing a new concept or word definition. For decreased short-term memory, coaching and repetition are very useful strategies that assist with recall. Memory also can be enhanced by involving the learner in devising ways to remember how or when to perform a procedure. Because many older adults experience test anxiety, try to explain procedures simply and thoroughly, reassure them, and if possible, give verbal rather than written tests.

2. Be aware of the effects of medications and energy levels on concentration, alertness, and coordination. Try to schedule teaching sessions before or well after medications are taken and when the person is rested. For example, the patient who has just returned from physical therapy or a diagnostic procedure will likely be too fatigued to attend to learning.

3. Be certain to ask what an individual already knows about a health-care issue or technique before explaining it. Repetition for reinforcement of learning is one thing; repeating information already known may seem patronizing.

4. Convincing older persons of the usefulness of what you are teaching is only half the battle for getting them motivated. You also may have to convince them that the information or technique you are teaching is correct. Anything that is entirely strange or that upsets established habits is likely to be far more difficult for them to learn. As perception slows, the mind has more trouble accommodating to new ways than the mind of a younger person. Find out about older persons' health habits and beliefs before trying to change their ways or teach something new. For example, many were taught as children that a bowel movement every day is necessary to prevent constipation. You need to know this before trying to teach them to change their dependency on using laxatives.

5. Arrange for brief teaching sessions because shortened attention span requires scheduling a series of sessions to provide for sufficient time for learning. In addition, if the material is relevant and focused on the here and now, older persons are more likely to be attentive to the information being presented.

6. Take into account that the process of conceptualizing and the ability to think abstractly become harder with aging. Conclude each teaching session with a summary of the information presented and allow for a question and answer period to correct any misconceptions (Figure 5–2).

PSYCHOSOCIAL NEEDS

1. Assess family relationships to determine how dependent the older person is on other members for financial and emotional support. In turn, explore the level of involvement by family members in reinforcing the lessons you are teaching and in giving assistance with self-care measures. Do they help the older person to function independently, or do they foster dependency? With permission of the patient, include family members in teaching sessions and enlist their support.

2. Determine availability of resources because a lack thereof can sabotage any teaching plan, especially if your recommendations include expecting older adults to do something they cannot afford to do or lack the means to do, such as buying or renting equipment, having transportation to get to therapy or teaching sessions, purchasing medications, and the like.

3. Encourage active involvement of older adults to improve their self-esteem and to stimulate them both mentally and socially. Teaching must be directed at helping them find meaningful ways to use their talents acquired over a lifetime. Establishing a rapport based on trust can provide them contact with others as a means to bolster their sense of self-worth.

4. Identify coping mechanisms. No other time in the life cycle carries with it the number of

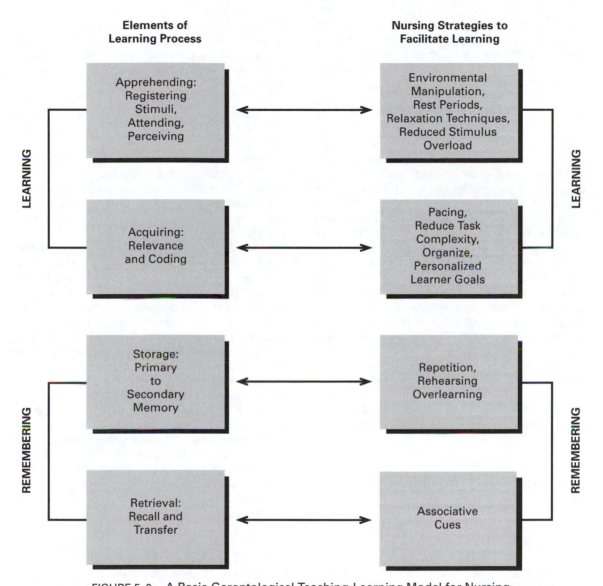

FIGURE 5–2. A Basic Gerontological Teaching-Learning Model for Nursing

SOURCE: Reprinted with permission from Rendon, D.C., Davis, D.K., Gioiella, E.C., & Tranzillo, M.J. (1986). The right to know, the right to be taught. *Journal of Gerontological Nursing, 12*(12), 36.

developmental tasks associated with adaptation to loss of roles, social and family contacts, and physical and cognitive capacities. Teaching must include offering constructive methods of coping.

The older person's ability to learn may be affected by the medium chosen for teaching. One-to-one instruction is a method that provides a non-

threatening environment for older adults to meet their individual needs and goals by helping them to compensate for their special deficits and promoting their active participation in learning. Group teaching also can be a beneficial approach for fostering social skills and maintaining contact with others through shared experiences. Self-paced instructional tools may be very appropriate, but it is important to know the client's previous learning techniques, mental and physical abilities, and comfort levels with certain approaches. Many older adults grew up in a time when audiovisual aids did not exist to the extent they do today, and those who have always learned by reading and discussion may not like mediated devices. Introducing new teaching methods and tools, such as use of computer and interactive video formats without adequate instructions on how to operate these technical devices, may inhibit learning by increasing anxiety and frustration levels and adversely affect self-esteem.

Games, role-playing, demonstration, and return demonstration can be used to rehearse problem-solving and psychomotor skills as long as these methods, and the tools used to complement them, are designed appropriately to accommodate the various developmental characteristics of this age group. These teaching methods stimulate learning and can offer opportunities to put knowledge into practice. Written materials, with attention paid to appropriateness in terms of literacy level and visual impairments in the elderly, are excellent adjuncts to augment, supplement, and reinforce verbal instructions (see Chapters 7, 11, and 12 for specific information on literacy and the design and use of instructional methods and materials).

THE ROLE OF THE FAMILY IN PATIENT EDUCATION

The role of the family is considered one of the key variables influencing patient care outcomes (Reeber, 1992). The primary motives in patient education for involving family members in the care delivery and decision-making process are to decrease the stress of hospitalization, reduce costs of care, and effectively prepare the client for self-care management outside the health-care setting. Family caregivers provide critical emotional, physical, and social support to the patient (Gilroth, 1990).

Under the most recent JCAHO accreditation standards, new demands have been placed on health-care organizations to show evidence that the family is included in patient education efforts. The standards mandate that the instruction of patients and significant others is an essential part in the provision of care. It is the responsibility of health-care professionals to assist both the patient and family to gain the knowledge and skills necessary to meet ongoing health-care needs (Hartman & Kochar, 1994). Critical pathways have become a popular and effective method to outline specific education needs of the patient and family. These pathways assist in prioritizing and meeting predetermined goals and objectives for learning. Such guidelines provide families with a better understanding of what needs to be learned and when (Barnes, 1995). Multidisciplinary collaboration is a major resource for ensuring continuity of patient and family teaching in and across health-care settings.

Including the family members in the teaching-learning process helps to guarantee a win-win situation for the client and the nurse educator. Family role enhancement and increased knowledge on the part of the family have positive benefits for both the learner and the teacher. Clients derive increased satisfaction and greater independence in self-care, and nurses experience increased job satisfaction and personal gratification in helping clients to reach their potentials and achieve successful outcomes (Barnes, 1995).

Orem's (1985) self-care deficit theory, Neuman's (1982) systems theory, Duvall's (1971) family theory, and Erikson's (1963) psychosocial development theory provide the conceptual frameworks for understanding the dynamics of family relationships and the importance of recognizing the developmental stages of the family as influential in achieving teaching-learning outcomes. There has been a great deal of attention given to the ways in which young and adolescent families function, but unfortunately minimal attention has been paid to the dynamics of the complex interactions that characterize the aging family (Phillips, 1989).

In patient education, the temptation on the part of the nurse is to teach as many family members as possible, but it is difficult to coordinate the instruction of a number of different people. The more individuals involved, the greater the potential for misunderstanding of instruction. The family must make the deliberate decision as to who is the most appropriate person to take the primary responsibility as the caregiver. The nurse educator must determine how the caregiver feels about the role of providing supportive care, how the caregiver feels about learning the necessary information, and what are the caregiver's learning style preferences, cognitive abilities, fears and concerns, and current knowledge of the situation. The caregiver needs information similar to what the patient is given to provide support, feedback, and reinforcement of self-care consistent with prescribed regimens of care. Sometimes the family members need more information than the patient to compensate for any sensory deficits or cognitive limitations the patient may have. Anticipatory teaching with family caregivers can reduce their anxiety, their uncertainty, and their lack of confidence. What the family is to do is important, but what the family is to expect also is essential information to be shared during the teaching-learning process (Haggard, 1989). The greatest challenge for caregivers is to develop confidence in their ability to do what is right for the patient. Education is the means to help them confront this challenge.

The family is the educator's greatest ally in preparing the patient for discharge and in helping the patient to become independent in self-care. The patient's family is perhaps the single most significant determinant of the success or failure of the education plan (Haggard, 1989). Rankin and Stallings's (1990) model for patient and family education serves as a foundation for assessing the family profile to determine the family's understanding of the actual or potential health problem(s), the resources available to them, their ways of functioning, and the educational backgrounds, lifestyles, and beliefs of family members.

Education is truly the most powerful tool nurse educators have to ensure safe discharge and the transfer of power to the patient-family dyad. It is imperative that attention be focused on both the assumed and expected responsibilities of family caregivers. The role of the family has been stressed under each developmental section throughout this chapter. Table 5-1 outlines the appropriate nursing interventions with the family at different stages in the life cycle.

SUMMARY

It is important to understand the specific and varied tasks associated with each developmental stage to individualize the approach to education in meeting the needs and desires of learners and their families. Assessment of physical, cognitive, and psychosocial maturation within each developmental period is crucial in determining the strategies to be used to facilitate the teaching-learning process. The younger learner is, in many ways, very different from the adult learner. Issues of dependency, extent of participation, the rate of and capacity for learning, and the situational and emotional barriers to learning vary significantly according to phases of development.

Readiness to learn in children is very subject centered and is highly influenced by their physical, cognitive, and psychosocial maturation. Motivation to learn in the adult is very problem centered and more oriented to psychosocial tasks related to roles and expectations of work, family, and community activities. For education to be effective, the nurse in the role of educator must create an environment conducive to learning by presenting information at the learner's level, inviting participation and feedback, and identifying whether parental and/or peer involvement is appropriate or necessary. Nurses, as the main source of health education, must determine what needs to be taught, when to teach, how to teach, and who should be the focus of teaching in light of the developmental stage of the learner.

References

Alford, D.M. (1982). Tips for teaching older adults. *Nursing Life, 2*(5), 60-63.

American Association of Colleges of Nursing. (1994). *AACN Issue Bulletin*. Washington, DC: American Association of Colleges of Nursing.

Babcock, D.E., & Miller, M.A. (1994). *Client education: Theory & practice*. St. Louis: Mosby–Year Book.

Banks, E. (1990). Concepts of health and sickness of preschool- and school-aged children. *Children's Health, 19*(1), 43-48.

Barnes, L.P. (1995). Finding the "win/win" in patient/family teaching. *MCN:American Journal of Maternal Child Nursing, 20*(4), 229.

Bille, D.A. (1980). Educational strategies for teaching the elderly patient. *Nursing & Health Care, 1*, 256-263.

Burgireno, J. (1985). Maximizing learning in the adult with SCI. *Rehabilitation Nursing, 10*(5), 20-21.

Burkett, K.W. (1989). Trends in pediatric rehabilitation. *Nursing Clinics of North America, 24*(1), 239-255.

Culbert, P.A., & Kos, B.A. (1971). Aging: Considerations for health teaching. *Nursing Clinics of North America, 6*(4), 605-614.

Day, M.C. (1981). Thinking at Piaget's stage of formal operations. *Educational Leadership, 39*, 44-47.

Duvall, E.M. (1971). *Family development,* 4th ed. Philadelphia: Lippincott.

Elkind, D. (1984). Teenage thinking: Implications for health care. *Pediatric Nursing, 10*(6), 383-385.

Ellison, S.A. (1985). Geriatric Oncology:A developmental approach. *Cancer Nursing,* Supplement 1, 28-32.

Erikson, E.H. (1963). *Childhood and Society,* 2nd ed. New York: Norton.

Erikson, E.H. (1968). *Identity: Youth and crisis.* New York: Norton.

Falvo, D.R. (1994). *Effective patient education: A guide to increased compliance,* 2nd ed. Gaithersburg, MD: Aspen.

Farrand, L.L., & Cox, C.L. (1993). Determinants of positive health behavior in middle childhood. *Nursing Research, 42*(4), 208-213.

Fey, M.S., & Deyes, M.J. (1989). Health and illness self care in adolescents with IDDM:A test of Orem's theory. *Advances in Nursing Science, 12*(1), 67-75.

Gessner, B.A. (1989). Adult education:The cornerstone of patient teaching. *Nursing Clinics of North America, 24*(3), 589-595.

Gilroth, B.E. (1990). Promoting patient involvement: Educational, organizational, and environmental strategies. *Patient Education and Counseling, 15*, 29-38.

Haggard, A. (1989). *Handbook of patient education.* Rockville, MD:Aspen.

Hallburg, J.C. (1976). The teaching of aged adults. *Journal of Gerontological Nursing, 2*(3), 13-19.

Hartman, R.A., & Kochar, M.S. (1994). The provision of patient and family education. *Patient Education and Counseling, 24*, 101-108.

Havighurst, R. (1976). Human characteristics and school learning: Essay review. *The Elementary School Journal, 77*, 101-109.

Heiney, S.P. (1991). Helping children through painful procedures. *American Journal of Nursing, 91*(11), 20-24.

Hussey, C.G., & Hirsh, A.M. (1983). Health education for children. *Topics in Clinical Nursing, 5*(1), 22-28.

Jackson, R.H., Davis, T.C., Murphy, P., Bairnsfather, L.E., & George, R.B. (1994). Reading deficiencies in older patients. *The American Journal of the Medical Sciences, 308*(2), 79-82.

Johnson-Saylor, M.T. (1980) Seize the moment: Health promotion for the young adult. *Topics in Clinical Nursing, 2*(2), 9-19.

Kennedy, C.M., & Riddle, I.I. (1989). The influence of the timing of preparation on the anxiety of preschool children experiencing surgery. *Maternal-Child Nursing Journal, 18*(2), 117-132.

Kick, E. (1989). Patient teaching for elders. *Nursing Clinics of North America, 24*(3), 681-686.

Knowles, M. (1990). *The adult learner: A neglected species,* 4th ed. Houston: Gulf.

Kotchabhakdi, P. (1985). School-age children's conceptions of the heart and its function. Monograph 15. *Maternal-Child Nursing Journal, 14*(4), 203-261.

Lambert, S.A. (1984). Variables that affect the school-age child's reaction to hospitalization and surgery: A review of the literature. *Maternal-Child Nursing Journal, 13*(1), 1-18.

Levine, M.D. (1983). *Developmental-behavioral pediatrics.* Philadelphia: Lippincott.

Morra, M.E. (1991). Future trends in patient education. *Seminars in Oncology Nursing, 7*(2), 143-145.

Neuman, B. (1982). *The Neuman system model.* Norwalk, CT:Appleton-Century-Crofts.

Orem, D. (1985). *Nursing: Concepts of practice,* 3rd ed. New York: McGraw-Hill.

Palmore, E. (1977). Facts on aging: A short quiz. *The Gerontologist, 17*(4), 1-5.

Perrin, E.C., Sayer, A.G., & Willett, J.B. (1991). Sticks and stones may break my bones . . . Reasoning about illness causality and body functioning in children who have a chronic illness. *Pediatrics, 88*(3), 608-619.

Petrillo, M., & Sanger, S. (1980). *Emotional care of hospitalized children,* 2nd ed. Philadelphia: Lippincott.

Phillips, L.R. (1989). Elder-family caregiver relationships: Determining appropriate nursing interventions. *Nursing Clinics of North America, 24*(3), 795-807.

Piaget, J. (1951). *Judgement and reasoning in the child.* London: Routlege and Kegan Paul.

Piaget, J. (1952). *The origins of intelligence in children.* New York: International Universities Press.

Piaget, J. (1976). *The grasp of consciousness: Action and concept in the young child.* Susan Wedgwood (Translator). Cambridge, MA: Harvard University Press.

Picariello, G. (1986).A Guide for teaching elders. *Geriatric Nursing, 7*(1), 38-39.

Pidgeon, V.A. (1977). Characteristics of children's thinking and implications for health teaching. *Maternal-Child Nursing Journal, 6*(1), 1-8.

Pidgeon, V. (1985). Children's concepts of illness: Implications for health teaching. *Maternal-Child Nursing Journal, 14*(1), 23-35.

Poster, E.C. (1983). Stress immunization: Techniques to help children cope with hospitalization. *Maternal-Child Nursing Journal, 12*(2), 119-134.

Rankin, S.H., & Stallings, K.D. (1990). *Patient education: Issues, principles, practices,* 2nd ed. Philadelphia: Lippincott.

Reeber, B.J. (1992). Evaluating the effects of a family education intervention. *Rehabilitation Nursing, 17*(6), 332-336.

Ryberg, J.W., & Merrifield, E.B. (1984). *Nurse Practitioner,* 9(6), 24-32.

Theis, S.L., & Merritt, S.L. (1994). A learning model to guide research and practice for teaching of elder clients. *Nursing and Health Care, 15*(9), 464-468.

Vulcan, B. (1984). Major coping behaviors of a hospitalized 3-year-old boy. *Maternal-Child Nursing Journal, 13*(2), 113-123.

Weinrich, S.P., & Boyd, M. (1992). Education in the elderly. *Journal of Gerontological Nursing, 18*(1), 15-20.

Weinrich, S.P., Boyd, M., & Nussbaum, J. (1989). Continuing education: Adapting strategies to teach the elderly. *Journal of Gerontological Nursing, 15*(11), 19-21.

Whitman, N.I., Graham, B.A., Gleit, C.J., & Boyd, M.D. (1992). *Teaching in nursing practice: A professional model,* 2nd ed. Norwalk, CT: Appleton & Lange.

CHAPTER 6

Motivation, Compliance, and Health Behaviors of the Learner

Eleanor Richards

CHAPTER HIGHLIGHTS

Motivation
    Motivational Factors
    Motivational Axioms
    Assessment of Motivation
    Motivational Strategies

Compliance

Compliance and Control

Health Behaviors of the Learner
    Health Belief Model
    Health Promotion Model
    Self-Efficacy Theory
    Theory of Reasoned Action
    PRECEDE-PROCEED Model
    Therapeutic Alliance Model
Selection of Models for Health Education
    Similarities and Dissimilarities of Models
    Educator Agreement with Model Conceptualizations
    Functional Utility of Models

Integration of Models for Use in Education

The Roles of Nurse as Educator in Health Promotion
    Facilitator of Change
    Contractor
    Organizer
    Evaluator

KEY TERMS

motivation	motivational axioms
compliance	noncompliance
adherence	hierarchy of needs
locus of control	educational contract
readiness to learn	motivational incentives
Health Belief Model	Health Promotion Model
Self-Efficacy Theory	Theory of Reasoned Action
PRECEDE-PROCEED Model	Therapeutic Alliance Model

OBJECTIVES

After completing this chapter, the reader will be able to

1. Define the terms *motivation*, *compliance*, and *adherence* relevant to behaviors of the learner.
2. Discuss motivation and compliance concepts/theories.
3. Identify incentives and obstacles that impact on motivation to learn.
4. Discuss axioms of motivation relevant to learning.
5. Assess levels of learner motivation.
6. Outline strategies that facilitate motivation and improve compliance.
7. Compare and contrast selected health behavior frameworks and their influence on learning.
8. Recognize the unique roles of the nurse as educator in health promotion.

The nurse as educator needs to understand what drives the learner to learn and what factors promote or hinder the acquisition and application of knowledge. Motivation and compliance, related yet different concepts, are central to the learning situation and are common denominators in many health behavior models.

Although the importance of motivation and compliance as they relate to learning is acknowledged in the literature, there is marginal incorporation of these concepts into educational plans. Educators frequently focus on the learner's level of motivation as an indicator of potential involvement in health education programs. Sands and Holman (1985) note that compliance is often used by researchers as a measure of outcomes of these programs. As early as 1974, Becker et al. found motivation to be significantly related to measures of compliance with a medical regimen.

Factors that determine health outcomes are complex. In a review of studies of health behavior, Ross and Rosser (1989) indicate that information alone does not account for changes in health behavior. Knowledge alone does not guarantee that the learner will engage in health-promoting behaviors, nor that the desired outcomes will be achieved. The most well thought-out educational program or plan of care will not achieve prescribed goals if the learner is not understood in the context of complex factors associated with motivation and compliance. A thorough understanding of the relationship between the reception of information and application of information and those factors that impede or promote desired health outcomes is essential for the nurse as educator.

This chapter presents the concepts of motivation and compliance as they relate to the learning situation with a focus on health behaviors. The discussion includes factors such as assessment of motivation, obstacles and facilitating factors for motivation and compliance, and motivational axioms. An overview and comparison of selected models of health behaviors is presented with a discussion of the role of nurse as educator in health promotion.

MOTIVATION

Motivation, from the Latin *movere*, means to set into motion. Motivation has been defined as a psychological force that moves a person toward some kind of action (Haggard, 1989) and as a willingness of the learner to embrace learning, with readiness as evidence of motivation (Redman, 1993). According to Kort (1987), it is the result of both internal and external factors and not the result of external manipulation alone. Implicit in motivation is movement in the direction of meeting a need or toward reaching a goal.

Lewin (1935), an early field theorist, conceptualized motivation in terms of positive or negative movement toward goals. Once an individual's equilibrium is disturbed, such as in the case of illness, forces of approach and avoidance may come into play. He noted that if avoidance endured in an approach-avoidance conflict, there would be negative movement away from a goal. His theory implies that there is a critical time factor relative to motivation. Ideally, the nurse educator's role is to facilitate the learner's approach toward a desired goal and to prevent untimely delays. The time factor is usually not a critical consideration in motivational models of health behavior or motivational research. For example, nursing staff may request an in-service program about clinical pathways. The in-service nurse educator may delay this request to the extent that the staff loses interest in the topic. Although untimely delays may be beyond the control of the educator, nevertheless, every effort should be made to capitalize on the staff's desire and readiness to learn.

Maslow (1943), another well-known early theorist, developed a theory of human motivation that is still widely used in the social sciences. The major premises of Maslow's motivation theory are integrated wholeness of the individual and a hierarchy of goals. Acknowledging the complexity of the concept of motivation, he notes that not all behavior is motivated and that behavior theories are not synonymous with motivation. There are many

determinants of behavior other than motives, and many motives can be involved in one behavior. Using the principles of hierarchy of basic needs—physiological, safety, love/belonging, self-esteem, and self-actualization—he notes the relatedness of needs, which are organized by their level of potency. Some individuals are highly motivated and others weakly motivated. When a need is fairly well satisfied, then the next potent need emerges. An example of hierarchy of basic needs is the potent need to satisfy hunger. This may be met by the nurse who assists the poststroke patient with feeding. The nurse-patient interaction may also satisfy the next potent needs, those of love/belonging and self-esteem.

There are relationships between motivation and learning, between motivation and behavior, and between motivation, learning, and behavior. There are many ways to view motivation in relation to learning. Redman (1993) categorizes theories of motivation that direct learning as behavioral reinforcers, need satisfaction, reduction of discomforting inconsistencies as a result of cognitive dissonance, allocating causal factors known as attributions, personality in which motivation is acknowledged to be a stable characteristic, expectancy theory encompassing value and perceived chance of success, and humanistic interpretations of motivation that emphasize personal choice. Each theory attempts to address the complex and somewhat elusive quality of motivation.

Motivational Factors

Factors that influence motivation can serve as incentives or obstacles to achieve desired behaviors. Both creating incentives and decreasing obstacles to motivation pose a challenge for the nurse as educator. The cognitive (thinking processes), affective (emotions and feelings), social, and behavioral domains of the learner can be influenced by the educator, who can act as a motivational facilitator or blocker.

Motivational incentives need to be considered in the context of the individual. What may be a motivational incentive for one learner may be a motivational obstacle to another. For example, a student who is assigned to work with an elderly woman may be motivated when the student holds older persons in high regard. Another student may be motivationally blocked by the emotional domain because previous experiences with older women, such as grandmother, were unrewarding.

Facilitating or blocking factors that shape motivation to learn can be classified into three major categories, which are not mutually exclusive: (1) personal attributes, which consist of physical, developmental, and psychological components of the individual learner; (2) environmental influences, which include the physical and attitudinal climate; and (3) learner relationship systems, such as those of significant other, family, community, and teacher-learner influence on motivation.

Personal Attributes

Personal attributes of the learner such as developmental stage, age, gender, emotional readiness, values and beliefs, sensory functioning, cognitive ability, educational level, actual or perceived state of health, and severity or chronicity of illness can shape an individual's motivation to learn. Functional ability to achieve behavioral outcomes is determined by physical, emotional, and cognitive dimensions. One's perception of disparity between current and expected states of health can be a motivating factor in health behavior and can drive readiness to learn.

The learner's views about the complexity or extent of changes that are needed can shape motivation. Values, beliefs, and natural curiosity can be firmly entrenched and enduring factors that can also shape desire to learn new behaviors. Other factors such as sensory input and processing of information and short-term and long-term memory can impact on motivation to learn. Emerging interest about male-female behavioral and learning differences indicates the need for in-depth research on gender-related characteristics affecting motivation to learn (see Chapter 8).

Environmental Influences

Physical characteristics of the learning environment, accessibility and availability of human and material resources, and different types of behavioral rewards influence the motivational level of the individual. Environment can create, promote, or detract from a state of learning receptivity. Pleasant, comfortable, and adaptable individualized surroundings can promote a state of readiness to learn. On the other hand, noise, confusion, inter-

ruptions, and lack of privacy can interfere with the capacity to concentrate and to learn.

The factors of accessibility and availability of resources include physical and psychological aspects. Can the client physically access a health facility, and once there, will the health-care personnel be psychologically available to the client? Psychological availability refers to the health-care system and whether it is flexible and sensitive to patients' needs. This includes factors such as promptness of services, sociocultural competence, emotional support, and communication skills. Attitude impacts on the engagement of the client with the health-care system.

The manner in which the health-care system is perceived by the client impacts on the client's willingness to participate in health-promoting behaviors. Behavioral rewards permeate the foundations of the learner's motivation. Rewards can be extrinsic, such as praise or acknowledgment from the educator or caretaker. Rewards can also be intrinsically based, such as feelings of a personal sense of fulfillment, gratification, or self-satisfaction.

Relationship Systems

Family/significant others in the support system, cultural identity, work/school and community roles, and teacher-learner interaction impact on an individual's motivation. The interactional aspects of motivation are perhaps the most salient because the learner exists in the context of interlocking relationship systems. Individuals are viewed in the context of family/community/cultural systems that have life-long impact on the choices that individuals make, including health-care seeking and health-care decision making. These significant-other systems may have even more of an impact on health outcomes than commonly acknowledged, and the health-promoting use of these systems needs to be taken into account by the nurse as educator.

All of these factors interact to address the motivation of the learner. They are not meant to be construed as comprehensive theory constructs but as forces that impact on motivation, serving to facilitate or block desire to learn.

Motivational Axioms

Axioms are premises on which an understanding of a phenomenon is based. The nurse as educator needs to understand the premises involved in promoting motivation of the learner. Motivational axioms are rules that set the stage for motivation. They are (1) state of optimum anxiety, (2) learner readiness, (3) realistic goal setting, (4) learner satisfaction/success, and (5) uncertainty-reducing or uncertainty-maintaining dialogue.

State of Optimum Anxiety

Learning occurs best when a state of mild anxiety exists. This is the optimum state for learning. In this state, one's ability to observe, focus attention, learn, and adapt is operative (Peplau, 1979). Perception, concentration, abstract thinking, and information processing are enhanced. Behavior is directed at a learning or challenging situation. Above this optimum level, at high or severe levels, the ability to perceive the environment, concentrate, and learn is reduced. A mild state of anxiety can be comfortably managed and is known to promote learning. As anxiety escalates, attention to external stimuli is reduced, the learner becomes increasingly self-absorbed, and behavior becomes defensively reactionary rather than being cognitively generated. For example, a patient who has been recently diagnosed with insulin-dependent diabetes and who has a high level of anxiety will not respond at an optimum level of retention of information when instructed about insulin injections. When the nurse as educator is able to aid the client in reducing anxiety, through techniques such as guided imagery, use of humor, or relaxation tapes, the patient will respond with a higher level of information retention.

Learner Readiness

Desire and readiness to move toward a goal are factors that influence motivation. Desire cannot be imposed on the learner. It can, however, be critically influenced by external forces and be promoted by the nurse as educator. Incentives are specific to the individual learner. An incentive to one individual can be a deterrent to another. Incentives in the form of reinforcers and rewards can be tangible or intangible, external or internal. As a facilitator to the learner, the nurse as educator offers positive perspectives and encouragement, which shape the desired behavior toward goal attainment. By making learning stimulating, making

information relevant and accessible, and creating an environment conducive to learning, educators can facilitate motivation to learn (see Chapter 4).

Realistic Goals

Goals that are within one's grasp, reasonable, and possible to be achieved are goals toward which an individual will work. Goals that are beyond one's reach are frustrating and counterproductive. Unrealistic goals with loss of valuable time can set the stage for the learner to "give up."

Setting realistic goals is a motivating factor. The belief that one can achieve the task set before him or her facilitates behavior toward that goal. Goals should parallel the extent to which behavioral changes are needed. Learning what the learner wants to change is a critical factor in setting realistic goals. Mutual goal setting between learner and educator reduces the negative impact of hidden agendas or the sabotaging of educational plans.

Learner Satisfaction/Success

The learner is motivated by success. Success is self-satisfying and feeds one's self-esteem. In a cyclical process, success and self-esteem escalate, moving the learner toward accomplishment of goals. When a learner feels good about step-by-step accomplishments, motivation is enhanced. For example, in the instructor-student relationship, evaluations can be a valuable method of promoting learner success. Clinical evaluations, when focused on demonstration of positive behaviors, can encourage movement toward performance goals. Focusing on successes as a means of positive reinforcement promotes learner satisfaction and a sense of accomplishment. On the other hand, focusing on weak clinical performance can reduce students' self-esteem.

Uncertainty Reduction or Maintenance

Uncertainty as well as certainty can be a motivating factor in the learning situation. Individuals have ongoing internal dialogues that can either reduce or maintain uncertainty. Individuals carry on "self-talk"; they "think things through." When one wants to change a state of health, behaviors will often follow a dialogue that examines uncertainty: "If I stop smoking, then my chances of getting lung cancer will be reduced." On the other hand, when the probable outcome of health behaviors is more uncertain, then behaviors may be uncertainty maintaining: "I am not sure that I need this surgery because the survival rate is no different for those who had this surgery when compared to those who did not." Some learners may maintain current behaviors, given probabilities of treatment outcomes, thus maintaining uncertainty.

Mishel (1990) reconceptualized the concept of uncertainty in illness. She views uncertainty as a necessary and natural rhythm of life, rather than an aversive experience. Uncertainty in sufficient concentration impacts on choices and decision making and can capitalize on receptivity or readiness for change. Premature uncertainty reduction can be counterproductive to the learner, who has not sufficiently explored alternatives. For example, when a staff nurse is uncertain about positions for catheterizing a debilitated female client and is presented with alternatives, then a thinking dialogue is carried out. If the decision to use a particular position is not premature, then uncertainty will promote exploration of alternative positions.

Assessment of Motivation

How does the nurse know when the learner is motivated? As a generic concept, assessment of motivation to learn has not been adequately addressed in the literature. Absence of adequate conceptually based measurement tools could be a factor.

Redman (1993) views motivational assessment as a part of general health assessment and states that it includes such areas as level of knowledge, client skills, decision-making capacity of the individual, and screening of target populations for educational programs. Leddy and Pepper (1993) view assessment of motivation in relation to capacity for change. Rankin and Stallings (1990) list several questions for the educator to pose in terms of the learner such as previous attempts, curiosity, goal setting, self-care ability, stress factors, survival issues, and life situations.

Motivational assessment of the learner needs to be comprehensive, systematic, and conceptually based. Cognitive, affective, physiological, experiential, environmental, and learning relationship variables need to be considered. Table 6–1 shows parameters for a comprehensive motivational assessment of the learner.

TABLE 6–1. Comprehensive parameters for motivational assessment of the learner

Cognitive Variables
- Capacity to learn
- Readiness to learn
  - Expressed self-determination
  - Constructive attitude
  - Expressed desire and curiosity
  - Willingness to contract for behavioral outcomes

Affective Variables
- Expressions of constructive emotional state
- Mild to moderate level of anxiety

Physiological Variables
- Capacity to perform required behavior

Experiential Variables
- Previous successful experiences

Environmental Variables
- Appropriateness of physical environment
- Social support systems
  - Family
  - Group
  - Work
  - Community resources

Educator-Learner Relationship System
- Prediction of positive relationship

These parameters incorporate Bandura's (1986) construction of incentive motivators, Ajzen and Fishbein's (1980) intent and attitude, Becker's (1974) and Pender's (1987) notion of likelihood of engaging in action, and Barofsky's (1978) focus on alliance in the learning situation. This proposed multidimensional guide allows assessment of the level of learner motivation. If responses to dimensions are positive, then the learner is likely to be motivated.

Assessment of learner motivation involves the judgment of the educator, since teaching-learning is a two-way process. Motivation can be assessed through subjective and objective means. A subjective means of assessing level of motivation is through dialogue. Through use of communication skills, the nurse can obtain verbal information from the client such as "I really want to maintain my weight" or "I want to have a healthy baby." Both of these statements indicate an energized desire with direction of movement toward an expected health outcome. Nonverbal cues can also indicate motivation, such as browsing through lay literature about healthy pregnancy. Likewise, a staff member or student nurse may express a verbal desire to know more about a specific advanced procedure. A nonverbal motivational cue could be expressed by the staff member or student nurse carefully observing a senior nurse or clinical specialist performing an advanced technique.

Measurement of motivation is another aspect to be considered. Subjective self-reports indicate level of motivation from the learner's perspective. Self-report measurements could be developed for educational programs. Objective measurement of motivation, an indirect measurement, can be quantified through observation of expected behaviors, the consequence of motivation. These behaviors can be observed in increments as the learner moves toward preset realistic health or practice goals.

Motivational Strategies

Incentives viewed as appeals or inducements to motivation can be either intrinsically or extrinsically generated. Incentives and motivation are both stimuli to action. Bandura (1986) associates motivation with incentives. He notes, however, that intrinsic motivation, although highly appealing, is elusive. Motivation rarely occurs without extrinsic influence. Green and Kreuter (1991) note that "strictly speaking we can appeal to people's motives, but we cannot motivate them" (p. 19). Extrinsic incentives are used for motivational strategizing in the educational situation.

Motivational strategies for the nurse as educator are extrinsically generated through the use of specific incentives. The critical question for the nurse as educator to ask is, "What is the specific behavior, under what circumstances, in what time frame desired by this learner?"

Strategizing begins with a systematic assessment of learner motivation, as seen in Table 6–1. When an applicable dimension is absent or reduced, then incentive strategizing is likely to move the individual away from the desired outcome. When considering strategies to improve learner motivation, Maslow's (1943) hierarchy of needs can also be taken into consideration. An appeal can be made to the innate need for the learner to suc-

ceed, known as achievement motivation (Atkinson, 1964).

In the educational situation, clear communication including clarification of directions and expectations is critical. Organization of material in a way that makes information meaningful to the learner, environmental manipulation, positive verbal feedback, and providing opportunities for success are motivational strategies proposed by Haggard (1989). Reducing or eliminating barriers to achieve goals is an important aspect of maintaining motivation.

One particular model developed by Keller (1987), the Attention, Relevance, Confidence, and Satisfaction (ARCS) Model, focuses on creating and maintaining motivational strategies used for instructional design. This model emphasizes strategies that the educator can use to effect changes in the learner by creating a motivating learning environment.

- **Attention** introduces opposing positions, case studies, and variable instructional presentations.
- **Relevance** capitalizes on the learners' experiences, usefulness, needs, and personal choices.
- **Confidence** deals with learning requirements, level of difficulty, expectations, attributions, and sense of accomplishment.
- **Satisfaction** pertains to timely use of a new skill, use of rewards, praise, and self-evaluation.

In motivational strategizing, it would also be beneficial to consider Damrosch's (1991) proposal that client health beliefs, personal vulnerability, efficacy of proposed change, and ability to effect the change are important in patient education efforts.

COMPLIANCE

Compliance is a term used to describe submission or yielding to predetermined goals. Defined as such, it has a manipulative or authoritative undertone in which the health-care provider or educator is viewed as the traditional authority, and the consumer or learner is viewed as submissive. The term has not been well received in nursing, perhaps due to the philosophical perspective that clients have the right to make their own health-care decisions and to not necessarily follow predetermined courses of action as set by health-care professionals.

Health-care literature suggests that compliance is the equivalent of the achieved goal to a predetermined regimen. Compliance, as an end unto itself, is different from motivational factors, which are a viewed as a means to an end.

> Compliance to a health regimen is an observable behavior and as such can be directly measured. Motivation, however, is a precursor to action that can be indirectly measured through behavioral consequences or results.

Commitment or attachment to a regimen is known as *adherence*, which may be long lasting. Both compliance and adherence refer to the ability to maintain health-promoting regimens, which are determined largely by a health-care provider. There is a subtle difference between compliance and adherence. It is possible for an individual to comply with a regimen and not necessarily be committed to it. For example, a patient who is experiencing sleep disturbances may comply with medication as directed for a period of 1 week. The patient may not continue to adhere to the regimen for an extended period of time even though there are continued sleep disturbances. In this situation, there is no commitment to follow through. Both *compliance* and *adherence* are terms used in the measurement of health outcomes and for the purpose of this chapter are used interchangeably.

Health-care literature has traditionally focused on compliance or adherence to a predetermined regimen. This phenomenon may be the result of an emphasis on cost-effective health care, for example, shorter length of hospital stay. The successes of educational programs in a fiscally responsible system will ultimately be linked to measurement of patient compliance relative to outcomes.

According to Eraker et al. (1984) and Levanthal and Cameron (1987), patient compliance to health regimens can be viewed from various theoretical perspectives: (1) biomedical, including patient demographics, severity of disease, and complexity of treatment regimen; (2) behavioral/social learning theory, using the behaviorist approach of rewards, cues, contracts, and social supports; (3) communication feedback loop of sending, receiving, comprehending, retaining, and acceptance; (4) rational belief theory, weighing the benefits of treatment and the risks of disease through the use of cost-benefit logic; and (5) self-regulatory systems, in which patients are seen as problem solvers whose regulation of behavior is based on perception of illness, cognitive skills, and past experiences that affect their ability to plan and cope with illness.

Compliance is an issue for all health-care disciplines. The major theories of compliance as described by Eraker et al. (1984) and Levanthal and Cameron (1987) are useful in explaining or describing compliance from a multidisciplinary approach including psychology and education. Fisher (1992) offered a pharmacist's perspective on the measurement of compliance to a medication regimen, with the communication model noted as the most effective for patient education. It is feasible for the nurse as educator to choose one or a combination of these theoretical perspectives with the goal of compliance to a specific health-promoting regimen.

COMPLIANCE AND CONTROL

The authoritative aspect of compliance infers that there is an attempt to control, in part, decision making on the part of the learner. Some models of compliance have attempted to balance the issue of control by using terms such as *mutual contracting* (Steckel, 1982) or *consensual regimen* (Fink, 1976).

One way to view the issue of control in the learning situation is through the concept of locus of control (Rotter, 1954) and health locus of control (Wallston et al., 1978). Through objective measurement, individuals can be categorized as "internals," whose health behavior is self-directed, or "externals," whereby others are viewed as more powerful in influencing health outcomes. Externals believe that fate is a powerful external force that determines life's course, whereas internals believe that they control their own destiny. For instance, an external might say, "Osteoporosis runs in my family, and it will 'catch up' with me." Whereas, an internal might say, "Although there is a history of osteoporosis in my family, I will have necessary screenings, eat an appropriate diet, and do weight-bearing exercise to prevent or control this problem."

Locus of control has been related to compliance with therapeutic regimens. Shillinger (1983) suggests that different teaching strategies are indicated for internals and externals. The literature, however, is inconclusive as to the nature of the relationship between compliance and internals versus externals. Oberle (1991) reviewed a decade of research on locus of control and concluded that the collective results of nursing studies yield little information useful in nursing practice. She noted that there were problems with nonexperimental designs, issues of reliability and validity, and the multidimensional nature of the construct of locus of control.

Hussey and Guilliland (1989) note that both locus of control and functional literacy level impact on compliance. Going beyond poor reading skills, "functional literacy is the idea of being able to function or act on content after reading it" (p. 607). This implies that reading skills, although important in assessing level of ability to comprehend written educational material or directions, do not measure one's ability to function or actually carry out regimens following presented content. Functional literacy level in relation to compliance also needs to be assessed by the nurse as educator (see Chapter 7).

Noncompliance describes resistance of the individual to follow a predetermined regimen. The literature is replete with studies that indicate high levels of patient noncompliance, with estimates of noncompliance estimated at 30% to 50% (Becker & Green, 1975; Sackett & Haynes, 1976). The question of why clients are noncompliant remains largely unanswered.

Recent research has shown that situational and personality characteristics play a significant role in determining compliance (Luker & Caress, 1989). The educator's self-awareness relative to the learner's personality characteristics and previous history of compliance to health regimens could play an important role in the educational process.

The expectation of total compliance in all spheres of behavior and at all times is unrealistic. At times, noncompliant behavior may be desirable and could be viewed as a necessary defensive response to stressful situations. The learner may use "time-outs" as the intensity of the learning situation is maintained or escalates. This mechanism of temporary withdrawal from the learning situation may actually be beneficial. The learner, following withdrawal, could reengage feeling renewed and ready to continue with an educational program or regimen. Viewed in this way, noncompliance is not an obstacle to learning and does not carry a negative connotation.

HEALTH BEHAVIORS OF THE LEARNER

Motivation and compliance are concepts relevant to health behaviors of the learner. The nurse as educator focuses on health education as well as the expected health behaviors. Health behavior frameworks are blueprints and, as such, are tools for the nurse as educator that can be used to maintain desired patient behaviors or promote changes. A familiarity with models and theories that describe, explain, or predict health behaviors will increase the range of health-promoting strategies for the nurse as educator. When these frameworks are understood, the principles inherent in each can be used either to facilitate motivation or to promote compliance to a health regimen. An overview of selected models and theories discussed are Health Belief Model, Health Promotion Model, Self-Efficacy Theory, Theory of Reasoned Action, PRECEDE-PROCEED Model, and Therapeutic Alliance Model.

Health Belief Model

The original Health Belief Model was developed in the 1950s from a social psychology perspective to examine why people did not participate in health-screening programs (Rosenstock, 1974). This model was modified by Becker (1974) to address compliance to therapeutic regimens.

The two major premises on which the model is built are the eventual success of disease prevention and curing regimens that involve the clients' willingness to participate and the belief that health is highly valued (Becker, 1990). Both of these premises need to be present for the model to be relevant in explaining health behavior. The model is grounded on the supposition that it is possible to predict health behavior given three major interacting components: individual perceptions, modifying factors, and likelihood of action (Figure 6-1).

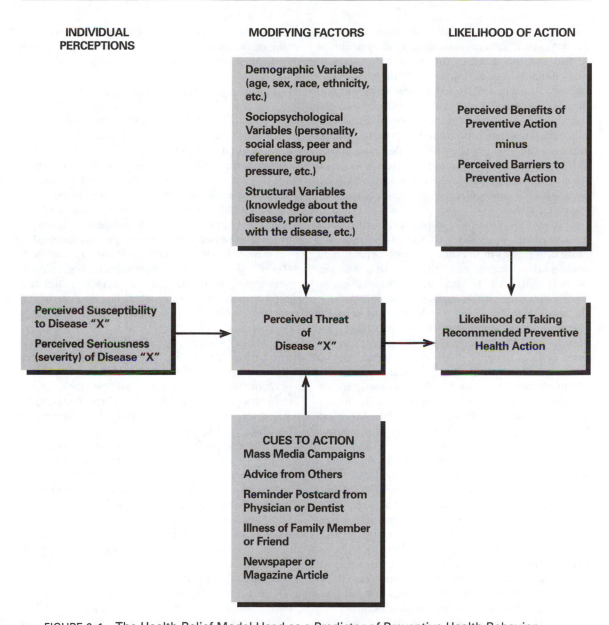

FIGURE 6–1   The Health Belief Model Used as a Predictor of Preventive Health Behavior

SOURCE: From M. Becker, R. Drachman, and J. Kirscht, A new approach to explaining sick-role behavior in low-income populations, 1974. *American Journal of Public Health, 64*(3), 206. Copyright by American Public Health Association. Reprinted with permission.

Figure 6–1 shows the direction and flow of the interacting components. Each is further divided into subcomponents. The individual perceptions component comprises perceived susceptibility or perceived severity of a specific disease. The modifying factors component consists of demographic variables (age, sex, race, ethnicity), sociopsychological variables (personality, locus of control, social class, peer and reference group pressure), and structural variables (knowledge about and prior contact with disease). These variables in conjunction with cues to action (mass media, advice, reminders, illness, reading material) impact on the subcomponent of perceived threat of the specific disease. The third major component, likelihood of action, consists of the subcomponents of perceived benefits of preventive action minus perceived barriers to preventive action. All the components are directed toward the likelihood of taking recommended preventive health action as the final phase of the model. In sum, individual perceptions and modifying factors interact. An individual appraisal of the preventive action occurs, which is followed by a prediction of the likelihood of action.

The Health Belief Model has been the predominant explanatory model since the 1970s for uncovering differences in preventive health behaviors as well as differences in preventive use of health services (Langlie, 1977). Used to predict preventive health behavior and to explain sick-role behavior, the model has been used widely in health behavior research across disciplines such as medicine, psychology, social behavior, and gerontology. It has also been widely used to study patient behaviors in relation to preventive behaviors and acute and chronic illnesses. Redeker (1988) reviewed the literature on health beliefs and adherence in chronic illness and uncovered studies focused on hypertension, coronary disease, diabetes, renal disease, pulmonary disease, and paraplegia.

There is support for this model found in nursing studies. For instance, Hahn (1993) examined health belief constructs regarding alcohol and other drug use, including perceived susceptibility, seriousness, barriers, benefits, and parental involvement. The findings showed, in a sample of 200 drug users, that they were more likely to perceive their children as susceptible to future alcohol and drug use when compared to nonusers. Hallal (1982) investigated the relationship of health beliefs, health locus of control, and self-concept to the practice of breast self-examination (BSE) in a sample of 207 adult women and found BSE to be correlated to health beliefs, with the highest correlation to perceived benefits.

Findings from studies such as these can be operationalized through educational programs specific to high-risk populations. Janz and Becker (1984) reviewed the Health Belief Model literature over a 10-year period and found that the model was robust in predicting health behaviors, with perceived barriers as the most influential factor. In light of this review, the nurse as educator needs to take into consideration the availability of barrier-free educational resources.

Health Promotion Model

The Health Promotion Model developed by Pender (1987) has been primarily used in the discipline of nursing (Figure 6–2). This model describes components and mechanisms that factor into health-promoting lifestyles. Actualizing health potential and increasing the level of well-being using approach behaviors rather than avoidance of disease behaviors delineate this model as a health promotion rather than a disease prevention model.

The sequence of factors is clearly outlined. Modifying factors (demographic, biologic, interpersonal, situational, and behavioral) directly impact on cognitive-perceptual factors such as importance of health, perceived control of health, perceived self-efficacy, definition of health, perceived health status, perceived benefits of health-promoting behaviors, and perceived barriers of health-promoting behaviors. The cognitive-perceptual factors directly impact on participation in health-promoting behaviors. Cues (triggers) to action directly impact on likelihood of engaging in health-promoting behaviors.

There are schematic similarities between the Health Belief Model and the Health Promotion Model, seen in a comparison of Figures 6–1 and 6–2. Both models describe the use of modifying factors that impact on perceptions and the likelihood of taking preventive or health-promoting actions. Cues to action impact directly or indirectly on the likelihood of action. Sequencing of factors, however, in each of the models shows some schematic dissimilarities.

In a nursing study, Johnson et al. (1993) found partial support for the Health Promotion Model. In their sample of 3000 adults, they discovered that modifying factors had strong direct effects on health-promoting behaviors. As proposed by the model, the modifying factors of age, income, education, and the selected biological characteristic of body mass had indirect effects on health-promoting lifestyles.

Research support for the Health Promotion Model has been shown by Lusk et al. (1995), who found significant differences in health-promoting lifestyles in a sample of 638 workers according to

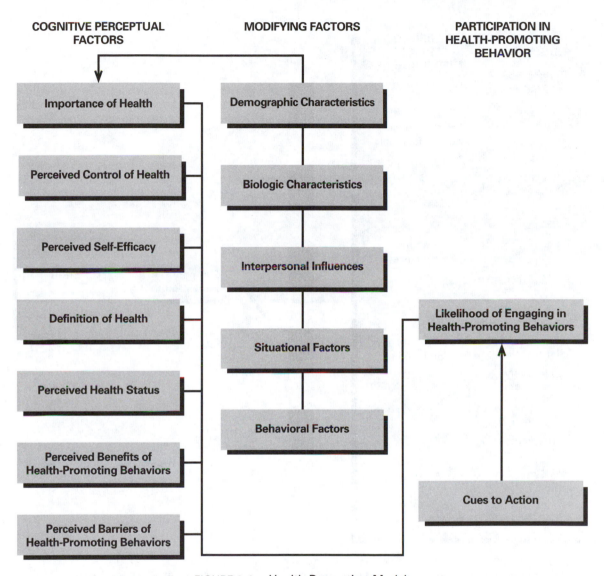

COGNITIVE PERCEPTUAL FACTORS

- Importance of Health
- Perceived Control of Health
- Perceived Self-Efficacy
- Definition of Health
- Perceived Health Status
- Perceived Benefits of Health-Promoting Behaviors
- Perceived Barriers of Health-Promoting Behaviors

MODIFYING FACTORS

- Demographic Characteristics
- Biologic Characteristics
- Interpersonal Influences
- Situational Factors
- Behavioral Factors

PARTICIPATION IN HEALTH-PROMOTING BEHAVIOR

- Likelihood of Engaging in Health-Promoting Behaviors
- Cues to Action

FIGURE 6–2. Health Promotion Model

job category (blue-collar, skilled trade, and white-collar). Blue-collar workers scored significantly lower on health-promoting lifestyles than workers in the other job categories. Significant differences in health-promoting lifestyles were also found for gender, exercise, and educational level, but not for marital status or ethnicity. These findings have implications for workplace educational program design.

Self-Efficacy Theory

Developed from a social-cognitive perspective, the Self-Efficacy Theory is based on a person's expectations relative to a specific course of action (Bandura, 1977a, 1977b, 1986). It is a predictive theory in the sense that it deals with the belief that one can accomplish a specific behavior. The belief of competency and capability relative to certain

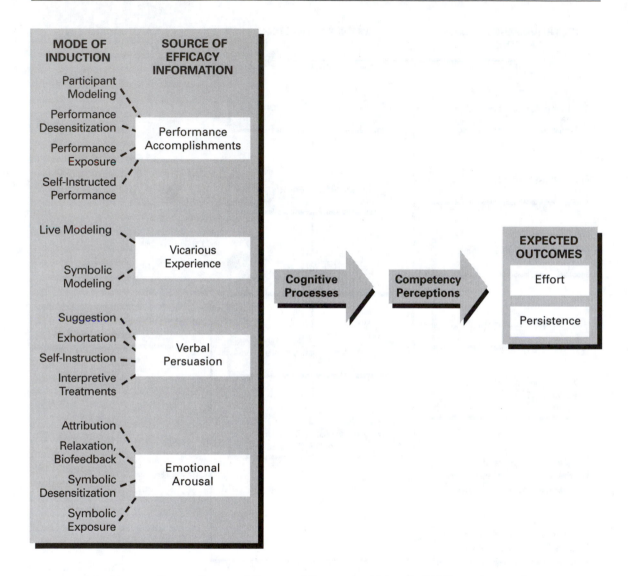

FIGURE 6–3.   Determinants of Expected Outcomes Using Self-Efficacy Perceptions

SOURCE: From Albert Bandura, *Social Learning Theory*, © 1977, p. 80. Reprinted by permission of Prentice-Hall, Upper Saddle River, New Jersey.

behaviors is a precursor to expected outcomes. Figure 6–3 shows an adaptation of Bandura's efficacy expectations model extended to include expected outcomes. In this adapted model, self-efficacy is used as an outcome determinant.

According to Bandura (1986), self-efficacy is cognitively appraised and processed through four principal sources of information: (1) performance accomplishment evidenced in self-mastery of similarly expected behaviors, (2) vicarious experiences such as observing successful expected behavior through the modeling of others, (3) verbal persuasion by others who present realistic beliefs that the individual is capable of the expected behavior, and (4) emotional arousal through self-judgment of physiological states of distress. Bandura (1986) notes that the most influential source of efficacy information is that of previous performance accomplishment. Efficacy expectations (expectations relative to a specific course of action) are induced through certain modes. Modes of induction include, but are not limited to desensitization, self-instruction, exposure, suggestion, and relaxation.

Self-efficacy has been useful in predicting the course of health behavior. Nursing literature has addressed linkages between self-efficacy and self-care. Moore (1990) used self-efficacy to teach self-care to the older adult. Lev (1995) used qualitative methodology to investigate the linkage between self-efficacy enhancing interventions and self-care in a sample of 73 patients receiving chemotherapy. Findings showed that interventions, particularly modeling and positive reinforcement, were potentially responsible for positive patient responses.

The use of the Self-Efficacy Theory for the nurse as educator is particularly relevant in developing educational programs. The behavior-specific predictions of the theory can be used for understanding the likelihood of individuals to participate in existing or projected educational programs. Educational strategies such as modeling, demonstration, and verbal reinforcement parallel modes of self-efficacy induction.

Theory of Reasoned Action

The Theory of Reasoned Action emerged from a research program that began in the 1950s and is concerned with prediction and understanding of any form of human behavior within a social context (Ajzen & Fishbein, 1980). It is based on the premise that humans are rational decision makers who make use of whatever information is available to them. Attitudes toward persons are not an integral part of this theory, rather the focus is on the predicted behavior. It is shown as a sequential model in Figure 6–4.

In a two-pronged linear approach, specific behavior is determined by (1) beliefs, attitude toward the behavior, and intention and (2) motivation to comply with influential persons known as referents, subjective norms, and intention. Intention to perform can be measured by relative weights of attitude and subjective norms.

In nursing research, Jemmott and Jemmott (1991) found support for the Theory of Reasoned Action in their study on AIDS risk behavior among 103 young, unmarried, sexually active black women. They found that attitude toward condom use was the strongest predictor, followed by increased support by referents for the intention to use condoms in the following 3 months. Knowledge of AIDS was not significantly related to attitude toward or actual use of condoms. Their findings indicate that attitudes and the influence of significant others need to be taken into consideration when intervening in risky sexual behavior.

This theory is useful in predicting health behaviors, particularly for educators who want to understand the attitudinal context within which behaviors are likely to change. Nurses as educators need to take beliefs, attitudinal factors, and subjective norms into consideration when designing educational programs relating to intent to change a specific health behavior.

PRECEDE-PROCEED Model

The PRECEDE-PROCEED Model emerged from an epidemiological perspective on health promotion in the hopes of combating leading causes of death (Green & Kreuter, 1991). The model acronym PRECEDE stands for Predisposing, Reinforcing, and Enabling Constructs in Educational Diagnosis and Evaluation, originally developed by Green et al. (1980). Green and Kreuter (1991) further refined the model to include a second component referred to as PROCEED, which means Policy, Regulatory, and Organizational Constructs in Educational and Environmental Development.

Health education, defined as the "voluntary participation of learners in determining their own health practices" (Green & Kreuter, 1991, p. 20), is the core of the model. Referring to the centrality of health education, Green and Kreuter (1991) state that the "organizational, economic, or other environmental supports for action are optional, depending on which of them is needed in combination with health education" (p. 14). The phases in the PRECEDE component identify priorities and objectives, while the phases in the PROCEED component address criteria for policy, and implementation and evaluation relative to a variety of diagnoses in the PRECEDE phases (Figure 6–5).

The model begins with population self-study/assessment relative to quality of life in phase 1 and ends with outcome evaluation in phase 9. Education is a key and pivotal dimension specifically addressed in phases 4 and 5. It is worthy to note that the educational diagnosis phase of this robust model (comprising predisposing, reinforcing, and enabling factors) synthesizes the Health Belief

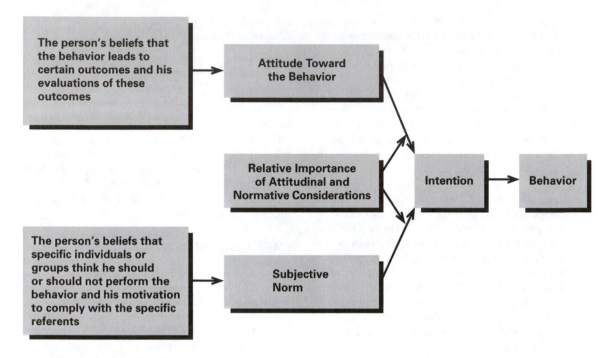

Note: Arrows indicate the direction of influence.

FIGURE 6–4.   Factors Determining a Person's Behavior

SOURCE: From I. Ajzen and M. Fishbein, *Understanding Attitudes and Predicting Social Behavior*, © 1980, p. 8. Reprinted by permission of Prentice-Hall, Upper Saddle River, New Jersey.

Model, Self-Efficacy Theory, and the Theory of Reasoned Action. The authors note that health behaviors are most influenced by the predisposing factors of knowledge, beliefs, values, attitudes, and confidence.

Mullen et al. (1987) compared the Health Belief Model, Theory of Reasoned Action, and the original PRECEDE Model for usefulness in predicting changes in health behavior in a random sample of 661 adults from ethnically diverse backgrounds and found that all three models were similar in predictive power. The strength of the PRECEDE-PROCEED model, however, is the inclusion of interventions from a population needs perspective.

Nurses as educators can use this model when considering implications for social policy change. There is particular relevance for community health nurses because the model notes that community is "the center of gravity." The design and development of health education programs for specific populations and the use of the perspec-

tive of community as client are within the scope of nursing practice and education.

Therapeutic Alliance Model

Barofsky's (1978) Therapeutic Alliance Model addresses a shift in power from the provider to a learning partnership in which collaboration and negotiation with the consumer are key. A therapeutic alliance is formed between the caregiver and receiver in which each participant in this affiliation is viewed as having equal power. The client is viewed as active and responsible with an outcome expectation of self-care. The shift toward self-determination and control over one's own life is fundamental to this model (Figure 6–6).

This model compares the components of compliance, adherence, and alliance. According to Barofsky, there is a needed change in treatment determinants from coercion in compliance and from conforming in adherence, to collaboration in

PRECEDE

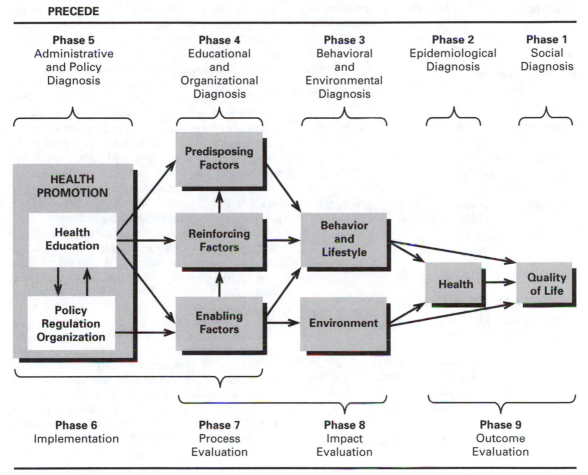

FIGURE 6–5.   The PRECEDE-PROCEED Model for Health Promotion Planning and Evaluation

SOURCE: From *Health Promotion Planning: An Educational and Environmental Approach* by Lawrence W. Green and Marshall W. Kreuter by permission of Mayfield Publishing Company. Copyright © 1991 by Mayfield Publishing Company.

alliance. The power in the relationship between the participants is equalized by alliance. The role of the patient is neither passive nor rebellious but active and responsible. The expected outcomes are not compliant dependence or counterdependence, but responsible self-care.

Not originally developed as an educational model, and not well-known in nursing, nevertheless its usefulness to the nurse as educator is acknowledged in the partnership of learning. This interpersonal model is appropriate in the educational process when shifting the focus from the patient as a passive-dependent learner to one of an active learner. It serves as a guide to refocus on collaboration rather than on compliance. The nurse as educator and the patient as learner form an alliance with the goal of self-care. Luker and Caress (1989) support the notion of therapeutic alliance in patient education and argue that "nurses have resisted equalizing their role with patients" (p. 715). Advocating the alternative of self-directed learning for the aim of self-care, they encourage the transfer of responsibility for learning from nurse to patient.

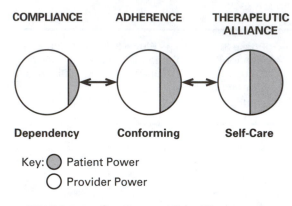

FIGURE 6–6. Continuum of the Therapeutic Alliance Model

SELECTION OF MODELS FOR HEALTH EDUCATION

Selection of models for educational use can be made with respect to (1) similarities and dissimilarities, (2) nurse as educator agreement with model conceptualizations, and (3) functional utility.

Similarities and Dissimilarities of Models

Models may be seen as so similar that there would be a negligible difference in choosing one over the other, or they may be seen as so dissimilar that one would be inappropriate for a specific educational purpose. A comparative analysis of the different frameworks reveals that the Health Belief Model and the Health Promotion Model are the most similar. Each uses the same salient factors of individual perceptions and modifying factors. The differences appear in the basic premises and the role of mediating factors. The Health Belief Model emphasizes susceptibility to disease and the likelihood of preventive action, while the Health Promotion Model emphasizes health potential and the likelihood of health-promoting behaviors.

The Self-Efficacy Theory and the Theory of Reasoned Action are similar in that they focus on the predictions or expectations of specific behaviors. Both of these theories lend themselves more

easily to less complex model testing than either the Health Belief Model or Health Promotion Model because the former are more linear in conceptualization. Specificity of behaviors may aid in targeting outcomes of educational programs.

The Health Belief Model, Health Promotion Model, Self-Efficacy Theory, and Theory of Reasoned Action are similar in that they acknowledge factors such as experiences, perceptions, or beliefs relative to the individual and factors external to the individual that can modify health behaviors. These frameworks also recognize the multidimensional nature, complexity, and probability of health behaviors. The PRECEDE-PROCEED model broadens this perspective to aggregates and populations.

All the models acknowledge the importance of the patient in decision making with respect to health behaviors. The differences are evident in patient focus, the relative importance of modifying factors, specificity of behavior, and outcomes.

The most dissimilar model is the Therapeutic Alliance Model. Although it is relatively narrow in scope, its simplicity and parsimony are a strength. When applied to the educational arena, the educator-learner relationship is the critical factor. Addressing potentially frustrating patient education situations such as noncompliance, Hochbaum (1980) noted that patient educators when "frustrated are unable to understand the apparently irrational and self-destructive action of their patients, and sometimes throw their hands up in despair, bedeviled by the seeming irrationality of the patient's behavior . . . but this behavior may be altogether rational from the patient's perspective" (p. 7). Understanding of the client as learner can be uncovered in the Therapeutic Alliance Model.

Educator Agreement with Model Conceptualizations

Nurses as educators have belief systems, which may or may not agree with some of the tenets of each of the models presented. Choice of model can be based on educators' level of agreement with salient factors in each framework. Likelihood of action is best addressed by either the Health Belief Model or Health Promotion Model. Attitude and intention are best viewed through the Theory of Reasoned Action. Belief in one's capabilities is best addressed by the Self-Efficacy Theory, and reduction of noncompliance through an educator-learner collaboration with use of the Therapeutic Alliance Model. The PRECEDE-PROCEED Model best fits with the beliefs that health education and health promotion are inseparable and that consent for voluntary change of people is necessary before attempts are made to change social systems. In scrutinizing each of the models, the attention of the educator may be drawn to other factors as well. The model or models that fit best with the educators' beliefs are more likely to be chosen.

Functional Utility of Models

Model selection for educational purposes can also be based on functional utility. Questions to be asked to determine functional utility are as follows: Who is the target learner? What is the focus of the learning? When is the optimal time? Where is the process to be carried out?

The question of who the learner is deals with whether the target learner is the individual, family, group, or community. The Health Belief Model, Health Promotion Model, Self-Efficacy Theory, and Theory of Reasoned Action are more likely to be used with individuals, families, and groups, with the focus on the individual. It is difficult to talk about collective self-perceptions, collective self-confidence, and collective intention to perform. Each of these factors is presented by the models in the context of the individual. The important notion for the nurse as educator to remember is the probability of individual variation. Another consideration in terms of the target learner is categorical groups, such as those considered at high risk and those diagnosed with acute or chronic illnesses.

The functional use of the models can also be determined by what is needed, when it should take place, and the setting in which the learning is to take place. What is needed is relative to the focus of the learning and addresses the content to be taught such as disease processes, specific disease, promotion of wellness, expectations of specific health practices, or focus on self-care. The PRECEDE-PROCEED Model is best used as a diagnostic framework for health education programs and health planning (Mullen et al., 1987).

The question of *when* is one of optimal timing and refers to the readiness of the learner, a mutually convenient time, and prevention of untimely

delays in moving toward a desired goal. Although considered important in the context of health education, this critical factor has received no specific reference in terms of health promotion models. This is a neglected factor in the models discussed, although it is apparent that determining optimal time can be a motivational incentive in terms of meeting health needs.

Addressing the question of *where* the educational process is to be carried out is another aspect of functional utility. The settings of home, workplace, school, institution, or specific community locations are options. All the models discussed lend themselves to these diverse settings. The one that is most specific to community locations is the PRECEDE-PROCEED Model, which deals with community-based populations (see Chapter 13).

INTEGRATION OF MODELS FOR USE IN EDUCATION

From the previous discussion, it is clear that the integration of various components of health promotion models is advantageous. When salient factors are taken into consideration in light of developmental stages of the learner, an integrated motivational model of learning in health promotion could emerge. Padilla and Bulcavage (1991) advocate a multitheory approach to promote health behaviors of the learner and note that theories can provide blueprints for interventions.

Salient health promotion factors that can be used in a multitheory approach to health education include but are not limited to level of knowledge, attitudes, values, beliefs, perceptions, level of anxiety, self-confidence, skills mastery, past experiences, intention, physiological capacity, sociocultural enablers, environment, educator-learner alliance, resources and reinforcements, mutual and realistic goal setting, hierarchy of needs, quality of life, and voluntary participation in learning.

Developmental stages of the learner incorporate principles of pedagogy (teaching children), andragogy (teaching adults), and gerogogy (teaching the aged) to meet the needs of the learner. A more comprehensive and holistic model for the nurse as educator emerges when learning is viewed along a unidirectional developmental continuum, in combination with salient health promotion factors. (For a discussion on educational approaches, see Chapter 5.)

An example of the multitheory approach is described by Bille (1980), who considers motivation, readiness to learn, selected concepts from theories of learning, and principles of gerogogy in the development of an educational plan for the older adult.

THE ROLES OF NURSE AS EDUCATOR IN HEALTH PROMOTION

Nurses as educators are in a position to promote healthy lifestyles. Combining content specific to the discipline of nursing, knowledge from educational theories, and health behavior models allows for an integrated approach to shaping health behaviors of the learner. Subroles of the nurse as educator include facilitator of change, contractor, organizer, and evaluator.

Facilitator of Change

The goal of the nurse as educator is to promote health. Health education and health promotion are integral. The nurse as educator is simultaneously a facilitator of change. When learning is viewed as an intervention, it needs to be considered in the context of other nursing interventions that will effect change. DeTornay and Thompson (1987) propose that explaining, analyzing, dividing complex skills, demonstrating, practicing, asking questions, and providing closure are effective in facilitating change in the learning situation.

Contractor

Contracting has been a popular means of facilitating learning. Informal or formal contracts can delineate and promote learning objectives. Similar to the nursing process, educational contracting involves stating mutual goals to be accomplished, devising an agreed-upon plan of action, evaluating the plan, and deriving alternatives (see learning contracts in Chapter 10). The plan of action needs to be as specific as possible and include the who, what, when, where, and how of the learning pro-

cess. Responsibilities that are clearly stated aid in evaluating the plan and directing plan revisions.

In light of our changing health-care system, there needs to be an emphasis on patient-nurse partnerships because patients are expected to take increasingly more responsibility and control in the decisions that affect their own health. Educational contracting is the key to informed decision making.

When education is viewed in the context of the client, rather than the client in the context of education, learning is individualized. The "fit" between the client as learner and the nurse as educator has the capacity to facilitate learning. The "goodness of fit" between these two educational participants can be a motivating factor. Do the client and educator share an understanding of backgrounds or language? Is there a mutual understanding of goal setting? Are health beliefs respected?

A contract involves a trusting relationship. In a mutually satisfying teacher-learner relationship system, trust is a key ingredient. The learner trusts that the nurse as educator possesses a respectable, current body of theoretically based and clinically applicable knowledge. The nurse needs to be approachable, trustworthy, and culturally sensitive because the learner's own health status is often valued as a private matter. In turn, the nurse trusts that when the client enters into an agreement, the learner will demonstrate behaviors that will be health promoting. Newman and Brown (1986) list elements of the relationship as follows: trust and respect, teacher assumes the student can learn and is sensitive to individual needs, and both feel free to learn and make mistakes.

Organizer

Organization of the learning situation, including manipulation of materials and space, sequential organization of content from simple to complex, and determining priority of subject matter, is a role of the nurse as educator. Organization of learning material decreases obstacles to learning (Haggard, 1989). Attendance at educational programs or individual sessions can be organized around the target learner as well as significant others to facilitate the learning process and promote motivation to learn.

Evaluator

Educational programs, like other health-care projects, need to be accountable to the learner or consumer of the health service. This is done by evaluation in the form of outcomes. Self-evaluation, patient evaluation, organization evaluation, and peer evaluation are not new concepts. Evaluative processes are an integral part of learning.

The nurse as educator is a role that has been challenged. Luker and Caress (1989) make the distinction between patient education and patient teaching, noting that the former is in the province of the clinical specialist. They also note that not all nurses are prepared to be patient educators. The specialist approach to education needs to be investigated in terms of health outcomes, as well as impact on professional role.

In the final analysis, application of knowledge that improves the health of individuals, families, groups, or communities is the evaluative measure of learning.

SUMMARY

Critical components of this chapter have included a discussion of concepts of motivation and compliance, assessment of level of learner motivation, identification of incentives and obstacles that impact on motivation and compliance, discussion of axioms of motivation relevant to learning, a comparison and contrast of selected health behavior frameworks and their influence on learning, an outline of specific strategies that facilitate motivation and compliance, and the recognition of the unique role of the nurse as educator in influencing learner motivation and compliance.

When information is imparted, accepted, and applied, the foundation is set for change in health behaviors. When people are motivated and know that they can make a difference in their own lives, then a barrier to health has been lifted.

References

Ajzen, I., & Fishbein, M. (1980). *Understanding attitudes and predicting social behavior.* Englewood Cliffs, NJ: Prentice-Hall.

Atkinson, J.W. (1964). *An introduction to motivation.* Princeton, NJ: Van Nostrand.

Bandura, A. (1977a). Self-efficacy: Toward a unifying theory of behavioral change. *Psychological Review, 84*(2), 191-215.

Bandura, A. (1977b). *Social learning theory.* Englewood Cliffs, NJ: Prentice-Hall.

Bandura, A. (1986). *Social foundations of thought and action: A social cognitive theory.* Englewood Cliffs, NJ: Prentice-Hall.

Barofsky, I. (1978). Compliance, adherence and the therapeutic alliance: Steps in the development of self-care. *Social Science and Medicine, 12*, 369-376.

Becker, M. (Ed.). (1974). *The health belief model and personal health behavior.* Thorofare, NJ: Slack.

Becker, M. (1990). Theoretical models of adherence and strategies for improving adherence. In S.A. Shumaker, E.B. Schron, & J.K. Ockene (Eds.), *The handbook of human health behavior* (pp. 5-43). New York: Springer.

Becker, M.W., Drachman, R.H., & Kirscht, J.P. (1974). A new approach to explaining sick-role behavior in low-income populations. *American Journal of Public Health, 64*(3), 205-216.

Becker, M.H., & Green, L.W. (1975). A family approach to compliance with medical treatment: A selective review of the literature. *International Journal of Health Education, 18, 173-182.*

Bille, D.A. (Dec. 1980). Educational strategies for teaching the elderly patient. *Nursing and Health Care 1,* 256-263.

Damrosch, S. (1991). General strategies for motivating people to change their behavior. *Nursing Clinics of North America, 26*(4), 833-843.

deTornay, R., & Thompson, M.A. (1987). *Strategies for teaching nursing,* 3rd ed. New York: Wiley.

Eraker, S.A., Kirscht, J.P., & Becker, M.H. (1984). Understanding and improving patient compliance. *Annals of Internal Medicine 100,* 258-268.

Fink, D.L. (1976). Tailoring in the consensual regimen. In D.L. Sackett & R.B. Haynes (Eds.), *Compliance with therapeutic regimens.* Baltimore: Johns Hopkins University Press.

Fisher, R.C. (1992). Patient education and compliance: A pharmacist's perspective. *Patient Education and Counseling, 19*, 261-271.

Green, L.W., & Kreuter, M.W. (1991). *Health promotion planning: An educational and environmental approach,* 2nd ed. Mountain View, CA: Mayfield.

Green L.W., Kreuter, M.W., Deeds, S.G., & Partridge, K.B. (1980). *Health education planning: A diagnostic approach.* Palo Alto, CA: Mayfield.

Haggard, A. (1989). *Handbook of patient education.* Rockville, MD: Aspen.

Hahn, E.J. (1993). Parental alcohol and other drug use (AOD) and health beliefs about parent involvement in AOD prevention. *Issues in Mental Health Nursing, 14,* 237-247.

Hallal, J.C. (1982). The relationship of health beliefs, health locus of control, and self-concept to the practice of breast self-examination in adult women. *Nursing Research, 31*(3), 137-142.

Hochbaum, G.M. (1980). Patient counseling vs. patient teaching. *Education for self-care.* Rockville, MD: Aspen.

Hussey, L.C., & Guilliland, K. (1989). Compliance, low literacy, and locus of control. *Nursing Clinics of North America, 24*(3), 605-610.

Janz, N.K., & Becker, M.H. (1984). The health belief model: A decade later. *Health Education Quarterly, 11*(1), 1-47.

Jemmott, L.S., & Jemmott, J.B., III. (1991). Applying the theory of reasoned action to AIDS risk behavior: Condom use among black women. *Nursing Research, 40*(4), 229-234.

Johnson, J.L., Ratner, P.A., Bottorff, J.L., & Hayduk, L.A. (1993). An exploration of Pender's health promotion model using LISREL. *Nursing Research, 42*(3), 132-138.

Keller, J.M. (1987). Development and use of the ARCS model of instructional design. *Journal of Instructional Development, 10*(3), 2-10.

Kort, M. (1987). Motivation: The challenge for today's health promoter. *The Canadian Nurse, 83*(9), 16-18.

Langlie, J.K. (Sept. 1977). Social networks, health beliefs, and preventive health behavior. *Journal of Health and Social Behavior, 18,* 244-260.

Leddy, S., & Pepper, J.M. (1993). *Conceptual basis of professional nursing.* Philadelphia: Lippincott.

Lev, E. (1995). Use of triangulation reveals theoretical linkages and outcomes in a nursing intervention study. *Clinical Nurse Specialist, 9*(6), 300-305.

Levanthal, H.C., & Cameron, L. (1987). Behavior theories and the problem of compliance. *Patient Education Counseling, 10,* 117-138.

Lewin, K. (1935). *A dynamic theory of personality.* New York: McGraw-Hill.

Luker, K., & Caress, A. L. (1989). Rethinking patient education. *Journal of Advanced Nursing, 14,* 711-718.

Lusk, S.L., Kerr, M.J., & Ronis, D.L. (1995). Health promoting lifestyles of blue-collar, skilled trade, and white-collar workers. *Nursing Research, 44*(1), 20-24.

Maslow, A.H. (1943). A theory of human motivation. *Psychological Review, 50*(4), 371-396.

Mishel, M.H. (1990). Reconceptualization of the uncertainty in illness theory. *Image: Journal of Nursing Scholarship, 22*(4), 256-262.

Moore, E.J. (1990). Using self-efficacy in teaching self-care to the elderly. *Holistic Nursing Practice, 4*(2), 22-29.

Mullen, P.D., Hersey, J.C., & Iverson, D.C. (1987). Health behavior models compared. *Social Science Medicine, 11,* 973-981.

Newman, F., & Brown, R. (1986). Creating optimal conditions for learning. *Educational Horizons, 64*(4), 188-189.

Oberle, K. (1991). A decade of research in locus of control: What have we learned? *Journal of Advanced Nursing, 16,* 800-806.

Padilla, G.V., & Bulcavage, L.M. (1991). Theories used in patient/health education. *Seminars in Oncology Nursing, 7*(2), 87-96.

Pender, N. (1987). *Health promotion in nursing practice,* 2nd ed. Norwalk, CT: Appleton-Lange.

Peplau, H.E. (1979). *The psychotherapy of Hildegard E. Peplau.* Texas: Atwood.

Rankin, S.H., & Stallings, K.D. (1990). *Patient education,* 2nd ed. Philadelphia: Lippincott.

Redeker, N. (1988). Health beliefs and adherence in chronic illness. *Image: Journal of Nursing Scholarship, 20*(1), 31-35.

Redman, B.K. (1993). *The process of patient education,* 7th ed. St. Louis: Mosby.

Rosenstock, I.M. (1974). Historical origins of the health belief model. In M.H. Becker (Ed.), *The health belief model and personal health behavior.* Thorofare, NJ: Slack.

Ross, M.W., & Rosser, B.R. (1989). Education and AIDS risks: A review. *Health Education Research, 4*(3), 273-284.

Rotter, J.B. (1954). *Social learning theory and clinical psychology.* Englewood Cliffs, NJ: Prentice-Hall.

Sackett, D.L., & Haynes, R.B. (1976). *Compliance with therapeutic regimens.* Baltimore: Johns Hopkins University Press.

Sands, D.S., & Holman, E.H. (1985). Does knowledge enhance patient compliance? *Journal of Gerontological Nursing, 11*(4), 23-29.

Shillinger, F. (1983). Locus of control: Implications for nursing practice. *Image: Journal of Nursing Scholarship, 15*(2), 58-63.

Steckel, S.B. (1982). Predicting, measuring, implementing and following up on patient compliance. *Nursing Clinics of North America, 17*(3), 491-497.

Wallston, K.A., Wallston, B.S., & DeVellis, R. (Spring 1978). Development of the multidimensional health locus of control (MHLC) scales. *Health Education Monographs,* 160-170.

CHAPTER 7

Literacy in the Adult Patient Population

Susan B. Bastable

CHAPTER HIGHLIGHTS

KEY TERMS

OBJECTIVES

After completing this chapter, the reader will be able to

1. Define the terms *literacy*, *low literacy*, *functional illiteracy*, *illiteracy*, *readability*, *comprehension*, and *numeracy*.
2. Identify the magnitude of the literacy problem in the United States.
3. Differentiate the characteristics of those individuals at risk for having difficulty with reading and comprehension of written and oral language.
4. Discuss common myths and assumptions about the illiterate person.
5. Identify clues that are indicators of reading and writing deficiencies.
6. Assess the impact of illiteracy and low literacy on patient motivation and compliance with health-care regimens.
7. Recognize the role of the nurse as educator in the assessment of patients' literacy skills.
8. Critically analyze readability and comprehension levels of printed materials using specific formulas and tests.
9. Describe specific guidelines for writing effective education materials.
10. Outline various teaching strategies useful in educating clients with low literacy skills.

Literacy of the U.S. population has been the subject of increasing interest and concern by educators as well as by government officials, employers, and media experts. Adult illiteracy continues to be a major problem in this country despite public and private efforts at all levels to address the issue through testing of literacy skills and developing literacy training programs. Today, the fact remains that many individuals do not possess the basic literacy abilities to function effectively in our technologically complex society. Many citizens of all ages have difficulty reading and comprehending information well enough to be able to perform such common tasks as filling out job and insurance applications, interpreting bus schedules and road signs, completing tax forms, or registering to vote. Ever since the early 1980s when President Reagan launched the National Adult Literacy Initiative, followed by the United Nations' declaration of 1990 as the International Literacy Year, illiteracy has become a common topic in the public media nationwide and worldwide (Belton, 1991; Wallerstein, 1992). Despite these facts, medical and nursing literature in this country and abroad has contained relatively little information until recently about the effects of patient illiteracy on health-care delivery.

With respect to the literacy problem, the nurse educator's attention specifically focuses on patient populations. Rarely do literacy levels become an issue in teaching staff nurses or nursing students because of their level of formal education. It may become a concern, however, if the audience for in-service programs includes less educated housekeeping and maintenance staff or if a member of the audience has been diagnosed with a learning disorder such as dyslexia. What must be of particular concern to the health-care industry are the numbers of consumers who are illiterate, functionally illiterate, or marginally literate. Researchers have discovered that people with poor reading and comprehension skills have disproportionately higher medical costs and more perceived physical and psychosocial problems than do literate persons (Jenks, 1992).

Health-care professionals traditionally have relied heavily on printed education materials as a cost-effective and time-efficient means to communicate health messages (Zion & Aiman, 1989). For years, nurses and physicians have assumed that written materials commonly distributed to patients were sufficient to insure informed consent for tests and procedures, to promote compliance with treatment regimens, and to guarantee adherence to discharge instructions. Only recently have health-care providers begun to recognize that the scientific and technical terminology inherent in the ubiquitous printed teaching aids is a bewildering set of written instructions little understood by the majority of patients. Unless education materials are written at a level appropriate for intended audiences, patients cannot be expected to be able or willing to accept responsibility for self-care. An essential prerequisite to implementing patient education programs is knowing a person's literacy skills. Yet assessment of literacy and recommendations for appropriate interventions for patients with poor literacy skills have largely been ignored (Luker & Caress, 1989).

This chapter examines the magnitude of the illiteracy problem, the factors that influence readability and comprehension of written health educational materials, the important role nurses play in assessing patients' literacy skills, and the impact of illiteracy on the health and well-being of the public. In addition, the formulas and tests used to evaluate readability and comprehension of printed tools are reviewed, specific guidelines are put forth for writing effective health education materials, and teaching strategies are recommended as a means for breaking down the barriers of illiteracy.

DEFINITION OF TERMS

Literacy is an umbrella term used to describe socially required and expected reading and writing abilities. There is no clear agreement about what it means to be literate in U.S. society. *Literacy* is defined by *Webster's New World Dictionary of American English* (1991) as the "ability to read and write" (p. 789). More specifically, literacy has been thought of as the relative ability to use printed and written material commonly encountered in daily living (Kirsch & Jungeblat, 1986). UNESCO (1987) termed a literate person as "one who can both read and write a short simple statement about everyday life." Others have defined literacy based on the number of grade levels of school completed or the equivalent on achievement tests. Many researchers have found, though, that the reported number of years of schooling attended is an inadequate predictor of a person's reading and writing skills (Doak et al., 1996; Jackson et al., 1991; Davis et al., 1990; Mathews et al., 1988; Powers, 1988). Many studies have been

flawed by the inconsistent and erroneous definitions of literacy, including equating literacy with academic achievement and years of schooling (Adams-Price, 1993). Performance on reading tests has become the conventional method used to measure grade-level achievement. The commonly accepted definition of *literacy* is the ability to read, understand, and interpret information written at the eighth grade level or above. On the other end of the spectrum, *illiteracy* is the total inability to read or write, which up until now has been relatively rare in our society and constitutes less than 5% of all adults in the U.S. population (Doak et al., 1985).

Literacy can be categorized into three general kinds of tasks: *prose tasks*, which measure reading comprehension and the ability to extract themes from newspapers, magazines, poems, and books; *document tasks*, which assess the ability of readers to interpret documents such as insurance reports, consent forms, and transportation schedules; and *quantitative tasks*, which assess the ability to work with numerical information embedded in written material such as computing restaurant menu bills, figuring out taxes, interpreting paycheck stubs, or calculating calories on a nutrition checklist (Adams-Price, 1993).

Low literacy, also termed marginally literate or marginally illiterate, refers to the ability of adults to read, write, and comprehend information between the fifth- and eighth-grade level of difficulty. Low-literate persons have trouble using commonly printed and written information to meet their everyday needs such as reading a TV schedule, taking a telephone message, or filling out a relatively simple application form.

Functional illiteracy means that adults have reading, writing, and comprehension skills below the fifth-grade level; that is, they lack fundamental education skills needed to function effectively in today's society. Functionally illiterate persons have very limited competency with communication via the written or spoken word and in many cases do not understand basic written instructions, audiovisual aids, or even tape recordings. They are unable to read well enough to understand and interpret what they have read or use the information as it was intended (Doak et al., 1996). For example, a functionally illiterate person may be able to read the words on a label of a can of soup that directs "Pour soup into pan. Add one can water. Heat until hot" but cannot comprehend the meaning and sequence of the words to carry through with these directions.

These operational definitions, at best, are approximations. Conventional grade-level definitions of literacy are considered conservative because even an adult with the ability to read at the eighth grade level will encounter difficulties functioning in our advanced society. However, although an individual may have poor reading skills, this does not necessarily imply a lack of intelligence. Low literacy or illiteracy cannot be equated with IQ level (Hussey & Guilliland, 1989). A person can be illiterate or low literate, yet intellectually be within at least normal IQ range.

Readability and comprehension are also words frequently used when determining levels of literacy. *Readability* is defined as the ease with which written or printed information can be read. It is a measure of those elements within a given text of printed material that influence with what degree of success a group of readers will be able to read the style of writing of a selected printed passage. Readability is commonly determined by using one or more readability measurement formulas.

Reading is a complex activity involving many variables with respect to both the reader and the actual written material (Mathews et al., 1988; McCabe et al., 1989; Owen, Johnson, et al., 1993). Table 7–1 shows examples of elements that affect readability.

Comprehension is the degree to which individuals understand what they have read. It is the ability to grasp the meaning of a message—to get the gist of it. A health-care professional can determine if comprehension of health instruction has occurred if patients are able to correctly demonstrate or recall in their own words the message that was received. If the elements of logic, language, and experience in health instruction are compatible with those of the patient's, the message will be clear, relevant, and achievable (Barnes, 1992a, 1992b). A mismatch will likely make the message confusing, incomprehensible, and useless to the patient. Comprehension is affected by the amount, clarity, and complexity of the information presented. The ability to read does not alone guarantee reading comprehension. For example, illness or other disruptive life situations have been found to significantly interfere with comprehension. Patterns of recall, that is, the length of time between information disclosure and the need to remember the information, as well as the nature of the information (how threatening) and the method of presentation also affect understanding (Silva & Sorrell, 1984).

Another term used when discussing literacy is *numeracy*, which is the ability to read and interpret numbers. Overwhelmingly, those with limited literacy also have limited skills in numeracy (Morgan, 1993).

Literacy Relative to Oral Instruction

It must be noted that very little attention has been paid to the role of oral communication in the assessment of illiteracy. Certainly, inability to comprehend the spoken word or oral instruction above the level of understanding simple words, phrases, and slang words should be considered an important element in the definition or assessment of literacy. Doak et al. (1985) address the fact that there is no universally accepted way to test the degree of difficulty with oral language. However, as these authors observed, ". . . it is believed that some of the same characteristics that are critical for written materials will also affect the comprehensibility of spoken language" (p. 40). Much more research needs to be done on "iloralcy," or the inability to understand simple oral language, as a generic concept of illiteracy.

TABLE 7–1. Examples of elements that affect readability

Material Variables	*Reader Variables*
Legibility (e.g., print size, spacing)	Health status
Organization and flow of content	Perceived threat of illness
Concept level	Effects of illness/stress
Length of text	Physical and mental energy
Sentence structure	Level of motivation
Level of vocabulary	Visual and auditory acuity
Relevance to the reader	Educational attainment
Jargon (medical terminology)	Background knowledge
Number of polysyllabic words	Ability to decipher language of message

Literacy Relative to Computer Instruction

The literacy issue has always been examined from the standpoint of readability of materials in print. Recently, computer literacy has become an increasingly popular topic and a new dimension of the issue of literacy. There is a bright future for the use of computers as an educational tool, but the potential has not yet been fully realized or appreciated. Those patients who are well educated and career oriented are already likely to be computer literate. As more resources are invested in computer technology and software programs by health-care organizations and agencies, computer literacy of the patient population will become an issue of increasing concern. Computers not only will be used to convey instructional messages but also will serve as a valuable tool to access additional sources of information (see Chapters 11 and 12). The opportunity to expand patients' knowledge base through telecommunications will require nurse educators to attend to computer literacy levels much in the same way they have begun to recognize the negative effects illiteracy and low literacy in using print materials has had on restricting the information base of consumers of health care. Evidence suggests that computer software programs can be highly suitable for low-literate patients as long as they have the basic capacity to use computers. The trend toward managed care and home care portends that computers will play an important role in patient teaching. Thus, nurses must begin to advocate for computer literacy in the public they serve (Doak et al., 1996; Bell, 1986).

SCOPE AND INCIDENCE OF THE PROBLEM

Based on available statistics, it is evident that the United States has significant literacy problems. With respect to the average level of literacy in our country, the United States ranks only forty-ninth among 159 members of the United Nations (Kozol, 1985). Experts differ in their estimates of exactly the number of U.S. adults who struggle with basic readability skills. Figures range from about 20 to 30 million people who are considered illiterate or functionally illiterate, that is, they cannot read or they read below the fifth-grade level. An additional 30 to 45 million persons are considered to be in the low-literacy category, that is, they read between the fifth- and eighth-grade level. Figures vary depending on the reporting agency, but the number of illiterate and low-literate persons is estimated to be a total of 50 to 75 million. Conservatively, this figure represents about one-fifth (20%) of the adult U.S. population (Doak et al., 1996; Fain, 1994b; Dixon & Park, 1990; Baydar et al., 1993; Fleener & Scholl, 1992; Zion & Aiman, 1989).

In cases of both illiteracy and low literacy, the level of readability is in terms of performance, not years of school attendance. Even though the mean reading education level of the U.S. population is at grade 12.6, the mean literacy level is at or below eighth grade. Many people read two to four grade levels below their reported level of formal education. This is because schools have a tendency to promote students for social and age-related reasons rather than for academic achievement alone, patients may report inaccurate histories of years of school attended, and reading skills may be lost over time through lack of practice (Yasenchak & Bridle, 1993; Jackson et al., 1991; Stephens, 1992; Miller & Brodie, 1994; Meade & Wittbrot, 1988). In addition, although most students taking the Scholastic Aptitude Tests (SATs) graduate from high school, their proficiency in reading and comprehension shows signs of declining (Thomison, 1991).

Thus, at least one out of five Americans lacks the literacy skills and knowledge to cope with the requirements of day-to-day living. For example, one needs to be able to read at the sixth-grade level to understand a driver's license manual, the eighth-grade level to follow directions on a frozen dinner package, and the tenth-grade level to read instructions on a bottle of aspirin (Doak et al., 1985). The literacy problem is so widespread that the government, in an effort to reduce traffic accidents, has substituted conventional printed road signs with ones using symbols (Loughrey, 1983).

Because of the difficulty inherent in defining and testing literacy and because few people with limited reading skills admit to having difficulty, the scope of the literacy problem may be much greater (Jolly et al., 1993). The above numbers are only estimates, and the rates have risen steadily over the years. Although many believe the numbers of illiterates are greater than the estimates, it is difficult to determine exact numbers because of the ever increasing complexity of the technological and informational demands of our society today. To be literate 100 years ago meant that people could read and write their own name. Today, being literate means that one is able to learn new skills, think critically, problem solve, and apply general knowledge to various situations (Fain, 1994a).

The trend toward an increased proportion of Americans with inadequate literacy levels for active participation in our advanced technological society is due most likely to factors such as the following (Baydar et al., 1993):

- A rise in the number of immigrants
- The aging of our population
- The increasing complexity of information
- An added number of people living in poverty
- Changes in policies and funding for public education
- A disparity in the literacy achievements of minority versus nonminority populations

All of these factors correlate significantly with the level of formal schooling attained and the level of literacy ability. Although it was stated previously that research indicates the number of years of schooling is not a good predictor of literacy level, there still remains a correlation between someone's educational background and the ability to read. According to the 1980 census, 38% of U.S. adults did not have a high school diploma, and 13% of high school seniors could not read and correctly answer basic test questions (Dixon & Park, 1990). As our society becomes more and more high tech, with new products and more complicated functions to perform, the basic language requirements needed for survival will continue to rise. A greater number of people are beginning to fall behind, unable to keep up with our increasingly sophisticated world.

Levels of literacy are often seen as indicators of the well-being of individuals, and the literacy problem has greater implications for the social and economic status of the country as a whole. Low levels of literacy have been associated with marginal productivity, high unemployment, minimum earnings, high costs of health care, and high rates of welfare dependency (Baydar et al., 1993). Illiteracy is considered to be an element contributing to many of the grave social issues confronting the United States today such as homelessness, teen pregnancy, unemployment, delinquency, crime, and drug abuse (Fleener & Scholl, 1992). Deficiencies in basic literacy skills compound to create devastating cumulative ignorance for these citizens, creating a social burden that is extremely costly for the American people. Reports indicate that poor basic literacy skills are evident in 69% of all those arrested, 85% of unwed mothers, 79% of welfare recipients, 85% of dropouts, and 72% of unemployed (Johnson & Layng, 1992). Illiteracy and low literacy are not necessarily the reasons for these ills, but the high correlation between literacy levels and social problems is a marker for disconnectedness from society in general (Jenks, 1992).

The decline in reading achievement scores across the United States suggests that the number of people capable of decoding words and comprehending health information written at the high school level and above actually may be dwindling. Those with minimal educational achievement are most likely to be at even greater risk for the conditions that many health education materials attempt to address (Manning, 1981).

THOSE AT RISK

Illiteracy has been portrayed "as an invisible handicap that affects all classes, ethnic groups, and ages" (Fleener & Scholl, 1992, p. 740). Illiteracy knows no boundaries and exists among persons of every race and ethnic background, socioeconomic class, and age category. It is true, however, that illiteracy is rare in the higher socioeconomic classes, for example, and that there are segments of the U.S. population that are more likely to be affected than others by lack of literacy skills. According to Jackson et al. (1991), those who have been identified as having poorer reading and comprehension skills than the average American include

- The economically disadvantaged
- The elderly
- Immigrants (particularly illegal ones)
- High school dropouts
- Racial minorities of blacks, Latinos, and Native Americans
- The unemployed

- Inner-city residents
- Southerners (Louisiana, Texas, and Mississippi report the highest rates of illiteracy in the nation)

With respect to demographics, statistics indicate that there are presently 38 million Americans living in poverty. Although the disadvantaged represent many diverse cultural and ethnic groups, including millions of poor white people, one-third of the disadvantaged in this country are minorities, and a larger percentage of minorities fall into the disadvantaged category. Within the next 10 years, the major growth in the population will come from the ranks of minority groups. By the year 2001, one out of every four people in the United States will belong to a racial or ethnic minority, and in 53 of the 100 largest cities, minorities will be the majority. The birthrate of Latinos, for example, is growing five times greater than the national average, and their population is expected to increase to almost 30 million by the twenty-first century (Morra, 1991).

Many minority and economically disadvantaged people are not benefactors of mainstream health education activities, which often fail to reach them. Overall, they are not active seekers of health information because they tend to have weaker communication skills and inadequate foundational knowledge on which to better understand their needs. Many are without enough fluency to make good use of written health education materials (Morra, 1991). Areas with the highest percentage of minorities and high rates of poverty and immigration also have the highest percentage of functionally illiterate people. When these people need medical care, they tend to require more resources, have longer hospital stays, and have a greater number of readmissions (Davis et al., 1990). The challenge now and in the future will be to find improved ways of communicating with these population groups and to develop innovative strategies in the delivery of medical and nursing care.

Of the approximately 30 million Americans over 65 years of age, older adults constitute 38% of the illiterate population (National Council on Aging, 1986). Those over 85 years of age are the fastest growing age group in the country. By the turn of the century, they will account for almost 5 million people. Children born today can expect to live to an average age of 83. Statistics indicate that our population is growing older as people live longer. As time goes on, the older population will be more educated and demand more services. In 1960, only 20% of older people were high school graduates, whereas by the year 2000, 64% will be educated at the high school level. Although these statistics portend for a more highly educated group of older adults in the future, the information explosion and rapid technological advances may cause them to fall behind relative to future standards of education.

Today, the illiteracy problem in the aged is due to the fact that not only did they have less education in the past but also reading skills once acquired have declined because of disuse. In addition, cognition and intellectual functioning are affected by aging (Alford, 1982; Jackson et al., 1994; Hallburg, 1976; Kick, 1989; Weinrich et al., 1989; Weinrich & Boyd, 1992). The vast majority of older people have some degree of cognitive changes and vision impairments, and about one-quarter have serious hearing loss. Along with these normal physiological changes, many suffer from chronic diseases, and large numbers are taking prescribed medications. All of these conditions can interfere with the ability to learn or impact negatively on thought processes, which contributes to the high incidence of illiteracy in this population group.

Beyond the issue of prevalency, illiteracy also presents unique psychosocial problems for the older adult. Because older persons tend to learn material more slowly than do young adults, especially with such tasks that require reading and writing, they may become more easily frustrated in a learning situation (Morra, 1991). Furthermore, many of them have developed ways to compensate for missing skills through their support network. Lifetime patterns of behavior have been set such that they may lack the motivation to improve their literacy skills (Anscher & Gold, 1991). Today and in the years to come, those involved with providing health education will be challenged to overcome these obstacles to learning in the aged.

Keeping in mind that illiteracy has been said to run in families from generation to generation, Baydar et al. (1993) conducted an interesting study on childhood and adolescent determinants of literacy in adulthood. These researchers used longitudinal data collected over 20 years from a sample of black children of teenaged mothers from the Baltimore area, which correlated with nationally representative data. Their aim was to identify early precursors of adulthood literacy levels that could define high-risk groups in each developmental period from early childhood to adolescence. They found that family environmental factors affecting the physical and emotional quality of the home environment (maternal education, family size in early childhood, maternal marital status, and income) as well as early childhood developmental levels (preschool cognitive and behavioral functioning) and educational background of the child (grade repetition or school suspension) were all predictive of literacy in young adulthood. Although most illiterate adults in this country are white, native-born, English-speaking Americans, a disproportionate number belong to other ethnic groups. In proportion to the population, functional or marginal illiterates number 16% white, 44% black, and 56% Latino citizens.

Although most illiterates have had some degree of formal education, the majority have not graduated from high school, are below 40 years of age, live in metropolitan areas, and over 40% are unemployed (Powers, 1988). Thus, those with less education, which often includes the groups of low-income persons, older adults, racial minorities, and people with ethnic origins for whom English is a second language, are likely to have more difficulty with reading and comprehending written materials as well as understanding oral instruction. This profile is not intended to stereotype illiterates but to give a broad picture of who most likely lacks literacy skills. It is essential that nurses and other health-care providers are aware of who might be susceptible to having literacy problems when carrying out assessments on their patient populations.

ASSESSMENT: CLUES, STEREOTYPES, AND MYTHS

Rarely do people voluntarily admit that they are illiterate. Most individuals with poor literacy skills have learned that it is dangerous to reveal their illiteracy because of fear that others such as strangers, friends, or employers would consider them dumb or incapable of functioning responsibly. The literature contains many examples of illiterates who have managed to keep their secret

from others and have successfully held jobs and survived in a world that requires literacy skills (Walker, 1987). Most people with limited literacy abilities are masters at concealment. Typically, they are ashamed by their limitation and attempt in clever ways to hide the problem. Often, they are resourceful and intelligent about trying to conceal their illiteracy and have developed remarkable memories to help them cope with family and career situations (Kanonowicz, 1993). Many have discovered ways to function quite well in society without being able to read by memorizing signs and instructions, by making intelligent guesses, or by finding employment opportunities that are not heavily dependent on reading and writing skills. As Fain (1994b) points out, illiterate patients "become very good actors, practiced in misdirection and evasion" (p. 16B).

An important thing to remember is that there are many myths about illiteracy. It is very easy for health-care providers to fall into the trap of wrongly labeling someone as illiterate or, for that matter, assuming that they are literate based on stereotypical images. Walker (1987) addressed some of the most common myths:

Myth #1: Illiterates are stupid and slow learners or incapable of learning at all. (In fact, many illiterates have normal or above normal intelligence quotients.)

Myth #2: Illiterates can be recognized by their appearance. (In fact, appearance alone is an unreliable basis for judgment because some very articulate, well-dressed people suffer from illiteracy.)

Myth #3: The number of years of schooling completed correlates with literacy skills. (In fact, grade level achievement does not correspond well to reading ability.)

Myth #4: All illiterates are foreigners, poor, of ethnic or racial minority, and/or from the South. (In fact, illiterate people come from very diverse backgrounds.)

Myth #5: Most illiterates will freely admit that they do not know how to read or do not understand. (In fact, most often they try to hide their reading deficiencies and will go to great lengths to avoid discovery, even when directly asked about their possible limitations. As Doak says, "People would rather tell you they have a venereal disease than that they can't read" [Jenks, 1992, p. 1069].)

So the question remains: How does one recognize an illiterate person? Identifying illiteracy is not easy because there is no stereotypical pattern. Nurses, because of their highly developed assessment skills and frequent contact with patients, are in an ideal position to determine the literacy levels of their clients. Knowing a person's ability to read and comprehend is critical in providing teaching-learning encounters that are beneficial, efficient, and cost-effective.

There are a number of informal clues to watch out for that are indicators of reading and writing deficiencies. Because of the prevalence of illiteracy, nurses should never assume that the patients they care for are literate. The caveat is not to rely on the obvious but to look for the unexpected. There are so many instances when a patient does not fit the stereotypical image of an illiterate that nurses and physicians never even considered the possibility. Overlooking the problem has the potential for grave consequences in treatment outcomes and has resulted in frustration for both the patient and the caregiver (Carr, 1988; Rossof, 1988; Frankel, 1987; Rudolph, 1994). Furthermore, health-care providers are hesitant to infer that a patient may have low literacy skills because there is an implication of personal inadequacy associated with the failure to have learned to read (Walker, 1987).

Since illiterate or semiliterate patients often have had many years of practice at disguising the problem, they will often go to elaborate lengths to hide the fact that they do not possess a skill already acquired by most 6-year-olds. The observant practitioner should always be on the lookout for possible signs of poor reading ability in a patient. During assessment, the nurse should take note of the following clues that illiterate patients may demonstrate (Loughrey, 1983; Fain, 1994b; Meade & Thornhill, 1989):

- Reacting to complex learning situations by withdrawal or complete avoidance.
- Using the excuse that they were too busy, too tired, or too sedated with medication to maintain attention span when given a booklet or instruction sheet to read.
- Claiming that they just did not feel like reading, that they gave the information to their spouse to take home, or that they lost, forgot, or broke their glasses.
- Camouflaging their problem by surrounding themselves with books, magazines, and newspapers to give the impression they are able to read.
- Circumventing their inability by insisting on taking the information home to read or having a family member or friend with them when written information is presented.
- Asking you to read the information for them under the guise that their eyes are bothersome, they lack interest, or they do not have the energy to devote to the task of learning.
- Showing nervousness as a result of feeling stressed by the threat of the possibility of "getting caught" or having to confess to illiteracy.
- Acting confused, talking out of context, or expressing thoughts that may seem totally irrelevant to the topic of conversation.
- Showing a great deal of frustration and restlessness when attempting to read, often mouthing words aloud (vocalization) or silently (subvocalization), substituting words they cannot decipher (decode) with meaningless words, pointing to words or phrases on a page, or exhibiting facial signs of bewilderment or defeat.
- Standing in a location clearly designated for "authorized personnel only."
- Listening and watching very attentively to observe and memorize how things work.
- Demonstrating difficulty with following instructions about relatively simple activities such as breathing exercises or with operating the TV, electric bed, call light, and other simple equipment, even when the operating instructions are clearly printed on them.
- Failing to ask any questions about the information they received.
- Revealing a discrepancy between what is understood by listening and what is understood by reading.

In summary, although it has been clearly pointed out that the level of completed formal education is an inaccurate presumption by which to predict reading level, it is certainly one estimate that nurses should incorporate into their methods of assessment. Negative feedback and clues from the patient in the form of puzzled looks, inappropriate behaviors, excuses, or irrelevant statements may give the nurse the gut feeling that the message being communicated is neither received nor understood (Meade & Wittbrot, 1988). Not only do illiterate patients become confused and frustrated in their attempts to deal with the complex system of health care, which is so dependent on written and verbal information, but also they become stressed in their efforts to cover up their disability.

Nurses, in turn, also can feel frustrated when patients with undiagnosed literacy problems seem at face value to be unmotivated and noncompliant in following self-care instructions. How many times nurses wonder why patients make caregiving so hard for themselves as well as for the provider. It is not unusual for nurses to conclude, "He's too proud to bend," "She's in denial," "He's just noncompliant—it's a control issue." Nurses must go beyond their own assumptions, look beyond a patient's appearance and behavior, and look for the less than obvious by conducting a thorough initial assessment of variables to uncover the possibility that a literacy problem exists (Rudolph, 1994). An awareness of this possibility and good skills at observation are key to diagnosing illiteracy or low literacy in the patient population. Early diagnosis will enable nurses to intervene appropriately to avoid disservice to illiterate patients, who need nurses' support and encouragement.

IMPACT OF ILLITERACY ON COMPLIANCE AND MOTIVATION

In addition to the fact that poor literacy skills impact on the ability to read as well as understand and interpret the meaning of written and verbal instruction, an illiterate or semiliterate person also struggles with other significant interrelated limitations with communication that negatively influence health-care teaching (Barnes, 1992a). The person's organization of thought, perception, vocabulary and language/fluency development, and

problem-solving skills are also adversely affected. Fleener and Scholl (1992) investigated characteristics of self-identified illiterates. For the functionally illiterate, the most common deficiencies found were in phonics, comprehension, and perception. Difficulties in perception were evident in the reversal of letters and words, miscalling letters, and adding and omitting letters. Also, a major problem was comprehension, the calling of words without knowing their meaning. Some individuals needed to read aloud to understand, and others read so slowly they lost the meaning of a paragraph before they had finished it. Still other subjects perceived difficulty in remembering as a factor in their lack of reading skill.

People with poor reading skills have difficulty analyzing instructions, assimilating and correlating new information, and formulating questions (Barnes, 1992a). They may be reluctant to ask questions because of the concern that their questions will be regarded as incomprehensible or irrelevant. Not only do they probably not know what to ask but also they do not want anyone to think of them as ignorant or lacking in intelligence. Hussey and Guilliland (1989) provide a poignant example of a young pregnant girl prescribed antiemetic suppositories to control her nausea. When she had no relief of symptoms, questioning by the nurse revealed that she was swallowing the medication. Obviously, not only did she not understand how to take the medicine, but also she probably had never seen a suppository and was not even able to read the word. She did not ask what it was, probably because she did not know what to ask in the first place, and also she may have been reluctant to question the treatment out of fear that she would be regarded as stupid.

If past experiences with learning have been less than positive, illiterates may prefer not knowing the answers to questions and withdraw altogether to avoid awkward and embarrassing learning situations. They may react to complicated, fast-paced instruction by discouragement and refusal to participate because their process of interpretation is so slow. Even when questioned about their understanding, persons with low literacy skills will most likely claim that the information was understood even when it was not (Doak et al., 1985).

Another characteristic of illiterate individuals is that they have difficulty synthesizing information in a way that fits into their behavior patterns. If they are unable to comprehend a required behavior change or cannot understand why it is needed, then any health teaching will be disregarded (Hussey & Guilliland, 1989). For example, cardiac patients who are told via verbal and written instructions to lose weight, increase exercise, decrease dietary fat, and begin taking medications may fail to comply because of lack of understanding of the information and how to go about incorporating these changes into their lifestyle.

Persons with poor literacy skills also think in only concrete, specific, and literal terms. An example of this limitation is the diabetic patient whose glucose levels were out of control even when the patient insisted he was taking his insulin as instructed—injecting the orange and then eating the fruit (Hussey & Guilliland, 1989).

The illiterate or semiliterate person also has difficulty handling large amounts of information and classifying it into categories. Patients who need to take several different medications at various times and in different dosages may either become confused with the schedule or ignore the instruction. Or, if asked to change their daily medication routine, a great deal of retraining is needed to convince them of the benefits of the new regimen.

Hussey & Guilliland (1989) also identified culture as another aspect of literacy. They define *cultural literacy* as "knowing how to communicate without having to explain" (p. 608). In conversation, an individual must be able to understand undertones, voice intonations, and in what context (slang, terminology, or customs) the message is being delivered.

Also, a major factor in noncompliance is the lack of adequate and specific instructions about prescribed treatment regimens. Poor literacy skills, seldom assessed by health-care personnel when teaching a patient about medications, limit the patient's ability to understand the array of instructions regarding medication labels, dosage scheduling, adverse reactions, drug interactions, and complications. No wonder those who lack vocabulary, organized thinking and the ability to formulate questions coupled with inadequate instruction are confused and easily frustrated to the point of taking medications incorrectly or refusing to take them at all.

Thus, functional illiteracy and low literacy significantly impact on motivation and compliance levels (see Chapter 6). What is often mistaken for noncompliance is instead the simple inability to comply. Although approximately 20% of adult patients are functionally illiterate, this statistic is overlooked by many health-care professionals as a major factor in noncompliance with prescribed regimens, follow-up appointments, and measures to prevent medical complications (Doak et al., 1996). A number of studies have correlated literacy levels with noncompliance (Hussey & Guilliland, 1989; Sands & Holman, 1985; Jolly et al., 1993; Hussey, 1994). Individuals with poor literacy skills that coincide with inadequate language skills have difficulty following instructions and providing accurate and complete health histories, which are vital to the delivery of good health care. The burden of illiteracy leads patients into noncompliance not because they do not want to comply, but because they are unable to do so (Rossof, 1988; Frankel, 1987).

ETHICAL AND LEGAL CONCERNS

Sources of printed education materials (PEMs) include health-care facilities, commercial vendors, government services, voluntary health agencies, nonprofit charitable organizations, pharmaceutical firms, and medical equipment supply companies. These materials are distributed primarily by nurses and physicians and are the major sources of information for patients participating in health programs in many settings. Written health information materials are intended to reinforce learning about health promotion, disease prevention, illness process, diagnostic procedures, drug and treatment modalities, rehabilitative course, and self-care regimens. However, many of these sources fail to take into account the educational level, preexisting knowledge base, cultural influences, language barriers, racial or ethnic status, or economic backgrounds of persons with limited literacy skills. Unless patients are competent in reading and comprehending the literature given to them, these tools are useless as adjuncts for health education and are neither a cost-effective nor time-efficient means for teaching and learning. Materials that are widely distributed, but little or not at all understood, pose not only a health hazard for the patient but also an ethical and legal liability for health-care providers. Meade and Wittbrot (1988) warn that materials that are too difficult to read or comprehend serve little purpose. Patient education cannot be considered to have taken place if the patient has not gained enough knowledge and requisite skills necessary for self-care. Indiscriminate or non-selective use of PEMs can result in complete or partial lack of communication between health-care providers and consumers.

Standards put forth in 1993 by the Joint Commission for Accreditation of Healthcare Organizations (JCAHO) now requires that "the patient and/or, when appropriate, his/her significant other(s) are provided with education that can enhance their knowledge, skills, and those behaviors necessary to fully benefit from the health care interventions provided by the organization" (JCAHO, 1993, p. 1030). This standard further specifies that education relevant to a person's health-care needs must be "understandable" to the patient and/or significant others. Therefore, PEMs must be written in ways that assist patients to understand their health problems and to undertake self-care regimens such as medications, diet and exercise therapies, and use of medical equipment (Bernier, 1993).

Furthermore, the federally mandated Patient's Bill of Rights has established the rights of patients to receive complete and current information regarding their diagnoses, treatments, and prognoses in terms they can understand (Glazer-Waldman et al., 1985). It is imperative that the reading levels of PEMs match the patients' reading abilities or vice versa. Compounding the need for appropriately written materials is the fact that research reveals that patients forget within 5 minutes about one-half of oral instruction they receive. Failure to retain information combined with inappropriate reading levels of materials used to reinforce or supplement verbal teaching methods may very well decrease compliance, increase morbidity, and encourage misuse of health-care facilities (Boyd, 1988).

Encouraging self-care through patient education for purposes of health promotion, disease prevention, health maintenance, and rehabilitation is not a new concept to either consumers or providers of health care. However, the constraints of the current health-care system in the United States have impinged on the professional ability of nurses to provide needed information to ensure

self-care that is safe and effective. Patient education has assumed an even more vital role in assisting patients to independently manage their own health-care needs given such factors as

- Early discharge
- Decreased reimbursement for direct care
- Increased emphasis of delivery of care in the community and home setting
- Greater demands on nursing personnel time
- Increased technological complexity of treatment
- Assumption by caregivers that printed information is an adequate substitute for direct instruction of patients

These trends do not allow sufficient opportunity for patients in various health-care settings to receive the necessary education they need for self-management after discharge. Most outpatient care such as that given in clinics, doctors' offices, and same-day surgery centers requires patients and their families to understand both written and oral instruction (Jackson et al., 1991). Consequently, professional nurses are relying to a greater extent than ever before on PEMs to supplement their teaching (Owen, Porter et al., 1993). The burden of becoming adequately educated falls on the shoulders of patients, their families, and significant others. Often unprepared because of shortened hospital stays or limited contact with health-care providers, patients have to assume a greater role in their own recovery and the maximization of their health potential (Stephens, 1992). It is only recently that research in the area of written health education materials in relation to patients' literacy skills has examined and attempted to answer even the most basic questions as the following:

Do patients read the education literature provided them?

Are they capable of reading it?

Can they comprehend what they read?

Are written materials appropriate and sufficient for the intended target audience?

In our increasingly litigious society, growing attention is being paid by health professionals regarding informed consent and teaching for self-care via verbal as well as written health-care instruction. The potential for misinterpretation of instructions not only can adversely affect treatment but also raises serious concern regarding the legal implications with respect to professional liability when information is written at a level incomprehensible to many patients (Powers, 1988). A properly informed consumer is not only a legal concern in health-care today but an ethical one as well (see Chapter 2).

READABILITY OF PRINTED EDUCATION MATERIALS

The purpose of many studies on literacy has been to document the disparity between the reading levels within the patient population and the estimated readability of printed health information. Since the health of people depends in part on their ability to understand information contained in food labeling, over-the-counter and prescription medication instructions, environmental safety warnings, discharge instructions, health promotion and disease prevention flyers, and the like, the focus of attention on identifying this discrepancy is more than warranted. There is numerous evidence in the literature that there is a significant gap between patients' reading and comprehension levels and the level of reading difficulty of PEMs.

Health-care providers are beginning to recognize that the reams of written materials relied on by so many of them to convey health information to consumers are essentially closed to the illiterate patient (Morgan, 1993). For example, look at the lines below.

Laeyo aoiou dxpo quto a uoixyo mnstr.

Mnstr laeyo dxpo guto tzny auoibxgo.

Do they make sense, or are you confused? If they appear unreadable, that is exactly what written teaching instructions look like to someone who cannot read (Loughrey, 1983).

A number of researchers have assessed specific population groups in a variety of health-care settings on the ability of patients to meet the literacy demands of written materials related to their care. All of these investigators used commonly accepted readability formulas to test patients' under-

standing of printed health information. Their findings revealed:

- Patients are better able to understand written materials prepared at grade level five than at grade level nine (Estey et al., 1991).
- Emergency department instructional materials (average tenth-grade readability) are written at a level of difficulty out of the readable range for most patients (Jolly et al., 1993; Powers, 1988).
- A significant mismatch exists between the reading ability of older adults and the readability levels of documents essential to their gaining access to health-related services offered through local, state, and federal government programs (Walmsley & Allington, 1982).
- A large discrepancy exists between average patient reading comprehension levels and the readability demand of PEMs used in ambulatory care settings (Davis et al., 1990).
- Standard institutional consent forms require college-level reading comprehension (Davis et al., 1990; Baker & Taub, 1983).
- A variety of education materials available from sources such as the government, health agencies, professional associations, universities, and industries are written beyond the reading ability of the majority of patients (Streiff, 1986; Spadero, 1983; Owen, Porter, et al., 1993; Glanz & Rudd, 1990; Swanson et al., 1990; Williams-Deane & Potter, 1992; Mathews et al., 1988; Holt et al., 1990; Smith & Adams, 1978; Richwald et al., 1988).
- An analysis of over 2000 health-care publications by Leonard and Cecelia Doak, well-recognized leaders in the field of patient literacy, found that the majority of PEMs are written in medical school language, which is at a level incomprehensible to the average person (Jenks, 1992).
- Of the American Cancer Society PEMs commonly used to deliver messages about cancer detection methods, lifestyle risks, and treatment modalties, more than half are written at the twelfth-grade level or above (Meade et al., 1992).

Thus, numerous investigators have demonstrated that PEMs for patients are written at grade levels that far exceed the reading ability of the majority of patients. Data results from these studies reveal that most patient education literature is written above the eighth-grade level, the average level falling between the tenth and twelfth grade, and many PEMs are above this upper range even though the average reading level of adults falls between the fifth- and eighth-grade levels and millions of people in our population read considerably below that level (Spadero, 1983). Furthermore, the education literature indicates that people typically read at least two grade levels below their highest level of schooling and prefer reading materials that are written below their school level (Mariner & McArdle, 1985). The conclusion that can be drawn is that PEMs serve no useful teaching purpose if patients are unable to understand them. Literacy levels of patients compared with literacy demands of PEMs, whether in hospital or community-based settings, are an important factor in the rehabilitation and recidivism of patients.

MEASUREMENT TOOLS TO TEST READABILITY OF WRITTEN MATERIALS

Health-care professionals continuously struggle with the task of effectively communicating highly complex and technical information to their consumers, who often lack sufficient background knowledge to understand sophisticated content of instruction relevant to their care. Whether they author or merely distribute printed education information, nursing and other health-care practitioners are responsible for ensuring the readability of the materials given to patients. If the readability of education materials matches the patients' literacy levels, consumers may be better able to understand and comply with treatment regimens, thereby reducing the number of readmissions and improving quality of life (Mathews et al., 1988). Because nurses rely heavily on PEMs to convey necessary information to their clients, the usefulness and efficacy of these materials in terms of readability must be determined.

Readability has been a concern of educators for years. In the 1940s, there was a great upsurge in the momentum by educators and reading specialists to develop systematic procedures by which to objectively evaluate reading materials. Today, over 40 formulas are available to measure the readability levels of PEMs.

According to George Klare, a noted authority on readability formulas, readers' interest in the subject of instructional material may also influence their comprehension. When interest is high, the formulas may overestimate text difficulty, and likewise, when interest is low, they may underestimate difficulty (Pichert & Elam, 1985). Fundamental to the readability of any particular piece of written material is the literacy skills of the reader.

Readability indices have been devised to determine the reading skill required to understand specific written information. Although they can predict a level of reading difficulty of material based on an analysis of sentence structure and word length, they do not take into account the "within" or inherent individual variables that affect the reader or the actual content of the materials (Mathews et al., 1988). Even though materials may have similar readability levels as measured by some formula, not all readers will have equal competence in reading them. For example, a patient with a long-standing chronic illness may already be familiar with vocabulary related to the disease and, therefore, may be able to read and understand new material much more easily than a newly diagnosed patient, even though they both may have equal reading skill with other types of material (Doak & Doak, 1985).

As assessment tools, readability formulas are useful but must be used with caution since the "match" between reader and material does not necessarily guarantee comprehension (McCabe et al., 1989). Readability formulas originally were designed as "predictive averages" to rank order the difficulty of books used in specific grades of school, not to determine exactly which factors contribute to the difficulty of a text. Educators should be careful in assuming that a patient can or cannot read instructional material simply because a formula-based readability score does or does not match the patient's educational level (Pichert & Elam, 1985). Therefore, while readability formulas are easily applied and have proved useful in determining the reading grade-level achievement of a person, when used alone they are not an adequate index of readability (Farkas et al., 1987). Pichert and Elam (1985) make the analogy that "using readability formulas to judge the quality of patient-education materials is like using a urine test to judge diabetes control" (p. 181). While both tests are valid and provide useful information, they also can be misleading, and one must be aware of the practical and theoretical limitations of these formulas for proper use in health education. Readability formulas are only one useful step in determining reading comprehension. Many researchers suggest using a multimethod approach to ascertain readability by applying a number of readability formulas to any given piece of written material as well as by taking into consideration the reader and material variables cited previously. Formula scores are only rough approximations of text difficulty. Human judgment is also needed in conjunction with formula-based estimates to determine the quality of PEMs.

To objectively evaluate reading materials, two basic methods exist: One method is based on ascertaining the average length of sentences and words (vocabulary difficulty) as exemplified by the various reading formulas; the second method is to measure patient comprehension and reading skills through the use of a number of standardized tests (see Appendix A). Both methods, although not ideal, are considered to have a sufficient enough relationship to reading ability to justify their use. The most widely used readability formulas, Spache, Flesch, Fog, Fry, and SMOG, as well as standardized achievement tests such as the CLOZE and WRAT methods, rate high on tests of reliability and predictive validity and do not require elaborate training to administer. In addition, the advent of computerized readability analysis has made evaluating reading materials much easier and quicker. All of these methods are most useful to nurse educators for designing and evaluating PEMs.

Readability formulas are mathematical equations, derived from multiple regression analysis, that describe the correlation between an author's style of writing and a reader's skill at decoding words as printed symbols (Manning, 1981). In many respects, a readability formula is like a reading test except that it does not test people, it tests written material (Fry, 1977). The first guideline to remember is that readability formulas should not be the only tool for assessment of PEMs. The second rule is to select readability formulas that have been validated on the reader population for whom the PEM is intended. Several formulas are geared to

specific types of material or population groups. Since there are so many readability formulas available for assessment of reading levels of PEMs, only those that are relatively simple to work with, are accepted as reliable and valid, and are in widespread use have been chosen for review.

What is unique about the *Spache Grade-Level Score* formula is that, unlike the other leading formulas, which focus largely on the evaluation of materials written for adults, this one is specifically designed to judge materials written for children at grade levels below fourth grade (elementary grades one through three). It should be avoided in assessing adult reading materials. Other formulas are available for evaluating primary materials (Lewerenz or Wilkinson), but they are lengthy and cumbersome (Spache, 1953). The elements used to estimate reading difficulty using the Spache formula are word length, sentence length, the percent of personal words or personal sentences, the number of syllables as well as the number of affixes (i.e., prefixes or suffixes) and prepositional phrases, and the number of words outside the Dale "Easy Word List" of 769 words required for formula calculation. See Appendix A for the method of formula analysis.

The *Flesch formula* was developed as an objective measurement of readability of materials between grade five and college level. It has been validated repeatedly over the more than 50 years in use for assessing news reports, adult education materials, and government publications. This formula is based on a count of two basic language elements: average sentence length in words of selected samples and average word length measured as syllables per 100 words of sample. The reading ease (RE) score is calculated by combining these two variables (Flesch, 1948; Spadero, 1983; Spadero et al., 1980). See Appendix A for the method of formula analysis.

The *Fog Index* by Gunning (1968) is appropriate for use in determining readability of materials from fourth grade to college level. The formula is calculated based on average sentence length and the percentage of multisyllabic words in a 100-word passage. It is considered one of the easier methods because it is based on a short sample of words (100), it does not require counting syllables of all words, and the rules are simple (Spadero, 1983; Spadero et al., 1980). See Appendix A for the method of formula analysis.

The contribution of the *Fry Readability Graph—Extended* is in the simplicity of its use without sacrificing accuracy as well as its wide and continuous range of testing readability of materials (especially books, pamphlets, and brochures) at the level of grade one through college. A few simple rules can be applied to the Fry Readability Graph to estimate the readability of a wide range of reading materials. The Fry Readability Graph plots two language elements—the number of syllables and the number of sentences in three 100-word selections (Fry, 1968; Fry, 1977; Spadero et al., 1980). See Appendix A for directions on how to use the Fry Readability Graph.

The *SMOG formula* by McLaughlin (1969) is recommended not only for its relative ease of computation (simple and fast) but also because it is one of the most valid tests of readability (Doak et al., 1996). Whereas other methods base the calculation of grade level on 50% to 75% comprehension, the SMOG method is based on 100% comprehension of material read; that is, if the SMOG formula tests reading material at grade seven, it means all readers able to read at a seventh-grade level should fully comprehend the material. If the same piece of writing were assessed by any of the other formulas, the material would be comprehended by only 50% to 75% of all persons reading at the seventh-grade level. Thus, when using the SMOG formula to calculate grade level of material, the SMOG results are usually about two grades higher than the grade levels calculated by the other methods (Spadero, 1983). The SMOG formula has been used extensively to judge grade-level readability of patient education materials. It is the most popular measurement tool because of its reputation for reading-level accuracy, its simple directions, and its speed of use, which is a particularly important factor if computerized resources for analysis of test samples are not available (Meade & Smith, 1991). The SMOG formula measures readability of PEMs from grade four to college level based on the number of polysyllabic words within a set number of sentences to define the grade level needed for complete comprehension. See Appendix A for the method of formula analysis and for an example of how to apply the SMOG formula to a short passage.

In summary, Doak and Doak (1987) recommend that all written materials should be tested for their readability at the time they are drafted or adopted by using one or more of the many available formulas. Pretesting PEMs before distribution is the way to be sure they fit the literacy level of the audience for which they are intended. It is imperative that the formulas used to measure grade-level readability of PEMs are appropriate for the type of material being tested in relation to the grade level of the target reader (Table 7-2).

The recent advent of *computerized readability software programs* has helped tremendously to facilitate the use of readability formulas. Some software programs are capable of applying a number of formulas to analyze one text selection. In addition, some software packages are able to identify difficult words in written passages that may not be understood by patients (McCabe et al., 1989). A variety of user-friendly, menu-driven commercial software packages such as PC Style (by Buttonware, Bellevue, WA, 1987), Grammatik IV (by Reference Software International, San Francisco, 1989), MNIRAP (Minnesota Interactive Readability Pro-

TABLE 7-2.   Appropriate readability formula choice

Formula	Selection Shorter than 300 Words	Selection Longer than 300 Words	Entire Piece	Grade Level
Spache score	Yes	Yes	Yes	1-3
Flesch formula	Yes	Yes	Yes	5 to college
Fog formula	Yes (minimum of 100 words)	Yes	Yes	4 to college
Fry Graph	Not recommended	Yes	Yes	1 to college
SMOG formula	Yes	Yes	Yes	4 to college

SOURCE: Adapted from Spadero (1980), p. 216.

gram from the Computer Center at the University of Wisconsin-LaCrosse, 1981), RightWriter (by QUE Software, Carmel, IN, 1991), Corporate Voice (by Scandinavian PC Systems, Baton Rogue, LA, 1992), and Microsoft Word for Windows (by Microsoft Corporation, Redmond, WA, 1991) can automatically calculate reading levels as well as provide advice on how to simplify text (Wong, 1992; Davis et al., 1990; Meade & Wittbrot, 1988; Mailloux et al., 1995). The reliability of computerized assessment of readability has been questioned, and it is advisable to take an average across several pieces of literature, using several different formulas and software programs when calculating estimates of readability (Mailloux et al., 1995).

MEASUREMENT TOOLS TO TEST COMPREHENSION AND READING SKILLS

In addition to the preceding five readability formulas, there are a number of standardized tests that have proved reliable and valid to measure comprehension and reading skills of patients, a relatively new concept in health education (Doak et al., 1996). Usually pre- and posttests used in institutional settings measure recall of knowledge rather than comprehension and reading skills. Rarely is a patient's understanding of information measured in the health-care system. However, patients' reading skills and ability to comprehend information are essential if health education materials are to serve a useful purpose, both from the standpoint of assisting patients to assume self-care as well as protecting the health professional from legal liability. The two most popular standardized methods to measure comprehension of written materials are the Cloze test and listening test. These tests can be used to determine how much a patient understands from reading or listening to a passage of text.

The *Cloze procedure* (derived from the term *closure*) has been specifically recommended for assessing health education literature. Although it takes more time and resources to compute than do readability formulas, the Cloze procedure has been validated for its adequacy in ranking reading difficulty of medical literature, which typically has a high concept load. This procedure is not a for-

mula that provides a school grade–type level of readability like the formulas already described, but it takes into consideration the context of a written passage. This technique is best used when reviewing the appropriateness of several texts of the same content for a particular audience. The Cloze procedure is designed so that every fifth word is systematically deleted from a portion of a text and the reader is asked to fill in the blanks. The task of the reader is to determine the missing words. One point is scored for every missing word correctly guessed by the reader. The Cloze score is the total number of blanks correctly filled in by the reader. To be successful, the reader must demonstrate sensitivity to clues related to grammar, syntax, and semantics. If the reader is able to fill in the blanks with appropriate words, this process is an indication of how well the material has been comprehended, that is, how much knowledge was obtained from the set surrounding the blank spaces and how well the information was used to supply the additional information (Doak et al., 1996; Dale & Chall, 1978). The underlying theory is that the more readable a passage is, the better it will be understood even when words are omitted. The resulting score can be converted to a percentage for ease in interpreting and analyzing the data (Pichert & Elam, 1985).

Instead of using packaged Cloze tests available from commercial sources, it is suggested that educators should devise their own tests so that the resultant scores will indicate a patient's comprehension of their own instructions. It is not suggested, however, that a Cloze test be administered to every patient, but rather to a representative sample of patients (Doak et al., 1996). Then problem words or sentences within these PEMs can be revised accordingly to make them more understandable. See Appendix A for an outline of the steps for constructing a Cloze test, how to score the test, and a sample Cloze test.

Because the Cloze procedure is a test of patients' ability to understand what they have read, be sure to be honest about the purpose of the test. You might state that it is important for them to understand what they are to do when on their own after discharge, so you want to be sure they understand the written instructions they will need to follow. Doak et al. (1985) found that most patients are willing to participate in the testing activity. They suggest that the following guidelines should be given to patients before taking the Cloze test:

1. Encourage them to read through the entire test passage before attempting to fill in the blanks.
2. Tell them that only one word should be written in each blank.
3. Let them know that it is all right to guess, but that they should try to fill in every blank.
4. Reassure them that spelling errors are all right just as long as the word they have put in the blank can be recognized.
5. Tell them that this is not a timed test. (However, if patients end up struggling to complete it, tell them not to worry, that it is not necessary for them to fill in all the blanks, and set the test aside to go on to something else less frustrating or less threatening).

The listening test also measures a reader's comprehension skills. But unlike the Cloze test, which may be too difficult for patients who read below the sixth-grade level—that is, those who likely lack fluency and read with hesitancy—the listening test is a good approach to determining what a low-literate patient understands and remembers when listening (Doak et al., 1996). The procedure for administering the listening test is to select a passage from instructional materials that takes about three minutes to read aloud and is written at approximately the fifth-grade level. Formulate eight to ten questions relevant to the content of the passage by selecting key points of the text. Read the passage to the patient at a normal rate. Ask the listener the questions orally and record the answers. To determine the percentage score, divide the number of questions answered correctly by the total number of questions. The instructional material will be appropriate for the patient's comprehension level if the score is approximately 75% (some additional assistance when teaching the material may be necessary for full comprehension). A score of 90% or above indicates that the material is too easy for the patient and can be fully comprehended independently. A score of less than 75% means that the material is too difficult and simpler instructional material will need to be used when teaching the patient (Doak et al., 1985). Doak et al. (1985, 1996) provide examples of sample passages and questions for a listening comprehension test.

The two most popular standardized methods to measure reading skill are the WRAT and the REALM tests. The *WRAT (Wide Range Achievement Test)* is a word recognition screening test. It is used to assess a patient's ability to recognize and pronounce a list of words out of context as a criterion for measuring reading skills. There are a number of word recognition tests available, but the WRAT requires the least time to administer (approximately 5 minutes as compared with 30 minutes or more for the other tests). Although it is limited to measuring only word recognition and does not test other aspects of reading such as vocabulary and comprehension of text material, it is a useful test for determining an appropriate level of instruction and for establishing a patient's level of literacy. This test is based on the belief that reading skill is associated with the ability to look at written words and put them into oral language, a necessary first step in comprehension. As designed, it only should be used to test people whose native language is English.

The WRAT tests on two levels: level I is designed for children 5 to 12 years of age, and level II is intended for testing persons over age 12. The WRAT scores are normed on age but can be converted to grade levels (Boyd, 1988). The WRAT consists of a graduated list of 100 words. The patient is asked only to pronounce the words from the list. The individual administering the test listens carefully to the patient's responses and scores those responses on a master score sheet. Next to those words that are mispronounced, a checkmark should be placed. When three words are mispronounced, indicating that the patient has reached his or her limit, the test is stopped. To score the test, the number of words missed or not tried is subtracted from the list of words on the master score sheet to get a raw score. Then a table of raw scores is used to find the equivalent grade rating (GR). For more information on this test, see Doak et al. (1985) and Jastak and Wilkinson (1984).

Another reading skills measure is the *REALM (Rapid Estimate of Adult Literacy in Medicine)* test. The REALM has advantages over the WRAT and other word tests because it measures a patient's ability to read medical and health-related vocabulary, it takes less time to administer, and the scoring is simpler. Although it offers less precision than other word tests because the raw score is converted to a range of grade levels rather than an exact grade level, it correlates well with the WRAT reading scores and it is quite acceptable to most patients. The procedure for administering the test is to ask patients to read words aloud from three word lists. Sixty-six medical and health-related words are arranged in three columns beginning with short easy words such as *fat, flu, pill*, and *dose* and ending with more difficult words such as *anemia, obesity, osteoporosis*, and *impetigo*. Patients are asked to begin at the top of the first column and read down, pronouncing all the words that they can from the three lists. The total number of words pronounced correctly is their raw score, which is converted to a grade ranging from third grade and below to ninth grade and above. For the REALM test, the scoring guide, and validation results summary, see Doak et al. (1996).

Readability formulas and standardized tests for comprehension and reading skills were never designed for the purpose of serving as writing guides. Patient educators may be tempted to write PEMs to fit the formulas and tests but doing so places emphasis on structure, not content, and comprehensibility of a written message may be greatly compromised. Pichert and Elam (1985) recommend that readability formulas should be used solely to judge material written without formulas in mind. Formulas are only methods to check readability, and standardized tests are only methods to check comprehension and word recognition. Neither are methods to guarantee good style in the form of direct, conversational writing.

ASSESSING SUITABILITY OF INSTRUCTIONAL MATERIALS

In addition to using formulas and tests to measure readability and comprehension, Doak et al. (1996) have addressed the dilemma of how to rapidly and systematically assess the suitability of instructional materials for a given population of patients. They recognize that ideally the way to evaluate instructional tools is with a sample of the intended audience, but limited time and resources may preclude such an approach. In response to this dilemma, they developed a suitability assessment of materials (SAM) instrument. Not only can SAM be used with print material and illustrations, but it has been designed to be applied to video- and audiotaped instructions as well. SAM yields a numerical

percent score, with materials tested falling into one of three categories: superior, adequate, or not suitable. The application of SAM can identify specific deficiencies in instructional materials that reduce their suitability. SAM includes factors and evaluation criteria to assess the content, literacy demand, graphics, layout and typography, learning stimulation and motivation, and cultural appropriateness of instructional materials being developed or already in use. For directions, score sheet, and a description of the evaluation criteria, see Chapter 4 of Doak et al. (1996).

SIMPLIFYING THE READABILITY OF PRINTED EDUCATION MATERIALS

Readability of written materials is dependent not only on actual reading skills, which can be measured by standardized tests, but also on those elements within a text such as technical format, concept demand, legibility, literacy level of the material, and accuracy and clarity of the message. It must never be forgotten that knowing the target audience in terms of their level of motivation, reading abilities, experiential factors, and cultural background is also of crucial importance in determining the appropriateness of printed health information as effective communication tools (Meade & Smith, 1991). Even good readers may fail to respond to important health education literature if they lack the motivation to do so or if the material is not appealing to them (Manning, 1981). Despite the well-documented potential of written materials to increase knowledge, compliance, and satisfaction with care, printed education materials are often too difficult for even motivated patients to read. Clearly, the technical nature of health education literature lends itself to high readability levels, often requiring college-level reading skills to fully comprehend. Even though printed materials are the most commonly used form of media, as currently written, they are the least effective means to reach a large proportion of the adult population who have marginal literacy skills (Glanz & Rudd, 1990). What the nurse in the role of patient educator must strive to achieve when designing or selecting health-based literature is a good and proper fit between the material and the reader.

Certainly the best solution for improving the overall comprehension and reading skills of patients would be to strengthen their basic general education, but this process will require decades to accomplish (Jackson et al., 1991). What is needed now are ways in which to write or rewrite educational materials commensurate with current comprehension and reading skills of patients. Nathaniel Hawthorne was once reported to have said, "Easy reading is damned hard writing" (Pichert & Elam, 1985), and he was correct in his perception that clear and concise writing is a task that takes effort and practice. It is possible, though, to reduce the disparity between the literacy demand of written instructional materials and the actual reading level of patients by attending to some basic linguistic, motivational, organizational, and content principles. Linguistics refers to the type of language and grammatical style used. Motivation principles focus on those elements that stimulate the reader, such as relevance and appeal of the material. Organizational factors have to do with layout and clarity. Content principles relate to load and concept density of information (Bernier, 1993). These elements will be examined as they relate to designing or revising instructional materials for the marginally literate reader.

Prior to writing or rewriting a text for easier reading, however, there are some preliminary planning steps that need to be taken to ensure that written material will be geared to the target audience (Doak et al., 1996):

1. Decide on what the patient(s) should *do* or *know*. In other words, what is the purpose of the instruction? What outcome(s) do you hope the patient will achieve?

2. Choose information that is relevant and needed by the patient to achieve the behavioral objectives. Limit or cut out altogether extraneous and "nice to know" information such as the history or detailed physiological processes of a disease. Include only survival skills and essential main ideas of *who*, *what*, *where*, and *when*, with new information related to what the reader already knows. Remember: A person does not have to know how an engine works in order to drive a car.

3. Select other media to supplement the written information such as pictures, demonstrations, models, audiotapes, and videotapes. Even poor readers will benefit from written material if combined with other forms of delivering a message. Consider the field of advertising, for example. Advertisers get their message across with words but often in combination with strong action-packed visuals.

4. Organize topics into chunks that follow a logical sequence. Prioritize to present the most important information first. If topics are of equal importance, proceed from the more general, as a basis on which to build, to the more specific. Begin with a statement of purpose. In a list of items, place key facts at the top and bottom because readers best remember information presented first and last in a series.

5. Determine what should be the reading level of the material. If the reader has been tested, preferably write two to four grades below the reading grade-level score. If the audience has not been tested, there is likely to be a wide range of reading skills within the group. When in doubt, write instructional materials at the fifth-grade level, which is the lowest common denominator, keeping in mind that the average reading level of the population is approximately fifth to eighth grade, 20% read below the fifth-grade level, and less than half read above the tenth-grade level. To cover a wide range of reading skills, it is also possible to develop two sets of instructions—one at a higher grade level and one at a lower grade level, allowing patients to select the one they prefer (Table 7–3). Once the reading level of a piece of written material is determined, it should be printed on the back of the document in coded form for easy reference.

There are numerous references in the literature regarding techniques for writing effective educational materials (Doak et al., 1996; Doak & Doak, 1987; Bernier, 1993; Wong, 1992). Recommendations have been put forth for developing written instructions that can be more easily understood by a wide audience. General guidelines for writing PEMs with clarity and completeness can be found in Chapter 12. Although there may be some overlap of information, the following strategies are specific with regard to simplifying written health information for patients with low literacy skills. The key factor in accommodating low-literate patients is to

TABLE 7–3. Example of lowered readability level

Ninth-Grade Level

Smoking contributes to heart disease in the following ways:

1. When you smoke, you inhale carbon monoxide and nicotine, which causes your blood vessels to narrow, your heart rate to increase, and your blood pressure to go up. All of these factors increase the workload for your heart.
2. Carbon monoxide stimulates your body to produce more red blood cells. The presence of more red cells means that your blood will clot more readily, leading to increased risk of coronary artery disease and stroke.
3. Carbon monoxide and nicotine may also increase your risk of atherosclerotic buildup by causing damage to your artery walls.
4. Smoking raises blood cholesterol level and has been known to cause irregular heartbeats.

Fourth-Grade Level

Smoking hurts your heart in many ways:

1. Smoking makes your heart beat faster, raises your blood pressure, and makes your blood vessels smaller. All these things cause your heart to work harder.
2. Smoking makes your blood clot easier. This increases your chance of having a heart attack or a stroke.
3. Smoking makes your cholesterol level go up. It may also damage your blood vessels.
4. Smoking may make your heartbeat less regular.

SOURCE: From Martha Wong, "Self-Care Instructions: Do Patients Understand Educational Materials?" Reprinted with permission of American Association of Critical-Care Nurses from *Focus on Critical Care*, Vol. 19, No. 1, February 1992, pp. 47–49.

write in plain, familiar language using an easy visual format. The following are some basic linguistic, motivational, organizational, and content principles to adhere to when writing PEMs.

1. Write in a conversational style with an active voice using the personal pronoun *you* and the possessive pronoun *your*. The message is more personalized, more imperative, more interesting, and easier to understand if instruction is written as "You should . . ." instead of "The patient should . . . ." *This rule is considered to be the* *most important technique to reduce the level of reading difficulty and improving comprehension of what is read.* Speaking directly to the reader through personal words and sentences engages the reader. For example:

LESS EFFECTIVE

People who sunburn easily and have fair skin with red or blond hair are most prone to develop skin cancer.

The amount of time spent in the sun affects a person's risk of skin cancer.[1]

MORE EFFECTIVE

If you sunburn easily and have fair skin with red or blond hair, you are more likely to get skin cancer.

How much time you spend in the sun affects your risk of skin cancer.

2. Use short words with only one or two syllables as much as possible. Rely on sight words, known as high-frequency words, such as *there, said, come, stop, house,* and *go,* that are recognized by almost everyone. The key is to choose words that sound familiar and natural and are easy to read and understand, like *shot* rather than *injection* and *use* instead of *utilize.* Avoid compound words, such as *lifesaver,* and words with prefixes or suffixes, such as *reoccur* or *emptying,* that create multisyllable words. Also, try to avoid technical words and medical terms, and substitute common, nontechnical, lay terms such as *stroke* instead of *cardiovascular accident.* Be careful to select substitutions carefully because they may have a different meaning for some people than for others or in one context versus another. For example, if the word *medicine* is replaced with the word *drug,* the latter may be interpreted as the illegal variety. Use of modest words is not considered "talking down" to patients, it is considered "talking to" them at a more comfortable level.

3. Spell words out rather than using abbreviations or acronyms. *That is* should be used instead of *i.e.* and *for example* rather than *e.g.* Abbreviations for the months of the year (e.g., *Sept.*) or the days of the week (e.g., *Wed.*) are a real problem for

[1]*Fry Now. Pay Later.* American Cancer Society pamphlet, No. 2611, 1985.

patients with limited vocabulary. Also do not use *CVA* or *PMS*, for example, unless these medical abbreviations are clearly defined beforehand in the text.

4. Use numbers sparingly and only when absolutely necessary. Statistics are usually meaningless and are another source of confusion for the low-literate reader.

5. Keep sentences short, preferably not longer than 20 words and less if possible, because they are easier to read and understand for readers with short-term memories. Avoid subordinate (dependent) clauses that make the reading more difficult. Long, complex sentences "turn off" the reader. Titles also should be short and convey the purpose and meaning of the material that follows.

6. Clearly define any technical or unfamiliar words by using apposite phrases or parenthetical expressions, for example, "bacteria (germ)." A glossary of terms is a helpful tool, but defining the terms and spelling out difficult words phonetically immediately following the unfamiliar word within the text are most recommended, for example, "Alzheimer's (pronounced Altz-hi-merz)." New vocabulary should be taught in small increments and reviewed frequently (Spees, 1991; Byrne & Edeani, 1984). Standal's (1981) method suggests identifying words whose meaning should be taught to the reader prior to introducing the instructional material to increase comprehensibility and to avoid having to make major revisions to a printed piece.

7. Use words consistently throughout the text. Avoid interchanging of words such as *diet*, *meal plan*, *menu*, *food schedule*, and *dietary prescription*, which only confuses the reader and can lead to misunderstanding of instruction.

8. Use advance organizers (topic headings or headers) and subheadings. They clue the reader into what is going to be presented and help focus the reader's attention on the message.

9. Limit the use of connectives such as *however*, *consequently*, *even though*, and *in spite of*.

10. Make the first sentence of a paragraph the topic sentence, and if possible, make the first word the topic of the sentence. For example:

LESS EFFECTIVE

> Even though overexposure to the sun is the leading cause, it isn't necessary to give up the outdoors in order to reduce your chances of developing skin cancer.[1]

MORE EFFECTIVE

> Enjoying the outdoors is still possible if you take steps to reduce your risk of skin cancer when in the sun.
>
> or
>
> Your chance of skin cancer can be reduced even when enjoying the outdoors.

11. Reduce concept density by limiting each paragraph to a single message or action. In the following example, the first paragraph contains six concepts. As rewritten, the second paragraph has been reduced to four concepts:

> A person who has had a stroke may or may not be able to return to his or her former level of functioning, depending on the extent and location of brain damage. Mental attitude, efforts of the rehabilitation team and the understanding of family and friends also affect the patient's progress. Recovery must be gradual, but it should begin the moment the patient is hospitalized. After the patient is tested to determine the extent of brain damage, rehabilitation such as physical, speech, and occupational therapy should begin. Family and friends should be told how to handle special problems the stroke victim may have, such as irrational behavior or difficulty communicating.[2]

> Returning to your normal life after a stroke is an important part of your recovery. Each stroke patient is different and your progress depends on where and how much the brain is damaged. Your rehabilitation must be gradual and therapy will begin to meet your needs while you are in the hospital. Your mental attitude, the treatment given by the medical team

[1] *Fry Now. Pay Later.* American Cancer Society, Inc., No. 2611, 1985.

[2] Adapted from American Heart Association (1983) *An Older Person's Guide to Cardiovascular Health*, National Center, 7320 Greenville Avenue, Dallas, TX: 75321. The information from this booklet is not current and is used for illustrative purposes only.

and the caring from your family and friends will help you handle special problems.

12. Include a summary paragraph to review in a different form what has already been presented. A question-and-answer format using the patient's point of view is an effective way to summarize information in single units using a conversational style. The following example is adapted from the American Cancer Society pamphlet entitled *Fry Now. Pay Later* (1985):

Q: Am I likely to get skin cancer?

A: If you have spent a lot of time in the sun and if you sunburn easily and have fair skin with red or blond hair, you have a greater chance of getting skin cancer than people with dark skin or people who have stayed out of the strong sunlight.

Q: How can I tell if I have skin cancer?

A: The only way to know for certain if you have a skin cancer is to see your doctor. Your doctor may want to take a sample of skin to test for cancer if you have a problem such as red, scaly patches, a mole that has changed, or an area of the skin that does not heal.

Q: How can I prevent skin cancer?

A: Stay out of direct sunlight between 11 A.M. to 2 P.M. When in the sun, cover up with clothing, a wide-brimmed hat, and use sunscreens that block out the sun's harmful rays.

Ask for feedback after patients have read your instructions. Either have patients explain the information in their own words or have them demonstrate the desired behavior. If patients can do this correctly, this is a good indication that the information is understood. Do not ask questions such as "Do you understand?" because you are likely to get a "yes" or "no" answer, not a substantive response.

13. Allow for plenty of white space in margins, and use generous spacing between paragraphs to reduce density. Uncrowded pages seem less overwhelming to the reader with low literacy skills.

14. Design layouts that encourage eye movement from left to right, as in normal reading. In simple drawings and diagrams, using arrows or circles that give direction is helpful, but do not add too many elements to a schematic.

15. Select a simple type style (serif) and a large font (14 or 18 print size) for ease of reading and to increase motivation to read. Avoid *italics*, *fancy lettering*, or all CAPITAL letters. Low-literate readers are not fluent with the alphabet and need to look at each letter to recognize a word. To facilitate decoding of words in titles, headings, and subheadings, use upper- and lowercase letters, which provide reading cues given by tall and short letters on the type line.

16. Highlight important ideas or terms with bold type or underlining.

17. If using color, employ it consistently throughout the text to emphasize key points or to organize topics. Color, if used appropriately, attracts the reader.

18. Limit the entire length of a document. The shorter, the better. It should be long enough just to cover the essential information. Too many pages will "turn off" even the most eager and capable reader.

19. Select paper that is attractive and on which the typeface is easy to read. Black print on white or yellow paper is most easily read. Dull finishes reduce the glare of light, while high-gloss paper reflects light into the eyes of the reader and is usually too formal and not in harmony with the purpose and informal tone of your message.

20. Use bold line drawings and simple diagrams. Basic visuals aid the reader to better understand the text information. However, use cartoons judiciously because they can trivialize the message and make it less credible. Be careful to use pictures that portray only the messages intended. For example, avoid using a picture of a pregnant woman smoking or drinking alcohol because this negative message is dependent on careful reading of the text to correct a faulty impression. The visuals should clearly show only those actions that you want the reader to do and remember. Use simple subtitles and captions for each picture. Also, be sure drawings are recognizable to the audience. For instance, if you draw a picture of the lungs, be certain they are within the outline of the person's body to accurately depict the location of the

TABLE 7–4.   Summary of guidelines for designing effective low-literacy printed materials

Content

Clearly define purpose of material.

Decide when and how the information will be used.

Use behavioral objectives that cover the main points.

Verify accuracy of content with experts.

Give "how to" information for learner to achieve objectives.

Present only the most essential information (3–4 main ideas: who, what, where, and when).

Relate new information to what audience already knows.

Present content clearly relevant to the audience.

Organization

Keep titles short, yet use words that clearly convey meaning of contents.

Provide table of contents for lengthy material.

Present most important information first.

Use topic headings (advance organizers).

Make first sentence of paragraphs the topic sentence.

Include only one idea per paragraph.

Use short, simple sentences that convey only one idea at a time.

Limit lists to no more than 7 items.

Present each idea in logical sequence.

Layout/Graphics

Select large, easily read print (at least 12-point type).

Write headings and subheadings in both lower- and uppercase letters.

Use bold type to emphasize important information.

Use lots of white space between segments of information.

Use generous margins.

Provide question-and-answer format for patient-nurse interaction.

Select leading (space between lines of type), type style (serif), and font (print size) for ease of reading.

Design a colorful, eye-catching cover that suggests the message contained in the text.

Linguistics

Keep sentences short (8–10 words).

Write in the active voice, and use the pronouns *you* and *your* to engage the reader.

Use 1- to 2-syllable words as much as possible.

Use words familiar and understandable to the target audience.

Avoid complex grammatical structures (i.e., multiple clauses).

Limit the number of concepts.

Focus content on what the audience should *do* as well as *know.*

Use positive statements.

Use questions throughout text to encourage active learning.

Provide examples the audience can use to relate to personal experiences/circumstances.

Avoid using double negatives.

Clearly define terms likely to be unclear to audience.

TABLE 7–4. *Continued*

Visuals

Include simple, culturally sensitive illustrations and pictures.

Use simple drawings, but only if they improve the understanding of essential information.

Choose illustrations and photographs free of clutter and distractions.

Convey a single message or point of information in each visual.

Use visuals that are relevant to the text and meaningful to the audience.

Use drawings recognizable to the audience that reflect familiar images.

Use adult rather than childlike images (avoid cartoons).

Use captions to describe illustrations.

Use cues such as arrows, underlines, circles, and color to give direction to ideas and to highlight the most important information.

Use appealing and appropriate colors for audience (for elderly, use black and white, and avoid pastel shades, especially blue, green, and violet hues).

Readability and Comprehension

Perform analysis with readability formulas and conprehension tests to determine reading level of material.

Write materials 2-4 grade levels below the determined literacy level of audience.

Pilot test brochure to determine readability, comprehensibility, and appeal before widespread use.

SOURCE: Adapted from Bernier (1993), p. 42, and from papers from the 16th Annual Conference on Patient Education, Nov. 17–20, 1994, Orlando, FL—sponsored by American Academy of Family Physicians and Society of Teachers of Family Medicine.

organ. The low-literate person may not know what they are looking at if the lungs are not put in context with the body's torso. However, pictures do not necessarily make the text easier to read if the readability level remains high. Be careful that visuals do not communicate cultural bias. (See Table 7-4 for a summary of guidelines.)

It does not take a great deal of effort, just know-how and common sense, to improve the readability and comprehensibility of instructional materials. The benefits are significant in terms of compliance and quality of care when marginally literate patients are given PEMs that effectively communicate messages they can read and understand. Readily understandable materials also reduce time and frustration on the part of the nurse educator as well as reducing possible litigation when better quality and more appropriate healthcare instructions are used. The important role of printed media to communicate health information should compel all writers of PEMs to use the techniques recommended in this chapter. As Doak and Doak (1987) so aptly summarize, "With so much to

be gained, the investments of a little time and thoughtful attention to the materials provided to patients can pay back dividends too important to ignore" (p. 8).

TEACHING STRATEGIES FOR LOW-LITERATE PATIENTS

Working with illiterate and marginally literate patients requires more than designing simple-to-read instructional literature. It also calls for using alternative and innovative teaching strategies to break down the barriers of illiteracy. Teaching clients with poor reading skills does not have to be viewed as a problem but rather as a challenge (Dunn et al., 1985). Existing teaching methods and tools can be adapted to meet the logic, language, and experience of the patient who has difficulty with reading and comprehension. Incidentally, many literate and highly motivated patients also can benefit from some of these same teaching strategies. Many authors (Walker, 1987; Wallerstein, 1992; Fain, 1994b; Meade & Thornhill, 1989; Dunn et al., 1985; Hussey, 1991) suggest the following tips as useful strategies for the nurse educator to employ:

1. *Establish a trusting relationship before beginning the teaching-learning process:* Start by getting to know the patients and helping to reduce their anxiety. Since many poor readers have a history of being defensive, the nurse educator must attempt to overcome their defense mechanisms by casting aside barriers such as any preconceived notions, including myths and stereotypes, of illiterates as poor or from racial or ethnic minority groups. Focus on patients' strengths, demonstrate your belief in them as responsible individuals, and be open and honest about what specifically needs to be learned to build up their confidence in their ability to perform self-care activities. Encourage family and friends to help reinforce patients' self-confidence. Remember, you cannot learn for the patient, but you can facilitate learning by providing guidance and support.

2. *Use the smallest amount of information possible to accomplish the predetermined behavioral objectives:* Stick to the essentials, paring down the information you teach to what the patient *must* learn. Prioritize behavioral objectives, and select only one or two concepts to present and discuss in any one session. Remember, patients with poor reading and comprehension skills are easily overwhelmed. Information about the historical background, general principles, and extraneous facts of a subject are not necessary for them to learn. Keep teaching sessions short, limiting them to no more than 20 to 30 minutes.

3. *Make points of information as vivid and explicit as possible:* Explain information in simple terms, using everyday language and personal examples relevant to the patient's background (Spees, 1991; Byrne & Edeani, 1984). Visual aids, such as signs and pictorials, should be large with readable print and only contain one or two messages to communicate information. For example, a sign reading "NOTHING BY MOUTH" or, worse yet, "NPO" should be changed to "Do Not Eat or Drink Anything" (remember to avoid using all capital letters and abbreviations). Color coding, ar-

rows, and common international symbols can be used effectively to give directions and draw attention to important information. For example, using different-colored floor tiles that lead to specific areas of the hospital and the use of other visual stimuli and pictorial cues are valuable for increasing independence and safety.

4. *Teach one step at a time:* Teaching in increments and organizing information into chunks help to reduce anxiety and confusion and permit time for patients to understand each item before proceeding to the next unit of information. Also, a block format gives patients a sense of order, a chance to ask questions, and an opportunity for you to assess their progress and reward them with words of encouragement, praise, and reinforcement every step of the way. Pacing of instruction also allows for more adequate time between sessions for learners to assimilate information.

5. *Use multiple teaching methods and tools requiring fewer literacy skills:* Oral instruction contains cues such as tone, gestures, and expressions that are not found in written materials. However, the spoken word lacks other signals such as punctuation and capital letters. Therefore, a person with poor reading skills is likely to have some difficulty with comprehending the spoken language as well as with reading. There is no accepted way to test the difficulty level of oral instruction unless a spoken message is first taped, then converted into a written form, and finally a readability formula applied to it. Therefore, exposing patients to repetition and multiple forms of the same message is recommended. Audiotaped instruction, used in combination with other visual resources such as simple lists, pictorials, and videotapes, can help to improve comprehension and reduce learning time. These media forms, as more permanent sources of information, can also be sent home for added reinforcement of health messages. Interactive computer programs allow patients to proceed at their own pace and can be programmed developmentally to match literacy skill levels.

6. *Allow patients the chance to restate information in their own words and to demonstrate any procedures being taught:* Encouraging patients to explain something in their own words may take longer and requires patience on the part of the educator, but feedback in this manner can reveal gaps in knowledge or misconceptions of information. Return demonstration, hands-on practice, role-playing real-life situations, and sharing personal stories in dialogue form are communication modes that provide you with feedback as to the patient's level of functioning. Trying to elicit feedback by asking questions of patients does not always work because low literates often do not have the right vocabulary or fluency to explain what they do and do not understand. As a reminder, do not ask questions that will elicit only a "yes" or "no" response because patients will likely respond in the affirmative, even when they have no clue as to what you are talking about, just so they do not have to admit their ignorance. Furthermore, they are unlikely to initiate asking questions of you for fear of embarrassment at not understanding instructions. Story typing, a strategy used for low-level readers, also is a helpful technique. While audiotaping, patients listen to your oral instruction, they repeat it back to you in their own words, and then the message (with corrections of any errors in procedural methods) is transcribed into a typed version using the patient's own phrases. In this way, patients can read the message themselves in familiar language as many times as necessary. Story typing is an especially effective technique in teaching functional skills such as administering medications, changing dressings, and the like.

7. *Keep motivation high:* It is important to recognize that illiterates may feel like failures when they cannot work through a problem. Reassure patients that it is normal to have trouble with new information, that they are doing well, and encourage them to keep trying. Recognition of progress being made, even in small increments, is motivating to the slow learner. Rewards, not punishments, are excellent motivators. Sticking to the basics and keeping the information relevant and succinct will maintain a patient's interest and willingness to learn.

8. *Build in coordination of procedures:* A way to facilitate learning is to simplify information by using the principles of tailoring and cuing. Tailoring refers to coordinating patients' regimens into their daily schedule rather than forcing them to adjust their lifestyle to a regimen imposed on them. Tailoring allows new tasks to be associated with old behaviors. For example, coordinating a medication schedule to patients' mealtimes does not drastically alter their everyday lifestyle and tends to increase motivation and compliance. Cuing involves the appropriate combination of time and situation using prompts and reminders to get a person to perform a routine task. For example, placing medications where they best can be seen on a frequent basis or keeping a simple chart to check off each time a pill is taken is a reminder to comply with taking medications as prescribed. Both of these principles are related to the behavior modification theory and are especially useful techniques to encourage compliance with medications. Because poor readers often cannot decipher schedules, tailoring and cuing assist them to adhere to time frames.

And last, but not least,

9. *Use repetition to reinforce information:* Repetition, at appropriate intervals, is a *key strategy* to use with low-literate clients. Each major point along the way must be reviewed repeatedly, and time must be set aside to remind learners of what has come before and to prepare them for what is to follow. Repetition, in the form of saying the same thing in different ways, is one of the most powerful tools to help patients understand their problems and learn self-care.

All of these teaching strategies are especially adapted to the individual needs of patients with low literacy skills. It is always a challenge to teach patients who, because of illness or a threat to their well-being, may be anxious, frightened, depressed, in denial, or in pain. Patient teaching is even more of a special challenge in today's health-care environment, when varying degrees of literacy compound the ability of a significant portion of the adult population to understand information vital to their health and welfare.

SUMMARY

The ability to learn from health instruction varies with patients depending on their intellectual skills, educational background, motivational levels, and reading and comprehension skills. The prevalence of functional illiteracy and low literacy is a major problem in the adult population of this country. Nurses, in the role of teachers and interpreters of health information, must always be alert to the potentially limited capacity of these patients to grasp the meaning of written and oral instruction. Nurse educators need to know how to identify patients with literacy problems, assess their needs, and choose appropriate interventions that create a supportive environment directed toward helping patients with poor reading and comprehension skills to better and more safely care for themselves. An awareness of the incidence of illiteracy, who is at risk, and the impact literacy levels have on motivation and compliance with self-management regimens is key to understanding the barriers to communication between nurses and patients.

The first half of this chapter focused on the magnitude of the illiteracy problem, the myths and stereotypes associated with poor literacy skills, the assessment of variables affecting reading and comprehension of information, and the readability levels of patient education materials. The remainder of this chapter examined in detail the measurement tools available, how to use them to test for readability and comprehensibility of patient education literature, the guidelines for writing effective education materials, and the specific teaching strategies to be used to match the logic, language, and experience of the low-literate patient. Data suggest that written materials are an important source of health information to reinforce and complement other methods and tools of instruction. PEMs are the most cost-effective and time-efficient means to communicate health messages. However, research findings suggest that there is a large discrepancy between the average reading skills of patients and the readability required of written instructional aids. Unless this gap is narrowed, printed sources of information will serve no useful purpose for illiterate and low-literate adult clients. Removing the barriers to communication between patients and health-care providers offers an ideal opportunity for nurse educators and other health professionals to work collaboratively together to improve the quality of care delivered to consumers. It is our mandated responsibility to teach in understandable terms so that patients can fully benefit from our health-care interventions.

References

Adams-Price, C.E. (1993). Age, education, and literacy skills of adult Mississippians. *The Gerontologist, 33*(6), 741-746.

Alford, D.M. (1982). Tips for teaching older adults. *Nursing Life, 2*(5), 60-63.

Anscher, M.S., & Gold, D.T. (1991). Literacy and laryngectomy: How should one treat head and neck cancer in patients who cannot read or write? *Southern Medical Journal, 84*(2), 209-213.

Baker, M.T., & Taub, H.A. (1983). Readability of informed consent forms for research in a Veterans Administration medical center. *J.A.M.A., 250*(19), 2646-2648.

Barnes, L.P. (1992a). The illiterate client. *MCN: American Journal of Maternal-Child Nursing, 17*(2), 99.

Barnes, L.P. (1992b). The illiterate client: Strategies in patient teaching. *MCN: American Journal of Maternal-Child Nursing, 13*(3), 127.

Baydar, N., Brooks-Gunn, J., & Furstenberg, F.F. (1993). Early warning signs of functional illiteracy: Predictors in childhood and adolescence. *Child Development, 64*(3), 815-829.

Bell, J.A. (1986). The role of microcomputers in patient education. *Computers in Nursing, 4*(6), 255-258.

Belton, A.B. (1991). Reading levels of patients in a general hospital. *Beta Release, 15*(1), 21-24.

Bernier, M.J. (1993). Developing and evaluating printed education materials: A prescriptive model for quality. *Orthopedic Nursing, 12*(6), 39-46.

Boyd, M.D. (1988). Patient education literature: A comparison of reading levels and the reading abilities of patients. *Advances in Health Education, 1*, 101-110.

Byrne, T., & Edeani, D. (1984). Knowledge of medical terminology among hospital patients. *Nursing Research, 33*(3), 178-181.

Carr, P. (1988). The secret behind John's smile. *Nursing 88*, 160.

Dale, E., & Chall, J.S. (1978). The Cloze procedure: Measuring the readability of selected patient education materials. *Health Education, 9*, 8-10.

Davis, T.C., Crouch, M.A., Wills, G., Miller, S., & Abdehou, D.M. (1990). The gap between patient reading comprehension and the readability of patient education materials. *The Journal of Family Practice, 31*(5), 533-538.

DiFlorio, I. (1991). Mothers' comprehension of terminology associated with the care of a newborn baby. *Pediatric Nursing, 17*(2), 193-196.

Dixon, E., & Park, R. (1990). Do patients understand written health information? *Nursing Outlook, 38*(6), 278-281.

Doak, L.G., & Doak, C.C. (July/August 1987). Lowering the silent barriers to compliance for patients with low literacy skills. *Promoting Health*, 6-8.

Doak, C.C., Doak, L.G., & Root, J.H. (1985). *Teaching patients with low literacy skills*, 1st ed. Philadelphia: Lippincott.

Doak, C.C., Doak, L.G., & Root, J.H. (1996). *Teaching patients with low literacy skills*, 2nd ed. Philadelphia: Lippincott.

Dunn, M.M., Buckwalter, K.C., Weinstein, L.B., & Palti, H. (1985). Teaching the illiterate client does not have to be a problem. *Family & Community Health, 8*(3), 76-80.

Estey, A., Musseau, A., & Keehn, L. (1991). Comprehension levels of patients reading health information. *Patient Education and Counseling, 18*, 165-169.

Fain, J.A. (1994a). Assessing nutrition education in clients with weak literacy skills. *Nurse Practitioner Forum, 5*(1), 52-55.

Fain, J.A. (1994b). When Your Patient Can't Read. *American Journal of Nursing, 94*(5), 16B and 16D.

Farkas, C.S., Glenday, P.G., O'Connor, P.J., & Schmeltzer, J. (1987). An evaluation of the readability of prenatal health education materials. *Canadian Journal of Public Health, 78*, 374-378.

Fleener, F.T., & Scholl, J.F. (1992). Academic characteristics of self-identified illiterates. *Perceptual and Motor Skills, 74*(3), 739-744.

Flesch, R. (1948). A new readability yardstick. *Journal of Applied Psychology, 32*(3), 221-233.

Frankel, D.H. (1987). Think horses, not zebras. *Lancet, 2*(8574), 1515-1516.

Fry, E. (1968). A readability formula that saves time. *Journal of Reading, 11*, 513-516, 575-579.

Fry, E. (1977). Fry's Readability Graph: Clarifications, validity, and extension to level 17. *Journal of Reading, 21*, 242-252.

Glanz, K., & Rudd, J. (1990). Readability and content analysis of print cholesterol education materials. *Patient Education and Counseling, 16*, 109-118.

Glazer-Waldman, H., Hall, K., & Weiner, M. (1985). Patient education in a public hospital. *Nursing Research, 34*, 184-185.

Gunning, R. (1968). The Fog Index after 20 years. *The Journal of Business Communications, 6*, 3-13.

Hallburg, J.C. (1976). The teaching of aged adults. *Journal of Gerontological Nursing, 2*(3), 13-19.

Holt, G.A., Hollon, J.D., Hughes, S.E., & Coyle, R. (1990). OTC labels: Can consumers read and understand them? *American Pharmacy, NS30*(11), 51-54.

Hussey, L.C. (1991). Overcoming the clinical barriers of low literacy and medication noncompliance among the elderly. *Journal of Gerontological Nursing, 17*(3), 27-29.

Hussey, L.C. (1994). Minimizing effects of low literacy on medication knowledge and compliance among the elderly. *Clinical Nursing Research, 3*(2), 132-145.

Hussey, L.C., & Guilliland, K. (1989). Compliance, low literacy, and locus of control. *Nursing Clinics of North America, 24*(3), 605-611.

Jackson, R.H., Davis, T.C., Bairnsfather, L.E., George, R.B., Crouch, M.A., & Gault, H. (1991). Patient reading ability: An overlooked problem in health care. *Southern Medical Journal, 84*(10), 1172-1175.

Jackson, R.H., Davis, T.C., Murphy, P., Bairnsfather, L.E., & George, R.B. (1994). Reading deficiencies in older patients. *The American Journal of the Medical Sciences, 308*(2), 79-82.

Jastak, S., & Wilkinson, G. (1984). *The Wide Range Achievement Test Revised: Administration manual*. Wilmington, DE: Jastak Associates.

Jenks, S. (1992). Researchers link low literacy to high health care costs. *Journal of the National Cancer Institute, 84*(14), 1068-1069.

Johnson, K.R., & Layng, T.V.J. (1992). Breaking the structuralist barrier: Literacy and numeracy with fluency. *American Psychologist, 47*(11), 1475-1490.

Joint Commission on Accreditation of Healthcare Organizations (1993). *Accreditation manuals for hospitals—1993*. Chicago: JCAHO.

Jolly, T., Scott, J.L., Feied, C.F., & Sandford, S.M. (1993). Functional illiteracy among emergency department patients: A preliminary study. *Annals of Emergency Medicine, 22*(3), 573-578.

Kanonowicz, L. (1993). National project to publicize link between literacy, health. *Canadian Medical Association Journal, 148*(7), 1201-1202.

Kick, E. (1989). Patient teaching for elders. *Nursing Clinics of North America, 24*(3), 681-686.

Kirsch, I.S., & Jungeblat, A. (1986). *Literacy: Profiles of America's young adults*. Princeton, NJ: ETS.

Kozol, J. (1985). *Illiterate America*. New York: Doubleday.

Loughrey, L. (1983). Dealing with the illiterate patient . . . You can't read him like a book. *Nursing 83, 13*(1), 65-67.

Luker, K., & Caress, A.L. (1989). Rethinking patient education. *Journal of Advanced Nursing, 14*(9), 711-718.

Mailloux, S.L., Johnson, M.E., Fisher, D.G., & Pettibone, T.J. (1995). How reliable is computerized assessment of readability? *Computers in Nursing, 13*(5), 221-225.

Manning, D. (1981). Writing readable health messages. *Public Health Reports, 96*(5), 464-465.

Mariner, W.K., & McArdle, P.A. (1985). Consent forms, readability, and comprehension: The need for new assessment tools. *Law, Medicine and Health Care, 13*(2), 68-74.

Mathews, P.J., Thornton, L., & McLean, L. (1988). Reading-level scores of patient education materials and the effect of teaching special vocabulary. *Respiratory Care, 33*(4), 245-249.

McCabe, B.J., Tysinger, J.W., Kreger, M., & Curwin, A.C. (1989). A strategy for designing effective patient education materials. *Journal of the American Dietetic Association, 89*(9), 1290-1295.

McLaughlin, G.H. (1969). SMOG-grading: A new readability formula. *Journal of Reading, 12*, 639-646.

Meade, C.D., Diekmann J., & Thornhill, D.G. (1992). Readability of American Cancer Society patient education literature. *Oncology Nursing Forum, 19*(1), 51-55.

Meade, C.D., & Smith, C.F. (1991). Readability formulas: Cautions and criteria. *Patient Education and Counseling, 17*, 153-158.

Meade, C.D., & Thornhill, D.G. (1989). Illiteracy in health-care. *Nursing Management, 20*(10), 14-15.

Meade, C.D., & Wittbrot, R. (1988). Computerized readability analysis of written materials. *Computers in Nursing, 6*(1), 30-36.

Miller, B., & Bodie, M. (1994). Determination of reading comprehension level for effective patient health-education materials. *Nursing Research, 43*(2), 118-119.

Morgan, P.P. (1993). Illiteracy can have major impact on patients' understanding of health care information. *Canadian Medical Association Journal, 148*(7), 1196-1197.

Morra, M.E. (1991). Future trends in patient education. *Seminars in Oncology Nursing, 7*(2), 143-145.

National Council on Aging. (1986). *Literacy education for the elderly.* Washington, DC: National Council on Aging.

Owen, P.M., Johnson, E.M., Frost, C.D., Porter, K.A., & O'Hare, E. (1993). Reading, readability, and patient education materials. *Cardiovascular Nursing, 29*(2), 9-13.

Owen, P.M., Porter, K.A., Frost, C.D., O'Hare, E., & Johnson, E. (1993). Determination of the readability of educational materials for patients with cardiac disease. *Journal of Cardiopulmonary Rehabilitation, 13*(1), 20-24.

Pichert, J.W., & Elam, P. (1985). Readability formulas may mislead you. *Patient Education and Counseling, 7*, 181-191.

Powers, R.D. (1988). Emergency department patient literacy and the readability of patient-directed materials. *Annals of Emergency Medicine, 17*(2), 124-126.

Richwald, G.A., Walmsley, M.A., Coulson, A.H., & Morisky, D.E. (1988). Are condom instructions readable? Results of a readability study. *Public Health Reports, 103*(4), 355-359.

Rossof, A.H. (1988). Non-compliant or illiterate? *Lancet, 1*(8581), 362.

Rudolph, R.S. (1994). What Mr. Connor couldn't say. *Nursing 94, 24*(6), 47-48.

Sands, D., & Holman, E. (1985). Does knowledge enhance patient compliance? *Journal of Gerontological Nursing, 11*, 23-29.

Silva, M.C., & Sorrell, J.M. (1984). Factors influencing comprehension of information for informed consent: Ethical implications for nursing research. *International Journal of Nursing Studies, 21*(4), 233-240.

Smith, T.P., & Adams, R.C. (1978). Readability levels of patient package inserts. *American Journal of Hospital Pharmacy, 35*, 1034.

Spache, G. (1953). A new readability formula for primary-grade reading materials. *Elementary School Journal, 53*(7), 410-413.

Spadero, D.C. (1983). Assessing readability of patient information materials. *Pediatric Nursing, 9*(4), 274-278.

Spadero, D.C., Robinson, L.A., & Smith, L.T. (1980). Assessing readability of patient information materials. *American Journal of Hospital Pharmacy, 37*, 215-221.

Spees, C.M. (1991). Knowledge of medical terminology among clients and families. *Image: Journal of Nursing Scholarship, 23*(4), 225-229.

Standal, T.C. (1981). How to use readability formulas more effectively. *Social Education, 45*, 183-186.

Stephens, S.T. (1992). Patient education materials: Are they readable? *Oncology Nursing Forum, 19*(1), 83-85.

Streiff, L.D. (1986). Can clients understand our instructions? *Image: Journal of Nursing Scholarship, 18*, 48.

Swanson, J.M., Forrest, K., Ledbetter, C., Hall, S., Holstine, E.J., & Shafer, M.R. (1990). Readability of commercial and generic contraceptive instructions. *Image: Journal of Nursing Scholarship, 22*(2), 96-100.

Thomison, J.B. (1991). Why Johnny is illiterate. *Southern Medical Journal, 84*(5), 547-548.

UNESCO. (1987). Illiteracy in America, 1986: Extent, causes, and suggested solutions. National Advisory Council on Adult Education, UNESCO.

United States. National Advisory Council on Adult Education. Literacy Committee (1987). *Illiteracy in America: Extent, causes, and suggested solutions.* Washington, DC: The National Advisory Council on Adult Education.

Walker, A. (1987). Teaching the illiterate patient. *Journal of Enterostomal Therapy, 14*(2), 83-86.

Wallerstein, N. (1992). Health and safety education for workers with low-literacy or limited-English skills. *American Journal of Industrial Medicine, 22*(5), 751-765.

Walmsley, S.A., & Allington, R.L. (1982). Reading abilities of elderly persons in relation to the difficulty of essential documents. *The Gerontologist, 22*(1), 36-38.

Webster's New World Dictionary of American English, 3rd college ed. (1991). New York: Simon & Schuster.

Weinrich, S.P., & Boyd, M. (1992). Education in the elderly. *Journal of Gerontological Nursing, 18*(1), 15-20.

Weinrich, S.P., Boyd, M., & Nussbaum, J. (1989). Continuing education: Adapting strategies to teach the elderly. *Journal of Gerontological Nursing, 15*(11), 19-21.

Williams-Deane, M., & Potter, L.S. (1992). Current oral contraceptive use instructions: An analysis of patient package inserts. *Family Planning Perspectives, 24*(3), 111-115.

Wong, M. (1992). Self-care instructions: Do patients understand educational materials? *Focus on Critical Care, 19*(1), 47-49.

Yasenchak, P.A., & Bridle, M.J. (1993). A low-literacy skin care manual for spinal cord injury patients. *Patient Education and Counseling, 22*(1), 1-5.

Zion, A.B., & Aiman, J. (1989). Level of reading difficulty in the American College of Obstetricians and Gynecologists patient education pamphlets. *Obstetrics & Gynecology, 74*(6), 955-960.

CHAPTER 8

Gender, Socioeconomic, and Cultural Attributes of the Learner

Susan B. Bastable

CHAPTER HIGHLIGHTS

Gender Differences

Socioeconomic Differences

Cultural Differences
   Definition of Terms
   Approaches to Delivering Culturally Sensitive Care
   Cultural Assessment
   General Assessment and Teaching Interventions
   The Four Major Culture Groups
      Latin American Culture
      Black American Culture
      Asian/Pacific Culture
      Native American Culture

KEY TERMS

gender differences	socioeconomic differences
culture	culturological assessment
ethnicity	historically underrepresented groups
ethnocentrism	cultural relativism
cultural assessment	acculturation
transcultural nursing	ethnomedical

OBJECTIVES

After completing this chapter, the reader will be able to

1. Identify gender-related differences in the learner based on social and hereditary influences on brain functioning and personality characteristics.
2. Recognize the impact of socioeconomics on determining health status and health behaviors.
3. Define the various terms associated with diversity.
4. Identify three approaches within clinical practice, academe, and research to prepare practitioners to function in a culturally sensitive manner.
5. Examine cultural assessment from the perspective of different models of care.
6. Distinguish between the beliefs and customs of the four major cultural groups in the United States.
7. Suggest teaching strategies specific to the needs of learners belonging to each of the four historically underrepresented groups.
8. Examine ways by which transcultural nursing serves as a framework for meeting the learning needs of various ethnic populations.

Gender, socioeconomic level, and cultural background have a significant influence on a learner's willingness and ability to respond to and make use of the teaching-learning situation. Two of the three factors, gender and socioeconomic status, have been given very little attention to date by nurse educators. The third factor, cultural and ethnic diversity, though, has been the focus of considerable study in recent years with respect to its impact on learning. Understanding diversity, particularly those variations among learners related to gender, socioeconomics, and culture, is of major importance when designing and implementing education programs to meet the needs of an increasingly unique population of learners.

This chapter explores how individuals respond differently to health-care interventions through examination of gender-related differences resulting from heredity or social conditioning in how the brain functions for learning, the impact of environment on the learner from a socioeconomic viewpoint, and the significant effects cultural norms have on the behaviors of learners from the viewpoint of the four major subcultures in the United States. In addition, models for cultural assessment and the planning of care are highlighted.

GENDER DIFFERENCES

Most of the information on gender differences with respect to learning can be found in the educational psychology literature. Nursing literature contains scant information about this subject from a teaching-learning perspective. There are, however, differences between males and females that affect their learning, and this issue needs to be addressed more closely. Two well-established facts exist: First, individual differences *within* a group are usually greater than differences *between* groups, and secondly, studies that compare the sexes seldom are able to separate out genetic differences from environmental influences on behavior.

Despite the sophistication of social sciences research, there remains a gap in knowledge of what the sexes would be like if mankind were devoid of behavioral conditioning. Since no person can survive outside a social matrix, individuals have already begun to be shaped by their environment right from birth. For example, our U.S. culture exposes girls and boys respectively to pink and blue blankets in the nursery, dolls and trucks in preschool, ballet and basketball in the elementary grades, and cheerleading and football in high school. These social influences continue to have an impact on the sexes throughout the life span. However, studies that show gender-related differences in intellectual functioning tend to overestimate their findings. The results of those studies that do not show gender differences usually fail to get published or little attention is paid to the results (Gage & Berliner, 1992). Thus, the extent to which learning is affected by differences between the sexes is still open to question.

Of course, men and women are different. But the question remains, how are they different when it comes to learning and to what can the differences be attributed? Biological and behavioral scientists have, to date, been unable to quantify the impact genetics and environment have on the brain. Opinions are rampant, and research findings are inconclusive. But the fact remains, there are sex differences as to how males and females act, react, and perform in situations affecting every sphere of life. In human relationships, for example, women's intuition tends to pick up subtle tones of voice and facial expressions, whereas men tend to be more insensitive to these communication cues; in navigation, women tend to have difficulty finding their way, while men seem to have a better sense of direction; in cognition, females excel in languages and verbalization, and men demonstrate stronger spatial and mathematical abilities. Scientists are beginning to believe that gender differences have as much to do with the biology of the brain as with the way people are raised (Gorman, 1992).

Some would argue that these examples are representative of stereotyping. Perhaps, but as generalizations there seems to be enough truth in these statements that neuroscientists have begun to suspect there are structural as well as functional differences in the brain of males and females. This suspicion has led to an upsurge in research into the mental lives of men and women. Thanks to technology, new imaging machines are revolutionizing the field of neuroscience. Functional magnetic resonance imaging (FMRI) and positron emission tomography (PET) are able to observe human brains in the very act of cognating, feeling, or remembering. Researchers already have reported that men and women use different clusters of neurons when they read than when their brains are "idling."

Provocative new studies are revealing that women engage more of their brains when thinking sad thoughts and, possibly, less of their brains when solving math problems. Functional brain data are yielding many new insights supporting the hypothesis that, in general, men and women have brains that work differently. For example, researchers reported recently that men and women employ different parts of their brains to figure out rhymes. In another study, although men and women were able to perform equally well in math problems, tests indicate that they seem to use the temporal lobes of the brain differently to figure out problems. In yet another study, when men and women subjects were asked to conjure up sad memories, the front of the limbic system in the brain of women glowed with activity eight times more than in men. These are just a few examples of some of the tentative, yet tantalizing, findings from research that are beginning to show that male and female identity is a creation of both nature and nurture. Along with genetics, life experiences and the choices men and women make in the course of a lifetime help to mold personal characteristics and determine gender differences in the very way the sexes think, sense, and respond (Begley et al., 1995).

Despite the differences in how men and women feel, act, process information, and perform on cognitive tests, scientists have been able to identify only a few gender differences in the brain structure of humans (Table 8–1). Most gender differences that have been uncovered are quite small statistically. Even the largest differences in cognitive function are not as significant as, for example, the differences found between male and female height. There is a great deal of overlap, otherwise ". . . women could never read maps and men would always be lefthanded. That flexibility within the sexes reveals just how complex a puzzle gender actually is, requiring pieces from biology, sociology, and culture" (Gorman, 1992, p. 44).

With respect to brain functioning, there is likely a mix between the factors of heredity and environment that accounts for gender inequities. The following is a list of cognitive abilities and any gender-related differences specific to each ability (Gage & Berliner, 1992):

General intelligence: Various studies have not yielded consistent findings on whether males and females differ in general intelligence. When mean differences have occurred, they are small. On IQ tests, during preschool years,

TABLE 8–1.   Gender differences in brain structure

	MEN	*WOMEN*
Temporal Lobe		
Regions of the cerebral cortex help to control hearing, memory, and a person's sense of self and time.	In cognitively normal men, a small region of the temporal lobe has about 10% fewer neurons than it does in women.	More neurons are located in the temporal region where language, melodies, and speech tones are understood.
Corpus Callosum		
The main bridge between the left and right brain contains a bundle of neurons that carry messages between the two brain hemispheres.	This part of the brain in men takes up less volume than a woman's does, which suggests less communication between the two brain hemispheres.	The back portion of the callosum in women is bigger than in men, which may explain why women use both sides of their brains for language.
Anterior Commissure		
This collection of nerve cells, smaller than the corpus collosum, also connects the brain's two hemispheres.	The commissure in men is smaller than in women even though men's brains average larger in size than women's brains.	The commissure in women is larger than in men, which may be a reason their cerebral hemispheres seem to work together on tasks from language to emotional responses.
Brain Hemispheres		
The left side of the brain controls language, and the right side of the brain is the seat of emotion.	The right hemisphere of men's brains tends to be dominant.	Women tend to use their brains more holistically, calling on both hemispheres simultaneously.
Brain Size		
Total brain size is approximately 3 pounds.	Men's brains, on average, are larger than women's.	Women have smaller brains, on average, than men because the anatomical structure of their entire bodies is smaller. However, they have more neurons than men (an overall 11%) crammed into the cerebral cortex.

SOURCE: Adapted from Begley et al. (March 27, 1995), p. 51.

girls score higher; in high school, boys score higher on these tests. Differences may be due to dropout rates in high school of low-ability boys. Thus, overall there are no dramatic differences between the sexes on measures of general intelligence.

Verbal ability: Girls learn to talk, to use sentences, and to use a greater variety of words earlier than boys. In addition, girls speak more clearly, read earlier, and do consistently better on tests of spelling and grammar. Originally, researchers believed females performed better than males on measures of verbal fluency, but

recent research has questioned this early superiority of females in the verbal domain. On tests of verbal reasoning, verbal comprehension, and vocabulary, the findings are not consistent, and the conclusion is that there are no significant gender differences in verbal ability.

Mathematical ability: During the preschool years, there appears to be no gender-related differences in ability to do mathematics. By the end of elementary school, however, boys show signs of excelling in mathematical reasoning, and the differences in math abilities of boys over girls become even greater in high school. New studies reveal that any male superiority likely is related to the way math is traditionally taught—as a competitive individual activity rather than a cooperative group learning endeavor. When the approach to teaching math is taken into consideration, there is only about a 1% variation in quantitative skills seen in the general population. In our culture, math achievement may be the result of different role expectations. The findings on math ability and achievement can also be extended to science ability and achievement because these two subjects are related.

Spatial ability: The ability to recognize a figure when it is rotated, to detect a shape embedded in another figure, or to accurately replicate a three-dimensional object is consistently done better by males than females. Of all possible gender-related differences in intellectual activity, the spatial ability of males is consistently higher than females and, thus, probably has a genetic origin. However, the magnitude of this sex difference accounts for only about 5% of the variation in spatial ability. Interestingly, women surpass men in the ability to discern and later recall the location of objects in a complex, random pattern. Scientists have reasoned that historically men may have developed strong spatial skills to be successful hunters, while women may have needed other types of visual skills to excel as gatherers and foragers of food (Gorman, 1992). Because differences that exist are declining and can be removed through special training, these factors make it unlikely that there is any strong gender explanation for the differences.

Problem solving: The complex concepts of problem solving, creativity, analytical skill, and cognitive styles, when examined, have led to mixed findings regarding gender differences. Men tend to try new approaches in problem solving and are "field independent," that is, less influenced by irrelevant cues and more focused on common features in certain learning tasks. Males also show more curiosity and significantly less conservatism than women in risk-taking situations. But in the area of human relations, women perform better at problem solving than men.

School achievement: Without exception, girls get better grades on the average than boys, particularly at the elementary school level. Scholastic performance of girls is more stable, less fluctuating, than that of boys.

Although there is no compelling evidence to suggest significant gender-linked differences in the areas of cognitive functioning mentioned above, there are findings that reveal sex differences when it comes to personality characteristics (Gage & Berliner, 1992). Most of the observed differences between the sexes in personality and affective behaviors are thought to be largely determined by culture but are, to some extent, a result of mutual interaction between environment and heredity:

Aggression: Males of all ages and in most cultures are generally more aggressive than females. The role of the gender-specific hormone testosterone is being investigated as a possible cause of the more aggressive behavior demonstrated by males. However, there is an ongoing disagreement between anthropologists, psychologists, sociologists, and scientists in other fields as to whether aggression is biologically based or environmentally influenced. Regardless, male and female roles differ widely in most cultures, with males being usually more dominant, assertive, energetic, active, hostile, and destructive.

Conformity and dependence: Females have been found generally to be more conforming and more influenced by suggestion, but the biases of some studies have made these findings open to suspect.

Emotional adjustment: The emotional stability of the sexes is approximately the same in childhood, but differences do arise in how emotional problems are manifested. There is some indication that adolescent girls and adult females have more neurotic symptoms than males, but this may be due to how society defines mental health in ways that coincide with male roles or because the tests to measure mental health usually have been designed by men.

Values and life goals: In the past, men have tended to show greater interest in scientific, mathematical, mechanical, and physically active occupations as well as to express stronger theoretical, economic, and political values. Women have tended to choose literary, social service, and clerical occupations and to express stronger aesthetic, social sense, and religious values. These differences have become smaller over time as women have begun to think differently about themselves and as society has begun to take a more "equal opportunity" viewpoint for both sexes.

Achievement orientation: Females are more likely to express achievement motivation in social skills and social relations, while men are more likely to try to succeed in intellectual or competitive activities. This is thought to be due to sex-role expectations that are strongly communicated at very early ages.

So how do the above observations on gender differences in intellectual functioning and personality relate to the process of teaching clients whom the nurse as educator encounters? Gender differences need to be investigated further for explanations of how and when females and males learn best. It is very difficult to differentiate between biological and environmental influences simply because these two factors are intertwined and influence each other. The cause, meaning, and outcome of these differences remain speculative at this time (Babcock & Miller, 1994).

The behavioral differences that are well documented to date include the fact that females have an accelerated biological timetable and, in general, are more prone to have verbal ability. In opposition, males lag behind females in biological development and attention span but tend to excel in visual-spatial ability and mathematical pursuits, and during adolescence, they surpass females in physical strength. With respect to gender differences and aging, men are biologically weaker, as suggested by life-span mortality rates. White females have a life expectancy of 79.1 years compared to 72.6 for white males (U.S. Bureau of the Census, 1991). However, less is known about women's health because women's health issues have been underrepresented in research efforts, although this trend is changing.

Women, overall, are likely to seek health care more often than men. It is suspected that one of the reasons women have more contact with the health-care system is that they tend to be the primary caretakers of their children, who need pediatric services. In addition, during childbearing years, women seek health services for care surrounding pregnancy and childbirth. Perhaps the reason that men tend not to rely as much as women on care from health providers is because of the sex role expectation by our society that men should be stronger. They also have a tendency to be risk takers and to think of themselves as more independent. Compounding the fact that men are less likely to pursue routine health care for purposes of health and safety promotion and disease and accident prevention, they typically face a greater number of health hazards, such as a higher incidence of automobile accidents, use of drugs and alcohol, suicide, heart disease, and engaging in dangerous occupations.

As health educators, nurses must become aware of the extent to which social and heredity-related differences between the genders affect health-seeking behaviors and influence individual health needs. It is imperative for nurses to have an understanding of the intellectual functioning and personality variables that affect how men and women learn, when they learn, what they are most adept at learning, and what they are interested in learning. As stated previously, there are areas in which males and females display different orientations and levels of success at communicating and learning, depending on their interests and past experiences in the biological and social roles of men and women in our society.

Women and men display a social culture that is distinct from one another. They use different symbols, belief systems, and ways to express themselves, much in the same manner that different ethnic groups have distinct cultures. According to Fern Johnson, Professor of Communications at the University of Massachusetts, for example, women tend to be good listeners who get the focus of the discussion onto the issues and off of themselves. They tend to engage in more reciprocity, less verbal jockeying, and show greater sensitivity to people, which are considered to be good traits for teamwork. Men, on the other hand, are better at controlling discussions (Genesee Hospital Development Unit, 1989). In the future, these gender differences may become less pronounced as the sex roles become more blended. But, for now, one especially must consider the impact of society on instilling certain characteristic learning behaviors in males and females, however stereotypical they may seem to be.

SOCIOECONOMIC DIFFERENCES

Socioeconomic status, in addition to gender differences, impacts on the teaching-learning process. Social and economic levels of individuals have been found to be significant variables affecting health status and in determining health behaviors. Presently, 38 million Americans are living in poverty. Disadvantaged people, those with low incomes, low educational levels, and/or social deprivation, come from many different ethnic groups, including millions of poor white people (Morra, 1991). Socioeconomic status relates to the variables of educational level, family income, and family structure, all of which seem to have an effect on health beliefs, health practices, and readiness to learn (VanHoozer et al., 1987).

The relationship between poverty, suboptimal cognitive development, and academic failure has been well established, but the mechanics and processes involved are highly complex and remain poorly understood (Campbell & Ramey, 1994). Although many educators, psychologists, and sociologists have recognized that there is a cause and effect relationship between low socioeconomic status, low IQ score attainment, and poor quality of life, they are hard-pressed to know what to do about breaking the cycle. So, too, are health-care providers, who recognize that those belonging to lower social classes have higher rates of illness, more severe illnesses, and reduced rates of life expectancy, all of which are costly to society in general and to the health-care system in particular.

Social class is measured by one or more of the following types of indices: occupation of parents, income of family, location of residence, and educational level of parents. A number of studies have compared IQ scores of fathers and their sons, with findings substantially indicating that intelligence levels decrease for both groups as the father's social class goes down. Data clearly show that certain levels of intelligence are typically found in certain occupations and not others. For example,

teachers, accountants, and engineers typically score above average in standardized tests of intelligence, while lumberjacks, teamsters, and cobblers score below average. Certain occupations not only require certain levels of academic aptitude, but they also attract people of a certain level of measured intelligence. Whatever the factors that keep particular groups from achieving at higher levels, these groups are likely to remain on the lower end of the occupational structure. This cycle has been coined the *poverty circle* (Gage & Berliner, 1992; Nagoshi et al., 1993). Gage and Berliner (1992, p. 61) describe it as follows:

> Parents low in scholastic ability and consequently in educational level create an environment in their homes and neighborhoods that produces children who are also low in scholastic ability and academic attainment. These children grow up and become parents, repeating the cycle. Like them, their children are fit only for occupations at lower levels of pay, prestige, and intellectual demand.

In addition, Baydar et al. (1993) studied family environmental factors such as maternal education, family size, maternal marital status, and family income as predictors of illiteracy in children and adolescents. They point out that low levels of literacy have been linked to low productivity, high unemployment, low earnings, high rates of welfare dependency, and teenage parenting, all of which are common measures of a society's economic well-being. People with low socioeconomic status, as measured by indicators such as income, education, and occupation, have increased rates of mortality compared to those with higher socioeconomic status. Although adverse health-related behavior and less access to medical care have been found to contribute to higher mortality rates, there is limited research on the effect socioeconomic status has on disability-free or active life expectancy (Guralnik et al., 1993).

The lower socioeconomic classes have been studied more than others probably because the health views of this group deviate the most from those viewpoints of health professionals who care for this group of individuals. People from the lower social stratum have been characterized as being indifferent to the symptoms of illness until poor health interferes with their lifestyle and independence. Their view of life is one of a sense of powerlessness, meaninglessness, and isolation from middle-class knowledge of health and the need for preventive measures, such as vaccination for their children (VanHoozer et al., 1987; Lipman et al., 1994; Winkleby et al., 1992).

It is very possible that the high cost of health care is one major factor affecting health practices of people in the lower socioeconomic classes. Individuals with adequate financial and emotional resources are able to purchase services and usually have support systems on which to rely to sustain them during recovery or augment their remaining functions after the course of an acute illness. Those individuals deprived of monetary and psychosocial resources are at much greater risk for failing to reach an optimal level of health and well-being.

Just as socioeconomic status can have a negative effect on illness, so too can illness have a devastating impact on a person's socioeconomic well-being. A catastrophic or chronic illness can lead to unemployment, loss of health insurance coverage or ineligibility for health insurance benefits, enforced social isolation, and a strain on social support systems. Without the socioeconomic means to counteract these threats to their well-being, these impoverished individuals are powerless to improve their situation. These multiple losses tax the individual, their families, and the health-care system.

Low-income groups are especially affected by changes in federal and state assistance for Medicare and Medicaid. The spiraling costs associated with illness and consequent overuse of the health-care system have resulted in increased interest on the part of the public and health-care providers to control costs. Today, there is more emphasis being given to health promotion, health maintenance, and disease prevention. The push for health-care reform in this country has resulted in efforts targeted toward the concept of managed care. Although health-care reform has not yet been realized at the national level, local and state legislators, hospital administrators, health-care providers, health insurers, and others are consolidating their attempts to make health-care reform a reality. For some, managed care means the reallocation of health-care dollars to selected groups who will share the monies as well as the risks of keeping people healthy. It also means the opportunity to contain costs and eliminate duplication or misuse of tertiary health-care services (Kinsey, 1995).

The current trends in health care, as a result of economic concerns, are directed toward teaching individuals how to attain and maintain health. The nurse plays a key role in educating the consumer about avoiding health risks, reducing illness episodes, establishing healthful environmental conditions, and how to access health-care services. The primary targets for these initial efforts at using public dollars to support managed care are the populations currently receiving medical assistance, such as low-income families in urban and rural areas. Kinsey (1995) believes that if planning is careful and collaborative between all parties concerned, including the consumer, managed care could yield positive outcomes. If health resources could become more accessible and appropriate for socioeconomically deprived individuals to stabilize and improve their health indices and maximize their family life, then true savings could be realized by society. However, these goals are contingent on many factors, such as collective public interest and deemphasis on profit motives, to find ways to ensure individual and family well-being and to improve the society's health overall. This author warns, however, that managed care, if not properly designed and carried out, could be a threat to the health of low-income groups if their needs are neglected.

Educational interventions by nurses for those who are socially and economically deprived have the potential for yielding short-term benefits in meeting these individuals' immediate health-care needs. However, more research must be done to determine if teaching can ensure the long-term benefits of helping deprived people develop skills to reach and sustain independence in self-care management. Nurse educators must be aware of the probable effects of low socioeconomic status on an individual's ability to learn as a result of suboptimal cognitive functioning, poor academic achievement, low literacy, high susceptibility to illness, and disintegration of social support systems. Low-income people are at greater risk for these factors that can interfere with learning, but one cannot assume that everyone at the poverty or near-poverty level is equally influenced by these threats to their well-being. Therefore, to avoid stereotyping, it is essential that each individual or family be assessed to determine their particular strengths and weaknesses for learning. In this way, teaching strategies unique to particular circumstances can be designed to assist socioeconomically deprived individuals in meeting their health-care needs. Most likely, the nurse educator will have to rely on specific teaching methods and tools similar to those identified as appropriate for intervening with clients who have low literacy abilities (see Chapter 7).

CULTURAL DIFFERENCES

By the year 2000, estimates indicate that more than one-quarter of the U.S. population will consist of people from culturally diverse groups. By the turn of the century, minorities will be the majority in 53 of the 100 largest cities (Morra, 1991). Also, future projections are for a continued increase in the number of legal and illegal immigrants and refugees coming into this country (Andrews, 1992). Therefore, in the immediate years to come, the major growth in the U.S. population and in the workplace will be from the ranks of historically underrepresented racial and ethnic groups. By the year 2080, ethnic minorities will account for over half (51%) of our total population. If predictions prove true, it will be the first time in U.S. history that minority subgroups will become the majority of the total population. According to demographic trends, when this historical milestone occurs, the racial and ethnic composition of this country is expected to be 23.4% Latinos, 14.7% blacks, and 12% Asian and others (Morra, 1991).

To keep pace with a society that is increasingly becoming culturally diverse, nurses will need to have sound knowledge of cultural values and beliefs of ethnic groups as well as be aware of individual practices and preferences (Price & Cordell, 1994; Spicer et al., 1994; Rooda & Gay, 1993). Health-care providers have experienced difficulties in caring for clients whose cultural beliefs are different from their own because these beliefs about health and illness vary considerably among cultural groups. Lack of cultural sensitivity by health-care professionals has resulted in the waste of millions of dollars annually through misuse of health-care services, the alienation of large numbers of people, and the misdiagnosis of health problems with often tragic and dangerous consequences. In addition, certain minority groups are beginning to demand culturally relevant health

care that respects their cultural rights and incorporates their specific beliefs and practices into the delivery of care. This expectation is in direct conflict with the unicultural, Western, biomedical paradigm taught in many nursing and other health-care provider programs across the country. Andrews (1992) suggests that there exists a serious conceptual problem within the nursing profession because nurses are presumed to understand and be able to meet the health-care needs of a culturally diverse population even though they do not have the formal educational preparation to do so.

Definition of Terms

Before examining the major cultural subgroups within the United States, it is imperative to define the following terms commonly used in dealing with the subject of culture:

Minority groups: The U.S. Bureau of the Census (1991) defines minority groups in this country as: blacks (African, Haitian, and Dominican Republic descents), Hispanics (Mexican, Cuban, Puerto Rican, and other Latino descents), Asians (Japanese, Chinese, Filipino, Korean, Vietnamese, Hawaiian, Guamian, Samoan, and Asian Indian descents), and American Indians (Eskimos and hundreds of tribes of Native Americans).

Historically underrepresented groups: A more politically sensitive and correct term used as a substitute for the word *minority.*

Culturological assessment: Defined by Leininger (1978) as a "systematic appraisal or examination of individuals, groups, and communities as to their cultural beliefs, values, and practices to determine explicit needs and intervention practices within the cultural context of the people being evaluated" (pp. 85-86).

Culture: A complex concept that is an integral part of each person's life and includes knowledge, beliefs, values, morals, customs, traditions, and habits acquired by each person as a member of a society.

Ethnicity: A dynamic and complex concept referring to "how members of a group perceive themselves and how, in turn, they are perceived by others. . . . When ethnic identity is strong, individuals maintain ethnic group values, beliefs, behaviors, perspectives, language, culture, and ways of thinking" (Price & Cordell, 1994, p. 163). Ethnicity specifies a population subgroup that has a common heritage of customs, characteristics, language, and common history (Rempusheski, 1989). Incorporated in culture is ethnicity—the biological and racial background of an individual that may be linked to culture or separate from it. For example, someone's ethnic background may be French, but because they emigrated to another country several generations ago, the person may identify with the culture of their adopted country (Falvo, 1994).

Ethnocentrism: A concept defined as the view "in which one's own group is the center of everything, and all others are scaled and rated with reference to it. . . . Each group thinks its own folkways the only right ones, and if it observes that other groups have other folkways, these excite its scorn" (Tripp-Reimer, 1982, p. 180).

Cultural relativism: Implies that "the values every human group assigns to its conventions arise out of its own historical background and can be understood only in the light of that background" (Tripp-Reimer, 1982, p. 181). As Tripp-Reimer explains, the definitions of ethnocentrism and cultural relativeness are two sides of the same coin, the first denoting the perspective of the health professional's culture and the second denoting the client's perspective.

Cultural assessment: "A systematic appraisal of beliefs, values, and practices conducted in order to determine the context of client needs and to tailor nursing interventions" (Tripp-Reimer & Afifi, 1989, pp. 613-614).

Acculturation: Describes an individual's adaptation to the customs, values, beliefs, and behaviors of a new country. The degree of acculturation is dependent on many factors such as time and willingness to assimilate to the traditions, values, and beliefs of another culture (Falvo, 1994). For example, some individuals may live in an adopted country for their entire lives but continue to cherish and practice the traditions, values, and beliefs of their original culture.

Transcultural nursing: Defined by Leininger (1978) as "a formal area of study and practice focused on a comparative analysis of different cultures and sub-cultures in the world with respect to cultural care, health and illness beliefs, values and practices with the goal of using this knowledge to provide culture-specific and culture-universal care to people" (p. 493). Transcultural nursing provides a framework for meeting the health-care needs of culturally diverse groups.

Ethnomedical: A concept of illness incorporating the relationship of humans with the universe, bridging culture with a sensitivity toward the traditional practices of specific ethnic groups (Mail et al., 1989).

Approaches to Delivering Culturally Sensitive Care

Given our rapidly changing world and the significant increased geographical mobility of people around the globe, the reality is that our health-care system and our educational institutions must respond by shifting from a dominant monocultural, ethnocentric focus to a more multicultural, transcultural focus. Tripp-Reimer and Afifi (1989, p. 613) describe the present situation from a historical perspective:

In the United States, the myth of the melting pot emerged largely from a combination of a cultural ideal of equality and a European ethnocentric perspective. This myth promoted the notion that all Americans are alike —that is, like white, middle-class persons. For many years, the notion that ethnicity should be discounted or ignored was prominent in the delivery of health care, including health teaching programs. . . . the majority of health education programs have been one of two types: those developed by whites for use with white patients, or pre-existing white programs adapted to an ethnic group by layering a thin veneer of cultural information over the white-based format. Recently, however, ethnicity has emerged as an important consideration for the effective delivery of health education programs.

The question posed by Leininger (1994) remains, "How can nurses competently respond to and effectively care for people from diverse cultures who act, speak, and behave in ways different than their own?" Studies indicate that health professionals are often unaware of all the complex factors influencing clients' responses to health care. In conducting a nursing assessment, six cultural phenomena need to be taken into account. These phenomena include communication, personal space, social organization, time, environment, and biological factors (Figure 8–1).

According to Anderson (1990), the cultural meanings that shape clients' experiences are not being taken into account when care is planned by practitioners. Strategies must be implemented to enhance the profession's ability to deliver care to culturally diverse populations in the United States as well as abroad (Hahn, 1995). A four-step approach is outlined by Price & Cordell (1994) to help nurses provide culturally sensitive patient teaching (Figure 8–2).

Hegyvary (1992) encourages the nursing profession to carefully consider the full meaning of diversity, not only as the reality of the future but as an exciting present-day challenge and opportunity for enrichment. Andrews (1992) suggests three approaches for the nursing profession to undertake to prepare its practitioners for the future:

1. Within clinical practice settings, nursing staff from culturally diverse backgrounds should be hired and promoted in increasing numbers. By design or by default, the nursing profession is made up of a very homogeneous membership. It is imperative that minority issues be explored and recommendations from the profession should be widely disseminated. There is need for continuing education programs to raise the awareness of staff nurses about their own culturally based values, beliefs, and practices as well as increase their knowledge base about culture-specific health-related beliefs and practices of others whom they are likely to encounter within their specialty areas of practice.

2. Within academic settings, steady progress has been made by undergraduate and graduate nursing programs to integrate cultural concepts into the nursing curricula. But more concentrated effort is needed from nurse educators who have formal, in-depth preparation in transcultural, cross-cultural nursing with perspectives from the related disciplines of anthropology and sociology. Teaching must focus on culturological assessment, biocultural variations in health and illness, and cultural differences in communication, religious beliefs, nutrition, aspects of aging, and the like. Teaching-learning strategies to integrate cultural concepts into the curriculum include simulated games, values clarification exercises, consciousness-raising encounter groups, and field experiences.

3. Within the field of research, cross-cultural studies in both basic and applied research domains are needed. Funding agencies and private foundations must be encouraged to support cross-cultural studies, most of which place heavy emphasis on qualitative research methods. The debate over quantitative versus qualitative research methodology should cease because a combination of methods provides useful data and allows researchers to achieve optimal results.

Cultural Assessment

The *Nurse-Client Negotiations Model* is for the purpose of cultural assessment and planning for care of culturally diverse people. However, the concepts advanced in this model are relevant for any nurse-client interaction regardless of the client's background and situation (Anderson, 1990). The Negotiations Model recognizes discrepancies that exist between notions of the nurse and client about health, illness, and treatments. This model attempts to bridge the gap between the scientific perspectives of the nurse and the popular perspectives of the client. Fundamental to understanding this model, one must recognize that there are three structural arenas of health care in most social systems within which sickness is reacted to and experienced. The concept of popular, professional, and folk arenas is used to compare medical systems as cultural systems. Each arena or domain possesses its own model for explaining health and illness (Kleinman, 1978):

The *popular arena* comprises the family context of sickness and care, including the social network and community perspective. In both

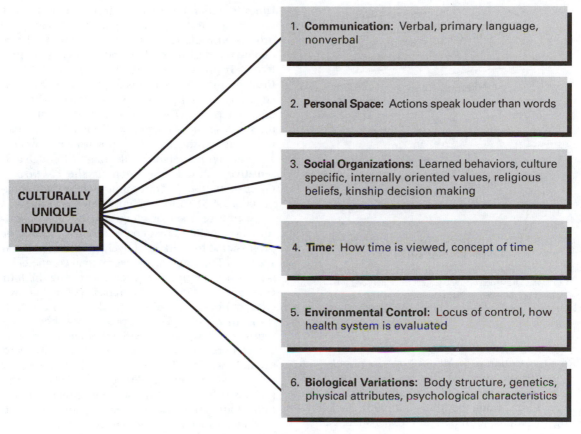

1. **Communication:** Verbal, primary language, nonverbal

2. **Personal Space:** Actions speak louder than words

3. **Social Organizations:** Learned behaviors, culture specific, internally oriented values, religious beliefs, kinship decision making

4. **Time:** How time is viewed, concept of time

5. **Environmental Control:** Locus of control, how health system is evaluated

6. **Biological Variations:** Body structure, genetics, physical attributes, psychological characteristics

CULTURALLY UNIQUE INDIVIDUAL

FIGURE 8–1.   Six Cultural Phenomena

SOURCE: Adapted from Giger, J.N. & Davidhizar, R.E. (1995), *Transcultural Nursing: Assessment and Intervention,* 2nd ed., p. 9. St. Louis: Mosby–Year Book.

Western and non-Western societies, approximately 70 to 90% of sickness is managed solely within this domain.

The *professional arena* consists of scientific medicine (Western and cosmopolitan) and professionalized healthy traditions as practiced by nursing, medical, and other health professionals.

The *folk arena* consists of nonprofessional healing specialists, often referred to as "healers."

According to the Negotiations Model, the nurse should not begin negotiation with the premise that there exists predefined problems for which there is an acceptable list of solutions. Instead, the nurse should find out clients' understanding of their situation, their interpretation of illness and symptoms, the symbolic meanings they attach to an event, and their notions about treatment. The goal is to actively involve clients in the learning process to acquire healthy coping mechanisms and styles of living. Negotiation implies a mutual exchange of information between the nurse and clients, whereby the nurse learns from the clients about their understanding of the particular situation, and in turn, the nurse explains to the clients about the professional scientific model. Together the nurse and clients then need to engage

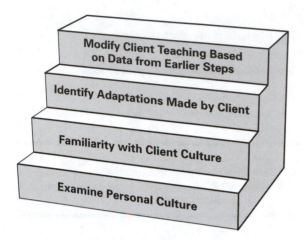

FIGURE 8–2. Four-Step Approach to Providing Culturally Sensitive Care

SOURCE: Reprinted with permission from Price, J.L. and Cordell, B. (1994). Cultural diversity and patient teaching. *The Journal of Continuing Education in Nursing, 25*(4), 164.

in a transaction to work out how the popular and scientific perspective can be reconstructed to achieve goals related to the individual client's interests. According to Anderson (1990), the following questions, although not exhaustive, can be used as a means for understanding the client's perspective or viewpoint and can serve as the basis for negotiation:

- What do you think caused your problem?
- Why do you think the problem started when it did?
- What does your sickness do to you? How does it work?
- How severe is your illness? Will it have a short- or long-term course?
- What kinds of treatments do you think you should receive?
- What are the most important results you hope to obtain from your treatments?
- What major problems does your illness cause you?
- What do you fear most about your illness?

The processes involved are known as cultural negotiation and cultural brokerage—acts of trans-

lation in which messages, instructions, and belief systems are linked or manipulated between the professional and layperson with respect to determining the health problem and the treatment preferred (Tripp-Reimer & Afifi, 1989; Jezewski, 1993). Crucial to the processes is to elicit and acknowledge the client's point of view regarding the illness experience. The integration of concepts from the social sciences is essential if nurses are to practice competently in a culturally sensitive manner.

Another model for conducting a thorough and sensitive cultural assessment is the *Culturally Competent Model of Care* proposed by Campinha-Bacote (1995). Cultural competence is defined as consisting of a set of congruent behaviors, attitudes, and policies that enable a system, agency, or professional to work effectively in a cross-cultural situation. Through this model, cultural competence is seen as a continuous process involving the four components of cultural awareness, cultural knowledge, cultural skill, and cultural encounters. *Cultural awareness* is the process of becoming sensitive to interactions with other cultural groups and requires nurses to examine their biases and prejudices toward others of another culture or ethnic background. *Cultural knowledge* is the process that refers to nurses' acquiring an educational foundation with respect to various cultural world views. *Cultural skill* involves the process of learning how to conduct an accurate cultural assessment. And lastly, *cultural encounters* encourage nurses to expose themselves in practice to cross-cultural interactions with clients of diverse cultural backgrounds. All four components are essential to deliver culturally competent nursing care (Figure 8–3).

Nurse educators who are competent in cultural assessment and negotiation likely will be the most successful at designing and implementing teaching programs. They also will be able to assist their colleagues in working with clients who may be considered "uncooperative," "noncompliant," or "difficult," help with identifying potential areas of cultural conflict, and devise teaching interventions that will minimize conflict. Nurses must understand how the reactions of practitioners influence labeling of clients' behaviors and, therefore, eventually impact on nurse-client interactions (Anderson, 1990). There is one very important caveat to remember:

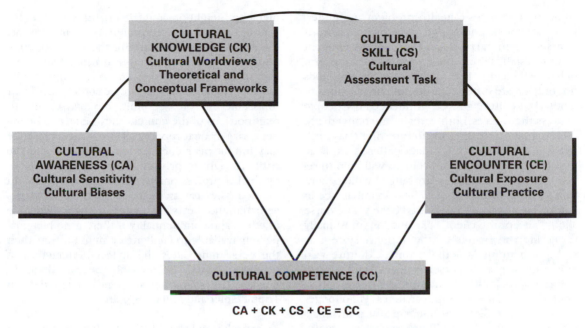

FIGURE 8–3. Culturally Competent Model of Care

SOURCE: Reprinted with permission from Campinha-Bacote, J. (1995), The quest for cultural competence in nursing care. *Nursing Forum,* *30*(4), 20.

Although it is crucial to understand cultural context in developing and carrying out effective health education programs, nurses must be especially careful not to over-generalize or stereotype clients on the basis of their cultural heritage. Just because someone belongs to a particular ethnic group does not necessarily mean they adhere to all the beliefs, values, customs, and practices of that ethnic group. As a note of caution, nurses should never assume a client's learning needs or preferred treatment programs simply based on the individual's ethnicity.

As Andrews and Boyle (1995) so aptly explained, "Sometimes cultural stereotyping may be perpetuated when a recipe-like approach to clients from specific cultural groups is used: i.e., there is a tendency by the nurse to view all members of a group homogenously and to expect certain beliefs or practices because of presumptions that may or may not apply to the client" (p. 50). Knowledge of cultural variations should serve only

as background cues for obtaining additional information through assessment.

General Assessment and Teaching Interventions

The nurse in the role of educator must implement successful teaching interventions using the universal skills of establishing rapport, assessing readiness to learn, and using active listening to assess and understand problems. Tripp-Reimer and Afifi (1989) point out the need for nurses to assess the established customs that influence the behavior one is attempting to change. The impact of cultural heritage is sometimes difficult to detect in our pluralistic society. As a component of the teaching process, assessment needs to be done to determine health beliefs, values, and practices, keeping in mind that belonging to an ethnic group does not always mean a person follows or "buys into" all of the traditions or customs of the group to which they have affiliation. Since culture affects the way someone perceives a health problem and understands its course and possible treatment options, it is essential to carry out a thorough assessment prior to establishing a plan of action for long-term behavioral change. Different cultural backgrounds not only create different attitudes and reactions to illness, but culture also can influence how people express themselves, both verbally and nonverbally, which may prove difficult to interpret (Haggard, 1989). For example, eliciting a patient's explanation for the etiology of a problem will help to reveal whether the cause is attributed by the patient to a spiritual intervention, a hex, an imbalance in nature, or other culturally based beliefs. The nurse should accept the client's explanation (most likely reflecting the beliefs of the support system as well) in a nonjudgmental manner. Culture also guides the way an ill person is defined and treated. For example, in some cultures, the belief is that once the symptoms disappear, illness is no longer present. This belief is problematic for individuals suffering from an acute illness such as a streptococcal infection, when a 1- or 2-day course of antibiotic therapy relieves the soreness in the throat. This notion is also problematic for the individual afflicted with a chronic disease that is manifested by periods of remission or exacerbation.

Readiness to learn must also be assessed from the standpoint of a person's culture because this is a key element in cross-cultural education. Patients and their families, for instance, may believe that behavior change is context specific, such that they will adhere to a recommended medical regimen while in the hospital setting but fail to follow through with the guidelines once they return to the home setting. In addition, the nurse and other health-care providers must be cautious not to assume that the values adhered to by professionals are equally important or cherished by the patient and significant others. Consideration must also be given to barriers that might exist, such as time, financial, and environmental variables, which may hinder readiness to learn (see Chapter 4). Finally, the client needs to believe that new behaviors are not only possible but also beneficial if behavioral change is to be long term.

If the client speaks a foreign language, whenever possible the client's primary language should be used. When the nurse does not fluently speak the same language, it is necessary to secure the assistance of a translator. Translators may be family members, neighbors and friends, other health-care staff, or professional interpreters. For many reasons, the use of family or friends for translation of communication is not as desirable as using professionally trained interpreters. For one thing, family members and friends may not be sufficiently fluent to assume the role. Secondly, they may choose to omit portions of the content they believe to be unnecessary or unacceptable. Thirdly, their presence may inhibit peer communication and violate the patient's right to privacy and confidentiality. It is optimal if professionally trained interpreters can be used. They can translate instructional messages verbatim, and they work under an established code of ethics and confidentiality. If there is no bilingual person available to facilitate communication, then the nurse must alter the style of interaction in teaching clients who are only partially fluent in English. The following strategies, adapted from Tripp-Reimer and Afifi (1989), are recommended:

- Speak slowly and distinctly, allowing for twice as much time as a typical teaching session would take.
- Use simple sentence structures, relying on a direct subject-verb pattern and an active rather than passive voice.
- Avoid technical terms (e.g., *heart* rather than *cardiac*, or *stomach* rather than *gastric*), medical jargon (e.g., *blood pressure* rather than *BP*), and American idioms (e.g., red tape, or "I heard it straight from the horse's mouth").
- Organize instructional material in the sequence in which the plan of action should be carried out.
- Make no assumptions that the information given has been understood. Ask for clients to explain in their own words the protocol, and if appropriate, request a return demonstration of a skill that has been taught.

The Four Major Culture Groups

Given the fact that there exist hundreds of ethnic minority subgroups in the United States, and many more worldwide, it is impossible to address the cultural characteristics of each one of them. The following is a review of the beliefs and health practices of the four major cultural groups in this country—the Latin Americans, black Americans, Asian Americans, and Native Americans, who are the historically underrepresented groups accounting for approximately one-quarter of our U.S. population. These groups are recognized by our government as disadvantaged due to low income, low education, and/or sociocultural deprivation. It must be remembered that one of the most important roles of the nurse as educator is to serve as an advocate for clients—as a representative of their interests. If nurses are to assume this role, then their efforts should be directed at making the health-care setting as similar to the client's natural environment as possible. To do this, they must be aware of clients' customs, beliefs, and lifestyles and be willing to take the responsibility for making adaptations in the institutional environment. For additional information on the four minority groups discussed or on particular tribes or subgroups not identified, see Cohen (1991), Kniep-Hardy and Burkhardt (1977), Shomaker (1981), Perry (1982), Galanti (1991), Horton and Freire (1990), and Smolan et al. (1990).

Latin American Culture

According to the U.S. Bureau of the Census (1991), Latinos are the fastest growing minority in the United States. Latinos now represent 9.6% of the total population of the United States. By the year 2000, they will constitute 11% of the population, and it is projected that in another 100 years they will make up approximately 25% of the population. There has been a tremendous increase in the numbers of Latinos since 1970 as a result of a higher birth rate in this group than the rest of the population, a significant increase in immigration, as well as improved census procedures. Latin Americans derive from diverse origins. The largest group are Mexicans, followed by Puerto Ricans, Central and South Americans, and Cubans. They are found in every state but are concentrated in just 10 states. California and Texas together have one-half of the Latino population, and other large concentrations are found in New York, New Jersey, Massachusetts, Florida, Illinois, Arizona, New Mexico, and Colorado. Nurse educators who practice in the Southwestern states are most likely to encounter Mexicans, those practicing in the Northeast states will most likely be caregivers for Puerto Ricans, and nurses in Florida will be delivering care to a large number of Cubans. Also, Latinos are more likely to live in metropolitan areas than non-

Latinos (Torres, 1994). While Latin Americans have many common characteristics, each subgroup has unique characteristics. For example, Latinos of Cuban as well as Central and South American origin compare much closer in education and economic levels to non-Latino whites than to other Latino Americans (Westberg, 1989).

Latinos have particular health-care needs that must be addressed. They are disproportionately affected by certain cancers, alcoholism, drug abuse, obesity, hypertension, diabetes, adolescent pregnancy, dental disease, and HIV/AIDS. Unlike in non-Latino whites, homicide, AIDS, and perinatal conditions rank in the top ten as causing mortality in Latinos. They are more prone to certain diseases, are less likely to receive preventive care, lack health insurance, and have less access to health care than other whites living in the United States.

Unfortunately, both the curricula in nursing schools nationwide and the literature in nursing with respect to patient education efforts of Latin Americans have paid little attention to the health-care needs of this minority group. Although Latinos are a culturally diverse group of people with varying health needs, avenues for including Latino health-care issues in nursing curricula have been minimal and especially need to be developed in schools located in areas with high concentrations of Latinos. Fluency in Spanish as a foreign language is a necessity, or at least highly recommended, when practitioners are responsible for delivering care to this growing, underserved, culturally diverse group. Spanish-speaking people represent 54% of all non-English speaking persons in the United States. In proportion to the U.S. population, Latinos are underrepresented in nursing education. Only 3% of all graduates of basic nursing programs are of Latino descent. There are far too few graduates to fulfill the increasing need for Latino health-care professionals. The inability of Latinos to become health professionals is not thought to be a result of low aspirations on their part. Many Latino high school students rank health/medical services, along with business and engineering, as one of their top ten career choices. But poor academic achievement of Latinos in high schools and colleges is associated with a number of factors related to socioeconomic and educational disadvantages.

Access to health care by Latinos is limited both by choice as well as by unavailability of health services. Only one-fifth of Puerto Ricans,

one-quarter of Cubans, and one-third of Mexicans see a physician during the course of a year. Even when Latinos have access to the health-care system, they may not receive the care they need. Difficulty in obtaining services, dissatisfaction with the care provided, and inability to afford the rising costs of medical care are the major factors that discourage them from using the health-care system. Latino families are 2½ times more likely to be below the poverty level than other groups in the United States. Economic disadvantage leaves little disposable income for paying out-of-pocket expenses for health care. When they do seek a regular source of care, many rely on public health facilities, hospital outpatient clinics, and emergency rooms (Westberg, 1989; Andersen et al., 1986).

The health beliefs of Latinos also affect their decision to seek traditional care. Many early studies dating back to the 1940s on Latino health beliefs and practices stressed exotic folklore practices, such as their use of herbs, teas, home remedies, and over-the-counter drugs for treating symptoms of acute and chronic illnesses. In addition, Latinos place a high degree of reliance on health healers, known as "curenderos" or "esperitistas," for health advice and treatment.

Early studies also reported that illnesses of Mexican Americans could be organized into the following categories (Markides & Coreil, 1986):

1. Diseases of "hot" and "cold," believed to be due to an imbalanced intake of foods or ingestion of foods at extreme opposites in temperature. In addition, cold air was thought to lead to joint pain, and a "cold womb" resulted in barrenness in women. Heating or chilling was the cure for parts of the body afflicted by disease.
2. Diseases of dislocation of internal organs, cured by massage or physical manipulation of body parts.
3. Diseases of magical origin, caused by "mal Ojo" or "evil eye," a disorder of infants and children as a result of a woman's looking admiringly at someone else's child without touching the child, resulting in crying, fitful sleep, diarrhea, vomiting, and fever.
4. Diseases of emotional origin, attributed to sudden or prolonged terror called "Susto."
5. Folk-defined diseases, such as "latido."
6. "Standard scientific" diseases.

Additional studies in the 1950s and 1960s focused primarily on mental health issues. These studies suggested the existence of an "epidemiological paradox," meaning that unlike other socioeconomically disadvantaged minority groups, Mexican Americans in particular were found to have low rates of psychiatric problems, probably explained by strong family ties that protected them against stress. More recent research concludes that Southwestern Latinos' health status is determined by key health indicators on infant mortality, life expectancy, and mortality from cardiovascular disease, cancer, and measures of functional health. This research reveals that the health of Latinos is much closer to that of whites than to blacks, with whom Latinos share similar socioeconomic conditions. Concerning the incidence of diabetes and infectious and parasitic diseases, however, Latinos are clearly at a disadvantage in relation to whites. Possible explanations for the relative advantages and disadvantages in health status of Latinos involve such factors as cultural practices favoring reproductive success, early and high fertility contributing to low breast cancer but high cervical cancer rates, dietary habits linked to low cancer rates but high prevalence of obesity and diabetes, genetic heritage, extended family support reducing need for psychiatric services, and low socioeconomic status contributing to increased infectious and parasitic diseases. As the Latino population becomes more acculturated, it is anticipated that there will be an increase in certain risk factors conducive to cardiovascular disease and certain cancers (Markides & Coreil, 1986).

Today, there is discrepancy in the literature about the extent and frequency to which Latinos use home remedies and folk practices. It has been found that 21% of the Latino population in the Southwestern United States uses herbs and other home remedies to treat illness episodes, which is twice the proportion reported in the total U.S. population. But some studies claim that the use of folk practitioners has declined and has practically disappeared. Knowing where people get their health information provides clues to practitioners as to how to reach particular population groups. One study indicated that Mexican Americans receive almost as much information from mass media sources (TV, magazines, and newspapers) as they do from physicians and nurses. This indicates that mass media could play an important role in disseminating information to a large portion of the Mexican American population.

Because of the centrality of the family in Latino peoples' lives, the extended family serves as the single most important source of social support to its members. There is a pattern of respect and obedience to elders as well as a pattern of male dominance. Caregivers' focus, therefore, needs to be on the family rather than on the individual. It is likely, for example, that a woman would be reluctant to make a decision about her or her child's health care without consulting her husband first. Changes are occurring, however, as Latino women are taking jobs outside the home. Also children are picking up the English language more quickly than their parents and are ending up in the powerful position of acting as interpreters for their parents. Reliance on family has been attributed to low utilization of health-care services. In addition, levels of education correlate highly with access to health care: that is, the less education possessed by the head of the household, the poorer the family's health status and access to health care (Westberg, 1989).

Teaching strategies   Only about half the number of Latinos have completed 4 years of high school or more and only 10% have completed college, as compared with 77% and 21%, respectively, for the rest of the population. The educational level of Latino clients needs to be taken into consideration when selecting instructional materials. Sophisticated teaching methods and tools would be inappropriate for those who have minimal levels of education. The age of the population can also affect health and patient education efforts. Since the Latino population is young as a total group (30% are under 20 years of age), the school system is an important setting for educating members of the Latino community. Morbidity, mortality, and risk factor data also provide clues to the areas in which patient education efforts should be directed. As cited earlier, Latinos face higher rates of diabetes, AIDS, obesity, alcohol-related illnesses, and mortality from homicide than the general population. These are all topics that should be targeted for educational efforts at disease prevention and health promotion.

Unfortunately, little data exist regarding patient education for Latino Americans. A few small

studies reviewed by Westberg (1989) have implications for patient education. In a study on the educational and emotional needs of Latino women who were hospitalized for prenatal care, the women revealed that they were so nervous in talking to physicians that they would forget to ask questions, and when they did, they would forget the doctor's answers; they found it difficult to talk with health professionals about their "private parts"; and they found it easiest to talk with those practitioners with whom they had met on prior visits. The findings of other studies indicate that education programs in the school system for Latino students on alcohol and drug abuse and on cardiovascular disease risk reduction proved successful if

- Cultural beliefs were observed.
- The educator was first introduced by an individual accepted and respected by the learners.
- Family members were included.
- The community was encouraged to take responsibility for resolving the health problems discussed.

Another study investigated the impact that the mass media of radio and television had on increasing health knowledge and awareness as well as stimulating responses in the Latino population to the problems communicated through these instructional tools. Researchers concluded that regular radio and TV broadcasts delivering public service announcements in Spanish can be an effective health education strategy.

The following general suggestions are useful when designing and implementing education programs for Latino Americans (Westberg, 1989):

1. Encourage Latinos to be involved in planning education programs.
2. Identify those Latinos in the community who are not currently recipients of health education services.
3. Consider developing outreach programs, like mass media segments, to reach the unmet needs of underserved Latinos.
4. Identify the Latin American subgroups (Mexicans, Cubans, and Puerto Ricans) in the community whose needs differ on health beliefs, language, and general health status so that

education programs are targeted to meet their distinct ethnic needs.

5. Be aware of individual differences within subgroups as to age, years of education, income levels, job status and degree of acculturation.

6. Take into account the special health needs of Latin Americans with respect to incidences of diseases and risk factors to which they are prone—diabetes, AIDS, obesity, alcohol-related illnesses, homicide, and accidental injuries.

7. Be aware of the importance of the family in order to direct education efforts to include all interested family members. Remember that Latino families are usually willing to provide support to each other and decision making usually rests with the male and elder authority figures in the family.

8. Provide adequate space for teaching to accommodate family members who typically accompany patients seeking health care.

9. Be cognizant of the importance of the Roman Catholic religion in the lives of Latinos when dealing with such issues as contraception, abortion, and family planning.

10. Demonstrate cultural sensitivity to health beliefs by respecting ethnic values and taking time to learn about Latino beliefs.

11. Consider other sources of care that the Latinos might be using, such as home remedies, before they enter or while they are within the health-care system.

12. Be aware of the modesty felt by some Latinos, especially women and girls, who may be particularly uncomfortable in talking about sexual issues in mixed company.

13. Display warmth, friendliness, and tactfulness when developing a relationship with Latinos because they expect health-care providers to be informal and interested in their lives.

14. Determine if Spanish is the most comfortable language for the client in which to converse and read. Many Latinos prefer to speak Spanish but are not proficient in reading this language.

15. Speak slowly and distinctly, avoiding the use of slang and idioms if the client has limited proficiency in English.

16. Do not assume that a nod of the head or a smile indicates understanding of what has been said. For Latinos who are not familiar with English and because they respect authority, it is not uncommon for them to display nonverbal cues that may be misleading or misinterpreted by the receiver. Ask clients to repeat in their own words what they have been told to determine their level of understanding.

17. If interpreters are used, be sure they speak the dialect used by the learner. Be certain the interpreter "interprets" rather than just "translates" so that the real meaning of instructions gets across. Also, be sure to talk to the client, not to the interpreter.

18. Provide written and audiovisual materials in Spanish. There are an increasing number of patient education materials available strictly in Spanish or prepared for a bilingual audience.

19. Locate the hotline telephone number in the community that provides a direct link to Spanish-speaking interpreters who can assist health-care providers in communicating with non–English-speaking patients.

A review of the literature indicates that much more must be learned about the Latin American population with respect to their cultural beliefs and their health and education needs. Given the limited knowledge available, it is evident that many members of this cultural group are not receiving the kind and amount of health services they desire and deserve. Nurse educators, particularly in those regions of the country densely populated with these ethnic subgroups, need to extend themselves to Latinos in a culturally sensitive manner to effectively and efficiently address the needs of this rapidly growing segment of the American population.

Black American Culture

At the present time, members of the black culture make up the largest historically underrepresented group in the United States, but this is expected to change in the near future due to the rapid growth of the Latino population. The cultural origins and heritage of black Americans are quite diverse. Their roots are mainly from Africa and the Caribbean Islands. They speak a variety of languages including French, Spanish, African dialects, and various forms of English. The one distinguishing factor of this group is the length of time many of these people have had to acculturate to the American "way of life," adapting to a number of the beliefs and practices of Western medicine. Quite a few black families have ancestry who settled in America dating back many generations. Although the cultural heritage of the black subgroups varies, it is possible to make some generalizations about their cultural beliefs and traditions, particularly those customs and beliefs of the more recent immigrants or those that were carried through the generations from colonial times, when blacks were held as slaves. It must be pointed out that there are few recent studies conducted specifically investigating the black American culture. Perhaps this is because their cultural heritage has been blended into the social fabric of America over time as blacks were exposed to whites with whom they lived and served (Spector, 1991).

Unfortunately, a disproportionate number of people from the black American culture are disadvantaged as a result of poverty and low educational attainment. Many black families are exposed to numerous risk factors simultaneously as a result of poor environmental conditions under which they live. Black children born to teenaged mothers, for example, were found to be approximately four times as likely to have low scores on achievement tests. Poor learning outcomes in these children have been linked to their exposure to poverty, low maternal educational level, absence of a father or father figure in the home, and the like. Another potential risk factor with respect to learning is urban residence. In a comparison of urban and rural communities, those living in urban areas were twice as likely to have behavioral and reading problems than those families living in rural settings. This prevalence is believed to be largely as a result of the variety of stressors (e.g., crowded and noisy living conditions) found in the urban setting. In addition, the urban school systems were found to provide less than optimal settings for the acquisition of skills and information (Luster & McAdoo, 1994).

Black Americans of African descent have been found by sociologists and anthropologists to have similarities with respect to the importance of extended family. Common to the black culture is the concept of extended family, consisting of several households, with the older adults often taking the leadership role within the family constellation. Respect for elders and ancestors is valued. They are held in high esteem because living a long life indicates that the individual had the opportunities to acquire much experience and knowledge. Decision making regarding health-care issues is often left to the elders. Family ties are especially strong between grandchildren and grandparents. It is not unusual for grandmothers to want to stay at the hospital bedside when their grandchildren are ill. This extended family network provides emotional, physical, and financial support to members during times of illness and other crises (Spector, 1991).

Beliefs, consisting of knowledge, opinions, and faith that dispose persons to demonstrate certain kinds of behavior, are not necessarily dependent on the degree to which they correspond to reality. The strength of a belief also is not dependent on its congruence with other beliefs held by the individual. In a study of black teenaged women in a prenatal clinic, their beliefs were shown to contribute to noncompliance relating to prevention of pregnancy. Although they believed contraception was appropriate, birth control pills and IUDs were considered unacceptable because they were felt to alter menstrual cycles and thus cause illness. The understanding of young black women of how contraceptives work, what they do, and how pregnancy occurs is handed down through a rich description of events by their mothers and other female relatives. Becoming a mother at a young age, although not highly desirable by this sample of black women, did have a fairly high level of acceptance in their cultural group. In fact, these women did not perceive negative sanctions within their culture if they did not meet the ideal norm of getting an education or job followed by marriage and children. Each of the black women believed their families would support them if they needed help (Horn, 1983).

Black people tend to have strong religious values, and these religious beliefs extend to their feelings about illness and health. A major folk practice, known as voodoo, consists of beliefs about spirits inhabiting the world: All animate and inanimate objects have good or evil spirits. A religious priest, witch doctor, or medicine man has the power to appease or release hostile spirits. Illness, or disharmony, is thought to be caused by evil spirits because a person failed to follow religious rules or the dictates of ancestors. Curative measures involve finding the cause of an illness—a hex or a spell placed on a person by another or the breaking of a taboo—and then finding someone with magical healing powers or witchcraft to rid them of the evil spirit(s). Some black American families also continue to practice home remedies such as the use of mustard plasters, taking of herbal medicines and teas, and wearing of amulets to cure or ward off a variety of illnesses and afflictions (Spector, 1991).

Teaching strategies   In teaching black Americans preventive and promotion measures, as well as caring for them during acute and chronic illnesses, the nurse must explore the belief systems of the client. Any folk practices or religious beliefs should be respected and allowed (if not harmful) and incorporated into the recommended treatment or health-care interventions used by Western medicine.

Asian/Pacific Culture

People from Asian countries and the Pacific Islands constitute this cultural group. As a result of the Korean War in the 1950s, the fall of Vietnam in 1975, and the successive disintegration of the governments of Laos and Cambodia, the West Coast region of the United States, in particular, has been settled by Southeast Asian refugees. As of approximately a decade ago, over 45,000 Vietnamese, Cambodians, and Laotians lived in the San Francisco Bay area alone, and 29,000 had officially resettled in Washington State (Schultz, 1982; Kubota & Matsuda, 1982). The states of New York, New Jersey, and Texas also have had a large influx of Asian peoples. In total, almost three-quarters of a million people of Asian/Pacific origin have immigrated into the United States in the last two decades. The Chinese, Filipinos and Japanese also are members of this Asian culture.

The medical system of the Asian/Pacific countries and the culture and religion of these peoples need to be understood to successfully deal with their health issues. The language barrier has proved to be the biggest problem in providing health-care services to these populations. Many misconceptions can occur because the Southeast Asian languages are not as technical as English. Although the Asian/Pacific people have been classified as one ethnic group by many researchers and census takers and many presume that the culture of all these people is the same, a wide variety of cultural, religious, and language backgrounds are represented. There are some similarities among members of the Asian/Pacific group, but there are also many differences. By understanding the basic philosophical tenets of the Southeast Asian clients, whether they are refugees or immigrants, or first-, second-, or third-generation Americans, nurses and other health-care practitioners are better prepared to *understand*, if not *accept,* their cultural differences and varied behavior patterns (Kubota & Matsuda, 1982).

According to Kubota and Matsuda (1982), the major philosophical orientation of the Asian/Pacific people is a blend of four philosophies—Buddhism, Confucianism, Taoism, and Phi. There are four common values that are strongly reflected in these philosophies:

1. Male authority and dominance
2. "Saving face" (conduct as a result of a sense of pride)
3. Strong family ties
4. Respect for parents, elders, teachers, and other authority figures

Based on studies from Kubota and Matsuda (1982) and Schultz (1982), the following is a brief review of the beliefs and health-care practices of the Asian/Pacific people:

Buddhism: The fundamental belief of Buddhism is that all existence is suffering. The continuation of life, therefore suffering, arises from desires and passions, and the ultimate solution lies in the cessation of personal desire. According to the Buddhist philosophy, no human beings are limited to a single existence terminating in death. Instead, everyone is reincarnated. "Ultimate salvation lies in the elimination of the self, which is to be gained by an understanding of the causality of things—a condition known as enlightenment, or *nirvana*, a state that cannot be described" (Kubota & Matsuda, 1982, p. 21). Cambodians, who in particular are strongly influenced by the Buddhist philosophy, strive to accumulate religious merits or good deeds to ensure a better life to come. They adhere to a deep belief in karma, whereby things done in this existence will help or hinder their ascension on the ladder to nirvana. Good deeds, sharing, donating, and being generous and kind are all ways to accumulate merits.

Confucianism: The moral values and beliefs of Southeast Asians are heavily influenced by the Confucianism philosophy. In this concept, the moral personality is the focus. Two predominant moral qualities, developed through cultivation of the personality, include humaneness (the attitude shown toward others) and a sense of moral duty and obligation (attitudes persons display toward themselves). The following principles guide the social behavior of people who adhere to Confucianism:

- *Patterns of authority*—five relationships run from inferior to superior to form a pattern of obligation and authority in the family as well as in social and political realms:

  1. Son (child) to father
  2. Wife to husband
  3. Younger brother to older brother
  4. Friend to friend
  5. Subject to ruler

  These patterns of authority and obligation influence decision making and social interactions. For example, a friend is to regard a friend as a younger or older brother. Women's subservience to men is reflected in a woman's behavior to always seek the advice of her husband when making decisions. This authority needs to be respected by nursing staff when, for instance, a woman refuses to choose a contraceptive method until she asks for her husband's advice and permission.

- *Man in harmony with the universe*—in the Confucian system, people are between heaven and earth, and life has to be in harmony with the universe. An example of this principle in action is when an Asian responds passively to new information, quietly accepting the information rather than actively seeking to understand and clarify it. Given this typical behavior, it is important for the nurse when instructing the client to ask for an explanation of the information to ascertain if it was understood.

- *Ancestor worship*—concern for the moral order of relationships, which is reflected in a deep reverence for tradition and prescribed rites. Great emphasis is placed on funerals, etiquette for mourning, and the sharing of a communal meal with the dead.

The Asian/Pacific culture values harmony in life and a balance of nature. Shame is something to be avoided, families are the center of life, elders are respected, and ancestors are worshiped and remembered. Children are highly valued because they carry on the family name and are expected to care for aging parents. The woman's role is one of subservience throughout her entire life—follow the advice of parents while unmarried, the husband's advice while married, and the children's advice when widowed. This subservient role is in direct conflict with U.S. social and family values, which expect women to take a more independent, assertive, and self-determined role.

Taoism: The Tao philosophy has its roots in the belief of two opposing magical forces in nature, the negative (Yin) and the positive (Yang), which affect the course of all material and spiritual life. The basic concepts of Chinese philosophy, the beliefs in Tao (the way of nature) and Yin and Yang (the principle of balance), stress that human achievement in harmony with nature should be accomplished through "nonaction." Common also is the idea that good health depends on the balance between hot and cold. Equilibrium of hot and cold elements produces good health. Drugs, natural elements, and foods are classified as either hot or cold. It is believed that sickness can be caused by eating too much hot or cold food. If a child has a stomachache, for example, the mother considers the diet. Hot foods are meats, sweets, and spices. Cold foods are rice and vegetables.

The Chinese adhere to strong family ties, respect for elders, and the authority of men as the head of the household, and sons are highly valued. Illness is believed to be the result of an imbalance in the forces of nature. Ill health is believed to be a curse from heaven, mental illness being the worst possible curse, because the individual was irresponsible in not obtaining the right amount of rest, food, and work.

Phi: Phi worship is a belief in the spirits of dead relatives or the spirits of animals and nature. Phi range from bad to good. If a place has a strong phi, the individual must make an offering before doing anything in that place, like building a house or tilling the land. If someone violates a rule of order, an atmosphere of bad phi can result in illness or death. Redemption can be sought from a phi priest as a hope of getting relief from suffering. Offerings are made and special rites are performed to rid the person of a bad phi. Worshipers of this philosophy respect elders and avoid conflict by doing things in a pleasant manner. Those who adhere to the phi philosophy are hospitable, generous, show respect to others in the way a person is addressed, and tend to prize hard work and ambition.

For people of the Asian/Pacific ethnic group, there are marked cultural differences that confront them when they live in the United States with respect to ways of life, ways of thinking, values orientation, social structure, and family interactions (Chao, 1994). Children tend to adapt quickly to acculturation, but the older generations tend to have difficulty. Their medical practices, like their other unique cultural practices, differ significantly from Western ways. The health-seeking behaviors of immigrants are crisis oriented, following the pattern in their homelands, where medical care was not readily available. They only tend to seek health care when seriously ill. Reinforcement is needed to encourage them to come for follow-up visits after an initial encounter with the health-care system. Sometimes they are viewed by practitioners as noncompliant when they do not do exactly what is expected of them, when they withdraw from follow-up treatments, or when they do not keep prearranged appointments.

Asians make great use of herbal remedies to treat fevers, diarrhea, and coughs. Dermabrasion, often misunderstood by U.S. practitioners, is a home remedy to treat a wide variety of problems such as headaches, cold symptoms, and fever and chills. In their traditional health-care system, they rely on folk medicine from healers, sorcerers, and monks. Western medicine is thought as "shots that cure," and Asian patients expect to get medicine (injections or pills) whenever they seek medical help in the United States. If no medication is prescribed, the person, if not given an explanation, may feel that care is inadequate and fail to return for future care. Common to many Southeast Asians is the idea that illnesses, just like foods, are classified as hot and cold, which coincide with the Yin and Yang philosophy of the principles of balance. If a disease is considered hot in origin, then giving cold foods is thought of as the proper treatment. Conflict and fear are the most likely responses to laboratory tests and having blood drawn because of the belief that removing blood makes the body weak and that blood is not replenished. Fear of surgery is a result of the belief that souls inhabit the body and may be released. Loss of privacy leading to extreme embarrassment and humiliation also is another major fear.

Teaching strategies   Respect is automatically endowed on most health-care providers and teachers because they are seen as knowledgeable. Asians are sensitive and formal people, and, therefore, a friendly and nonthreatening approach to them is necessary before giving care. They must be given permission to ask a question but are not offended by questions from others. Language barriers are usually the first and biggest obstacle to overcome in dealing with people of Asian descent. Translators can be used to facilitate interactions. The learning style of Asians is essentially passive—no personal opinions, no confrontations, no challenges, and no outward disagreements—and learning is done by repetition and rote memorization of information. It must be remembered that decision making is a family affair, and family members need to be included, especially the male authority figure, in the process of deciding the best solution for a situation. Nurses and other health-care practitioners should be aware that in the Asians' wish to "save face" for themselves and others, they avoid being disruptive and will agree to what is said so as not to be offensive. They are easily shamed, so patients must be reassured and told what is considered acceptable behavior by Western moral and legal standards. Nods of the head do not necessarily mean agreement or understanding. Questions directed to them need to be asked in several ways to confirm that they understand any instructional messages given.

Native American Culture

The U.S. Bureau of the Census (1991) identified nearly 1.7 million people who were of Native American or native Alaskan descent living in the United States. Of these, approximately one million were eligible for health services provided by the federal government. Medical care to the Native American people has a long history. As far back as 1832, the War Department undertook a smallpox vaccination campaign for tribes of Native American people, largely to protect military troops from infection. In 1849, health-care responsibility was transferred to the newly created Bureau of Indian Affairs. In 1954, the Department of Health, Education and Welfare of the U.S. Public Health Service (USPHS) took over jurisdiction. Today the Indian Health Service (IHS) of the USPHS maintains responsibility for providing health care to over 500 distinct tribes of Native Americans and native Alaskans (Mail et al., 1989). The largest of the Native American tribes are the Navajo, Cherokee, Sioux, Chippewa, and Pueblo, who reside primarily in the northwestern, central, and southwestern regions of the United States.

The current challenge to health-care practitioners is to integrate Western medicine with traditional non-Western tribal folk medicine to provide cross-cultural health education to Native Americans in reservation-based communities across the nation. To do so, nurses must understand contemporary Native American cultural patterns, including theories of disease causality and associated therapies. It is also essential for nursing professionals to become focused on a more "ethnomedical" orientation delineating the nature and consequences of illness problems and disease interventions rather than adhering to the biomedical orientation of defining diseases and illness interventions. In the ethnomedical context, the concept of illness incorporates the relationship of humans with their universe—a concept that bridges culture with a sensitivity toward the daily practices inherent within specific ethnic groups. The challenge for the nurse educator is to understand the world perspective of contemporary Native American people that sets them apart from non–Native Americans (Mail et al.,1989).

As outlined by Primeaux (1977), the following include the major characteristics of the Native American culture:

1. A spiritual attachment to the land
2. An intimacy of religion and medicine
3. The importance of strong ties to family, other relatives, and the tribe
4. The view that children are an asset, not a liability
5. A belief that supernatural powers exist in animate as well as in inanimate objects
6. A desire to remain Native American and avoid acculturation, thereby retaining own culture and language
7. A lack of materialism, time consciousness, and a desire to share with others

Unless the awareness of non–Native American health-care workers is raised, these common characteristics are likely to be overlooked by them when care is being provided to the Native American client. Although Anglo-American culture and Western health-care practices have been integrated to some extent into the Native American way of life, the above characteristics still predominate today to set Native Americans apart as a unique cultural group.

There remains for the Native American a close connection between religion and health. When a family member becomes ill, witchcraft is still perceived by some tribes as the real cause of illness. In traditional societies, witchcraft functions to supply answers to perplexing or disturbing questions. Witchcraft also serves as an explanation for personal insecurities, intragroup tensions, fears, and anxieties. Witches, with their supernatural powers, have served as convenient scapegoats on which to blame the misfortunes in life. It also has provided tribes with a mechanism for social control. It is hypothesized that as the cultural practices of witchcraft were increasingly denigrated by missionaries and bureaucrats, substitutions such as compulsive drinking and frequent use of narcotics (peyote) became a culturally sanctioned outlet for aggressive impulses and frustrations. These behaviors were seen as less disruptive than demonstrating overt hostilities. This is one of the many proposed theories to explain the prevalence of substance abuse by Native Americans. Some Native American tribes still practice witchcraft but tend to deny it as a reality because of the negative stereotype and stigma attached to it by outsiders. Nevertheless, the intimacy between religion and medicine exists and is exhibited in the form of "sing" prayers and ceremonial cure practices. However, few nurses would think of providing space and privacy for several relatives to be able to conduct a ceremony for a hospitalized family member.

Some Native American tribal beliefs also require incorporating the medicine man (Shaman) into the system of care given to patients. It is important to realize that the central and formal aspects of Native American medicine are ceremonial, embracing the notion of a supernatural power. Although the ceremonies do vary from tribe to tribe, the ideas of causation and cure are common to all Native Americans. The ritual is determined by the signs and symptoms of an illness. Sometimes rituals are performed by family members. Cornmeal, from the sacred food of corn, is one item that is frequently used in a variety of curative ceremonies. The nurse must demonstrate legitimate respect for such ritualistic symbols and ceremonial activities (Primeaux, 1977).

To be considered really poor in the Native American world is for someone to be devoid of relatives. The family and tribe are of utmost importance, a belief that children learn from infancy (Primeaux, 1977). It is not unusual for many family members, sometimes large groups of 10 to 15 people, to arrive at the hospital and camp out on the hospital grounds to be with their sick relative. Talking is unnecessary, but being there is highly important for everyone concerned. Hospital personnel have often labeled this behavior as useless and disruptive and deem the patient and family to be uncooperative. Grandmothers, in particular, have great importance to a sick child. It is frequently the grandmother who must give permission for a child to be hospitalized and treated. The Native American kinship system, in fact, allows for a child to have several sets of grandparents, aunts, uncles, cousins, brothers, and sisters. Sometimes a number of women substitute as a mother figure for a child, which may cause role confusion for the non–Native American health-care provider.

Children are given a great deal of freedom and independence to learn by their decisions and live by the consequences of their actions. Their entire childhood years consist of experiential learning to develop skills and self-confidence to function as adults. They may appear "spoiled," but in fact they are taught self-care and respect for others at a very early age. Outside of their private domain, Native American children tend not to be very competitive or assertive. This behavior can be seen in children in the public school system. To call attention to oneself is interpreted by Native Americans as "showy" and inappropriate. Children are doted on by family members, and in turn, they have high regard for their elders. In fact, the older adults in Native American communities are highly respected and looked to for advice and counsel.

Another characteristic of Native Americans is that they generally are not very future oriented; they take one day at a time and do not feel they have control over their own destiny. This attitude or way of thinking has proved to be a significant obstacle when health educators have attempted to provide preventive care. Time is on a continuum with no beginning and no end. Native Americans tend not to live by clocks and schedules. In fact, many Native American homes do not have clocks, and family members eat meals and do other activities when they please. They are more casual in their approach to life than many non–Native American people. This lack of time consciousness and pressure is a crucial factor to be remembered by health-care providers when a prescribed regimen calls for the patient to follow a medication, exercise, or dietary schedule. Inattention to time also can interfere with their keeping scheduled appointments, although lack of funds rather than time seems to be the main cause of missed appointments.

Another aspect of time is reflected in their belief that death is just a part of the life cycle—a much healthier and more accepting attitude toward dying than that held by most Anglo-Americans. Their grief process is culturally very different. Funerals are accompanied by large feasts and the sharing of gifts with relatives of the deceased. There is no belief in a life hereafter as a reward for a lifetime of good deeds while on earth. Life after death is an opportunity to join the world of long-ago ancestors. Their view of death is closely related to their opinion about the appropriate disposal of amputated limbs. Because diabetes is so prevalent in the Native American population, it is important to know that they usually want to reclaim an amputated body part for proper burial.

Sharing is another core value of the Native Americans. The concept of "being" is fundamental, and there is little stress on achievement or the worth of material wealth. Individuals are valued much more highly than material goods. Overall, Native Americans are a proud, sensitive, cooperative, passive people, devoted to tribe and family, and willing to share possessions and self with others. They are very vulnerable when it comes to their pride and dignity. They can be easily offended by nonsensitive caregivers. In terms of human relationships, it is important to note that Native Americans believe that to look someone in the eye is considered disrespectful. Some tribes feel that looking into the eyes of another reveals and may even steal someone's soul. Since a friendly handshake and eye contact are acceptable and even expected in the Anglo-American culture, it must be acknowledged that these gestures do not have the same meaning for the Native American. In fact, eye contact by Anglo-American definition is interpreted to mean that someone is paying attention, is interested, or understands. Non–Native American health-care workers, therefore, may consider lack of eye contact to mean that these patients are shiftless, shifty, uninterested in learning, or inattentive, when in fact all along they were taking in the message of instruction being given. If asked, they can often repeat verbatim what someone just said to them. As Primeaux (1977) so aptly comments, "Perhaps the notion of being spoken *to* rather than *with* has importance here" (p. 94).

The health problems faced by Native Americans are undergoing significant change. Whereas in the first half of the twentieth century acute and infectious diseases were prevalent and were the principal cause of death, today, as a result of increased life expectancy, Native Americans are succumbing to many lifestyle diseases and chronic conditions. Chief among the causes of morbidity and mortality are heart disease, cancer, diabetes, and drug and alcohol abuse—all of which to some extent are amenable to educational intervention.

Teaching strategies   Patient educators need to focus on giving information about these diseases and risk factors and emphasize the teaching of skills related to changes in diet and exercise, as well as help people to build positive coping mechanisms to deal with emotional problems (Hosey & Stracqualursi, 1990). For the most part, acute and infectious diseases, with the exception of a recurrence in tuberculosis, are no longer a major cause of illness and death because of the availability of drug therapy, early case finding, improved sanitary conditions, and better provision of health education. Another factor has been the availability of Community Health Representatives (CHRs), indigenous community outreach workers who have played a significant role in case finding, early diagnosis, and reinforcement of patient and other health education recommendations. As Mail et al. (1989) stated: "Involving the CHR in patient education is an important cross-cultural consideration, because this is the individual who will reinforce behavior changes with the community and home" (p. 97).

Although all Native Americans share some of the core beliefs and practices of their culture, each tribe is unique in its customs and language. Finding the ways and means to integrate Western medicine with the traditional Native American folk medicine in caring for the varied needs of this population group presents a challenge to the nurse educator as well as a learning opportunity for the recipient of health education services.

SUMMARY

This chapter explored the impact of gender, socioeconomic status, and cultural beliefs on both the ability and willingness of clients to learn health-care measures. The in-depth examination of these three factors serves as an explanatory model for certain behaviors observed or potentially encountered in a teaching-learning situation. Even though the emphasis of this chapter was on patients or the general public from various ethnic groups with whom nurse educators interact, an understanding of gender differences, socioeconomic influences, and cultural characteristics can be a useful source of information as well when teaching nursing students or staff who may come from a variety of backgrounds and orientations.

The most important aspect to remember from reading this chapter is the care one must take not to stereotype or generalize common characteristics of a group to all members associated with that particular group. If the nurse does not know much about a culture, that is OK. The important point is to ask clients about their beliefs, not just assume they abide by the tenets of a certain cultural group. In that way, nurses can avoid offending the learner. The educator must be cautious to treat each learner as an individual and ascertain the extent to which they ascribe to, exhibit beliefs in, or adhere to ways of doing things that impact on learning. Both men and women live in a double environment—an outer layer of natural resources and climate and an inner layer of culture and innate strengths and weaknesses—which influences how human beings perceive and respond to their world (Griffith, 1982). Nurses as professionals should constantly strive to improve the delivery of care to all people regardless of their gender orientation, ethnic origin, creed, nationality, or socioeconomic background (Holtz & Bairan, 1990). Yet there is much more for nurses to know about how these three factors of gender, socioeconomics, and culture affect the teaching-learning process before we can competently, confidently, and sensitively deliver care to satisfy the needs of our socially, intellectually, and culturally diverse clientele.

References

Anderson, J.M. (1990). Health care across cultures. *Nursing Outlook, 38*(3), 136-139.

Andersen, R.M., Giachello, A.L., & Aday, L.A. (1986). Access of Hispanics to health care and cuts in services: A state-of-the-art overview. *Public Health Reports, 101*(3), 238-252.

Andrews, M.M. (1992). Cultural perspectives on nursing in the 21st century. *Journal of Professional Nursing, 8*(1), 7-15.

Andrews, M.M., & Boyle, J.S. (1995). Transcultural nursing care. In *Transcultural concepts in nursing care,* 2nd ed. Philadelphia: Lippincott.

Babcock, D.E., & Miller, M.A. (1994). *Client education: Theory and practice*. St. Louis: Mosby–Year Book.

Baydar, N., Brooks-Gunn, J., & Furstenberg, F.F. (1993). Early warning signs of functional illiteracy: Predictors in childhood and adolescence. *Child Development, 64*, 815-829.

Begley, S., Murr, A., & Rogers, A. (March 27, 1995). Gray matters. *Newsweek*, 48-54.

Campbell, F.A., & Ramey, C.T. (1994). Effects of early intervention on intellectual and academic achievement: A follow-up study of children from low-income families. *Child Development, 65*, 684-698.

Campinha-Bacote, J. (1995). The quest for cultural competence in nursing care. *Nursing Forum, 30*(4), 19-25.

Chao, R.K. (1994). Beyond parental control and authoritarian parenting style: Understanding Chinese parenting through the cultural notion of training. *Child Development, 65,* 1111-1119.

Cohen, D. (Ed.). (1991). *The circle of life: Rituals from the human family album.* New York: HarperCollins.

Falvo, D.R. (1994). *Effective patient education: A guide to increased compliance,* 2nd ed. Gaithersburg, MD: Aspen.

Gage, N.L., & Berliner, D.C. (1992). *Educational Psychology,* 5th ed. (chaps. 3 & 5). Boston: Houghton Mifflin.

Galanti, G.A. (1991). *Caring for patients from different cultures.* Philadelphia: University of Pennsylvania Press.

Genesee Hospital Developmental Unit. (1989). Women's language: A manner of speaking. *ASHA, 34.*

Giger, J.N., & Davidhizar, R.E. (1991). *Transcultural nursing: Assessment and intervention.* St. Louis: Mosby–Year Book.

Gorman, C. (January 20, 1992). Sizing up the sexes. *Time*, 42-51.

Griffith, S. (1982). Childbearing and the concept of culture. *Journal of Obstetrics, Gynecological, and Neonatal Nursing, 11*(3), 181-184.

Guralnik, J.M., Land, K.C., Blazer, D., Fillenbaum, G.G., & Branch, L.C. (1993). Educational status and active life expectancy among older blacks and whites. *New England Journal of Medicine, 329*(2), 110-116.

Haggard, A. (1989). *Handbook of patient education.* Rockville, MD: Aspen.

Hahn, M. (November 1995). Providing health care in a culturally complex world. *Advance for Nurse Practitioners*, 43-45.

Hegyvary, S.T. (1992). From diversity to enrichment. *Journal of Professional Nursing, 8*(5), 261.

Holtz, C., & Bairan, A. (1990). Personal contact: A method of teaching cultural empathy. *Nurse Educator, 15*(3), 13, 23, & 28.

Horn, B. (September 1983). Cultural beliefs and teenage pregnancy. *Nurse Practitioner*, 38-39.

Horton, M., & Freire, P. (1990). *We make the road by walking.* Philadelphia: Temple University Press.

Hosey, G.M., & Stracqualurski, F. (1990). Designing and evaluating diabetes education material for American Indians. *The Diabetes Educator, 16*(5), 407-414.

Jezewski, M.A. (1993). Culture brokering as a model for advocacy. *Nursing & Health Care, 14*(2), 78-85.

Kinsey, K.K. (1995). Risky business: Managing the health care of urban low-income families. *Holistic Nursing Practice, 9*(4), 41-53.

Kleinman, A. (1978). Concepts and a model for the comparison of medical systems as cultural systems. *Social Science & Medicine, 12*, 85-93.

Kniep-Hardy, M., & Burkhardt, M.A. (1977). Nursing the Navajo. *American Journal of Nursing, 77*(1), 95-96.

Kubota, J., & Matsuda, K.J. (1982). Family planning services for southeast Asian refugees. *Family & Community Health, 5*(1), 19-25.

Leininger, M. (1978). *Transcultural nursing: Concepts, theories and practices.* New York: Wiley.

Leininger, M. (1994). Transcultural nursing education: A worldwide imperative. *Nursing & Health Care, 15*(5), 254-257.

Lipman, E.L., Offord, D.R., & Boyle, M.H. (1994). Relation between economic disadvantage and psychosocial morbidity in children. *Canadian Medical Association Journal, 151*(4), 431-437.

Luster, T., & McAdoo, H.P. (1994). Factors related to the achievement and adjustment of young African American children. *Child Development, 65*, 1080-1094.

Mail, P.D., McKay, R.B., & Katz, M. (1989). Expanding practice horizons: Learning from American Indian patients. *Patient Education & Counseling, 13*, 91-102.

Markides, K.S., & Coreil, J. (1986). The health of Hispanics in southwestern U.S.: An epidemiological paradox. *Public Health Reports, 101*(3), 253-265.

Morra, M.E. (1991). Future trends in patient education. *Seminars in Oncology Nursing, 7*(2), 143-145.

Nagoshi, C.T., Johnson, R.C., & Honbo, K.A. (1993). Family background, cognitive abilities, and personality as predictors of education and occupational attainment across two generations. *Journal of Biosocial Science, 25*(2), 259-276.

Perry, D.S. (1982). The umbilical cord: Transcultural care and customs. *Journal of Nurse-Midwifery, 27*(4), 25-30.

Price, J.L., & Cordell, B. (1994). Cultural diversity and patient teaching. *Journal of Continuing Education in Nursing, 25*(4), 163-166.

Primeaux, M. (1977). Caring for the American Indian patient. *American Journal of Nursing, 77*(1), 91-94.

Rempusheski, V.F. (1989). The role of ethnicity in elder care. *Nursing Clinics of North America, 24*(3), 717-724.

Rooda, L., & Gay, G. (1993). Staff development for culturally sensitive nursing care. *Journal of Nursing Staff Development, 9*(6), 262-265.

Schultz, S.L. (1982). How Southeast-Asian refugees in California adapt to unfamiliar health care practices. *Health & Social Work, 7*(2), 148-156.

Shomaker, D.M. (1981). Navajo nursing homes: Conflict of philosophies. *Journal of Gerontological Nursing, 7*(9), 531-536.

Smolan, R., Moffitt, P., & Naythons, M. (1990). *The power to heal: Ancient arts and modern medicine,* New York: Prentice Hall Press.

Spector, R.E. (1991). *Cultural diversity in health and illness,* 3rd ed. Norwalk, CT: Appleton & Lange.

Spicer, J.G., Ripple, H.B., Louie, E., Baj, P., & Keating, S. (1994). Supporting ethnic and cultural diversity in nursing staff. *Nursing Management, 25*(1), 38-40.

Torres, S. (1994). A challenge to nursing education: Meeting the health care needs of the Hispanic community. *Deans Notes: A Communication Service to Nursing School Deans, Administrators, and Faculty, 15*(5).

Tripp-Reimer, T. (1982). Barriers to health care: Variations in interpretation of Appalachian client behaviors by Appalachian and non-Appalachian health professionals. *Western Journal of Nursing Research, 4*(2), 179-191.

Tripp-Reimer, T., & Afifi, L.A. (1989). Cross-cultural perspectives on patient teaching. *Nursing Clinics of North America, 24*(3), 613-619.

U.S. Bureau of the Census. (1991). *Statistical abstract of the United States: 1991,* 111th ed. Washington, DC: U.S. Bureau of the Census.

VanHoozer, H.L., Bratton, B.D., Ostmoe, P.M., et al. (1987). *The teaching process: Theory and practice in nursing.* Norwalk, CT: Appleton-Century-Crofts.

Westberg, J. (1989). Patient education for Hispanic Americans. *Patient Education and Counseling, 13*, 143-160.

Winkleby, M.A., Jatulis, D.E., Frank, E., & Fortmann, S.P. (1992). Socioeconomic status and health: How education, income, and occupation contribute to risk factors for cardiovascular disease. *American Journal of Public Health, 82*(6), 816-820.

CHAPTER 9

Special Populations

Kay Viggiani

CHAPTER HIGHLIGHTS

KEY TERMS

disability	rehabilitation
sensory deficits	visual and hearing impairments
learning disability	input and output disabilities
developmental disability	attention deficit disorder
brain injury	spinal cord injury
dysarthria	expressive and receptive aphasia
psychoeducation	mental illness
adaptive computing	chronic illness
habilitation	

OBJECTIVES

After completing this chapter, the reader will be able to

1. Describe how visual and hearing deficits require adaptive intervention.
2. Identify the various teaching strategies that are effective with learning disabilities.
3. Describe the different physical and mental disabilities for appropriate adaptation of the teaching-learning plan.
4. Enhance the teaching-learning process for someone with a communication disability.
5. Discuss the impact of a chronic illness on people and their families and how it affects the teaching-learning process.
6. Describe adaptive computing and its application for people with disabilities.

Teaching others to be independent in self-management of their lives is a critical and challenging role for the nurse in any setting and with any population of individuals. However, the teaching-learning process is especially challenging when dealing with patients, and in some instances even nursing staff, nursing students, or hospital personnel, who have altered functional status due to a disabling condition affecting their physical, cognitive, or sensory capacities. The educational component of the practice of nursing becomes paramount in importance as the nurse's efforts are directed toward assisting the disabled and their significant others to maintain already established patterns of living or develop new ones to accommodate changes in functional ability. The terms *habilitation* and *rehabilitation* are frequently used to differentiate approaches for both developmental and acquired types of disabilities. "Habilitation includes all the activities and interactions that enable an individual with a disability to develop new abilities to achieve his or her maximum potential, whereas rehabilitation is the relearning of previous skills, which often requires an adjustment to altered functional abilities and altered lifestyle" (Burkett, 1989, p. 239). Thus, habilitation and rehabilitation are futuristic processes that focus on helping the disabled learn to live with their disability in their own environment through identification and use of tools that allow them to cope with the ramifications of their altered functional status.

Unfortunately, an increasing number of individuals are faced with having to deal with a disability caused by an injury, a disease, or a birth defect that is permanent and has long-term consequences on their mode of living. Nurses and other health-care providers need to be prepared to provide those services that will meet the demands of a broad range of clients whose problems and situations are the result of a developmental or acquired disability. Specifically with respect to patient populations, the teaching-learning process is an integral element in the habilitation and rehabilitation of disabled clients who need assistance in making the transition from being a recipient of care to assuming a self-care role. Certainly the disabled patient's family members and significant others are also major players in the habilitation and rehabilitation experience. Education of the client and family is the key factor in preparing them for self-care as they make the transition from the hospital or extended-care facility to the home setting. In a recent study, Weeks (1995) supports the idea that family caregivers need and want information on how to best assist their newly disabled adult family member. An appropriate educational program can foster independence in the client and family by helping them to acquire new information, develop new skills, make changes required to achieve competencies in functional activities, assume behaviors that will aid in recovery and the prevention of future disability, and adapt to future situations (Diehl, 1989).

The information in this chapter focuses specifically on patient populations, but the principles of teaching and learning can be extrapolated to apply to other categories of learners, for example, when the nurse educator is responsible in the position of in-service educator, faculty member, or staff development coordinator for teaching hospital personnel or nursing students who may have a physical or learning disability. The purpose of this chapter is to provide an overview of some of the more common disabilities, to address the learning problems inherent in population groups with various types of deficits, to highlight the role of the nurse as educator in designing and implementing specific teaching strategies that can be used to overcome communication difficulties, and to suggest ways in which nurse educators can incorporate appropriate adaptations into their teaching plans to accommodate the needs of disabled patients and their families. A resource list is provided in Appendix B as a further reference to the reader who may be seeking additional information about a specific disability.

This chapter on special populations is a unique addition to this book on the role of the nurse as educator because few other publications address the subject or suggest nursing interventions involving teaching self-care measures to individuals with a wide range of disabilities.

If we stopped for a moment to conjure up a mental picture of the disabled, what would we envision? The people in this special population group may look like the average person, and then again, they may not. Some will have overt physical disabilities, while others may have a cognitive or mental impairment that on the surface may make them indistinguishable from anyone else. But the one thing that they will have in common is a problem that makes learning more difficult for them. For the purpose of this chapter, the term *disability* is defined as "the inability to perform some key life functions and is often used interchangeably with functional limitations" (Dittmar, 1989, p. 7).

On July 26, 1990, President George Bush signed into law the Americans with Disabilities Act (ADA). The definition of disability under the ADA is "a physical or mental impairment which substantially limits one or more of the major life activities of the individual." A "major life activity" includes functions such as caring for oneself, standing, lifting, reaching, seeing, hearing, speaking, breathing, learning, and walking. This significant legislation extends civil rights protection to an estimated 43 million Americans with disabilities. The first part of the law, effective January 1992, mandated accessibility to public accommodations. In July 1992, the second part of the law went into effect requiring employers to make "reasonable accommodations" in hiring people with disabilities (Merrow, 1994). Thus, the ADA legislation makes it illegal to discriminate on the basis of a disability in the areas of employment, public service, public accommodations, transportation, and telecommunications. This statute provides the foundation on which all facets of society will be free of discrimination, including the health-care system. Therefore, we can expect to find people with disabilities in every setting in which nurses practice such as schools, clinics, hospitals, nursing homes, and occupational and home-care settings. Persons with special needs caused by a disability will expect nurses and other health-care professionals to provide appropriate instruction adapted to their needs.

The role of the nurse in teaching the disabled client is an evolving one, as more than ever before, clients expect and are expected to assume greater responsibility as self-care agents. The focus is on wellness and strengths (not limitations) of the individual. The family is increasingly involved in their disabled member's rehabilitation efforts, and individuals with disabilities are expecting and demanding to be a part of community life. Because of the complex needs of the disabled as a special population group, the nurse's role out of necessity must be an integral part of an interdisciplinary team effort by physicians, social workers, physical therapists, psychologists, occupational and speech therapists, and the like in planning for the care of disabled persons and their families, in dealing with educational issues, and in designing and promoting an environment conducive to learning (Diehl, 1989).

THE NURSE AS EDUCATOR'S ROLE IN ASSESSMENT

Application of the teaching-learning process is for the purpose of promoting changes in clients that support their optimal recovery and a return to living in the community. Learning must take place in the cognitive, psychomotor, and affective domains to assist disabled individuals to make the necessary adaptations. Prior to teaching, assessment is always the first step in determining the needs of clients with respect to the nature of their problems, the short- and long-term consequences of their disability, the effectiveness of the coping mechanisms they employ, and the type and extent of sensorimotor, cognitive, perceptual, and communication deficits experienced by clients. The nurse must determine the extent of clients' knowledge with respect to their disability, the amount and type of new information needed for a change in behavior, and clients' readiness to learn. At this initial stage, it is imperative that the nurse educator not only obtain feedback from the clients, but also use assessment skills of observation, testing, and interviewing of family members and significant others as well as taking into account the findings of the team of health-care professionals. Diehl (1989) outlines the following questions to be asked when determining the disabled person's readiness to learn:

1. Do the individual and family members demonstrate an interest in learning by requesting information or posing questions in an effort at problem solving or determining their needs?
2. Are there barriers to learning such as low literacy or vision or hearing impairments? If so, is the client willing and able to use supportive devices?

3. What learning style best suits the client in processing information and applying it to self-care activities?
4. Is there congruence between the goals of the client and family?
5. Is the environment conducive to learning?
6. Does the client value learning of new information and skills as a means to achieve functional improvement? Does the client correlate learning with the opportunity to regain an optimal level of functioning?

The prerequisite to the role of the nurse as teacher and provider of care is to serve as a mentor to patients and family in coordinating and facilitating the multidisciplinary services required to assist disabled persons to attain optimal functioning. The family and significant others, as the disabled person's support system in the community, must be invited right from the beginning to take an active part in learning information as it applies to assisting with self-care activities for their loved ones.

TYPES OF DISABILITIES

The disabilities affecting millions of Americans can be categorized into two major types: mental and physical. These disabilities may have a neurological, physiological, or cognitive basis, can affect thinking processes, and may involve sensorimotor/neuromuscular functioning. The origin of these disabilities is a result of injury, disease, heredity, or congenital defect. For purposes of simplification to review the more common disabilities encountered by the nurse in practice, the following categories have been chosen: sensory deficits, learning disabilities, developmental disability, mental illness, physical disabilities, and communication disorders. Included within each category are the specific teaching strategies that should be used to meet the needs of the learner who has a particular disability.

Sensory Deficits

Hearing Impairments
People with impaired hearing, both the deaf and the hard of hearing, have a complete loss or a reduction in their sensitivity to sounds. *Hearing impairment* is a term used to describe any type of

hearing loss, the etiology of which may be related to either conductive or sensorineural problems resulting from congenital defect, trauma, or disease. Currently about 10% of Americans have some degree of hearing loss, ranging from mild to profound, and approximately 1.8 million people in this country are deaf. For those who are deaf, "being a recipient of health care services is similar to being in a foreign country without fluency in the native language" (Harrison, 1990, p. 113). Regardless of the degree of hearing loss, any person with a hearing impairment faces communication barriers that interfere with efforts at patient teaching. Hearing loss poses a very real communication problem because deaf and hearing-impaired individuals may also be unable to speak or have limited verbal abilities and often have poor vocabularies. The average literacy skill of deaf adults is approximately at the fourth grade reading comprehension level. Their writing skills may also be weak. This low-level literacy, known as functional illiteracy, results from the fact that their primary language is not English but American Sign Language (ASL). Even though the incidence of literacy problems is significant within the hearing-impaired population, most of them are quite independent in carrying through with activities of daily living.

Individuals who are deaf will have different skills and needs depending on the type of deafness and how long they have been without a sense of hearing. For those individuals who have been deaf since birth, they will not have had the benefit of language acquisition and, therefore, may not possess understandable speech and often will have limited reading and vocabulary skills as well. Most likely, their primary modes of communication will be sign language and lipreading. If deafness has occurred after language has been acquired, they may speak quite understandably and have some facility with reading, writing, and lipreading. If deafness has occurred in later life, often caused by the process of aging, they will probably have poor lipreading ability, but their reading and writing skills should be within average range, depending on their educational and experiential background. If aging is the cause of hearing loss, visual impairments may also be a compounding factor. Because vision and hearing are two common sensory losses in the older adult, these deficits pose major communication problems when teaching older clients (Whitman et al., 1992).

Deaf and hearing-impaired persons, like other individuals, will require health care and health education information at various periods during their life. Although you as the nurse educator will encounter many differences among people who are deaf, there is one common denominator—they will always rely on their other senses for information input, especially their sense of sight. For patient education to be effective, then, communication must be visible. Because there are several different ways to communicate with a person who is deaf, one of the first things you need to do is ask your deaf client to identify communication preferences. Sign language, written information, lipreading, and visual aids are some of the common choices. It is true that one of the simplest ways to transfer information is through visible communication signals such as hand gestures and facial expressions; however, this method will not be adequate for any lengthy teaching sessions. The following modes of communication are suggested as ways to decrease the barriers of communication and facilitate teaching and learning for hearing-impaired patients in any setting in which you may practice:

Sign language: For most deaf people whose native language is ASL, sign language is often the preferred mode of communication. If you do not know ASL, you need to obtain the services of a professional interpreter. Sometimes a family member or friend of the patient skilled in signing also is willing and available to act as a translator during teaching sessions. However, prior to enlisting the assistance of an interpreter, always be certain to obtain the patient's permission because information communicated regarding health issues may be considered personal and private. If the information to be taught is confidential, it is advised that family or friends should not be enlisted as an interpreter. Hiring a certified language interpreter is often the best strategy. If a professional interpreter is requested by a deaf patient in a health facility receiving federal funds, it is required by federal law (Section 504 of the Rehabilitation Act of 1973, PL 93-112) that one be secured. If the patient cannot provide the names of interpreters, contact the Registry of Interpreters of the Deaf (RID) in your state. This registry will offer an up-to-date list of qualified sign language interpreters. When working with an interpreter, be sure to stand or sit next to the interpreter, talk at a normal pace, and look and talk directly to the deaf person when speaking. When considering the services of an interpreter, be certain that the deaf individual is the one who has made the choice.

Lipreading: One common misconception among hearing persons is that all deaf people can read lips. This is a potentially dangerous assumption (DiPietro, 1979). Only about forty percent of English sounds are visible on the lips. Therefore, only a skilled lip-reader will obtain any real benefit from this form of communication. If the individual can lip-read, it is not necessary to exaggerate your lip movements because this action will distort the movements of the lips and interfere with interpretation of your words. If lipreading is preferred, you must be sure to provide sufficient lighting on your face, remove all barriers from around your face such as gum, pencils, hands, and surgical masks. Beards, mustaches, and protruding teeth also present a challenge to the lip-reader. Because less than half of the English language is visible on the lips, supplement this form of communication with signing or written materials.

Written materials: Written information is probably the most reliable way to communicate, especially when understanding is critical. In fact, always write down the important information as a supplement to the spoken word even when the person is versed in lipreading. Written communication is the safest approach, even though it is time-consuming and sometimes stressful. Keeping in mind that the average reading comprehension of deaf adults is at the fourth grade level, be certain to provide printed patient education materials that match the readability level of your audience. When putting information in writing for your client who is deaf, keep the message as simple as possible. For instance, instead of writing, "When running a fever, take two aspirin," revise your message to read, "For a fever of 100.5°F or more, take two aspirin." Remember that a person with low reading skills often interprets words literally; therefore, the word *running* could be confusing because it is often used in

the context of someone who is "running to the store," for example (see the guidelines for writing or revising educational materials for low-literacy patients in Chapter 7). Visual aids such as simple pictures, drawings, diagrams, models, and the like are also very useful media as a supplement to increase understanding of written materials.

Verbalization by the client: Sometimes deaf clients will choose to communicate through speaking, especially if you have established a rapport and a trusting relationship with them. Often the tone and inflection of their voice will be different than normal speech, so you must give yourself time for listening carefully. Listen without interruptions until you become accustomed to the person's particular voice intonations and speech rhythms. If you still have trouble understanding what a client is saying, try writing down what you hear, which may help you to get the gist of the message.

Sound augmentation: For those patients who have a hearing loss but are not completely deaf, hearing aids are a useful device. Clients who have already been fitted for a hearing aid should be encouraged to use it, and you should be sure it is readily accessible, fitting properly, turned on, and the batteries in working order. If the client does not have a hearing aid, with permission of the patient and family you should make a referral to an auditory specialist, who can determine if this is an appropriate device for your patient. Another means by which sounds can be augmented is by cupping your hands around the client's ear or using a stethoscope in reverse, that is, the patient puts the stethoscope in his or her ears, and you talk into the bell of the instrument (Babcock & Miller, 1994). If the patient can hear better out of one ear than another, always stand or sit nearest to the side of the "good" ear. Be sure to slow your speech, provide adequate time for the patient to process your message and to respond, and avoid shouting.

Telecommunications: Telecommunication devices for the deaf (TDD) are an important resource for patient education. Television decoders for closed-caption programs are an important tool for further enhancing communication. Caption films for patient education also are available free of charge through Modern Talking Pictures and Services (see Appendix B). Under federal law, these devices are considered to be "reasonable accommodations" for deaf and hearing-impaired persons.

In summary, the following guidelines suggested by Navarro and Lacour (1980, p. 26) should be applied when using any of the aforementioned modes of communication:

- Be natural:
  - Don't be rigid and stiff or attempt to over-articulate your speech.
  - Use simple sentences.
  - Be sure to get the person's attention by a light touch on the arm before you start to talk.
  - Face the patient and stand no more than 6 feet from the patient when trying to communicate.
- Be considerate and refrain from
  - Talking and walking at the same time.
  - Bobbing your head excessively.
  - Talking with your mouth full or while chewing gum, etc.
  - Turning your face away from the deaf person while communicating.
  - Standing directly in front of a bright light, which may cast a shadow across your face, or glare directly into the patient's eyes.
  - Placing an IV in the hand the patient will need for sign language.

No matter what methods of communication for teaching you and your client decide to choose, it is important you confirm that your health messages have been received and understood. It is essential that patient comprehension is validated in a nonthreatening manner. It is not unusual in attempts to avoid embarrassing or offending one another, patients as well as health-care providers will acknowledge with a smile or a nod in response to what either one is trying to communicate when, in fact, the message is not understood at all. To ensure that the health education requirements of deaf or hearing-impaired patients are being met,

the nurse educator must find effective strategies to communicate the intended message clearly and precisely while at the same time demonstrating acceptance of individuals by making accommodations to suit their needs (Harrison, 1990). Patients who have lived with a hearing impairment for a while usually can tell you what modes of communication work best for them.

Visual Impairments

In the United States, a person is determined to be legally blind if vision is 20/200 or less in the better eye with correction or if visual field limits in both eyes are within 20 degrees diameter. People lose their vision and may be rendered legally blind for a variety of reasons: infections, accidents, poisoning, or congenital degeneration such as retinitis pigmentosa (Figure 9–1). Most recently, blindness in AIDS patients as a result of infection has been associated with the end stages of this disease. Also, visual impairment is common among older persons. According to the 1990 census, there are more than 2.5 million severely visually impaired individuals over the age of 65. The four leading eye diseases associated with the aging process are macular degeneration, cataracts, glaucoma, and diabetic retinopathy (Figure 9–1). Severe visual impairment after correction with glasses is defined as the inability to read newspaper print. Using this standard, studies of nursing home residents indicate that about 30% to 50% are considered to be visually impaired (Nelson, 1991).

If you suspect that patients are legally blind but have not been evaluated by a low-vision specialist, you should put them in contact with the local Blind Association. Patients may require assistance in negotiating the complex system of obtaining services from the local Commission for the Blind and Visually Handicapped (see Appendix B). Fortunately, there are many devices available to help legally blind persons maximize their remaining vision. Patients who are without sight most likely have had services and are familiar with what adaptations work best for them. However, depending on patients' situations and the circumstances under which you are teaching, you may want to further investigate their background to assure yourself that you are using the most appropriate format and tools for communicating with visually impaired clients.

Major diseases causing serious vision impairment that cannot be corrected with conventional spectacles or lenses are cataract, macular degeneration, glaucoma, and diabetic retinopathy. People who have advanced stages of these diseases have difficulty performing ordinary visual tasks, like reading.

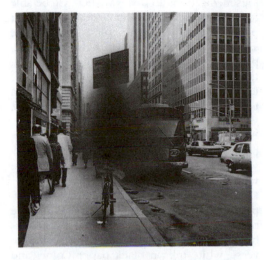

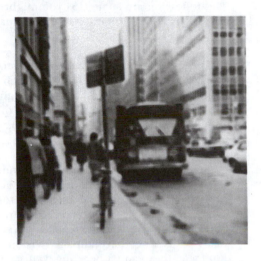

MACULAR DEGENERATION—The deterioration of the macula, the central area of the retina, results in an area of decreased central vision. Peripheral, or side, vision remains unaffected. This is the most prevalent eye disease.

CATARACT—An opacity of the lens results in diminished acuity but does not affect the field of vision. There are no blind spots, but the person's vision is hazy overall, particularly in glaring light.

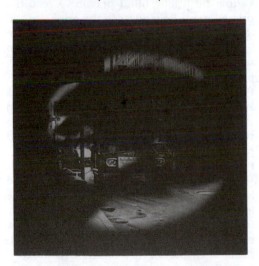

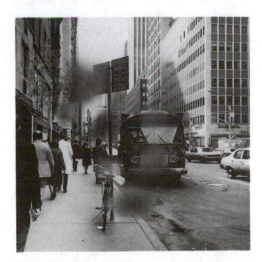

GLAUCOMA—Chronic elevated eye pressure in susceptible individuals may cause atrophy of the optic nerve and loss of peripheral vision. Early detection and close medical monitoring can help reduce complications.

DIABETIC RETINOPATHY—Leaking of retinal blood vessels in advanced or long-term diabetes can affect the macula or the entire retina and vitreous, producing blinding areas.

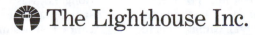 The Lighthouse Inc.

FIGURE 9–1.   Photo Essay on Partial Sight (Low Vision)

SOURCE: Reprinted courtesy of The Lighthouse Inc., New York, New York.

The following are some tips you might find helpful in caring for a blind or visually impaired patient:

- Secure the services of a low-vision specialist, who can prescribe optical devices such as a magnifying lens (with or without a light), a telescope, a closed-circuit TV, or a pair of sun shields, any of which will enable you to adapt your teaching material to meet the needs of your particular client.

- Persons who have long-standing blindness have learned to develop a heightened acuity of their other senses of hearing, taste, touch, and smell. Usually their listening skills are particularly acute, so avoid the tendency to shout. Just because they have impaired vision does not mean they cannot hear you well. Unlike a sighted person, the blind cannot attend to nonverbal cues such as hand gestures, facial expressions, and other body language. Before approaching a visually impaired person, always announce your presence, identify yourself, and explain clearly why you are there and what you are doing. Since their memory and recall also are better than most sighted persons, you can use this talent to maximize learning (Babcock & Miller, 1994). When conveying messages, rely on their auditory and tactile senses as a means to help them assimilate information from their environment.

- When explaining procedures, be as descriptive as possible. Expound on what you are doing, and explain any noises associated with treatments or the use of equipment. Allow the patient to touch, handle, and manipulate equipment (Whitman et al., 1992). Use the patient's sense of touch when you are in the process of teaching psychomotor skills as well as when the client is learning to return demonstrate.

- Because blind persons are unable to see shapes, sizes, and the placement of objects, again tactile learning is an important technique to use when teaching. For example, they can identify their medications by feeling the shape, size, and texture of tablets and capsules (Whitman et al., 1992). Gluing pills to the tops of bottle caps and putting medications in different sized or shaped containers will aid in blind persons' ability to identify various medications. In this way, they will be able to be more self-sufficient in following their prescribed regimens. Keeping items in the same place at all times will help them independently locate their belongings. Arranging things in front of them in a regular clockwise fashion will facilitate learning to perform a task that must be accomplished in an orderly, step-by-step manner.

- When using printed or handwritten materials, often enlarging the print (font size) or handwriting is an important first step for those who have diminished sight.

- Color is a key factor in whether a visually impaired person can distinguish objects. Be sure to assess on which medium your client sees better—black ink on white paper or the reverse, white ink on black paper. Colors and varying hues of color, other than black and white, are more difficult to discriminate by the older person with vision problems.

- Proper lighting is of utmost importance in assisting the legally blind person to read the printed word. Regardless of the print size and the color of the type and paper used, if the light is insufficient, the visually impaired person will have a great deal of difficulty reading print or working with objects.

- Providing contrast is a very helpful technique. For example, using a dark placemat with white dishes or serving black coffee in a white cup will allow persons with visual problems to better see items in front of them.

- Providing a template (writing guide) for signing their name or writing checks and addressing envelopes is a way to encourage independence.

- Large-print watches and clocks with either black or white backgrounds are available through the local chapter of the Blind Association.

- Audiotapes and cassette recorders are very useful tools. Today, many health education texts as well as other printed health information materials are available as "talking books" and can be obtained through the Library of Congress, Washington, D.C., or through your state library for the blind and visually handicapped. It is important to remember that these services are also available for people with other disabilities as well. Oral instruction can be audiotaped so that blind patients can listen to the information as often as they wish at another time and place. Repetition allows the opportunity for memorization to reinforce learning.

- The computer is a popular and useful tool for this population of learners. Although costly, there are computers that have synthetic speech as well as Braille keyboards.
- Most blind associations either have a Braille library or can direct you to appropriate resources for information written in Braille. If your client can read Braille and you have a large amount of printed material for patient education, local blind associations may Braille the materials so they can be used by the visually impaired learner.
- If you are assisting the person who is blind to ambulate, remember to always use the "sighted guide" technique, that is, allow the person to grasp your forearm while you walk about one-half step ahead of them. Another resource person to help with ambulation is an orientation and mobility instructor. These specialists are available in most school districts and the local Association for the Blind.

Diabetes education consumes a great deal of a nurse educator's teaching time because of the incidence of this disease in the American population. Diabetic retinopathy is a major cause of blindness, and thus, it is likely you will be teaching visually impaired diabetic patients who are also in need of diabetes education. This situation presents a unique challenge to the nurse. Persons who have lost their sight due to diabetic retinopathy probably have already mastered some of the necessary skills to care for themselves; however, it is also possible for visually impaired persons to be diagnosed at a later time with diabetes. In either case, at some point in the course of their lives, these persons will need to learn how to use appropriate adaptive equipment. In 1993, a task force, consisting of representatives from groups of diabetes educators and rehabilitation teachers for the blind, met and developed a document entitled *Adaptive Diabetes Education for Visually Impaired Persons* (ADEVIP). ADEVIP provides consistent practice guidelines for the care of diabetics who are visually handicapped. Fortunately, there also has been continuous improvement in the equipment used for self-monitoring of blood glucose levels. Available now are easy-to-use monitors with large display screens or voice instructions. Just as there are several devices for monitoring blood glucose levels, there also are available several different nonvisual adaptive devices for measuring insulin. It is evident that the teamwork between diabetes educators and rehabilitation specialists has led to the development of useful mechanisms that allow blind diabetic patients the opportunity to care for themselves and achieve both a successful medical and rehabilitation outcome (Baker, 1993).

Learning Disabilities

What exactly constitutes a learning disability has been the subject of a great deal of controversy over the years. Educators and psychologists have debated this very issue (Dykman et al., 1983; Kirk & Kirk, 1983; Knowles & Knowles, 1983; McLoughlin & Natick, 1983; Ysseldyke & Algozzine, 1983). In 1981, the National Joint Committee on Learning Disabilities defined *learning disabilities* as "a generic term that refers to a heterogeneous group of disorders manifested by significant difficulties in acquisition and use of listening, speaking, reading, writing, reasoning or mathematical abilities" (Hammill et al., 1981, p. 336). These disorders are intrinsic to the individual and presumed to be due to central nervous dysfunction (Kirk & Kirk, 1983). To date, this definition still stands as the accepted working definition for purposes of assessment, diagnosis, and categorization of an array of perceptual processing deficits. Other general terms for a learning disability are minimal brain dysfunction, attention deficit disorder (ADD), dyslexia, and hyperactivity.

An estimated 10% to 15% of the U.S. population in general is considered to be learning disabled, while approximately 6% to 10% of school-aged children are diagnosed with a learning disability, and an additional 20% have some degree of learning disability (Greenberg, 1991). In the past, a learning disability was thought to be a problem only involving children. However, evidence supports the belief that most individuals do not "outgrow" the problem. The rate of learning disabilities in adults is probably similar to the rate in children. Astin et al. (1988) discovered that 6% of all college freshmen were reported as having at least one learning disability, twice the rate in the previous 10 years. The majority of people with learning disabilities have language and/or memory deficits. If you compound their problem with the stresses and anxieties caused by illness and subsequent hospitalization or the pressures of having to perform in an academic setting, you can be assured they find themselves in a situation that is not at all conducive to learning.

Individuals with learning disabilities appear normal and have been found to have at least average if not superior (gifted) intelligence. Some very famous and successful people in the history of our world have been thought to have had a learning disability—Leonardo daVinci, Woodrow Wilson, George Patton, Winston Churchill, Nelson Rockefeller, and Albert Einstein. Even though there is a large discrepancy between a learning disabled person's intellectual abilities and their performance levels, those who exhibit this discrepancy are not necessarily learning disabled. Table 9–1 lists common myths and corresponding facts about learning disabilities. Learning disabilities are not caused by retardation, emotional disturbances, physical impairments (blindness or deafness), or environmental deprivation such as lack of educational opportunity or cultural diversity (Greenberg, 1991).

The factors that may affect learning in a learning disabled person are memory, language, motor, and integrative processing disabilities. These factors fall under two general headings: "input" and "output" disabilities. *Input disabilities,* which refer to the process of receiving and recording information in the brain, include visual perceptual, auditory perceptual, integrative processing, and memory disorders. *Output disabilities,* which refer to the process of orally responding and performing physical tasks, include language and motor disorders. Although these problems and their associated characteristics are frequently in reference to disabled children in particular, many of the characteristics of these problems can apply as well to an older person who has not been diagnosed as learning disabled until later in adulthood. It is important to remember that a learning disabled individual can experience one type of learning disability or a combination thereof. Greenberg (1991) outlines the following characteristics of these learning disability problems and the teaching strategies useful in assisting the learning disabled to acquire behaviors required for autonomy in self-care.

TABLE 9–1. Myths and facts

Myth: Children are labeled "learning disabled" because they can't learn.

Fact: They can learn, but their preferred learning modality must be identified.

Myth: Children who have a learning disability must be spoken to more slowly.

Fact: Actually, those who learn auditorily may become impatient with slower speech and stop listening; those who learn visually would benefit more from seeing the information.

Myth: Children who are learning disabled just have to try harder.

Fact: Telling these children to try harder is a turnoff. They already do try hard.

Myth: Children outgrow their disabilities.

Fact: Children do not outgrow their disabilities. They develop strategies to compensate for and minimize their disabilities.

Myth: Children with learning disabilities should be treated like everyone else.

Fact: That treatment would be unfair; they would not get what they need.

Myth: Nearly all children with a learning disability are boys.

Fact: Boys are more often referred for proper identification of learning disabilities because they are more overt in acting out their frustrations.

SOURCE: Copyright 1991 The American Journal of Nursing Company. Reprinted from *MCN: American Journal of Maternal Child Nursing,* Sept/Oct, 1991, Vol. 16, No. 5. Used with permission. All rights reserved.

Input Disabilities

Visual perceptual disorders   This type of disability results in an inability to read or difficulty with reading (dyslexia). Letters of the alphabet may be seen in reverse or rotated order, for example, *d* is *b* and *p* is *q* or *g*. Letters also may be confused with one another such as *was* being perceived as *saw*. In addition, the individual may have trouble focusing on a particular word or group of words. There may be a "figure ground" problem, too, such that the person is unable to attend to a specific object within a group of objects, such as finding a cup of juice on a food tray. Furthermore, judging distances or positions in space or dealing with special relationships may prove difficult, resulting in the person's bumping into things, being confused about left hand–right hand or up and down, or being unable to throw a ball or do a puzzle.

People with visual perceptual deficits tend to be auditory learners. Visual stimulation should be kept to a minimum. Visual materials such as pamphlets or books are ineffective unless the content is explained orally or the information is read aloud. If visual items are used, only one item should be given at any one time with a sufficient period in between times to allow for the information to be focused on and mastered. Since those with visual perceptual deficits usually learn best through hearing, using records and audiotapes (with or without earphones) and verbal instruction are keys in helping them learn. Recall and retention of information can be assessed by oral questioning, allowing learners to express back to you in oral form what they understand and remember about the content that has been presented.

Auditory perceptual disorders   This type of disability is characterized by the inability to distinguish subtle differences in sounds, for example, "blue" and "blow" or "ball" and "bell." There also may be a problem with auditory "figure ground" such that sounds of someone speaking cannot be identified clearly when others are speaking in the same room. Auditory "lags" also may occur whereby sound input cannot be processed at a normal rate. Parts of conversations may be missed unless one speaks at a speed that allows the disabled person time to process the information. During instruction, it is important to limit the noise level and eliminate distractions in the background. Using as few words as possible and repeating them when necessary (using the same words to avoid confusion) are a useful strategy. Direct eye contact helps keep the learner focused on the task at hand. Visual teaching methods such as demonstration–return demonstration, gaming (e.g., puppetry), modeling, and role-playing as well as visual instructional tools such as written materials, pictures, charts, films, books, puzzles, printed handouts, and the computer are the best ways to communicate information. Using hand signs for key words when giving verbal instructions and allowing the learner hands-on experiences and opportunities for observation are useful techniques. Directions for learning via these methods and tools should be in written form. The visual learner may intently watch your face for the formation of words, expressions, eye movements, and hand gestures. Awareness to these details may have developed as a compensatory strategy to aid comprehension. If the learner does not understand something being taught, frustration exhibited by irritability and inattentiveness may be demonstrated.

Individuals with either visual or auditory perceptual problems often rely on tactile learning as well. They enjoy doing things with their hands, want to touch everything, prefer writing and drawing, engage in physical exploration, and enjoy physical movement through sports activities.

Integrative processing disorders   Recording information in the brain requires that the information be organized and processed if it is to be used correctly. An inability to sequence or abstract visual, auditory, or tactile stimuli is characteristic of this type of disability. A child who has difficulty sequencing information may read and understand the word *dog* as *god* because the letters *d, o,* and *g* are processed in the incorrect order. Thought sequencing also may progress from the middle to the end rather than normally starting at the beginning. On the other hand, abstraction is the inability to infer meaning from words or phrases; that is, the specific intended meaning of words or thoughts is misunderstood. For example, a person who has difficulty with abstractions may interpret "window shopping" or "blowing smoke" in the literal rather than the figurative sense. Those with an integrative processing disability need specific explanations, and you should avoid using confusing phrases, puns, or sarcasm. Frequently ask the person to repeat or demonstrate what was learned to immediately clear up any misconceptions.

Short- or long-term memory disorders   Once information is recorded and integrated in the brain, it must be stored and ready for retrieval. Normally, most people can retrieve information fairly quickly and without much effort from either their short-term or long-term memories. Short-term memory refers to information that is remembered as long as one is attending to it, for example, being able to remember what you have been told recently or taking a telephone order and then being able to write it down completely shortly after you have hung up the phone. Long-term memory consists of information that has been repeated and stored and becomes available whenever you think about it, such as being able to remember someone's telephone number (or your own for that matter) over a long period of time. For those with short-term memory deficits, they may be unable to recall what they learned an hour before, but they may be able to recall the information at a later point in time. People with both short- and long-term memory disabilities need brief, frequent, repetitive teaching sessions for constant reinforcement of information.

Output Disabilities

Language disorders   There are two types of oral language—spontaneous (initiating a conversation) and demand (asking a question). With spontaneous language, persons select a topic, organize their thoughts, and choose the correct words to orally express themselves. Demand language is when someone else starts a conversation and poses questions for another person to answer. For persons with either type of language disability, the greatest gift you can give them is time—time to process internal thoughts, to find words, and then to speak for the purpose of initiating a conversation or responding with answers to questions. In response to demand language, the language disabled person may panic and answer, "Huh?" or "What?" or "I don't know." If you detect this response pattern, allowing sufficient time either to process the information received or to formulate a response will reduce barriers to communication as a result of anxiety and frustration. Although there is no one way to ensure results, the following are some adaptive techniques:

- Provide information on tape, or give a student the option of taking the test orally with a tape recorder.
- Use hand signs for key words when giving verbal directions.
- Use hands-on experience or observation.
- Highlight important information.
- Use a computer.
- Capitalize on teachable moments.
- Use puzzles.

- Appeal to all senses—auditory, visual, and tactile.
- Use mnemonics (Table 9–2).
- Use a cognitive map (Figure 9–2).
- Use an active reading strategy such as SQ3R (skim, question, read, rehearse, revise).

Motor disorders   Learning psychomotor tasks will be difficult if the individual has problems with performing gross and fine motor tasks. Often people with this type of disability will avoid such tasks because of inadequate motor skills. For example, they will shy away from using writing as a form of communication because it requires fine motor coordination to accomplish. Instead of forcing them to handwrite, using a tape recorder to allow them to demonstrate their knowledge of information is a good substitute. Depending on the disabled person's auditory and visual strengths, computers, typewriters, and preprinted materials may prove helpful tools for teaching and learning. Safety also is always a concern for those with gross motor difficulties because they are prone to clumsiness, stumbling, or falling. The environment should be kept as uncluttered as possible to avoid injury and embarrassment.

Attention Deficit Disorder

The ability to pay attention is an important prerequisite to success in school and work. Any difficulty with attending skills can have an adverse affect on learning. The American Psychiatric Association holds that *attention deficit disorder* is an appropriate term to use because in these persons difficulties are prominent and almost always present. Three major subtypes of ADD are attention deficit disorder with hyperactivity (ADDH), attention deficit disorder without hyperactivity (ADDNOH),

---

TABLE 9–2. Mnemonics

P	artner
R	esponsible
E	nthusiastic
C	oach
E	valuation
P	atience
T	eacher
O	pen minded
R	ole model

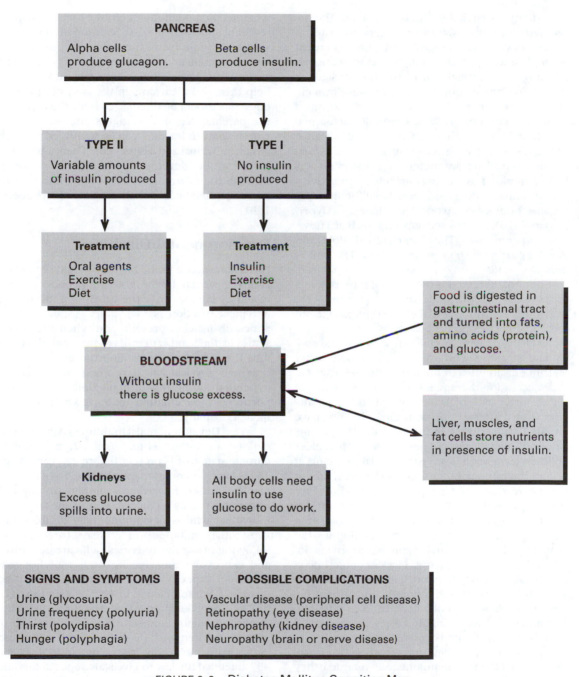

FIGURE 9–2. Diabetes Mellitus Cognitive Map

and attention deficit disorder, residual type. The onset of ADD is before the age of 7 years. Estimates of the presence of ADD range from 1.2 to 2.0 percent of all school-aged children. The exact cause is unknown. The primary characteristics are signs of inattention and impulsivity that are developmentally inappropriate. The child often fails to finish projects, seems not to listen, is easily distracted, and has difficulty concentrating. Other thoughts, sights, or sounds keep getting in their way, especially when the task is difficult or uninteresting. The child acts before thinking, switches from activity to activity, requires much supervision, and has difficulty with organization of time, work, and belongings. Hyperactivity (ADDH) often accompanies the inattentiveness and impulsivity. The older child and adolescent may be extremely restless and fidgety. The child's behavior tends to be haphazard, poorly organized, and not goal directed. ADD residual type is sometimes used to identify older adolescents who were previously identified as ADDH at a younger age but who no longer exhibit hyperactivity.

ADD is present in children with average ability and in those who are gifted. ADD and other learning disabilities frequently occur together. Often, medication therapy is the treatment of choice for children with ADD. Before embarking on any educational intervention with these children, have an open discussion with the child and the parents to determine what works best for them. Most older children have been involved in special programs at school that, among other things, help the child use specific learning strategies consistently, which is of primary importance. Provide new information in a quiet environment. For example, that may often mean using another place for the teaching session than the child's hospital room. When giving instructions or assigning a task, give directions one at a time, and divide the work into small parts. Reward achievement, and ignore inappropriate behavior. Eliminate as much distraction as possible. Encourage the older child to keep a notebook and to write the instructions down.

In summary, it is important to stress that learning disabled people are not mentally retarded; they just learn differently. They may have one or more disabilities ranging from mild to severe. The challenge is to determine how the client learns best and then to adapt your teaching strategies to meet their preferred style of learning—auditory, visual, or tactile. The most reliable way to determine what accommodations need to be made in your teaching approach is to ask learning disabled individuals about problems they encounter in processing information and what they find to be the most appropriate instructional methods and tools to help them with learning. In the case of children, questions should be directed to both the child and the parents. Persons' strengths and weaknesses with respect to learning can be identified through direct, individualized assessment. Then, a teaching plan can be developed to promote learning through use of strategies that compensate for or minimize the effect of their disability (Greenberg, 1991).

Developmental Disability

Parental response to the birth of a child with a disability is similar to the grieving process experienced by families after the death of a loved one. A typical reaction is, "Why me?" (Fraley, 1992). Shock or disbelief prevails, and when the reality settles in, the family attempts to integrate the child into the family structure. Enormous amounts of time and physical and psychological energy are expended during this difficult time. A large proportion of these children are born with a developmental disability.

The Developmental Disabilities Act of 1978 defined a *developmental disability* as a severe chronic state that is present before 22 years of age and is likely to continue indefinitely. The disability may be caused by either a mental or physical impairment or by a combination of the two. The individual who is developmentally disabled has substantial limitations in at least three of the following major life activities: self-care, receptive and expressive language learning, mobility, self-direction, capacity for independent living, and economic self-sufficiency. In 1975, Public Law (PL) 94-142, the Education of all Handicapped Children's Act, established state grant money to provide all children with disabilities with a free and appropriate public education. Then in 1986, PL 99-457 amended the law to give states special funding for educating all eligible preschool children with disabilities, ages 3 through 5, to help states develop early intervention programs for infants and toddlers (birth through age 2), and to require states to use qualified providers of special education and related services. In 1990, PL 101-476 made additional changes to the law, including a name change to Individuals with Disabilities Education Act, or IDEA. Under Part B of IDEA, all eligible preschool and school-aged children and youths with disabilities are entitled to receive a free and appropriate education, including special education and related services. According to the Fifteenth Annual Report to Congress (U.S. Department of Education, 1993), nearly 5 million children received services under IDEA. The manner in which the mentally retarded are provided services has gone through transformation in much the same way as the care of the mentally ill. Mandated early intervention and inclusion have increased the presence of the children and young adults in all facets of society, including hospitals and outpatient clinics. Many nurses are limited in their ability to provide holistic care for this population. Most nursing staff lack prior experience and often feel uncomfortable caring for these children. This becomes acute when the nurse is faced with trying to help the child understand particular treatments or tasks. Especially because the real experts in caring and working with these children are their parents, it is a wise nurse who invites the parents to participate and assist the nursing staff during their child's hospitalization. However caution should prevail, as the hospitalization may be their only respite from an arduous care schedule.

When planning a teaching intervention, keep in mind the client's developmental stage, not their chronological age. If the child does not communicate verbally, the nurse should note if there are certain nonverbal cues, like gestures, signing, or other symbols that are used for communication purposes. Most mentally retarded children are incapable of abstract thinking. Most can comprehend simple explanations, but concrete examples must be given. For example, instead of saying, "Lunch will be here in a few minutes," show a clock and point to the time. For children scheduled to have surgery, giving them a surgical mask to play with will help dispel fears they may have when entering the operating room. Remember that facial expression and voice tone are more important than words spoken. Be sure the family explains any nonverbal cues for a yes or no response, and then try to ask questions in a manner requiring a yes or no answer. Lavish any positive behavior with great praise. Keep the information simple, concrete, and repetitive. Be consistent, but firm, setting appropri-

ate limits. Be careful not to dominate any teaching session, but let the children actively participate and have a sense of accomplishment. Assign simple tasks with simple directions. Show what is to be done, rather than relying on verbal commands. Give only one direction at a time. A reward system works very well. Stickers with familiar childhood characters placed on their bed or pajamas remind the child of a job well done. "Children with developmental deviations have the potential for greater variability in their responses to hospitalization than their unaffected peers" (Vessey, 1988, p. 54).

Mental Illness

Until about 1886, the mentally ill were restrained in iron manacles. With the advent of pharmacotherapy in the 1950s, the life of a person with a mental illness began to change. The discovery of the various neuroleptic and antidepressant drugs was a major contribution to the improved quality of life for the mentally ill. Previously dependent clients were now able to live outside of an institution. For the last 25 years, the care of the mentally ill has been moving into the community health centers, and clients are spending less time confined to a mental health facility and more time in the community, at work, home, and play. In spite of all the great strides made in the treatment of mental illness, the mentally ill person still faces the problems of stigma. Nurse educators may need to explore teaching strategies that have been successful in the field of mental health. Education programs for the mentally ill are few and far between. Their needs for learning are great but they are often not given the same opportunities for educational programs as those persons with physical disabilities.

Although the obstacles appear overwhelming, recent research has demonstrated the value of a family psychoeducational approach (Fowler, 1993). This approach has made a significant impact on chronically mentally ill patients and their families by providing support, information, and management strategies. In 1988, Goldman and Quinn defined *psychoeducation* as "the education or training of a person with a psychiatric disorder in subject areas that serve the goal of treatment and rehabilitation." MacFarlane (1983) reports a number of studies that have supported the value of family psychoeducation. These programs have been successful in helping patients and their families manage their illness without frequent hospitalizations. Patients and families are provided with information as well as support and management strategies. It is not unreasonable to expect similar success when a nurse needs to provide information on other health promotion or disease prevention topics. In at least two other situations (Harmon & Tratnack, 1992; Goldman & Quinn, 1988), a family psychoeducation program was implemented using both a structured and experiential approach. In both programs, the "students" were diagnosed with a chronic mental illness. The patient education programs were deemed successful when the participants and their caregivers reported a significant increase in knowledge of the illness and of resources available. Although these studies were concerned with improving the overall treatment of mental illness, particularly schizophrenia, they may be applicable in other teaching situations. As previously noted, this population is living in the community, and it is likely you may find your next hospitalized patient requiring information regarding a physical illness, like diabetes or myocardial infarction.

Harmon and Tratnack (1992) offered the following suggestions when designing a psychiatric patient education program (adaptations may be needed depending on the setting):

- Use a didactic method. Convey the information in a nonthreatening, nonconfrontational manner. Length of lecture must be adjusted to the participants. These authors found 30 minutes to be the patient's limit of concentration.
- Use various teaching methods to reinforce and hold the person's interest, such as flip charts, blackboards, handouts, and checklists.
- Explain in plain English in a way that is compatible with the client's background, excluding jargon.
- Use good humor.
- Provide break times. After every 30 minutes of lecture, a 15-minute break was provided. This is a good time to practice a skill in a very informal manner.
- Recognize the importance of the setting. "Breaks" should be in a separate lounge area.

Motivating the patient with a chronic mental illness can be challenging. A certificate of recognition was given to each patient who completed this program, which proved to be a powerful motivator. They also used a point system. Psychiatric patient education is currently in the process of becoming a standard part of the milieu. It is clear that the family psychoeducational model has had a positive effect on the quality of life of the chronically mentally ill by providing useful information. Independence and self-management remain a goal for this special population, as with all others. Therefore, the nurse as educator will need to consider the strategies from all specialties to meet the challenge of teaching the person with a mental illness.

Physical Disabilities

Spinal Cord Injury

One of the major physical disabilities afflicting our population is spinal cord injury. The spinal cord–injured population has benefited directly from our advanced technologies. Not only are people surviving, they are living a greatly improved quality of life. Before 1945, the survival prognosis for people with paraplegia or quadriplegia was very poor (Zejdlik, 1992). By the 1970s, there were regional spinal cord injury centers established across the country. With more sophisticated techniques and equipment came improved mobility, less complications, and better restoration of musculoskeletal functions (Norris et al., 1982). Residual impairment from spinal cord injury affects all areas of life—physical, social, psychological, vocational, and spiritual. Typically, spinal cord–injured persons are males between the ages of 15 and 30 years old (Stover & Fine, 1986).

Spinal cord injury is sudden and devastating, both to the person and the family. The adjustment is difficult and continuous. During the rehabilitation phase of the hospitalization, all interventions are driven by the goal of independent living. As mentioned, spinal cord injuries occur most frequently in young adult males. Normally, this is a difficult stage of development, and families are already struggling with the young adult's need for independence. Very often when the person is ready for discharge, the home environment is unstable, as the family is also attempting to readjust to the disability. It is quite possible the family may be at a different phase of adjustment. At the same time, both the disabled person and the family are faced with the task of redefining roles. Fink (1967), a psychologist, described four sequential phases of recovery: shock, defensive retreat, acknowledgment, and adaptation. With the shortened lengths of stay for both the critical and the rehabilitation phase of hospitalization, the newly injured person and the family have less time to reach the adaptation phase. Many families will share that the adjustment is ongoing, with new challenges greeting them everyday. Initially, most spinal cord injury centers provide comprehensive rehabilitation. However, the skills required to maintain physical equilibrium are many. Often the quantity of information is overwhelming, and the spinal cord–injured persons find themselves plagued with frequent hospital readmissions. The most common problems are urinary tract infections and skin breakdown. Very often the knowledge is there, but it is just a matter of individualizing the approach to make it fit the person's lifestyle.

Much of the rehabilitation as it relates to patients' functional living is actually done by trial and error. It is wise to remember that most teenagers' concerns center on their friends, especially the boyfriend or girlfriend. So even if they are taught something, it is possible they will be unable to focus on the extensive information being offered. Before developing strategies that allow learners to bypass the disability, the nurse must consider some common obstacles. These might be within or related to the learner's ability to participate in the learning process. In this circumstance, learner readiness is important. Readiness is the learner's ability in terms of physical and mental development. Readiness in both respects is necessary for effective teaching (Lubkin, 1995; Haggard, 1989). As most nurses know, presenting important health-related information is only half the challenge. The other half is patients' ability to accept and use the information to change or improve their health status. Denial is the most frequent obstacle to learning readiness in the young spinal cord–injured male. Although the object of this denial is often the bowel program, it frequently reappears whenever the task seems overwhelming. Although denial may be an effective coping mechanism, it can also interfere with learning readiness.

Another obstacle to learning readiness is the lack of physical endurance. This may be especially apparent in the older client. In this situation, it may be prudent to involve a friend or family member to ensure a relief person will be able to take over when the client's energy level is inadequate. In her work with rehabilitation patients, Jacque L. Vance (1992) cited secondary gains of retained behaviors or attitudes as an obstacle to learning readiness. Seen frequently when the learning leads to role changes related to dependence or independence, in this situation either clients or caregivers may view new information as a threat to their role as patient or caregiver. For example, it is now possible for a person with quadriplegia to drive. If the client has been transported by a good friend for several years, the friend may view this new independence as a serious threat to his or her role as caregiver. It would be imperative for the nurse to deal with this issue from the beginning and if warranted refer both for counseling. Lack of readiness will occur when any physical or emotional limitations are present. A nursing diagnosis of noncompliance would be inappropriate when the underlying etiology is learner readiness. Before the teaching plan is implemented, every attempt should be made to determine the client's readiness to learn.

All too often the need for sharing is overlooked. Patients and their families need to have a positive vision of the future, and feelings of isolation are quick to overcome them. One of the ways to remedy this problem is by using the group approach to teaching, whereby recovered spinal cord–injured persons are included in some of the teaching sessions. In this way, newly injured persons benefit from the "trials and errors" of those who have gone before them. It is critical to understand that significant others and children need support throughout this experience too. Everyone has to work through the injury at their own pace. It is imperative that at whatever juncture the nurse encounters a person with a spinal cord injury, a careful assessment of the patient's learning readiness be carried out first. Next the family and, most important, the immediate caregiver, who may or may not be a family member, must be involved. With the appropriate support and knowledge, the client and family will be successful in learning and maintaining independence.

Brain Injury
A fall, car accident, gunshot wound, or a blow to the head are just a few examples of potential

causes of traumatic brain injury. There are more than two million traumatic brain injuries (TBI) per year in the United States; 500,000 of them are serious enough to require hospital admission (Interagency Head-Injured Task Force, 1989). *Closed head injury* refers to nonpenetrating injury. *Open head injury* refers to penetrating injury resulting in brain tissue exposure and disruption of normal protective barriers. Most of this population, aged 15 to 24 years, were previously healthy and active young people. Often, these persons suffer from behavior and personality changes, as well as an impairment in cognitive ability. "Disturbances in learning and memory, rate of information processing, and adaptive or executive functions are common cognitive sequelae" (Tate et al., 1991, p. 117). There is also a growing number of older individuals surviving a closed head injury. The same or similar cognitive deficits also afflict this population. The amount of deficits usually depends on the severity and location of the injury. Cognitive impairments may include poor attention span, slowness in thinking, confusion, difficulty with short-term and long-term memory, distractibility, impulsive and socially inappropriate behaviors, poor judgment, and mental fatigue, as well as difficulty with organization and problem solving. Difficulty in the area of reading and writing may also be present. In addition, the person may have acquired a hearing loss. As might be expected, communication will more than likely be an issue.

The treatment of people with severe brain injury is most often divided into three stages: (1) acute care (in an intensive care unit), (2) acute rehabilitation (in an inpatient brain-injured rehabilitation unit), and (3) long-term rehabilitation after discharge (at home or in a long-term care facility). At every stage, there are many hurdles to conquer. Once the person's life is assured and the physical condition improves, the patient is discharged from the acute care unit. It is at this point someone not familiar with traumatic brain injuries might wonder why a person who looks healthy and independent still needs rehabilitation. This is why from the very beginning families need to be kept up to date on their loved one's prognosis. Throughout the rehabilitation process, family teaching must be consistent and thoughtful, as most of the residual impairments are not visible, with the exception of the sensorimotor deficits. The communication, cognitive-perceptual, and behavioral changes may

be dramatic. "The combined effects of these multiple deficits following a TBI create tremendous psychosocial consequences for patients and their families. Especially in the early stages of the injury, patients are not able to handle normal routine social situations" (Grinspun, 1987, p. 63). However, the most difficult area for the family is the fact that their family member will probably never be the same person again. In fact, the personality change presents the biggest burden for the family. Studies have shown that the level of the family stress is directly related to personality changes and the relative's own perception of the symptoms arising from the head injury (Grinspun, 1987).

Although most of the literature deals with the importance of family inclusion during the rehabilitation period, it is clear that brain-injured persons will always need the involvement of their family. Again, this is an area where the benefits of participation in family groups is immeasurable. Considerable strength is gained from group participation, and learning is accomplished because of a friendly, informal approach. Learning needs for this population center on the issue of client safety and family coping. Safety issues are related to cognitive and behavioral capabilities. Families are faced with a life-changing event and will always require ongoing support and encouragement to take care of themselves. Of particular importance for brain-injured persons and their friends and family is the need for unconditional acceptance.

Recovery may take several years, and most often the person is left with some form of impairment. Tate et al. (1991) reported a frequency of 70% for each of the symptoms of personality change, slowness, and poor memory in the head-injured population. Table 9–3 lists some "dos" and "don'ts" for effective teaching of the person with a brain injury.

Communication Disorders

"Communication is a universal process by which human beings exchange ideas, impart feelings and express needs" (Adkins, 1991, p. 74). Communication occurs in a variety of ways, including drama, music, literature, and art. It is verbal and nonverbal, and there is a sending and receiving component. Stroke, or cerebrovascular accident, is the most common cause of impaired communication. As is true with the many other disabilities discussed in

TABLE 9–3. Guidelines for effective teaching of the brain-injured patient

Do	*Don't*
Use simple rather than complex statements	Stop talking or trying to communicate
Use gestures to complement what you are saying	Speak too fast
Give step-by-step directions	Talk down to the person
Allow time for responses	Talk in the person's presence as though he or she is not there
Recognize and praise all efforts to communicate	Give up (instead seek the assistance of a speech-language pathologist)
Ensure the use of listening devices	
Keep written instructions simple, with a small amount of information on each page	

this chapter, a stroke is a major crisis for both the person and the family. Many of the strategies discussed under the heading of spinal cord injury are applicable to an educational program for the person with a stroke. This discussion will cover some useful strategies appropriate for working with a person with impaired communication such as aphasia.

Strokes are a major cause of impaired communication. Each year 150 to 200 per 100,000 Americans suffer a stroke (McCourt, 1993). It is a more common occurrence in older adult men and in the black population. Perceptual deficits such as neglect and denial as well as spatial disturbances may also affect a person's ability to communicate (Olson, 1991). One of the most common residual deficits of a stroke is a problem with language. Language is not only speaking but also involves conveying and comprehending thoughts and ideas, as well as understanding and using symbols sequentially and grammatically (Boss, 1986). Aphasia is a communication problem, either with speaking, writing, or understanding. *Aphasia* may be defined as a multiple modality loss of language ability, usually caused by damage to the dominant hemisphere (Adkins, 1991). When you prepare to work with someone with aphasia, it is necessary to determine which type of aphasia—expressive or receptive—is present. If your involvement with the client is during the early stage, the speech therapist would be a good teammate.

The function of language primarily resides in the left hemisphere of the brain. Expressive aphasia occurs when there is an injury to the inferior frontal gyrus, just anterior to the facial and lingual areas of the motor cortex, known as Broca's area (Table 9–4). Most often when the injury is to the

dominant cerebral hemisphere (usually the left), the result is expressive aphasia. About 97% of the population has a dominant left hemisphere. Because Broca's area is so near the left motor area, the stroke leaves the person with right-sided paralysis. Wernicke's area of the brain (Table 9–4) is located in the temporal lobe and is needed for auditory and reading comprehension. When this area is affected, persons are left with receptive aphasia. Although their hearing is unimpaired, they are still unable to understand the significance of the spoken word. It is important to remember that although these persons are unable to communicate verbally, it does not mean there are intellectual impairments. The inability to communicate verbally is one of the most frustrating experiences. Speech therapy should be one of the earliest interventions, and the nurse will need to incorporate those strategies into the teaching-learning plan. Every effort must be made to establish communication at some level. Remember, regardless of how severe the communication deficit, it is almost always possible to have stroke patients communicate within their own environment in some manner and to some extent.

Encouragement and explanation will go a long way in ensuring client participation and recovery. Keep your teaching sessions filled with praise, and always acknowledge the client's frustration. Keep distractions to a minimum. Be sure the radio and television are turned off so you have the full attention of the client. Always have one person speak at a time. Speak slowly, and be sure to stand where the client is able to see your face (Norman & Baratz, 1979). In teaching people with aphasia, it is easy to overestimate their understanding of speech. Often they will smile and agree when they

TABLE 9–4. Clinical features of aphasia

Type	Involved Anatomy	Expression	Auditory Comprehension	Written Comprehension	Naming	Word/Phrase Repetition	Ability to Write
Broca's (motor, expressive)	Precentral gyrus, Broca's area	Nonfluent, telegraphic, may be mute	Subtle deficits	Subtle deficits	Impaired	Impaired	Impaired
Wernicke's (receptive, sensory)	Superior temporal gyrus	Fluent but content inappropriate	Impaired	Impaired	Severely impaired	Impaired	Impaired
Global (mixed)	Frontal-temporal area	Nonfluent	Severely impaired	Impaired	Severely impaired	Impaired	Severely impaired
Conductive (central)	Arcuate fasciculus	Fluent	Intact	Intact	Impaired	Severely impaired	Impaired
Anomic (amnesic)	Angular gyrus	Fluent	Intact	Intact	Severely impaired	Intact	Subtle deficits
Transcortical sensory (TCSA)	Periphery of Broca's and Wernicke's areas (watershed zone)	Fluent	Impaired	Impaired	Impaired	Intact	Severely impaired
Transcortical motor (TCMA)	Anterior, superior, or lateral to Broca's area	Nonfluent, speech initiation difficult	Intact	Subtle deficits	Impaired	Intact	Impaired

SOURCE: Reprinted by permission from Schofield Bronstein, Judith M. Popvich, and Christina Stewart-Amidei, *Promoting Stroke Recovery: A Research-Based Approach for Nursing*, Table 11-1. St. Louis: Mosby-Year Book, 1991.

are only understanding about half of the message. Providing enough time and constantly checking to be sure the message is understood without chastising the client is the challenge. Blanco (1982, p. 34) suggests the following general guidelines:

- Don't use baby talk.
- Speak in normal tones.
- Speak in short, slow, simple sentences.
- Allow the person time to answer.

Be patient, slow the person's response down, and involve the family. While working with a person with this type of language deficit, the nurse should also be aware that it may extend into the reading modality. Little is known about this disability or how many stroke patients suffer from the inability to read. In a reported study carried out by Loughrey (1992), a small group of patients with aphasia were able to improve their reading ability. Two methods of reteaching reading were utilized. A multisensory technique as well as a visual-verbal technique was implemented; both were successful in improving the subject's ability to recognize and use their newly acquired words. Although teaching reading is not a usual nursing responsibility, the nurse educator may choose to encourage the family to try and help their loved one relearn reading using these promising techniques.

Expressive Aphasia

In the event structured speech therapy is not available, the nursing staff will need to develop their own plan of care. When working with expressive aphasia, you might try having the person recall word images, first by naming commonly used objects (e.g., spoons, knives, forks) and then those objects in his immediate environment (e.g., bed, table). Another strategy is having the person repeat words spoken by the nurse. It is wise to begin with simple terms and work progressively to the more complex. These exercises may be carried out frequently during the day, keeping the sessions short. Most people tire when sessions are longer than 30 minutes. Often their speech will become slurred, and they will experience mental fatigue. In a following section you will find some helpful information regarding adaptive computing. People with expressive aphasia will find computers a wonderful tool to assist in their efforts to communicate.

Receptive Aphasia

When working with someone with receptive aphasia, you need to establish a means for nonverbal communication. Usually the tone of voice, facial expressions, gestures, and even pantomime will be effective in conveying a message. Most often, these persons are unaware of their impairment and will speak in what sounds like a correct statement, but on examination the words do not make sense. Speak slower and slightly louder to the person with receptive aphasia, as auditory stimulation seems to be effective. When comprehension and memory span increase, the person will begin to respond appropriately. Aphasic persons also have trouble with retention and recall. It seems old personal memories return first and recent events take longer to reappear.

"It is a lonely, isolated world for those who cannot communicate with other human beings" (Jennings, 1981, p. 39). As we attempt to work with and engage in a teaching-learning intervention, we must be aware of our own attitudes. The effort to communicate with someone without our usual speech and language is one of the more frustrating experiences. Be sure to take time out and reflect on the rewards of assisting the client and family in overcoming this barrier.

Dysarthria

Many people with degenerative disorders, such as Parkinson's disease, multiple sclerosis, and myasthenia gravis also have dysarthria. *Dysarthria* is a problem with the voluntary muscle control of speech. It is the consequence of damage to the central or peripheral nervous system and affects the same muscles used in eating and speaking. The result is unintelligible speech. "The degree of unintelligibility will be directly related to the severity of the dysarthria" (Dreher, 1981, p. 347). There are several types of dysarthria. It can be flaccid, spastic, ataxic, hypokinetic, or mixed. The difference in symptoms for each depends not on the underlying disease but on the site in the nervous system that the disease strikes (Dreher, 1981). Although the incidence of the various types is unknown, it is certain this category of communication problems will increase as the medical treatment for the various brain diseases improves and people live longer. Those who do survive will need help in overcoming all the residual social and communication problems. Currently Parkinson's disease is managed very well with medication, and there is ongoing research in the medical management of multiple sclerosis and myasthenia gravis. The intervention of a physical therapist may help improve the function of various muscles used for speech. There are also some mechanical devices such as a prosthetic palate, which is used to control hypernasality. Another useful tool is sign language, which may be used if the person's arm and hand muscles are unaffected. The nurse should work with the speech therapist to determine if any of the other nonverbal aids would be appropriate, such as communication boards or a portable electronic voice synthesizer. With the advent of the adaptive computer, the possibilities are limitless. To improve communication with the dysarthric person, Dreher (1981) makes the following suggestions:

- Be sure the environment is quiet, because you are listening to a person whose speech muscles are weak and uncoordinated. A careful listener may discern a consistent pattern in the sound errors.
- Ask the speaker to repeat unclear parts of the message. Concentration and intention aid clarity.
- Do not simplify your message. Dysarthria does not affect comprehension.
- Ask questions that need only short answers, to prevent exhausting the dysarthric with the great effort to shape sounds.
- Encourage the person to use more oral movement to produce each syllable, to slow the overall rate of speaking, and to speak louder.
- Ask the patient who is extremely unintelligible to gesture, write, or point to messages on a communication board.

Laryngectomy

The American Cancer Society reports that there are 30,000 laryngectomees in the United States. Most of these people return to society as useful citizens. Cancer of the larynx is five times more common in men than in women, and it occurs most often in persons over 60 years of age.

Until recently, *esophageal speech* was the primary method for speaking after a laryngectomy. Esophageal speech involves taking air into the upper part of the esophagus and adapting its normal sphincters to vibrate like vocal cords. With practice, the new voice sounds quite natural. Motivation and persistent effort are essential in learning this new kind of speech. Encouragement and support of the family as well as the clients are essential for success. About 75% of all clients who have their larynx removed acquire some sort of speech, and most people return to work in 1 to 2 months.

Tracheoesophageal speech is a more rapid restoration of speech. The speech is closer to normal in rate and phrasing, and it is more pleasing than with an electrolarynx. On the other hand, it means the person must rely on a prosthesis, and the tracheoesophageal fistula may undergo stenosis. The tracheoesophageal puncture (TEP) was first successfully performed in 1980. In this procedure, a tracheoesophageal puncture is made to create a tracheoesophageal fistula large enough to permit the insertion of a valve prosthesis (Figure 9–3). The prosthesis is a hollow silicone tube open at the tracheal end and closed with a horizontal slit at the laryngopharyngeal end. When the person talks, air pressure opens the closed end, permitting air to enter the laryngopharynx. When the person stops talking, the laryngopharyngeal end closes, preventing saliva from draining into the trachea. Since air is diverted from the trachea into the esophagus, this form of speech is referred to as tracheo-esophageal speech (Phipps et al., 1995). The stoma needs to be occluded during speech. Education of the person and family includes what to do if the prosthesis comes out.

If an individual is unable to learn esophageal speech in 60 to 90 days after surgery, a speech aid such as a vibrator or an *electronic artificial larynx* is recommended. It is a battery-powered, handheld device with a vibrating diaphragm that a person with a laryngectomy presses against the soft tissues of the neck. The newer ones permit a natural type of speech.

As previously noted, many of the people with laryngectomies are older and they often have a difficult time adjusting. If they are unable to use any of the aforementioned interventions, the nurse needs to be vigilant about preventing "silent suffering" and social isolation. It is essential that contact

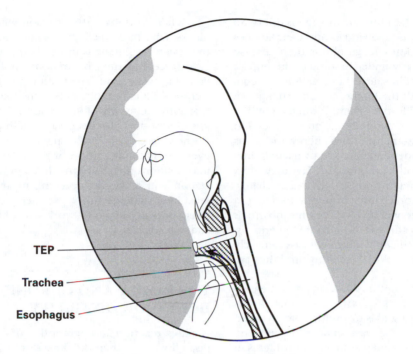

FIGURE 9–3. Tracheoesophageal Puncture

with other people remains intact. If none of the assistive speech devices work, then other means of nonverbal communication need to be adopted. Measures to improve communications with a person with a laryngectomy are listed by speech pathologist, Barbara Dreher (1981):

- Seek a quiet environment because esophageal speech is quieter and less intelligible than normal speech.
- Watch the speaker's lips because articulation is the same as before and mouth movements give clues.
- Do not alter your message. The laryngectomee's comprehension should be the same as before surgery.
- If you don't understand the speaker, repeat what you think the person said, and ask for more information.
- Encourage the laryngectomee who has not yet learned esophageal speech, or can't learn it, to write or gesture to communicate.

Losing the ability to communicate can be an isolating, depressing experience. It is of particular concern in this day and age of increased technology, when it is easy to lose sight of the human touch as the universal means of communication.

Chronic Illness

Lubkin (1995) states that chronic illness constitutes our nation's number one medical malady. It is impossible within the confines of this chapter to cover specific teaching strategies for each chronic illness. Unlike acute illnesses, which usually have a clearly defined beginning and end, chronic illness is permanent. It is never completely cured. It requires the full involvement of its victims. Every aspect of their life is affected—physical, psychological, social, economical, and spiritual. Since successful management of a chronic illness is a lifelong process, the development of good learning skills is a matter of survival. The learning process for individuals with a chronic illness begins with rehabilitation at the moment of the disability. So from the onset, those individuals and their families need to acquire knowledge about their disease and arrive at an early understanding of the impact on their lives. Families need information and education to deal with the limitations and changes in their loved one's lifestyle. There is often a conflict between feelings of dependence and the need to be independent. Sometimes the energy and focus of maintaining independence are overwhelming, both physically and emotionally. Living with a chronic illness often includes a loss and or change in roles. When people suffer from role loss (e.g., a father who is no longer able to keep his job), their self-esteem is also affected. If there are lingering issues surrounding the individual's role loss and self-esteem, it is best to hold off teaching until they are resolved.

Controlling symptoms is a major time-consuming activity of those with a chronic illness such as myasthenia gravis or multiple sclerosis. In a study of people with myasthenia gravis, concerning regimens and regimen-associated problems in adults, Hood (1990) discovered that persons with this disorder follow regimens to maximize their physical strength. When they encountered adverse effects with their regimens, they figured out methods to lessen regimen-associated problems. This information would support the work of Strauss et al. (1984, p. 16), who identified the following eight key problem areas experienced by the chronically ill patients:

1. Prevention of medical crisis and the management of problems once they occur.
2. Control of symptoms.
3. Carrying out of prescribed regimens and the management of problems attendant on carrying out the regimens.
4. Prevention of, or living with, social isolation causes lessened control with others.
5. Adjustment to changes in the course of the disease, whether it moves downward or has remission.
6. Attempts at normalizing both interactions with others and style of life.
7. Funding (finding the necessary money to pay for treatments or to survive despite partial or complete loss of employment).
8. Confronting attendant psychological, marital, and family problems.

When working with a person with a chronic illness, who must manage a sometimes complex therapeutic regimen (as in a diabetic regimen), it is easy to see how the label of noncompliance might enter the assessment. The truth is, the person with a chronic illness requires more than just teaching, that is, the acquiring of information. Acquisition of knowledge does not necessarily help people gain the new skills needed to deal with the problems of everyday life. Integration of the new knowledge into solutions that will provide them with normalization will make the learning meaningful and, most important, useful. Nurses need to remember to encourage people to work with their regimen and individualize it.

THE FAMILY AND CHRONIC ILLNESS OR DISABILITY

Families' reaction and perception of the illness or disability rather than the illness or disability itself influence all aspects of adjustment. Families are usually the care providers and the support system for the disabled person, and they need to be included in all the teaching-learning interactions. The literature has documented that family participation does have a profound impact on the success of a client's rehabilitation program. Rehabilitation nurses have learned to assess clients and families' learning needs and then develop a teaching plan. When the client and family are assessed, it is important to note what the family considers a priority learning need. Most often it will be related to the family member's perceived lifestyle change (will I be able to garden? go for lunch with friends?). It is important that the nurse assist the client and family to identify problems and develop mutually agreed upon goals. Adaptation is key. Communication between and among family members is crucial. If a family has open communication, the nurse is in a good position to help the family mobilize to gain emotional and educational support. The client and family educational process needs to take into consideration where the family is at in coping with their family member's disability. "Having a disabled individual within the family unit requires that all other members adapt to a new family structure" (Fraley, 1992, p. 108). A chronic illness or disability can either destroy or

TABLE 9–5.   Relieving external tensions in client and family education

Problem	Response
Family Dynamics	
Client or family member feels overwhelmed	Goal setting: Help family refocus on tasks at hand. Review goals that have been attained to boost morale.
Anxiety and fear of performing complex procedures	Establish an atmosphere of acceptance. Don't be in a hurry. Offer opportunities for talk and questions. Reassure client and family that they have made the right treatment choice.
Emotions associated with chronic or terminal conditions	Provide opportunities to express feelings. Offer referrals to community resources.
Caregiver burnout and illness	Simplify client management where possible (e.g., scheduling drug doses to reduce nighttime treatment). Remain accessible. Remember: When caregiver needs are not being met, resentments increase. Provide information on respite care.
Client fatigue, especially with chronic illness	Help the client identify individual tolerance for tiredness in planning for as much active participation in the family life as possible.
Young clients are frequently overwhelmed by complex emotions about their illness and therapy	Encourage both children and adolescents to use artwork to express their feelings. Suggest support groups. Offer support to parents and siblings who must alter their family lifestyle.
Geriatric Considerations	
An increase in the number of drugs taken daily (on average 4 or more a day) increases the potential for adverse reactions	Use only one pharmacy so that one source keeps track. Continually evaluate all drugs taken for need, safety, compatibility, potential adverse reactions, and expiration dates.
Decreased visual acuity	Use teaching materials with large, bold type. Encourage the use of a magnifying glass.

SOURCE: Adapted by permission from *Mosby's Home Health Nursing Pocket Consultant.* St. Louis: Mosby-Year Book, 1995.

strengthen family unity. Siblings and children of the disabled may be at a different stage of acceptance. Denial may be present during the initial diagnosis of a disability. Later on as the client and family realize the permanency and the consequence of the illness or disability, the nurse may witness periods of anger, guilt, depression, fear, and hostility. As these feelings dissipate, readjust the lesson to fit; flexibility is vital to a successful outcome. Be sure to treat each family member as unique and recognize that some family members never adjust. Table 9–5 lists some of the most common sources of tension in client and family educators as adapted from LaRocca, 1994.

Nurses need to value their teaching role when they work with the family of a disabled member. Unlike families dealing with an acutely ill member,

families with permanently disabled members will have intermittent contact with the health-care system throughout their lives. Therefore, whenever teaching sessions are required, the families' availability should be a primary consideration. Given adequate support and resources, families with a chronically ill family member can adapt, make adjustments, and live healthy, happy, full lives.

ADAPTIVE COMPUTING

The growth of modern technology has invaded all areas of our lives. Without a doubt, the personal computer has become the technology that has had the greatest impact. As Max Cleland states, "The real disabled people of the future are going to be those who don't have a computer to use" (Green & Brightman, 1990). Until recently, however, computers have been inaccessible to individuals with a disability, and yet when adaptive computing has been made available, disabled individuals have experienced dramatic changes in their lives. Computers with the appropriate adaptations have liberated people from social isolation and feelings of helplessness to feelings of self-worth and independence. Adaptive computing is relatively new; it refers to the professional services and the technology (both hardware and software) that make computing technology accessible for persons with disabilities (Merrow & Corbett, 1994). Since the enactment of the ADA in 1990 the diversity of our client population has grown to include more individuals with disabilities in every practice setting from community health, schools, occupational health, and of course, rehabilitation nursing. As nurses' understanding of adaptive computing is enhanced, so will their ability to advocate, recommend, and assist persons to attain the appropriate equipment and training. Adaptive computing not only enables independence, it is also a useful tool for health promotion activities. Just about every type of disability mentioned in this chapter could benefit from the use of an adaptive computer. Merrow and Corbett (1994) discovered that the health-care literature includes a number of research studies describing the use of computers with various populations such as the older adult, the physically disabled in long-term rehabilitation, the blind and visually impaired, and people with quadriplegia.

Assessment of Potential Barriers to Access

Although the personal computer has been proved to change the life of a person with even the most severe disability, the fact remains that it is a very individualized process. Personalized computer solutions are those that respond to a person, not to the particular disability (Green & Brightman, 1990). Merrow and Corbett (1994) identified six barriers to computer access:

1. The environment, which includes the room, the table/desk the computer sits on, and the actual hardware (the physical computer). For example, can the person in a wheelchair fit the wheelchair under the desk?

2. Input, the devices that are responsible for getting information into the computer (the keyboard or the mouse). People with no useful movement in their arms may benefit from a head pointer or a mouth stick.

3. Output devices, or the part of the computer responsible for sending the information back out to you, the monitor and printer. Aside from the obvious problem posed for the person with a visual impairment, the person with a learning disability or an acquired brain injury may also have a problem interpreting output. The solution may be as simple as slotted paper that permits the reading of one line at a time, reducing the glare, or decreasing the rate of text scrolling.

4. Documentation, the "written" text that describes how to operate the hardware or software. The problem is that it is often written in computerese. Some cognitive or physical disabilities present a barrier to accessing the instructions. For example, a person may not be able to physically handle a computer manual, but a manual in a spiral-bound book would be accessible. A person with a learning disability may do well with instructions if they are auditory or pictorial.

5. Support, which comes in two forms: cognitive and human support. For example, one of the participants in the Links and Frydenberg study (1989) was unwilling to attempt a word processing course, so she was assigned a simpler software program first; once it was mastered, she progressed and completed the program. Human support is someone who sets up the equipment and is also around to help answer questions and troubleshoot. For example, several agencies and organizations provide this service, as well as training.

6. Training, which needs to be supplied regarding the use of the hardware, software, and adaptations. Merrow and Corbett (1994) stated that training is probably the second greatest obstacle in adaptive technology. The greatest obstacle is finding out what devices are available and which devices fit an individual's need.

Types of Adaptations

Whether the area of impairment is mobility, hearing, seeing, communicating, or a learning disability will determine the type of adaptation. If the problem is in the area of input, then the person needs to investigate and find the best keyboard or mouse adaptation. Head pointers and mouth sticks have already been mentioned, and there are many others, including voice recognition systems. Joysticks and trackballs are often utilized to simulate mouse movements. They are ideal mouse alternatives because they can be positioned in unique places and activated with different parts of the body, such as the chin or even the mouth. A trackball looks like a mouse turned upside down. It is very useful for people who do not have a wide range of movement in their arms or hands.

People with communication problems, especially those who are unable to speak or whose speech is difficult to understand, can use the computer and are able to add a whole new dimension to their lives. Within the last 10 years, the technology for impaired speech has made great strides. There are several software packages available (see Appendix B). Visual feedback systems are devices that enable the computer to display graphic representation of spoken sounds. In this way, a person can work to match the correct displayed speech pattern. Computer-based electronic augmentative communication aids help people to use a synthetic voice to speak out loud (Green & Brightman, 1990).

Hearing-impaired and deaf persons can benefit from adaptive computing. The greatest challenge, however, usually is not the computer, but training on the computer.

The visually impaired and those who are blind can benefit from adaptive computing. As previously noted, there is a wide range between a person with low vision and a person who is blind. It is obvious that the problem falls into the category of output, in other words, the monitor and the printer. There are many types of adaptive devices that enable individuals with vision impairment to use a personal computer, everything from large-size monitors to large-print software. For people who are unable to see the screen at all, a solution may be to have the computer "speak" the screen contents. Another solution for computer users who are blind and especially for individuals who are deaf is tactile output. The images on the screen are converted into Braille or a device known as Opt-a-con, which gives the person an exact tactile representation of the letters and lines.

Learning disability problems can often be solved with some creative software package. For example, "Outliners," a type of thought processor, are programs that help people organize their ideas. They are very helpful in writing papers or reports. Sometimes the Outliners' software can be used in place of a word processor. Some experts feel the software may be the best place to start almost any kind of writing.

Every computer-based solution is the result of a carefully planned, individually determined process. Individuals with a disability are the experts on what works best for them. However, there are some guidelines to be considered when selecting the best adaptive computer. The best computer solution for individuals with disabilities will allow for independent and effective use. Other criteria include affordability, portability, flexibility, and simplicity of learning. If these criteria are met, then the adaptive computer is probably in compliance with the ADA's "reasonable accommodations." O'Leary et al. (1991) reviewed the literature and determined that there were certain characteristics of the older adult that would probably ensure successful computer usage. They determined that the client must

- Be oriented.
- Have an attention span and short-term memory exceeding 5 minutes.
- Not be agitated or combative.

Adaptive computing is here to stay. While computer technology will probably be forever changing, the process for ensuring individualized computer solutions will remain much the same. When that process is pursued, the benefits will prove to be enormous. It is exciting to reflect on the positive, possibly life-changing effect the personal computer will have on the lives of individuals with a disability. It has the potential of changing what it means to be disabled. Within the role of nurse as teacher is the client advocate component.

As client advocate, the nurse can work with the multidisciplinary team, including the computer specialist, to enable special populations to participate in all of life's experiences. Because of what adaptive personal computers will be able to do, people with disabilities will be more among us. Just think of all the opportunities for client teaching, health promotion, and counseling when a person using a modem is able to gain access to telecommunication.

SUMMARY

The shock of any disability, whether it occurs at the beginning of life or toward the end, has a tremendous impact on individuals and their families. At the onset and all through the habilitation or rehabilitation process, the patient and family are met with new information to be learned, as successful habilitation or rehabilitation means acquiring knowledge and applying it to their situation. Inner strength and courage are attributes needed to face each new day, as the effort to live a "normal" life is never over. The physical, social, emotional, and vocational implications of living with a disability necessitate the nurse as educator to be well prepared to meet any member of this special population right where they are in their struggle to live independently.

References

Adkins, E.R.H. (1991). Nursing care of the client with impaired communication. *Rehabilitation Nursing, 16*(2), 74-76.

Astin, A., Green, K., Korn, W., Schalit, M., & Berg, E. (1988). *American freshman national norm for 1988.* Los Angeles: University of California.

Babcock, D.E., & Miller, M.A. (1994). *Client education: Theory and practice.* St. Louis: Mosby.

Baker, S.S. (1993). Teamwork between the health care community and the blind rehabilitation system. *Journal of Visual Impairment and Blindness, 87*(9), 349-352.

Blanco, K.M. (1982). The aphasic patient. *Journal of Neurosurgical Nursing, 14,* 34-37.

Boss, B.J. (1986). The neuroanatomical and neurophysiological basis for learning. *Journal of Neuroscience Nursing, 18*(5), 256-264.

Bronstein, K.S., Popovoch, J., & Stewart-Amidei, C. (1991). *Promoting stroke recovery: A research-based approach for nurses.* St. Louis: Mosby–Year Book.

Burkett, K.W. (1989). Trends in pediatric rehabilitation. *Nursing Clinics of North America, 24*(1), 239-255.

Diehl, L.N. (1989). Client and family learning in the rehabilitation setting. *Nursing Clinics of North America, 24*(1), 257-264.

DiPietro, L. (1979). *Deaf patients, special needs, special responses.* Washington, DC: National Academy of Gallaudet College.

Dittmar, S. (1989). *Rehabilitation nursing.* St. Louis: Mosby–Year Book.

Dreher, B. (1981). Overcoming speech and language disorders. *Geriatric Nursing, 2,* 345-349.

Dykman, R.A., Ackerman, P.T., Holcomb, P.J., & Boudreau, A.Y. (1983). Physiological manifestations of learning disability. *Journal of Learning Disabilities, 16*(1), 46-53.

Fink, S.L. (1967). Crisis and motivation: A theoretical model. *Archives of Physical Rehabilitation, 48,* 492-597.

Fowler, L. (1993). *Psychoeducational family program: Patients, their families and significant other.* Kings County Hospital Center Psychiatric Day Hospital, Psychoeducational Family Conference.

Fraley, A.M. (1992). *Nursing and the disabled: Across the life span.* Boston: Jones and Bartlett.

Goldman, C.R., & Quinn, F.L. (1988). Effects of patient education program in the treatment of schizophrenia. *H & CP: Hospital & Community Psychiatry, 39*(3), 282-286.

Green, P., & Brightman, A.J. (1990). *Independence day: Designing computer solutions for individuals with disability.* Allen, TX: DLM.

Greenberg, L.A. (1991). Teaching children who are learning disabled about illness and hospitalization. *MCN: American Journal of Maternal Child Nursing, 16*(5), 260-263.

Grinspun, D. (1987). Teaching families of traumatic brain-injured adults. *Critical Care Nursing Quarterly, 10*(3), 61-72.

Haggard, A. (1989). *Handbook of patient education.* Rockville, MD: Aspen.

Hammill, D.D., Leigh, J.E., McNutt, G., & Larsen, S.C. (1981). A new definition of learning disabilities. *Learning Disability Quarterly, 4,* 336-342.

Harmon, R.B., & Tratnack, S.A. (1992). Teaching hospitalized patients with serious persistent mental illness. *Journal of Psychosocial Nursing, 30*(7), 33-36.

Harrison, L.L. (1990). Minimizing barriers when teaching hearing-impaired clients. *MCN: American Journal of Maternal Child Nursing, 15*(2), 113.

Hood, L.J. (1990). Myasthenia gravis: Regimens and regimen-associated problems in adults. *Journal of Neuroscience Nursing, 22*(16), 358-364.

Interagency Head-Injured Task Force. (1989). *Interagency Head-Injured Task Force Report*. Bethesda, MD: National Institute of Neurological Disorders and Stroke, National Institutes of Health.

Jennings, S. (1981). Communicating with your aphasic patients. *Journal of Practical Nursing, 31*, 22-23.

Kirk, S.A., & Kirk, W.D. (1983). On defining disabilities. *Journal of Learning Disabilities, 16*(1), 20-21.

Knowles, B.S., & Knowles, P.S. (1983). A model for identifying learning disabilities in college-bound students. *Journal of Learning Disabilities, 16*(1), 39-42.

LaRocca, J.C. (1994). *Handbook of home care IV therapy*. St. Louis: Mosby–Year Book.

Loughrey, L. (1992). The effects of two teaching techniques on recognition and use of function words by aphasic stroke patients. *Rehabilitation Nursing, 17*(3), 134-137.

Links, C., & Frydenberg, H. (1989). Microcomputer skills training program for the physically disabled in long term rehabilitation. *Physical & Occupational Therapy in Geriatrics, 6*(3/4), 133-140.

Lubkin, I.M. (1995). *Chronic illness: Impact and interventions*. Boston: Jones and Bartlett.

MacFarlane, W., ed. (1983). Family therapy in schizophrenia. New York: Guilford Press.

McCourt, A.E. (1993). *The specialty practice of rehabilitation: A core curriculum*, 3rd ed. Skokie: Rehabilitation Nursing Foundation of the Association of Rehabilitation Nurses.

McLoughlin, J.A., & Natick, A. (1983). Defining learning disabilities: A new and cooperative direction. *Journal of Learning Disabilities, 16*(1), 21-23.

Merrow, S.L., & Corbett, C. (1994). Adaptive computing for people with disabilities. *Computers in Nursing, 12*(4), 201-209.

Navarro, M.R., & Lacour, G. (1980). Helping hints for use with deaf patients. *Journal of Emergency Nursing, 6*(6), 26-28.

Nelson, K. (1991). *Projected increase in the prevalence of severe visual impairment among elderly Americans*. New York: American Foundation for the Blind.

Norman, S., & Baratz, R. (1979). The brain-damaged patient: Approaches to assessment, care, and rehabilitation. Understanding aphasia, pt. 4. *American Journal of Nursing, 79*, 2135-2138.

Norris, W.C., Wharton, G., Noble, C., & Strickland, S. (1982). The spinal injury learning series: An experimental test. *Archives of Physical Medicine, Rehabilitation, 63*(6), 243-248.

O'Leary, S., Mann, C., & Perkash, I. (1991). Access to computers for the older adults: Problems and solutions. *American Journal of Occupational Therapy, 45*(7), 636-642.

Olson, E. (1991). Perceptual deficits affecting the stroke patient. *Rehabilitation Nursing, 16*(14), 212-213.

Phipps, W.J., Cassmeyer, V.L., Sands, J.K., & Lehman, M.K. (1995). *Medical surgical nursing*, 5th ed. St. Louis: Mosby.

Stover, S.L., & Fine, P.R. (Eds.). (1986). *Spinal cord injury: The facts & figures*. Birmingham, AL: University of Alabama at Birmingham.

Strauss, A.L., Corbin, J., Fagerhaugh, S., et al. (1984). *Chronic illness and quality of life*, 2nd ed. St. Louis: Mosby.

Tate, R.L., Fenelon, B., Manning, M.L., & Hunter, M. (1991). Patterns of neuropsychological impairment after severe blunt injury. *Journal of Nervous and Mental Disease, 179*(3), 117-126.

Vance, J.L. (1992). Learning readiness in rehabilitation patients. *Rehabilitation Nursing, 17*(3), 148-149.

Vessey, J. (1988). Care of the hospitalized child with a cognitive developmental delay. *Holistic Nursing Practice, 2*(2), 48-54.

Weeks, S.K. (1995). What are the educational needs of prospective family caregiver of newly disabled adults? *Rehabilitation Nursing, 20*(5), 256-260.

Whitman, N.I., Graham, B.N., Gleit, C.J., & Boyd, M.D. (1992). *Teaching in nursing practice: A professional*. Norwalk, CT: Appleton and Lange.

Ysseldyke, J., & Allgozzine, B. (1983). LD or not LD: That's not the question! *Journal of Learning Disabilities, 16*(1), 29-31.

Zejdlik, C.P. (1992). *Management of spinal cord injury*, 2nd ed. Boston: Jones and Bartlett.

PART III

Techniques and Strategies of Teaching and Learning

CHAPTER 10

Educational Objectives

Susan Bastable
Cynthia Sculco

CHAPTER HIGHLIGHTS

Characteristics of Goals and Objectives

The Debate About Using Behavioral Objectives

Writing Behavioral Objectives

Common Mistakes When Writing Objectives

Taxonomy of Objectives According to Learning Domains
   The Cognitive Domain
   The Affective Domain
   The Psychomotor Domain

Development of Teaching Plans

Use of Learning Contracts
   Components of the Learning Contract
   Steps to Implement the Learning Contract

KEY TERMS

goals
taxonomic hierarchy
behavioral objectives
affective domain
cognitive domain
psychomotor domain

teaching plans
transfer of learning
intrinsic and augmented feedback
learning contracts
selective attention

OBJECTIVES

After completing this chapter, the reader will be able to

1. Identify the difference between goals and objectives.
2. Recognize opposing viewpoints regarding use of behavioral objectives in education.
3. Demonstrate the ability to write behavioral objectives accurately and concisely using the three components of condition, performance, and criterion.
4. Cite the most frequent errors made in objective writing.
5. Distinguish between the three domains of learning.
6. Explain the instructional methods appropriate for teaching in the cognitive, affective, and psychomotor domains.
7. Develop teaching plans that reflect internal consistency between elements.
8. Describe the importance of learning contracts as an alternative approach to structuring a learning experience.
9. Recognize the role of the nurse educator in formulating objectives for the planning, implementation, and evaluation of teaching and learning.

In previous chapters, the characteristics and attributes of the learner with respect to learning needs, readiness to learn, and learning styles have been addressed. Clearly, assessment of the learner is an essential first step in the teaching-learning process to determine what the learner needs to know, when and under what conditions the learner is most receptive to learning, and how the learner actually learns best. Before a decision can be made about selecting the content to be taught or choosing the instructional methods and materials to be used for the learner to accomplish a change in behavior, the educator must first decide what the learner is expected to accomplish. Analyzing client needs, by identifying the gaps in the learner's knowledge, attitudes, or skills, is a prerequisite to formulating behavioral objectives that serve to guide subsequent planning, implementation, and evaluation of teaching and learning.

Historically, noted educators and education psychologists of this century have developed approaches to writing and classifying behavioral objectives that offer teachers assistance in organizing instructional content for learners functioning at various levels of ability. Mager (1984) has been the primary educator credited with developing a system for writing behavioral objectives that serves to help teachers make appropriate instructional decisions as well as to assist learners in understanding what they need and are expected to know. The underlying principle has been, if one does not know where they are going, how will they know when they have arrived? In addition, the taxonomic system of Bloom et al. (1956) for categorizing learning objectives according to a hierarchy of behaviors has been the cornerstone of teaching for almost a half century.

The two dimensions to the preparation of behavioral objectives include the technique of writing objectives and the ordering of these behaviors according to their type and complexity. Both the formulation of objectives and the concept of taxonomy pertain to the nature of the knowledge to be learned, the behaviors most relevant and attainable for a particular learner or group of learners, and the sequencing of knowledge and experiences for learning.

The skill in preparing and classifying behavioral objectives is a necessary function of the educator's role, whether teaching patients and their families in health-care settings, teaching staff nurses in in-service and continuing education programs, or teaching nursing students in academic institutions. The importance of understanding the systems of writing and categorizing behavioral objectives for the purpose of specifying learner outcomes is imperative if data yielded from educational efforts are to be consistent and measurable.

Additionally, the knowledge and utilization of these techniques are becoming essential because of the need to quantify and justify the costs of teaching others in an ever-increasing cost-containment environment.

This chapter examines the role of behavioral objectives for effective teaching; describes how to write clear and precise behavioral objectives; explores the levels of achievement in the taxonomic hierarchy of cognitive, affective, and psychomotor domains; and outlines the development of teaching plans and learning contracts. All of these elements provide a framework for the successful instruction of the learner.

CHARACTERISTICS OF GOALS AND OBJECTIVES

As a basis for discussion and prior to differentiating between what is a goal and what is an objective, it is important to clarify the meaning of the terms *educational or instructional objectives* and *behavioral or learning objectives*. Although often used synonymously, these sets of terms can be distinguished from one another. Educational or instructional objectives are used to identify the intended outcomes of the education process, whether in reference to an aspect of a program or a total program of study. Behavioral or learning objectives, on the other hand, make use of the modifier *behavioral* or *learning* to denote that they are action oriented rather than content oriented and learner centered rather than teacher centered.

The terms *goal* and *objective* are often used interchangeably, albeit incorrectly because there does exist a real difference between the two terms, a distinction that must be clearly understood by nurse educators. Time span and specificity are the two factors that differentiate goals from objectives and vice versa (Haggard, 1989).

A *goal* is the final outcome of what is achieved at the end of the teaching-learning process. Goals are global and broad in nature and serve as long-term targets for both the learner and the teacher. Goals are the desired outcomes of learning that are realistically achievable in weeks or months. Goals are considered multidimensional in that a number of objectives are subsumed under or incorporated into an overall goal.

An *objective*, in contrast, is a specific, single, unidimensional behavior. Objectives are short-term in nature and should be achievable at the conclusion of one teaching session or within a matter of a few days following a series of teaching sessions. According to Mager (1984), an objective describes a performance learners should be able to exhibit before they are considered competent. An objective is the intended result of instruction, not the process or means of instruction itself. Objectives are statements of specific or short-term behaviors that lead step-by-step to the more general, overall long-term goal. Subobjectives reflect an aspect of a main objective and are also written as specific statements of short-term behaviors that lead to the achievement of the primary objective. Objectives and subobjectives specify what the learner will be able to do as a result of being exposed to one or more learning experiences. Objectives must be achieved before the goal can be reached. They must be observable and measurable to be able to determine if they have been met by the learner. Objectives can be thought of as advance organizers, statements that inform the learner of what is expected from a cognitive, affective, or psychomotor perspective to meet the intended outcome (Babcock & Miller, 1994). Objectives are derived from a goal and must be consistent with and related to that goal.

Together, objectives and goals form a map giving directions (objectives) as to how to arrive at a particular destination (goal). For example, a goal might be that a diabetic patient will learn to manage diabetes. To accomplish the goal, which has been agreed on by the nurse and the patient, specific objectives must be outlined to address such changes in behavior as the need to learn diet therapy, insulin administration, exercise regimens, stress management, and glucose monitoring. The objectives to accomplish the goal become the blueprint for attaining the desired outcomes of learning. The successful achievement of predetermined objectives is, in part, the result of appropriate instruction. Certainly, many other factors, such as learner motivation and ability to perform, are also key to the successful demonstration of specific behaviors before overall competence by the learner can be declared.

If the teaching-learning process is to be successful, the setting of goals and objectives must be a mutual decision on the part of both the teacher and the learner. Both parties must participate in the decision-making process and "buy into" the immediate objectives and ultimate goals. Involving the learner right from the start in creating goals and objectives is absolutely crucial. Otherwise, time and effort on the part of the educator and learner may be wasted because learners may choose to reject the content if it is deemed from their perspective to be unimportant, irrelevant, unapplicable, or something already known. Goal and objective setting for any educational experience should be as much a responsibility of the learner as of the teacher. Blending what the learner wants to learn with what the teacher has assessed the learner needs to know into a common set of objectives and goals provides for an educational experience that is mutually accountable, respectful, developmental, and fulfilling (Reilly & Oermann, 1990).

Objectives and goals must also be clearly written, realistic, and learner centered. If they do not precisely state what the learner is expected to do in the short and long term, then there are no clear guideposts to follow or an obvious end result to strive for in the learning process. If goals and objectives are too difficult to achieve, the learner will become easily discouraged, which dampens motivation and interferes with the ability to comply. For instance, a goal that expects a patient to maintain a salt-free diet is likely to be impossible to accomplish or adhere to over an extended period of time. However, establishing a goal of maintaining a low-salt diet with the objectives of learning to avoid eating and preparing foods high in sodium is a much more realistic and achievable expectation of the learner. Goals and objectives must be directed to what the learner is expected to be able to do, not what the teacher is expected to teach. Educators must be sure not only that their teaching remains objectives oriented but also that the objectives are learner centered to keep both them and the learners targeted on results, not on the act of teaching.

THE DEBATE ABOUT USING BEHAVIORAL OBJECTIVES

There are definite arguments put forth by educators for and against the use of behavioral objectives for teaching and learning. Certainly behavioral objectives are not a panacea for all the problems encountered in the planning, implementation, and evaluation of education (Reilly & Oermann, 1990). The following, outlined by Arends (1994), Reilly and Oermann (1990), Haggard (1989), and Durbach et al. (1987) are some common arguments by educators against using behavioral objectives:

- The understanding by experienced educators of learners' needs is so sophisticated that the exercise of writing behavioral objectives is superfluous.
- The practice of writing specific behavioral objectives leads to reductionism, a format that reduces behavioral processes into equivalents that do not reflect the sum total of the parts.
- Objective writing is a time-consuming task, requiring more effort for development than is warranted by their effect on an instructional program, such that the cost benefit does not justify the amount of time required to formulate them.
- The preparation of objectives is merely a pedagogic exercise often expressing the teacher's expectations of the outcome of teaching and precluding the opportunity for learners to seek their own objectives.
- Predetermined objectives, with emphasis on precise and observable learner behaviors, forces teachers and learners to attend only to specific objectives, which stifle creativity and interfere with the freedom to learn and to teach.
- The writing of specific objectives is incompatible with the complex field of study such as nursing because the number of possible objectives for almost any subject or topic could be innumerable.
- Behavioral objectives are unable to capture the more intricate cognitive processes that are not readily observable and measurable.

The rationale for using behavioral objectives, however, far outweighs the arguments against their use. The following considerations justify the need for writing behavioral objectives. Careful construction of objectives

- Helps to keep educators' thinking on target and learner centered.

- Communicates to others, both learners and health-care team members alike, what is planned for teaching and learning.
- Helps learners understand what is expected of them so they can keep track of their progress.
- Forces the educator to organize educational materials so as not to get lost in content and forget the learner's role in the process.
- Encourages educators to question their own motives—to think deliberately about why they are doing things and analyze what positive results will be attained from accomplishing specific objectives.
- Tailors teaching to the learner's particular circumstances and needs.
- Serves as guideposts for teacher evaluation and documentation of success or failure.
- Aids in focusing attention not on what is taught but on what the learner will come away with once the teaching-learning process is completed.
- Orients the teacher and learner to the specific end result of instruction.
- Makes it easier for the learner to actually visualize performing the required actions.

Robert Mager (1984), a recognized authority on preparing behavioral objectives, further points out three major advantages to writing explicit objective statements:

1. They provide a sound basis for the selection or design of instructional content, methods, and materials.
2. They provide the learner with the means to organize their efforts and activities toward accomplishing the intent of instruction.
3. They allow for a determination as to whether an objective has, in fact, been accomplished.

As Mager (1984) states, "If you don't know where you're going, it is difficult to select a suitable means for getting there" (p. 5); that is, before the educator prepares instruction, before materials and teaching methods are selected, before choosing the means to evaluate if learning has occurred, it is important to clearly and concisely state just what the intended results of instruction are to be. To paraphrase his thinking, mechanics do not select repair tools until they know what has to be fixed; surgeons do not choose instruments until they know what operation is to be performed; and builders do not buy construction materials before drafting a blueprint.

Haggard (1989) summarizes the questions that arise if objectives are not always written: How will anyone else know what objectives have been set? How will the educator evaluate and document success or failure? How will learners keep track of their progress? The writing of objectives is not merely a mechanical task but a synthesizing process. The process of developing behavioral objectives not only helps educators explore their own knowledge, values, and beliefs about the entire spectrum of teaching and learning, but it encourages them to examine the experiences, values, motivations, and knowledge of the learner as well. The time and effort expended in writing objectives represent a thoughtful deliberation about the knowledge, attitude, and skill requirements needed by the learner in meeting the desired level of competency. As the educator and learner work together to compose objectives and goals that focus on what is to be accomplished in the short and long run, the process provides direction that helps the educator identify the time that will be needed for teaching, the clues as to how the learner best acquires information, what teaching methods will work most effectively, and how best to evaluate the learner's progress. The additional advantages of stating well-written objectives is that the process not only encourages the educator to seriously contemplate what is worth teaching and what is worth spending time to accomplish but also can serve to highlight the value of an existing instructional program and can further provide the basis for improving a current teaching plan. Thus, the setting of objectives and goals is considered by many educators to be the initial, most important consideration in the education process (Haggard, 1989).

WRITING BEHAVIORAL OBJECTIVES

Well-written behavioral objectives give learners very clear statements about what is expected of them and assist teachers in being able to measure learner progress. Over the past three decades, Robert Mager's (1984) approach to writing behavioral objectives has been widely accepted among educators. His message to educators is that for objectives to be meaningful, they must precisely, clearly, and very specifically communicate the teacher's instructional intent (Arends, 1994).

According to Mager (1984), the format for writing concise and useful behavioral objectives includes the following three important characteristics:

1. *Performance:* Describes what the learner is expected to be able to *do* or *perform* to demonstrate the kinds of behaviors the teacher will accept as evidence that objectives have been achieved. Activities performed by the learner may be visible, such as "writing" or "listing," or invisible, such as "identifying" or "recalling."
2. *Conditions:* Describes the testing situation or constraints under which the behavior will be observed or the performance is expected to occur.
3. *Criterion:* Describes how well or with what accuracy the learner must be able to perform for the behavior to be considered acceptable; the standard, quality level, or amount of performance defined as satisfactorily demonstrating mastery.

A fourth component must also be included that describes the "who" to ensure that the behavioral objective is learner centered. For education in health care, the learner may be the patient, family members or significant others of the patient, staff nurses, or student nurses. Thus, behavioral objectives are statements that communicate *who* will *do what* under *what conditions* and *how well* (Cummings, 1994).

The preceding characteristics translate into the following questions: (1) What should the learner be able to do? (2) Under what conditions should the learner be able to do it? (3) How well must the learner be able to do it? Although it is not essential to include the second and third listed characteristics, the more complete the statements of objectives, the better the objectives will serve to communicate exactly what is expected of the learner and what is the intent of instruction.

A simple mnemonic for easily remembering Mager's components of a behavioral objective is the STP approach (Arends, 1994): student behavior (S), testing situation (T), and performance criteria

(P). To link the behavioral objective together, the following three steps are recommended: Begin by identifying the testing situation (condition), then state the learner and the learner's behavior (performance), and conclude by stating the performance level (criterion).

For example: "Following a 20-minute teaching session on hypoglycemia (*condition*), Mrs. Smith will be able to identify (*performance*) three out of four major symptoms of low blood sugar (*criterion*)."

Table 10–1 outlines the three-part method of objective writing, and Table 10–2 gives samples of well-written and poorly written objectives.

When writing behavioral objectives using the format suggested by Mager (1984), the recommendation is to use precise action words (verbs as labels, known as verbals) that are open to few interpretations when describing learner performance. Verbs that signify an internal state of thinking, feeling, or believing should be avoided because they are difficult to measure or observe (Redman, 1993). It is impossible to identify all behavioral terms that may be used in objective writing. The important thing to remember in selecting verbs to describe performance is that they are specific, can be observed or measured, and are action oriented. The lists in Table 10–3 give examples of verbals that, on the one hand, are too broad, ambiguous, and imprecise to evaluate and, on the other hand, are specific and relatively easy to measure (Gronlund, 1985).

COMMON MISTAKES WHEN WRITING OBJECTIVES

In formulating behavioral objectives, there are a number of common pitfalls that can easily be made by the novice as well as by the seasoned educator. The most frequent errors in writing objectives are

- To describe what the instructor rather than the learner is expected to do.
- To include more than one expected behavior in a single objective (avoid using the compound word *and*—e.g., the learner will select and prepare).

TABLE 10–1.   The three-part method of objective writing

Condition (Testing Situation)	Performance (Learner Behavior)	Criterion (Quality of Accuracy)
	The learner will be able to:	
Without using a calculator	solve	5 out of 6 problems
Using a model	demonstrate	the correct procedure
Following group discussion	list	at least two reasons
After watching a video	select	with 100% accuracy

TABLE 10–2.   Samples of written objectives

Well-written Objectives

After watching a demonstration on suctioning, the staff member will be able to correctly suction a tracheostomy
   tube using aseptic technique.

Following a class on hypertension, the patient will be able to state three out of four causes of high blood pressure.

On completing the reading materials provided on the care of a newborn, the mother will be able to express any
   concerns she has about caring for her baby after discharge.

Poorly Written Objectives

The patient will be able to prepare a menu using low-salt foods *(condition and criterion missing)*.

Given a list of exercises to relieve low back pain, the patient will understand how to control low back pain
   (performance not stated in measurable terms, criterion missing).

To demonstrate crutch walking postoperatively to the patient *(teacher-centered)*.

TABLE 10–3.   Verbals with many or few interpretations

Terms with Many Interpretations (Not Recommended)	Terms with Few Interpretations (Recommended)	
to know	to apply	to explain
to understand	to choose	to identify
to appreciate	to classify	to list
to realize	to compare	to order
to be familiar with	to contrast	to predict
to enjoy	to construct	to recall
to value	to define	to recognize
to be interested in	to describe	to select
to feel	to demonstrate	to state
to think	to differentiate	to verbalize
	to distinguish	to write

SOURCE: Adapted from Gronlund, N.E. (1985). *Stating Objectives for Classroom Instruction*, 3rd ed. New York: Macmillan.

- To forget to include all three components of condition, performance, and criterion.
- To use terms for performance that are subject to many interpretations, not action oriented, and difficult to measure.
- To write an objective that is unattainable given the ability level of the learner.
- To write objectives that do not relate to the stated goal.
- To clutter an objective by including unnecessary pieces of information.
- To be too general so as not to clearly specify the expected outcome.

TAXONOMY OF OBJECTIVES ACCORDING TO LEARNING DOMAINS

A taxonomy is a mechanism used to categorize things according to their relationships to one another. In science, for example, taxonomies are devices used to classify plants and animals in a systematic and logical fashion (Arends, 1994). In the late 1940s, psychologists and educators became concerned about the need for defining levels of behavior according to their type and complexity (Redman, 1993). Bloom et al. (1956) developed a very useful taxonomy, known as the *Taxonomy of Educational Objectives,* as a tool for systematically classifying behavioral objectives. This taxonomy, which became widely accepted as a standard aid for planning as well as evaluating learning, is divided into three broad categories or domains: cognitive, affective, and psychomotor.

The objectives in each domain are ordered in a taxonomic form of hierarchy. Behavioral objectives are classified into low, medium, and high levels with simple behaviors listed first (designated by numbers 1.0 or 2.0) and the more complex behaviors listed last (designated by numbers 5.0 or 6.0). Subobjectives are listed under the main objective and are designated by numbers that range in between whole numbers (e.g., 2.1, 3.9, 5.6, or 6.8). Inherent in the concept of hierarchy is that learners must successfully achieve behaviors at the lower levels of the domains before they are able to adequately learn behaviors at the higher levels of the domains.

The Cognitive Domain

The cognitive domain is known as the "thinking" domain. Learning in this domain involves the acquisition of information and refers to the learner's intellectual abilities, mental capacities, and thinking processes. Objectives in this domain are divided into six levels, each specifying the cognitive process ranging from the simple (knowledge) to the more complex (evaluation), as listed and described in the following section (Bloom et al., 1956).

Levels of Cognitive Behaviors

Knowledge (1.00–1.99): ability of the learner to memorize, recall, define, recognize or identify specific information, such as facts, rules, principles, conditions, and terms, presented during instruction.

Comprehension (2.00–2.99): ability of the learner to demonstrate an understanding or apprehension of what is being communicated by translating it into a different form or recognizing it in a translated form, such as grasping an idea by defining it or summarizing it in his or her own words (knowledge is a prerequisite behavior).

Application (3.00–3.99): ability of the learner to use ideas, principles, abstractions, or theories in particular and concrete situations, such as figuring, writing, reading, or handling equipment (knowledge and comprehension are prerequisite behaviors).

Analysis (4.00–4.99): ability of the learner to recognize and structure information by breaking it down into its constituent parts and specifying the relationship between parts (knowledge, comprehension, and application are prerequisite behaviors).

Synthesis (5.00–5.99): ability of the learner to put together parts and elements into a unified whole by creating a unique product that is written, oral, pictorial, and so on (knowledge, comprehension, application, and analysis are prerequisite behaviors).

Evaluation (6.00–6.99): ability of the learner to judge the value of something, such as an es-

TABLE 10–4.   Commonly used verbs according to domain classification

Cognitive Domain

Knowledge: choose, circle, define, identify, label, list, match, name, outline, recall, report, select, state
Comprehension: describe, discuss, distinguish, estimate, explain, generalize, give example, locate, recognize, summarize
Application: apply, demonstrate, illustrate, implement, interpret, modify, order, revise, solve, use
Analysis: analyze, arrange, calculate, classify, compare, conclude, contrast, determine, differentiate, discriminate
Synthesis: categorize, combine, compile, correlate, design, devise, generate, integrate, reorganize, revise, summarize
Evaluation: appraise, assess, conclude, criticize, debate, defend, judge, justify

Affective Domain

Receiving: accept, admit, ask, attend, focus, listen, observe, pay attention
Responding: agree, answer, conform, discuss, express, participate, recall, relate, report, state willingness, try, verbalize
Valuing: assert, assist, attempt, choose, complete, disagree, follow, help, initiate, join, propose, volunteer
Organization: adhere, alter, arrange, combine, defend, explain, express, generalize, integrate, resolve
Characterization: assert, commit, discriminate, display, influence, propose, qualify, solve, verify

Psychomotor Domain

Perception: attend, choose, describe, detect, differentiate, distinguish, identify, isolate, perceive, relate, select, separate
Set: attempt, begin, develop, display, position, prepare, proceed, reach, respond, show, start, try
Guided response mechanism and complex overt response: align, arrange, assemble, attach, build, change, choose, clean, compile, complete, construct, demonstrate, discriminate, dismantle, dissect, examine, find, grasp, hold, insert, lift, locate, maintain, manipulate, measure, mix, open, operate, organize, perform, pour, practice, reassemble, remove, repair, replace, separate, shake, suction, turn, transfer, walk, wash, wipe
Adaptation: adapt, alter, change, convert, correct, rearrange, reorganize, replace, revise, shift, substitute, switch
Origination: arrange, combine, compose, construct, create, design, exchange, reformulate

SOURCE: Adapted from Gronlund, N.E. (1985). *Stating Objectives for Classroom Instruction,* 3rd ed. New York: Macmillan.

This level indicates a movement beyond denial toward voluntary acceptance, which can lead to feelings of pleasure or enjoyment as a result of some new experience (receiving is a prerequisite behavior).

Valuing (3.00–3.99): ability of the learner to regard or accept the worth of a theory, idea, or event, demonstrating sufficient commitment or preference to be identified with some experience seen as having value and a definite willingness and desire to act to further that value (receiving and responding are prerequisite behaviors).

Organization (4.00–4.99): ability of the learner to organize, classify, and prioritize val-ues by integrating a new value into a general set of values, to determine interrelationships of values, and to harmoniously establish some as dominant and pervasive (receiving, responding, and valuing are prerequisite behaviors).

Characterization (5.00–5.99): ability of the learner to integrate values into a total philosophy or world view, showing firm commitment and consistency of responses to the values by generalizing certain experiences into a value system or attitude cluster (receiving, responding, valuing, and organization are prerequisite behaviors).

Table 10-4 is a list of verbs commonly used in writing affective-level behavioral objectives.

say, design, or action, by applying appropriate standards or criteria (knowledge, comprehension, application, analysis, and synthesis are prerequisite behaviors).

Table 10–4 lists verbs commonly used in writing cognitive-level behavioral objectives.

Examples of Behavioral Objectives in the Cognitive Domain

Analysis level: "After reading handouts provided by the nurse educator, the family member will calculate the correct number of total grams of protein included on average per day in the family diet."

Synthesis level: "Given a sample list of foods, the patient will devise a menu to include foods from the four food groups (dairy, meat, vegetables and fruits, and grains) in the recommended amounts for daily intake."

Teaching in the Cognitive Domain

A variety of teaching methods and tools exist for the primary purpose of developing cognitive abilities. The methods most often used to stimulate learning in the cognitive domain include lecture, one-to-one instruction, and computer-assisted instruction (see Chapter 11). Verbal, written, and visual tools are all particularly successful in supplementing the teaching methods to help learners master cognitive content. Content knowledge can be gained by exposure to all types of educational experiences, including the process methods used primarily for affective and psychomotor learning. Cognitive knowledge, however, is an essential prerequisite for the learner to engage in other educational activities such as group discussion or role-playing. Otherwise, what results is "pooled ignorance." For example, clients cannot adequately learn through group discussion if they do not possess an accurate and at least a basic knowledge level of the subject at hand to draw on for purposes of discourse. Participating in a group discussion experience is not the same thing as engaging in a brainstorming session. Brainstorming does not necessarily require prior knowledge of information about issues or problems to be explored.

Cognitive domain learning is the traditional focus of most teaching. In education of patients, nursing staff, and students, emphasis remains on the sharing of facts, theories, concepts, and the like. Cognitive processing, that is, the means through which knowledge is acquired, has taken precedence over psychomotor skill development and the learning of affective behaviors (Ellis, 1993). Perhaps this is because educators typically feel more confident and more skilled in being the "giver of information" rather than being the facilitator and coordinator of learning. Lecture and one-to-one instruction are the most often used, albeit abused, teaching methods. Both of these instructional approaches, when taught in a typical fashion, are directed almost exclusively at the cognitive domain.

The Affective Domain

The affective domain is known as the "feeling" domain. Learning in this domain involves an increasing internalization or commitment to feelings expressed as emotions, interests, attitudes, values, and appreciations. While the cognitive domain is ordered in terms of complexity of behaviors, the affective domain is divided into categories that specify the degree of a person's depth of emotional responses to tasks. It represents the degree to which feelings or attitudes toward complex phenomena are incorporated into one's personality or value system (Redman, 1993; Arends, 1994). Objectives in this domain are divided into five categories, each specifying the associated level of affective responses as listed and described in the following section (Bloom et al., 1956; Krathwohl et al., 1964).

Levels of Affective Behavior

Receiving (1.00–1.99): ability of the learner to show awareness of an idea or fact or a consciousness of a situation or event in the environment. This level represents a willingness to selectively attend to or focus on data or to receive a stimulus.

Responding (2.00–2.99): ability of the learner to respond to an experience, at first obediently and later willingly and with satisfaction.

Examples of Behavioral Objectives in the Affective Domain

> *Receiving level:* "During a group discussion session, the patient will admit to any fears he may have about needing to undergo a repeat angioplasty."

> *Characterization level:* "Following a series of in-service education sessions, the staff nurse will display consistent interest in maintaining strict hand-washing technique to control the spread of nosocomial infections to patients in the hospital."

> *Responding level:* "At the end of one-to-one instruction, the child will verbalize feelings of confidence in managing her asthma using the Peak Flow Tracking Chart."

Teaching in the Affective Domain

A variety of teaching methods have been found to be reliable in helping the learner acquire elements of the affective domain. Questioning, case study, role-playing, simulation gaming, and group discussion sessions are examples of instructional methods that can be used to prepare nursing staff and students as well as patients and their families to incorporate values and explore attitudes, interests, and feelings in the process of developing affective behaviors. Role modeling of desired behaviors by the educator is also a powerful tool for affective teaching.

Nurse educators have been encouraged to attend to the needs of the whole person by recognizing that learning is subjective and values driven (Schoenly, 1994). For practicing nurses, affective learning is especially important because they are constantly faced with ethical issues and value conflicts. In addition, our increasingly pluralistic society requires nurses to respect the racial and ethnic diversity in the population groups served by health-care providers. Advancing technology also places nurses in advocacy positions when patients, families, and other health-care professionals are grappling with treatment decisions. In turn, patients and family members also are faced with making moral and ethical choices as well as learning to internalize the value of complying with prescribed treatment regimens and incorporating health promotion and disease prevention practices into their daily lives.

The environment in which teaching and learning take place is important to the successful achievement of affective behavioral outcomes. A trusting relationship and an open, empathetic, accepting attitude by the educator toward the learner are necessary to secure client interest and involvement in learning. Unfortunately, equal weight is not usually given to teaching in the affective domain. The educator's focus more often emphasizes cognitive processing and psychomotor functioning with little time set aside for exploration and clarification of learner feelings, emotions, and attitudes (Ellis, 1993; Rinne, 1987).

Schoenly (1994) examined affective teaching strategies that can be used to assist learners in acquiring affective domain behaviors. Once appropriate objectives and an accepting climate have been established, the following educational interventions can be selected and implemented:

Questioning: Although the lecture method is usually identified with helping the learner gain cognitive skills, the technique of careful questioning during the lecture process can assist in meeting objectives in the affective domain. Affective questioning increases interest and motivation to learn about feelings, values, beliefs, and attitudes regarding a topic under study. Low-level affective questions are directed at stimulating learner awareness and responsiveness to a topic, midlevel affective questioning assists in determining the strength of a belief or the internalization of a value, and high-level affective questioning probes for information about the depth of integration of a value.

Case study: This method can assist the learner in developing problem-solving and critical thinking skills through exploration of participant attitudes, beliefs, and values. Using learning groups with the reader assuming the role of a key player in the situation (nurse, family member, patient) rather than as a neutral observer will help in eliciting affective behavioral responses.

Role-playing: This method provides an excellent opportunity to practice new behaviors and explore feelings, attitudes, and values, to problem-solve, and to resolve personal problems associated with human circumstances.

Role-playing allows the learner to "walk in someone else's shoes," but without the actual risk, to gain empathy for the reality of another's situation. Being an observer during role-playing can sensitize the learner to the phenomenon, while active participation in role-playing energizes the learner to attend and respond to the phenomenon under consideration.

Simulation gaming: Process games, controlled by the participants and with flexible rules, are more appropriate for accomplishing affective behavioral objectives than content games, which are characterized by structured roles and specific rules and are better for cognitive learning. Simulation gaming promotes active involvement of the learner in goal-directed, although not necessarily competitive, activities. Debriefing following gaming is an important aspect of the technique to provide the opportunity for guidance in the application and assimilation of the experience.

Group discussion: This method provides the opportunity for clarifying personal values as well as exploring social values and moral issues. Value clarification involves identifying and sharing personal values for the purpose of increasing self-awareness and self-discovery. Values inquiry involves investigating the value systems of various ethnic groups. Both approaches provide the chance for in-depth learning of affective behaviors.

The affective domain encompasses three levels that govern attitudes and feelings: The intrapersonal level includes personal perceptions of one's own self, such as self-concept, self-awareness, and self-acceptance; the interpersonal level includes the perspective of self in relation to other individuals; and the extrapersonal level involves the perception of others as established groups. All three levels are important in affective skill development and can be taught through a variety of methods specifically geared to affective-domain learning (Richards & Vicary, 1985).

Affective learning is a part of every type of educational experience even though the primary focus for learning may be on either the cognitive or psychomotor domain. Learner feelings or emotions cannot help but be aroused to some extent when exposed to all types of new educational experiences (Bucher, 1991). Without a doubt, learning is a multidimensional process that can occur formally or informally in structured or unstructured settings (Andrusyszyn, 1989). Evaluation of learning is just as complex a process. However, evaluation of affective behavior is more difficult than determining cognitive and psychomotor skill acquisition. This is because affective behaviors are not usually overt and clearly observable. They are less tangible and more challenging to measure. Bucher (1991) suggests using the Likert scale as a means of discovering learner attitudes relative to a particular learning experience.

The Psychomotor Domain

The psychomotor domain is known as the "skills" domain. Learning in this domain involves acquiring fine and gross motor abilities with increasing complexity of neuromuscular coordination to carry out physical movement such as walking, handwriting, manipulation of equipment, or carrying out a procedure. In contrast to the affective domain, psychomotor skills are easy to identify and measure because they include primarily movement-oriented activities that are relatively observable. Psychomotor learning, including perceptual-motor tasks, can be classified in a variety of ways (Harrow, 1972; Simpson, 1972; Moore, 1970). Simpson's system seems to be the most widely recognized as relevant to client teaching. Objectives in this domain, according to Simpson (1972), are divided into seven levels as listed and described in the following section.

Levels of Psychomotor Behavior

Perception (1.00–1.99): ability of the client to show sensory awareness of objects or cues associated with some task to be performed. Cues relevant to a situation are attended to, symbolically translated, and selected to guide action, gain insight, and receive feedback. This level involves reading directions or observing a process with attention to steps or techniques inherent in a process.

Set (2.00–2.99): ability of the learner to exhibit readiness to take a particular kind of action, such as following directions, through expressions of willingness, sensory attending, or body language favorable to performing a motor act (perception is a prerequisite behavior).

Guided response (3.00–3.99): ability of the learner to exert effort via overt actions under the guidance of an instructor to imitate an observed behavior with conscious awareness of effort. Imitating may be performed hesitantly but with compliance to directions and coaching (perception and set are prerequisite behaviors).

Mechanism (4.00–4.99): ability of the learner to repeatedly perform steps of a desired skill with a certain degree of confidence, indicating mastery to the extent that some or all aspects of the process become habitual; the steps are blended into a meaningful whole and are performed smoothly with little conscious effort (perception, set, and guided response are prerequisite behaviors).

Complex overt response (5.00–5.99): ability of the learner to automatically perform a complex motor act with independence and a high degree of skill without hesitation and with minimum expenditure of time and energy; performance of an entire sequence of a complex behavior without the need to attend to details (perception, set, guided response, and mechanism are prerequisite behaviors).

Adaptation (6.00–6.99): ability of the learner to make modifications or adaptations in a motor process to suit the individual or various situations, indicating mastery of highly developed movements that can be suited to a variety of conditions (perception, set, guided response, mechanism, and complex overt response are prerequisite behaviors).

Origination (7.00–7.99): ability of the learner to create new motor acts, such as novel ways of manipulating objects or materials, as a result of an understanding of a skill and developed ability to perform skills (perception, set, guided response, mechanism, complex overt response, and adaptation are prerequisite behaviors).

See Table 10-4 for verbs commonly used in writing psychomotor-level behavioral objectives.

Examples of Behavioral Objectives in the Psychomotor Domain

Guided response level: "After watching a 15-minute video on the procedure for self-examination of the breast, the client will perform the exam on a model with 100% accuracy."

Set level: "Following demonstration of proper crutch walking, the patient will attempt to crutch walk using the correct three-point gait technique."

Teaching of Psychomotor Skills

When teaching psychomotor skills, it is important for the educator to remember to keep skill instruction separate from a discussion of principles underlying the skill (cognitive component) or a discussion of how the learner feels about carrying out the skill (affective component). Psychomotor skill development is very egocentric and usually requires a great deal of concentration as the learner works toward mastery of a skill. It is easy to interfere with psychomotor learning if the teacher asks a knowledge (cognitive) question while the learner is trying to focus on the performance (psychomotor response) of a skill. For example, while a staff member is learning to properly suction a patient, it is not unusual for the teacher to ask, "Can you give me a rationale for why suctioning is important?" or "How often should suctioning be done for this particular patient?" These questions demand a cognitive response during the psychomotor performance.

As another example, while the patient is learning to self-administer parenteral medication, the teacher may simultaneously ask the patient to cognitively respond to the question "What are the actions or side effects of this medication?" or "How do you feel about injecting yourself?" These questions demand a cognitive and an affective response during psychomotor performance. Although it is not unusual for the teacher to intervene with questions in the midst of a learner's performing, it is definitely an inappropriate teaching technique. What the educator is doing, in fact, is asking the learner to demonstrate at least two different behaviors at the same time. This can result in, if nothing else, frustration and confusion and probably will result as well in failure to achieve any of the behaviors successfully. Questions related to the cognitive or affective domains should take place before or after the learner's involvement with practicing a psychomotor skill (Oermann, 1990).

In psychomotor skill development, the ability to perform a skill is not equivalent to learning a skill. Performance is a transitory action, while learning is a more permanent behavior as a result of repeated practice and experience (Oermann, 1990). The actual learning of a skill requires practice to allow the individual to repeat the performance time and again with accuracy, coordination, and out of habit. Practice does make perfect, and as such, repetition leads to perfection and reinforcement of the behavior. The riding of a bicycle is a perfect example. When one first attempts to ride a bicycle, movements tend to be very jerky, and the act requires a lot of concentration. Once the skill is learned, bicycle riding becomes a smooth, automatic operation that requires minimal attention to the details of fine and gross motor movements acting in concert to allow the learner to achieve the skill of riding a bicycle. Some behaviors that are learned do not require much reinforcement, even over a long period of disuse, whereas other behaviors once learned need to be rehearsed or relearned to perform them at the level of skill once achieved.

The amount of practice required to learn any new skill varies with the individual, depending on many factors. Oermann (1990) and Bell (1991) have addressed some of the more important variables:

Readiness to learn: The motivation to learn affects the degree of perseverance exhibited by the learner in working toward mastery of a skill.

Past experience: If the learner is familiar with equipment or techniques similar to that being needed to learn a new skill, then mastery of the new skill may be achieved at a faster rate. The effects of learning one skill on the subsequent performance of another related skill is known as *transfer of learning* (Gomez & Gomez, 1984). For example, if someone has already had experience with downhill skiing, then learning cross-country skiing should come more easily and with more confidence because the required coordination and equipment are similar. Or, to use an example in teaching health-care skills, if a family member already has had experience with aseptic technique in changing a dressing, then learning to suction a tracheostomy tube using sterile technique should not require as much time to master.

Health status: Illness state or other physical or emotional impairments in the learner may impact on the time it takes to acquire or successfully master a skill.

Environmental stimuli: Depending on the type and level of stimuli as well as the learning style (degree of tolerance for certain stimuli), distractions in the immediate surroundings may interfere with skill acquisition.

Anxiety level: The ability to concentrate can be highly affected by how anxious someone feels. Nervousness about performing in front of someone is particularly a key factor in psychomotor skill development. High anxiety levels interfere with coordination, steadiness, fine muscle movements, and concentration levels when performing complex psychomotor skills. It is important to reassure learners that they are not necessarily being "tested" during psychomotor skill performance. Reassurance and support reduce anxiety levels related to the fear of not meeting expectations of themselves or of the teacher.

Developmental stage: Certainly, a young child's fine and gross motor skills as well as cognitive abilities are at a different level than those of an adult. The older adult, too, will likely exhibit slower cognitive processing and increased response time (needing longer time to perform an activity) than younger clients.

Practice session length: During the beginning stages of learning a motor skill, short and carefully planned practice sessions and frequent rest periods are valuable techniques to help increase the rate and success of learning. These techniques are thought to be effective because they help prevent physical fatigue and restore the learner's attention to the task at hand.

Performing motor skills is not done in a vacuum. The learner is immersed in a particular environmental context full of stimuli. Learners must select those environmental influences that will assist them in achieving the behavior (relevant stimuli) and ignore those that interfere with a specific performance (irrelevant stimuli). This process of recognizing and selecting appropriate and inappropriate stimuli is called *selective attention* (Gomez & Gomez, 1984).

Motor skills should be practiced first in a laboratory setting to provide a safe and nonthreatening environment for the novice learner. However, Gomez and Gomez (1987) suggest also arranging for practice sessions to be done in the clinical or home setting to expose the learner to actual environmental conditions. This technique is known as "open" skills performance learned under changing and unstable environments. In addition, research findings indicate that progress in mastery of a psychomotor skill can be accomplished just as effectively through self-directed study as with teaching in a structured laboratory situation (Love et al., 1989). However, contact with the teacher during practice sessions is an important element for successful psychomotor learning. Although educator workload necessitates finding cost-effective and time-efficient ways to teach skill development, mediated instruction should not be used as a substitute, only a supplement, for instructor input (Baldwin et al., 1991).

In addition to using demonstration and return demonstration, mediated instruction, and self-directed study as teaching methods for psychomotor learning, mental imaging or mental practice has surfaced as a viable alternative approach to teaching motor skills. Research indicates that learning psychomotor skills can be enhanced through use of imagery. Mental practice is similar to the type of practice athletes use when preparing to perform in a sports competition (Eaton & Evans, 1986; Doheny, 1993; Bachman, 1990).

Another hallmark of psychomotor learning is the type and timing of the feedback learners receive. Psychomotor skill development allows for immediate feedback such that learners have an idea on the spot of the results of their performance. During skill practice, learners receive *intrinsic* feedback that is generated from within the self, giving learners a sense of or a feel for how they have performed. They may sense that they either did quite well or that they felt awkward and need more practice. In addition, the teacher has the opportunity to provide *augmented* feedback by sharing with learners an opinion or conveying a message through body language about how well they performed (Oermann, 1990). The immediacy of the feedback, together with the self-generated and teacher-supplemented feedback, makes this a unique feature of psychomotor learning. An important point to remember is that it is all right to make mistakes in the process of teaching or learning a psychomotor skill. Unlike cognitive skill development, where errorless learning is the objective, in psychomotor skill development a mistake made is an opportunity to demonstrate how to correct an error and to learn from the not-so-perfect initial attempts at performance.

Learning is a very complex phenomenon. The cognitive, affective, and psychomotor domains, although representing separate behaviors, are to some extent interrelated. Movement-oriented activities require an integration of related knowledge and values (Oermann, 1990). For example, the performance of a psychomotor skill often requires a certain degree of cognitive knowledge or understanding of information, such as the scientific principles underlying a practice or why a skill is important to carry out. Also, there may be an affective component to performing the movement dimension for the psychomotor behavior to be integrated as part of the learner's overall experience and ability to attain the ultimate goal of independence in self-care or practice delivery.

DEVELOPMENT OF TEACHING PLANS

After mutually agreed on goals and objectives have been written, it should be clear what the learner is to learn and the teacher is to teach. Predetermined goals and objectives serve as a basis for developing a teaching plan. Organizing and presenting information in the format of an internally consistent teaching plan require skill by the nurse educator. Developing an action plan to achieve the goals and objectives set forth requires a determination of the actual purpose, content, methods and tools, sequence, timing, and evaluation of instruction. The teaching plan should clearly and concisely describe the various elements of the education process.

The three major reasons for constructing teaching plans are

1. To force the teacher to examine the relationship among the steps of the teaching process to ensure a logical approach to teaching, which can serve as a map for organizing and keeping instruction on target.
2. To communicate in writing and in an outline format exactly what is being taught, how it is being taught and evaluated, and the time allotted for accomplishment of the behavioral objectives. As such, not only is the learner aware of and can follow the action plan, but just as importantly, other health-care team members are informed and can contribute to the teaching effort with a consistent approach.
3. To legally document that an individual plan for each learner is in place and is being properly implemented.

Teaching plans can be presented in a number of different formats, but no matter what format is chosen, all the various elements of the teaching process should be included. A complete teaching plan consists of eight basic parts (Ryan & Marinelli, 1990):

1. The purpose
2. A statement of the overall goal
3. A list of objectives (and subobjectives, if necessary)
4. An outline of the related content
5. The method(s) of presentation
6. The time allotted for the teaching of each objective
7. The instructional resources (materials/tools) needed
8. The method of evaluation of learning

The major criterion for judging a teaching plan is whether it facilitates a relationship between its parts. A sample teaching plan format is shown in Figure 10–1. This format is suggested because the use of columns allows the educator, as well as anyone else who is using it, to see all the parts of the teaching plan at one time and provides the best structure for monitoring internal consistency of the plan. A different format can be used to meet institutional requirements or the preference of the user, but all parts must be included for the teaching plan to be considered comprehensive and complete.

When constructing a teaching plan, the educator must be certain, above all else, that internal consistency exists within the plan (Ryan & Marinelli, 1990). A teaching plan is said to be internally consistent when all eight parts of the plan are related to one another as well as to the domain for learning previously selected and identified in the overall purpose for teaching. Internal consistency requires adherence to two major aspects of the plan. The first aspect ensures that the domain of learning remains the same throughout the teaching plan, from the purpose all the way through to the end process of evaluation. The following example is adapted from Ryan and Marinelli's (1990) self-study module on *Developing a Teaching Plan:*

For example: If the educator has decided to teach to the psychomotor domain, then the goal, objectives and subobjectives, related content, and so on should be reflective of the psychomotor domain.

Purpose: To provide the client with the information necessary for monitoring blood glucose.

Goal: The client will demonstrate the ability to test for blood glucose on a regular basis.

Objective: Following a 20-minute teaching session, the client will be able to use a reagent strip, Chemstrip bG, to determine blood glucose level with 100% accuracy.

Subobjective: The client will be able to assemble all equipment necessary to test for blood glucose using a reagent strip without assistance.

The purpose, goal, objective, and subobjective are reflective of the psychomotor domain and are therefore internally consistent. The decision about what domain should be the focus of the teaching plan must be made prior to developing the plan and should remain consistent throughout the plan. Thus, if the purpose is written with a focus on the cognitive domain, then the remaining seven parts should be reflective of the cognitive domain. The same holds true for the affective domain. The

PURPOSE:

GOAL:

Objectives and Subobjectives	Content Outline	Method of Presentation	Time Allotted (in min.)	Resources	Method of Evaluation

FIGURE 10–1. Sample Teaching Plan

overall design of the teaching plan must match the domain of learning selected as identified below:

DOMAIN	TEACHING DESIGN
Cognitive	Topic centered
Affective	Feeling centered
Psychomotor	Performance centered

The second aspect of internal consistency identified by Ryan and Marinelli (1990) is related to the content to be presented. The educator must determine the complexity and detail of the material that is to be taught depending on the data obtained during assessment of the learner, such as the client's readiness to learn, learning needs, and learning style as well as other factors such as the resources and time available for teaching and learning.

The amount and depth of information to be taught depend on the learning level of the client. The focus for teaching a low-level learner would be to concentrate on the "need to know" information to ensure that a skill can be performed safely, compared to a high-level learner who can handle and who may desire additional "nice to know" information. Whoever the client may be, the content to be taught for each objective must be directly related to the objective. If subobjectives are included in the plan, then the same rule applies; that is, the content to be taught for each subobjective is directly related to the subobjective.

The method of presentation chosen also should be appropriate for the information being taught. If, for example, the purpose is to teach a client to self-administer medication from an asthma inhaler (psychomotor domain), perhaps some discussion will be necessary and relevant, but the primary method of teaching should be demonstration and return demonstration. Conversely, lecture and programmed instruction are appropriate teaching methods if the purpose of teaching, for example, is to impart knowledge of what constitutes a low-fat diet (cognitive domain).

The time set aside for the teaching and learning of each objective and subobjective must be specified. How much time is needed for instruction and acquisition of a skill depends on learner attributes, the type and complexity of the behavior, the depth of content, and the resources to be used to supplement teaching and assist with learning. Each teaching session should be no more than 20 to 30 minutes in length. In this period of time, one or more objectives may be accomplished or partially accomplished. Additional teaching sessions may be required for the learner to attain expected outcomes.

The resources to be used also should appropriately match the content and teaching methodology. If the purpose is to teach breast self-examination, then written or audiovisual materials or an anatomical model of the breast would be useful instructional tools. It is also important for the educator to keep in mind what resources would be an appealing, comfortable, and convenient medium for the learner. A variety of resources may be necessary to maintain the learner's attention and to serve as reinforcers of information. An important consideration is the literacy level of the learner. Giving a low-literate person technical reading materials will only frustrate and confuse the learner and defeat the plan for teaching. Conversely, giving too simple material to a highly literate person may lead to boredom and inattention to instruction.

Finally, the method of evaluation should match the domain in which learning is to take place. For example, if the behavioral objective is for the learner to be able to identify (cognitive) three major symptoms of an impending heart attack, then the evaluation method must test that knowledge by requiring the learner to state, list, or circle (or some other cognitive term) three of the most important symptoms of a heart attack. Evaluation methods must measure the desired learning outcomes to determine if and to what extent the learner achieved the expectations for learning.

In summary, just as with a nursing care plan, all elements of a teaching plan need to "hang together." The goal must be reflective of the purpose, the objectives are dependent on and must derive from the goal, the instructional content is dependent on and must be derived from the objectives, the teaching methodology is dependent on and must be related to the content, and so forth. If, for instance, content outlined in the plan is not related to any of the objectives, then the content is either unnecessary or another objective must be written as a basis for including the extra content. Likewise, if a teaching plan has no content relative to a particular stated objective or subobjective, then additional content must be included or the objective or subobjective eliminated, if appropriate. Also, during the teaching process, if the learner indicates in some way an interest in or demonstrates a need for knowing more than the original plan addressed, then the plan can be revised accordingly. Whether a plan is adhered to or revised, it must, above all else, reflect internal consistency. (See Figure 10–2 for a sample teaching plan.)

USE OF LEARNING CONTRACTS

The concept of learning contracts is a relatively new but increasingly popular approach to teaching and learning that can be implemented with any audience of learners—patients and their families, nursing staff, or nursing students. In the strictest sense, a contract is a formal legal agreement governing the terms of a transaction over a specified period of time between two or more parties (O'Reilly, 1994). In education, a learning contract is defined as a written (formal) or verbal (informal) agreement between the teacher and the learner that delineates specific teaching and learning activities that are to occur within a certain time frame. Learning contracts are a mutually negotiated agreement, usually in the form of a written document drawn up by the teacher and the learner, that specifies what the learner will learn, how learning will be achieved and within what time allotment, and the criteria for measuring the success of the venture (Keyzer, 1986).

Inherent in the learning contract is that there is some type of reward for upholding the contractual agreement (Wallace & Mundie, 1987). For patients and families, the reward may be recognition of their success in mastery of a task to move closer to independence in self-care and a higher quality of life. For staff nurses, the reward might be having the privilege granted to practice in a chosen setting or at an advanced level. For nursing students, the reward may be in terms of being allowed continued progression through a program of study. Rewards may be tangible, such as a certificate or award in recognition of successful attainment of an outcome, or intangible, such as outward praise from the teacher or an intrinsic sense of satisfaction in accomplishing a predetermined goal.

Contract learning has been introduced in education as an alternative and an innovative approach to structuring a learning experience that embodies the principles of adult learning. The origin of contract learning is derived from humanistic theory that acknowledges the person as an autonomous being whose efforts are continuously aimed at self-determination and self-actualization. The central view of the humanistic educational theory is that knowledge is a process, not a product (Mazhindu, 1990). As such, according to Kreider and Barry (1993), contract learning emphasizes how a body of knowledge will be acquired (process plan), not how a body of knowledge will be transmitted (content plan). Learning contracts are considered to be an effective teaching strategy for empowering the learner because they emphasize self-direction, mutual negotiation, and mutual evaluation of established competency levels. A number of terms have been used to describe this approach, such as independent learning, self-directed learning, and learner-centered or project-oriented learning.

Learning contracts stress shared accountability for learning between the teacher and the learner. The method of contract learning actively involves the learner at all stages of the teaching-learning process, from assessment of learning needs and identification of learning resources to the planning, implementation, and evaluation of learning activities. Since learning contracts are a unique way of presenting information to the learner and are the essence of an equal and cooperative partnership, they challenge the traditional teacher-client relationship through a redistribution of power and control. Allowing learners to negotiate a contract for learning shifts the control and emphasis of the learning experience from a traditionally teacher-centered focus to a learner-centered focus. Active involvement of the learner increases feelings of commitment and fosters accountability for self-directed learning (Wallace & Mundie, 1987).

The purpose of learning contracts is to encourage active participation by the learner, improve teacher-client communication, and enhance learner expressiveness and creativity. Learning contracts, whether they are formal or informal, can be used to facilitate personal development of the learner. In the case of staff and student nurses, this approach to learning also can enhance professional development as well. Learning contracts serve as a vehicle for fulfilling the internal needs of

PURPOSE: To provide patient with information necessary for self-administration of insulin as prescribed

GOAL: The patient will be able to perform insulin injections independently according to treatment regimen

Objectives	Content Outline	Method of Presentation	Time Allotted (in min.)	Resources	Method of Evaluation
Following a 20-minute teaching session, the patient will be able to:					
Identify the five sites for insulin inject-ion with 100% accuracy (cognitive)	Location of five anatomical sites Rotation of sites	1:1 instruction	2	Anatomical chart	Circle 5 anatomical locations on an anatomical chart
Demonstrate proper techniques according to procedure for drawing up insulin from a multidose vial (psycho-motor)	Accepted technique according to procedure Reading syringe unit dose markings	Demonstration	5	Alcohol sponges Sterile SQ needles and insulin syringes Multidose vial of sterile water	Return demonstration
Give insulin to self in thigh area with 100% accuracy (psychomotor)	Procedure for injecting insulin SQ at 90-degree angle using aseptic technique	Demonstration	10	Human model SQ needle and syringe Multidose vial of sterile water Alcohol sponges	Return demonstration
Express any concerns about self-administration of insulin (affective)	Summarize common concerns Exploration of feelings	Discussion	3	Video Written handouts	Question and answer

FIGURE 10–2. Sample Teaching Plan for Self-Administration of Insulin

the learner and the external needs of an organization (Keyzer, 1986). Learners are given the opportunity to change behavior and reach their human potential through an approach that fosters choice and growth-promoting independence and allows for self-paced learning. Clearly defined expectations reduce learner anxiety, decrease frustration, increase levels of personal satisfaction, encourage the development of self-directed learning habits, increase the rate and quality of learning, and provide a defined basis for evaluation of the learner. Learning contracts also can be used to facilitate discharge of patients to the home setting. In complex cases involving the care of a patient by a large number of multidisciplinary team members, a contract provides cohesion and an excellent communication tool between the patient, family caretakers, and the health-care team (Cady & Yoshioka, 1991). The major advantage of contract learning is that it provides structure while simultaneously providing the flexibility required to meet the various learning needs of individuals (Wallace & Mundie, 1987; Mazhindu, 1990).

Components of the Learning Contract

A complete learning contract includes the following four major components (Wallace & Mundie, 1987):

1. *Content*—specifies the precise behavioral objectives to be achieved. Objectives must clearly state the desired outcomes of learning activities. Negotiation between the educator and the learner determines the content, level, and sequencing of objectives according to learner needs, abilities, and readiness.
2. *Time frame*—specifies the length of time needed for successful completion of the objectives. The target date for completion should reflect a reasonable period in which to achieve expected outcomes depending on the learner's abilities and circumstances.
3. *Performance expectations*—specifies the conditions under which learning activities will be facilitated, such as instructional strategies and resources.
4. *Evaluation*—specifies the criteria used to evaluate achievement of objectives, such as

skills checklists, care standards or protocols, and agency policies and procedures of care that identify the levels of competency expected of the learner.

In addition to the above four components, it is important to include the terms of the contract. Role definitions describe the teacher-learner relationship with respect to clarifying the expectations and assumptions about the roles each will play. The educator is responsible for coordinating and facilitating all phases of the contract process. In the case of nursing staff and student nurse learning, the educator plays a major role in the selection and preparation of preceptors and acts as a resource person for both the learner and the preceptor.

Steps to Implement the Learning Contract

Wallace and Mundie (1987) outlined the steps to implement a learning contract. Although they specifically addressed the implementation of contract learning with regard to the orientation of new staff nurses, the following steps apply to establishing and carrying out a learning contract for any type of learner:

Step 1 *Determine specific learning objectives:* Identify what the learner must be able to do within an allotted time frame.

Step 2 *Review the contracting process:* It is vital that learners have a complete understanding of what contract learning is all about as well as their role in the process. Because learning contracts have not been widely used until recently, most people are unfamiliar with this teaching-learning strategy.

Step 3 *Identify the learning resources:* Introduce the learner to instructional resources available such as self-study materials and audiovisual tools.

Step 4 *Assess the learner's competency level and learning needs:* The entire process of negotiation of a contract is based on the learner's current abilities and learning needs. The educator initiates the assessment of the learner and collects data primarily through interview, observation, and pretesting to formulate objectives.

Step 5 *Define roles:* Before planning learning experiences and negotiating a contract, the roles of the learner and the educator must be clearly established regarding expectations of each.

Step 6 *Plan the learning experiences:* Determine the content, learning resources to be used, the skills that must be demonstrated, and the amount of time to pursue learning through assisted or self-study to meet the predetermined objectives.

Step 7 *Negotiate the time frame:* Based on appropriate sequencing of behaviors, from simplest to most complex, establish a target date for completion of each objective.

Step 8 *Implement the learning experience:* Take into consideration individual variation in the level of ability to do self-directed study and any other variables that may play a factor in completion of the specified learning activities. For patients, progress in learning may be influenced by changes in their health status. For staff nurses, the constant pressures of providing patient care services place constraints on time available for educational activities. For any learner, the education process is influenced by readiness to learn and how well the information to be learned is organized and communicated.

Step 9 *Renegotiation:* The type and level of complexity of behavioral objectives and the target dates set forth for accomplishing these objectives may be renegotiated at any point along the continuum of the learning experience to meet the needs of the learner.

Step 10 *Evaluation:* Periodic (formative) and final (summative) evaluation of the learner's progress and the actual learning experience itself is a shared responsibility between the learner and the educator. Preestablished performance criteria, agreed on prior to the initiation of the learning process, serve as the means to ascertain achievement of outcomes based on predetermined and prenegotiated behavioral objectives.

Step 11 *Documentation:* Evidence of achievement of learning objectives is determined jointly by the learner and the educator (and preceptors if used for nursing staff and students). When an objective is satisfactorily met according to written performance expectations, each party cosigns the date completed in the appropriate column. (See Figure 10–3 for a sample form of a learning contract.)

SUMMARY

The major portion of this chapter focused on differentiating goals from objectives, preparing accurate and concise objectives, classifying objectives according to the three domains of learning, and the teaching of cognitive, affective, and psychomotor skills using appropriate instructional interventions. The writing of behavioral objectives as to type and complexity is fundamental to the education process. Objectives serve as a guide to the educator in the planning, implementation, and evaluation of teaching and learning.

Assessment of the learner is a prerequisite to formulating objectives. Prior to selecting the content to be taught and the methods and materials to be used for instruction, there must be a clear understanding of what the learner is expected to be able to do. Appraisal should be based on a mutual determination between the educator and the client as to what needs to be learned, under what conditions learning can best occur, and the teaching and evaluation methods most preferred. Objectives setting must be a partnership effort by the learner and the educator for any learning experience to be successful and rewarding in the achievement of expected outcomes.

In addition, this chapter outlined the development of teaching plans and learning contracts. Teaching plans provide the blueprint for organizing and presenting information in a coherent manner. Above all else, a teaching plan must reflect internal consistency of its parts. Learning contracts are an innovative and unique alternative to structuring a learning experience based on adult learning principles. Contracts are designed to provide for self-directed study, thereby encouraging active involvement and accountability on the part of the learner. The communication of desired behavioral outcomes and the mechanisms for accomplishing behavioral changes in the learner are essential elements in the decision-making process with respect to both teaching and learning.

| Name of Learner: |
| Name of Educator: |
| Name of Preceptor (if applicable): |
| Date of Contract Negotiated: |
| Terms of Contract: |

Objectives	Activities	Evaluation	Target Date	Completion Date
Lists cognitive, affective, and psychomotor behaviors mutually agreed on and intended to be achieved	Lists teaching-learning strategies and resources to be used to achieve the objectives	Lists the criteria to be used to measure learning demonstrated		

Signatures: _____ **(Learner)** _____ **(Educator)** _____ **(Preceptor)**

FIGURE 10–3. Sample Learning Contract

References

Andrusyszyn, M.A. (1989). Clinical evaluation of the affective domain. *Nurse Education Today, 9*(2), 75-81.

Arends, R.I. (1994). *Learning to teach,* 3rd ed. New York: McGraw-Hill.

Babcock, D.E., & Miller, M.A. (1994). *Client education: Theory and practice.* St. Louis: Mosby–Year Book.

Bachman, K. (1990). Using mental imagery to practice a specific psychomotor skill. *Journal of Continuing Education in Nursing, 21*(3), 125-128.

Baldwin, D., Hill, P., & Hanson, G. (1991). Performance of psychomotor skills: A comparison of two teaching strategies. *Journal of Nursing Education, 30*(8), 367-370.

Bell, M.L. (1991). Learning a complex nursing skill: Student anxiety and the effect of preclinical skill evaluation. *Journal of Nursing Education, 30*(5), 222-226.

Bloom, B.J., Englehart, M.S., Furst, E.J., Hill, W.H., & Krathwohl, D.R. (1956). T*axonomy of educational objectives: The classification of educational goals,* Handbook 1: Cognitive domain. New York: David McKay.

Bucher, L. (1991). Evaluating the affective domain. *Journal of Nursing Staff Development, 7*(5), 234-238.

Cady, C., & Yoshioka, R.S. (1991). Using a learning contract to successfully discharge an infant on home total parenteral nutrition. *Pediatric Nursing, 17*(1), 67-70 and 74.

Cummings, C. (1994). Tips for writing behavioral objectives. *Nursing Staff Development Insider, 3*(4), 6 and 8.

Doheny, M.O. (1993). Mental practice: An alternative approach to teaching motor skills. *Journal of Nursing Education, 32*(6), 260-264.

Durbach, E., Goodall, R., & Wilkinson, K. (1987). Instructional objectives in patient education. *Nursing Outlook, 35*(2), 82-83 and 88.

Eaton, S.L., & Evans, S.B. (1986). The effect of nonspecific imaging practice on the mental imagery ability of nursing students. *Journal of Nursing Education, 25*(5), 193-196.

Ellis, C. (1993). Incorporating the affective domain into staff development programs. *Journal of Nursing Staff Development, 9*(3), 127-130.

Gomez, G.E., & Gomez, E.A. (1984). The teaching of psychomotor skills in nursing. *Nurse Educator, 9*(4), 35-39.

Gomez, G.E., & Gomez, E.A. (1987). Learning of psychomotor skills: Laboratory versus patient care setting. *Journal of Nursing Education, 26*(1), 20-24.

Gronlund, N.E. (1985). *Stating objectives for classroom instruction,* 3rd ed. New York: Macmillan.

Haggard, A. (1989). *Handbook of patient education.* Rockville, MD: Aspen.

Harrow, A.J. (1972). A *taxonomy of the psychomotor domain: A guide for developing behavioral objectives.* New York: David McKay.

Keyzer, D. (1986). Using learning contracts to support change in nursing organizations. *Nurse Education Today, 6*(8), 103-108.

Krathwohl, D.R., Bloom, B.J., & Masia, B.B. (1964). *Taxonomy of educational objectives: The classification of educational goals.* Handbook II: The affective domain. New York: David McKay.

Kreider, M.C., & Barry, M. (1993). Clinical ladder development: Implementing contract learning. *Journal of Continuing Education in Nursing, 24*(4), 166-169.

Love, B., McAdams, C., Patton, D.M., Rankin, E.J., & Roberts, J. (1989). Teaching psychomotor skills in nursing: A randomized control trial. *Journal of Advanced Nursing, 14*(11), 970-975.

Mager, R. F. (1984). *Preparing instructional objectives,* revised 2nd ed. Belmont, CA: Lake Publishing.

Mazhindu, G.N. (1990). Contract learning reconsidered: A critical examination of implications for application in nurse education. *Journal of Advanced Nursing, 15*(1), 101-109.

Moore, M.R. (1970). The perceptual-motor domain and a proposed taxonomy of perception. *Audio Communications Review, 18*, 379-413.

Oermann, M.H. (1990). Psychomotor skill development. *Journal of Continuing Education in Nursing, 21*(5), 202-204.

O'Reilly, D. (1994). Communication and effective learning: Negotiated study and learning contracts. *Nursing Times, 90*(9), i-viii.

Redman, B.K. (1993). T*he process of patient education,* 7th ed. St. Louis: Mosby–Year Book.

Reilly, D.E., & Oermann, M.H. (1990). *Behavioral objectives: Evaluation in nursing,* 3rd ed. Pub. No. 15-2367. New York: National League for Nursing.

Richards, B., & Vicary, J.R. (1985). The affective domain in health occupations education. *Nursing Management, 16*(7), 52-54.

Rinne, C. (1987). The affective domain: Equal opportunity in nursing education. *Journal of Continuing Education in Nursing, 18*(2), 40-43.

Ryan, M., & Marinelli, T. (1990). *Developing a teaching plan.* Unpublished Self-Study Module, College of Nursing, State University of New York Health Science Center at Syracuse.

Schoenly, L. (1994). Teaching in the affective domain. *Journal of Continuing Education in Nursing, 25*(5), 209-212.

Simpson, E.J. (1972). The classification of educational objectives in the psychomotor domain. In M.T. Rainier (Ed.), *Contributions of behavioral science to instructional technology: The psychomotor domain,* 3rd ed. Englewood Cliffs, NJ: Gryphon Press, Prentice Hall.

Wallace, P.L., & Mundie, G.E. (1987). Contract learning in orientation. *Journal of Nursing Staff Development, 3*(4), 143-149.

CHAPTER 11

Instructional Methods
Selection, Use, and Evaluation

Kathleen Fitzgerald

CHAPTER HIGHLIGHTS

KEY TERMS

instructional method	simulation
lecture	role-playing
one-to-one instruction	role-modeling
group discussion	self-instruction
demonstration	computer-assisted instruction
return demonstration	distance learning
gaming	instructional strategies

OBJECTIVES

After completing this chapter, the reader will be able to

1. Define the term *instructional method*.
2. Explain the various types of instructional methods.
3. Describe how to use each method effectively.
4. Identify the strengths and limitations of each method.
5. Discuss the variables that influence the selection of a method.
6. Recognize strategies to enhance teaching effectiveness.
7. Explain how to evaluate the method(s) used.

After an excellent presentation, have you ever heard someone comment, "Now, there is a born teacher!"? This comment would seem to indicate that effective teaching comes automatically. In reality, teaching effectively is a learned skill. Development of this skill requires knowledge of the educational process including the instructional methods available and how to use them with a variety of learners and settings. Stimulating and effective learning experiences are designed, not accidental.

Instructional strategy is the overall plan for a learning experience. It involves the use of one or several methods of teaching and overall encompasses both the content and the process that will be used to achieve the desired outcomes of instruction (Rothwell & Kazanas, 1992). *Instructional methods* are the techniques or approaches the teacher uses to bring the learner into contact with the content to be learned. Methods are a *way,* an *approach,* or a *process* to communicate information, whereas *instructional materials* or *tools* are the actual *vehicles* by which information is shared with the learner. Some examples of methods are lecture, small-group discussion, demonstration and

return demonstration, role modeling, role-playing, gaming, simulation, computer-assisted instruction, self-learning modules, and individual instruction techniques. Books, videos, and posters are examples of materials and tools. It is important for this distinction to be made between the terms *methods* and *tools* because they are often used interchangeably by educators and not dealt with as distinctly separate entities when planning an educational activity.

This chapter will review the types of instructional methods available and how to choose and use them efficiently and effectively. It will also identify the strengths and limitations of each method, the variables influencing the selection of various techniques, and how to evaluate the methods used to improve the delivery of instruction. Because the educator is the one who is responsible for the instructional design and presentation and plays a major role in successful learning, specific teaching strategies will be suggested for enhancing the learning process. Throughout, examples will be drawn from both patient and staff education because the nurse is expected to teach a variety of learners in a variety of settings.

TYPES OF INSTRUCTIONAL METHODS

When learners know what is expected of them, they learn regardless of the methods or tools used for teaching (Haggard, 1989). However, the teacher functions in a vital role by providing guidance and support for learning. In addition, the use of appropriate methods to meet the needs of learners should not be underestimated. There is no one perfect method for all learners and learning experiences. Whatever the method chosen, it will usually be most effective if it is used in conjunction with other strategies and tools to enhance learning and improve teaching-learning productivity. Even though a teacher may use one method predominately over another, it is rarely adhered to in a pure fashion and is really a combination of various methods. Using the lecture as the primary format with the opportunity for question and answer periods and short discussion sessions interspersed is a good example of this. Decisions as to what methods to use will be based on such variables as how active the learner is or wishes to be and how much control the teacher chooses to exert over the learning experience. Audience size, diversity (e.g., age, educational background, culture), preferred learning style, and the setting for teaching are also important considerations.

Instructional methods can be categorized in many different ways. Rationale for classification is determined according to whether the learner's role is active or passive, the technique is student or instructor centered, or the focus is on content versus process knowledge. For the purposes of this discussion, traditional teaching methods, with which most people are familiar, will be examined first, followed by nontraditional methods of instruction. The traditional methods include lecture, group discussion, one-to-one instruction, demonstration, and return demonstration. These methods tend to have more teacher input and control during encounters with the learner than the less traditional formats, which include gaming, simulation, role-playing, role-modeling, self-instruction activities, computer-assisted instruction, and distance learning. Teachers' roles in these nontraditional approaches are more as designers and facilitators than as verbal presenters and the givers of information. Both traditional and nontraditional methods can be used either with the individual learner or with groups of learners.

Traditional Methods

Lecture

Lecture can be defined as a highly structured method by which the teacher verbally transmits information directly to groups of learners for the purpose of instruction. It is one of the oldest and most often used methods. In its purest form, the lecture format allows for only minimal exchange between the teacher and the learner, but it can be an effective method of teaching in the lower-level cognitive domain to impart content knowledge. It is useful to demonstrate patterns, highlight main ideas, or present unique ways of viewing information. It is an efficient, cost-effective method for getting large amounts of information across to a large number of people all at the same time as well as within a relatively reasonable time frame. For example, the lecture might be used to introduce an agency's mission statement to new staff orientees or to explain diabetes mellitus to a group of laypeople. It should not be used, however, to give people the same information that they could read independently at another time and place. It is the lecturer's expertise, both in theory and experience, that can substantially contribute to the learner's understanding of a subject. Lecture is also useful in providing foundational background information as a basis for subsequent group discussions and is a means to summarize data and current research findings not available elsewhere (Whitman et al., 1992). In addition, the lecture can be easily supplemented with handout materials and other audiovisual aids.

With respect to its limitations, the lecture method is ineffective in influencing affective and psychomotor behaviors. This method does not provide for much stimulation of learners, and there is little opportunity for learner involvement. They are passive recipients of the information being presented. The focus, instead, is very instructor centered, and thus the most active participant is frequently the most knowledgeable—the teacher. Because the lecture does not account for individual differences in background, attention span, or learning style, all learners are exposed to the same information regardless of ability or need. This is particularly evident in patient groups where cognitive abilities and stages of coping with some topics are at variable levels. This diversity within groups makes it difficult and challenging, if not impossible, for the teacher to effectively target the needs of all the learners in the audience. In addition, although the method is considered cost-effective, cost-effectiveness should not be determined just by calculating the teacher-student ratio of contact hours during class. Teacher preparation time, how often the material needs to be presented, and the follow-up time used to individualize learning and evaluate outcomes must also be taken into account.

Despite the limitations of this method, there are specific strategies to strengthen the impact of a lecture. Each lecture should include an introduction, body, and conclusion. During the introduction, learners should be presented with an overview of the behavioral objectives pertinent to the lecture topic along with an explanation as to why these objectives are significant.

Engage learners' attention by an informal survey or stating the objectives as questions that will be answered during the body of the lecture. Use humor and your personality to help to establish rapport with your audience. If this is one of a series of lectures, you need to make a connection with the overall subject to the topic being presented as well as its relationship to previous topics presented and the presentations that will follow.

The next portion of the lecture is the body, or the actual delivery of the content. Careful preparation is needed so that the important aspects are covered in an accurate, logical, cohesive, and interesting manner. Examples should be used throughout to enhance the salient points you wish to make, but extraneous facts and redundant examples should be edited so as not to reduce the impact of your message. Since the lecture format tends to be very passive for learners, the effectiveness of your presentation can be enhanced if you mix it with other methods, such as discussion or question and answer sessions. Use of audiovisual materials such as a video, overheads, or slides also adds variety to your presentation. Make sure all audiovisual equipment is functional and that you know how to use it before the beginning of the lecture. A technical malfunction will be disconcerting for both you and your audience. If you are nervous or inexperienced, practice before a mirror, a video camera, or a constructive colleague. Outline your presentation on cards, overheads, or slides. Reading a printed copy of the entire presentation is exceedingly boring to your audience. Vary your presentation style and tone of voice to avoid monotony. Move around the stage or room. Your enthusiasm, expertise, and interest in the topic can also be used to capture and hold the group's attention. Be sure to keep within the time allotted to you. Lectures of long duration will result in loss of attention and boredom on the part of the learner.

The final section of the lecture format is the summary or conclusion. At this juncture, review the major concepts presented. It is very important that your lecture not exceed the prescribed time so that you do not have to end because time has run out. Try to leave some leeway for questions and summary information. If you are using a microphone in a large group, be sure to repeat the questions so the rest of the audience can hear them. If time runs short, state that you will only be able to answer a few queries but invite immediate follow-up by meeting with interested individuals alone or in a smaller group or by suggesting relevant readings.

Group Discussion

Group discussion, by definition, is a method of teaching whereby learners get together to exchange information, feelings, and opinions with each other and the teacher. Discussion is one of the most commonly employed instructional techniques. The activity is learner centered and subject centered. Group size can vary, but most group discussion techniques can be used with as few as 3 people and as many as 15 to 20 people. Group discussion is an effective method for teaching in the affective as well as the cognitive domains.

The most important element to focus on is the preset behavioral objectives when using this method. These objectives are the learning goals of the interaction and should be presented at the beginning of each session. Careful adherence to them prevents the discussion from becoming an aimless wandering of ideas or a forum for the strongest group member to voice opinions and feelings. The teacher's role is to act as a facilitator in keeping the discussion on focus and in tying points together. The instructor must be well versed in the subject matter to field questions, to move the discussion along in the direction intended, and to give appropriate feedback.

Teacher involvement and control of the process vary with the needs of the group. Group discussion requires the teacher to be able to tolerate less structure and organization than other traditional methods such as lecture or one-to-one instruction. The group must have some knowledge of the content before this method can be effective. Otherwise the discussion is based on "pooled ignorance." An experienced group of staff may need little input while they work out a complex patient problem. A new group of patients or family members with little understanding of a topic will need to access information directly from the teacher or another source before they can knowledgeably participate in the problem-solving process. The teacher's responsibility is to make sure every member of the group has interpreted information correctly because failure to do so will lead to conclusions based on faulty data. Patient groups need to be prescreened. While diversity within a group is beneficial, a large range in literacy skills, states of anxiety, and experiences with acute and chronic conditions may lead to difficulty in meeting any one member's needs.

Also, it is important for the teacher to maintain the trust of the group. Everyone must feel safe and comfortable enough to express their point of view. Respectful attention and tolerance toward others should be modeled by the teacher and required of all group members. This does not preclude correcting errors or disagreements. A clear message must be given that while personal opinions may be debatable, the inherent value of what each member has to say and their right to participate is guaranteed.

The major advantage of group discussion is that it stimulates learners to think about issues and problems and exchange their own experiences, thereby making learning more active. It provides opportunities for sharing of ideas, receiving peer support, fostering a feeling of belonging, giving guidance, and reinforcing previous learning. Discussion is effective in assisting learners to identify resources and to internalize the topic being discussed by helping them to reflect on its personal meaning. Active learning leads to greater retention of information (Haggard, 1989).

The group discussion method is economically beneficial from a time-efficiency perspective. Teaching people in groups rather than individually allows the teacher to reach a number of learners at the same time. With health-care costs rising, this method should be considered as an efficient and effective method to teach groups with similar objectives such as preparation for childbirth or cardiac bypass surgery. Through group work, members share common concerns and receive reinforcement from each other. The idea that "we're all in the same boat" or "If you can do it, I can do it" serves to stimulate motivation for learning as a result of peer support. Group size, a major consideration in group teaching, should be determined by the purpose or task to be accomplished (Whitman et al., 1992). Although a large group has the potential for greater diversity because members will vary in experiential and knowledge background, there will be less chance for everyone to participate and for individual needs to be met (Anderson, 1990). Arnold and Boggs (1989) suggest that a group size of six to eight members is ideal to achieve diversity of ideas and yet allow for balanced interaction among members. Groups larger in number than this can be broken down into smaller units to promote greater interaction by all members and to better attend to the skill development of each individual.

Group discussion has proved particularly helpful to patients and families dealing with chronic illness. It is a forum to share content information for cognitive growth and also an opportunity to learn self-efficacy. This increase in confidence levels of patients and families helps in their ability to handle an illness (Lorig & Gonzalez, 1993). The process helps people learn how to respond to situations, improve their coping mechanisms, and explore ways to incorporate needed changes into their lives. Group discussion is most effective during the accommodation stage of psychological adjustment to chronic illness because the interactions help reduce isolation and foster identification with others who are in similar circumstances (Fredette, 1990). Group discussion also benefits other types of learners. For example, following a panel presentation by persons living with AIDS, a discussion session was an effective way to break down the negative stereotypes on the part of some health-care workers (Peters & Connell, 1991).

The opportunity afforded all members to be active participants is the major benefit of group discussion, but this method can also lead to difficulties if one or two members tend to dominate the discussion or digress from the objectives. Shy learners may refuse to become involved or will need a great deal of encouragement to participate, while digressing or dominating learners will need to be tactfully redirected in a manner that lessens their influence on the group without damaging the trust of other group members. Harsh or sarcastic treatment resulting in insults breaks down the relationship between the teacher and the learners as well as relationships among learners, which creates an environment unsuitable for learning. One helpful approach is to tell the group at the beginning of the session that the goal is to hear from all members by asking for their input and points of view during the actual discussion period. Persons who digress should be requested to hold questions that can be handled privately at the end of class because these are important but unique to their circumstances. The discussion method may prove especially difficult and disconcerting for the novice teacher when faced with a group that does not easily interact.

From a financial perspective, it must be noted that group discussion requires the teacher's presence during each session to act as facilitator and resource person. Also, it often takes more time to transmit information via this method than other methods such as lecture. In addition, third-party payment for some types of group patient education programs may be difficult to obtain when the traditional fee-for-service reimbursement is not available. However, these programs may be economically valuable in preventing hospitalization or reducing time in acute care. Documenting these benefits based on measurable outcomes is very important.

One-to-One Instruction

The one-to-one method of instruction is one in which the teacher delivers individual instruction designed specifically for a particular learner. It is an opportunity to communicate ideas and feelings primarily through oral exchange, although nonverbal messages can be conveyed as well. This method should never be a lecture delivered to an audience of one to meet the teacher's goals. This experience should actively involve the learner and be based on the unique learning needs of the individual. One-to-one instruction begins with assessment of the learner and the mutual setting of objectives to be accomplished.

One-to-one instruction can be tailored to meet objectives in all three domains of learning. For example, teaching an individual to give insulin would address both the cognitive and psychomotor domains. Coaching an expectant mother so she feels she has enough control in using the techniques learned in birth preparation classes is an example of instruction primarily in the affective domain.

Mutual goal setting by teacher and learner is very important. It has been proved that patient education and counseling in chronic illness will result in better outcomes when the learner plays an active role in discussing alternatives and in setting the objectives and goals for learning (Kaplan et al., 1989).

Contracting, which clearly spells out the role and expectations of the teacher as well as the learner, is one effective way to facilitate mutual goal setting. Contracts should be written in specific terms and evaluated by both participants (see an explanation of learning contracts in Chapter 10). Anytime teaching is done on a one-to-one basis, instructions should be specific and followed by immediate response from the learner and feedback from the teacher. Allowing learners the opportunity to state their understanding of information gives the teacher an opportunity to evaluate the extent of learning. Also, communicating to learners what further information is forthcoming allows them to connect what they have just learned with what they will be learning. For example, the nurse educator teaching a patient about hypoglycemia might say, "Now that you understand what causes low blood sugar, we will talk about how to tell when you have it and what to do if you experience it after discharge."

The process of one-to-one instruction involves moving learners from repeating the information to applying what they have learned. In the above example regarding hypoglycemia, you might give the person a hypothetical situation as close to the patient's lifestyle as possible and let the person work through how to respond to it. This technique is called rehearsal (Redman, 1993). For instance, you might ask a busy executive who has diabetes how he would respond to feeling shaky and sweaty at 2:00 P.M. on a day when a meeting runs late and he misses lunch. Be sure to clearly state that this is not a test but rather a dress rehearsal for life situations. You can change the scenarios with further questioning to help learners plan how they could prevent such a situation in the future. This technique gives learners a chance to use the information at a higher cognitive level. It also gives the nurse educator a chance to evaluate learning in a nonthreatening manner.

With the one-to-one method of instruction, questioning is an excellent strategy. It can be used to diagnose at what point to begin teaching the learner. It can also be used to reinforce information, as well as a means to evaluate the learner's knowledge in order to plan for the next learning activity (Magenty & Magenty, 1982). Questioning should not be interpreted by the learner as a test of knowledge but rather as a way to exchange information and stimulate thinking. Two problems can occur with questioning. Questions can be too ambiguous such that the learner does not know what you are asking, or they can contain too many facts for the person to process effectively (House et al., 1990). Watch your learner's nonverbal reactions, and rephrase the question if you detect either of these problems. If the learner seems confused, it is helpful to state that perhaps you did not ask the question in a clear manner. This will guard against the learner feeling guilty or discouraged if a question was incorrectly answered.

It is important to give learners time to process information and respond to your questions. Sometimes teachers are uncomfortable waiting in silence for an answer or are impatient and attempt to correct an answer before learners complete their response. Questioning will be ineffective as a technique when learners are not given enough time to process information. Preliminary interruption may further interfere with the learner's thinking process and create a tense atmosphere.

Many nurse educators conduct individualized teaching of other nurses or student learners in the clinical setting. Clinical instruction is not a discrete instructional method but rather a very complex setting in which to teach experientially. A variety of methods other than one-to-one instruction can be used. Role-modeling, demonstration, return demonstration, and discussion are but a few. One-to-one instruction may be part of orientation, student preceptorship, or a continuing education activity. The learner is singularly guided in the actual practice setting, which may be a hospital, mental health center, the home of a patient, or any other setting in which nursing care is delivered. Each learning experience needs specific objectives that are tailored to the individual's needs. These objectives should be known to both the instructor and the learner. The "Performance Based Development System" was designed to determine a newly hired nurse's competency (del Bueno et al., 1990). This is a structured assessment of an individual's competency completed before planning of clinical experiences. Very focused clinical activities can then be planned with the staff nurse, nurse educator, and clinical manager.

Preceptors who assume clinical teaching roles may need to be taught how to teach effectively because they usually are expert clinicians but may not necessarily be expert teachers. Workshops and coaching sessions may be an effective way to do this. Evaluation is difficult, especially when there is difficulty separating the learning phase from the testing phase. This is the difference between formative and summative evaluation. Formative evaluation is done during the learning phase to mark learner progress and give feedback for growth. Summative evaluation is the testing phase and a final assessment. It includes assessment of patterns rather than single events.

One-to-one instruction has many advantages. The major benefit is the ability to individualize teaching. This method is an ideal intervention for initial assessment and continued evaluation of the learner in all three domains of learning. It is especially suitable for teaching those who are educationally disadvantaged or who have been diagnosed with low-level literacy skills or learning disabilities. The teaching can be paced and the content tailored to meet individual needs. Understanding of content can be determined on a regular ongoing basis followed by immediate feedback from the teacher.

The major drawback of one-to-one instruction is the isolation of the learner from others who may have similar needs or concerns. Learners are deprived of the opportunity for identification with others through the sharing of ideas, thoughts, and feelings with those who may be in like circumstances. New staff nurses being oriented to an agency or patients recently diagnosed with cancer can benefit from group interaction to explore mutual concerns. Caution in using the one-to-one method also must be exercised to avoid having learners feel "put on the spot" because they are the only ones who are the object of teaching—the sole focus of attention. The educator, too, must be careful in the use of questioning because learners may interpret this technique as a "test" of their knowledge and skills. In addition, it is not unusual for the educator to make the mistake of cramming too much information into each session, which can result in the learner feeling overwhelmed and anxious.

Economically, this is a very labor-intensive method and should be well tailored to make the expense worthwhile in terms of learner outcomes. One-to-one teaching of patients and families is often an inefficient approach to learning because the educator is reaching only one individual at a time. Clinical orientation of staff and students and continuing education for staff development are vital but costly when carried out on a one-to-one basis. The cost is in payroll dollars and in short-term nonproductivity of the employee being oriented (del Bueno et al., 1990).

Demonstration and Return Demonstration

It is imperative to begin by making a clear distinction between the methods of demonstration and return demonstration. Demonstration is a method by which the learner is shown by the teacher how to perform a particular skill. Return demonstration is the method by which the learner attempts to perform the skill with cues from the teacher as needed. These two methods require different abilities by both the teacher and the learner. Each is effective in teaching psychomotor domain skills. They also may enhance cognitive and affective learning, for example, when helping someone develop interactive skills to be used in crisis intervention or assertiveness training.

Prior to giving a demonstration, learners should be informed of the purpose of the procedure, the sequential steps involved, the equipment being used, and what they will be expected to do. Equipment should be tested beforehand to be sure it is complete and in working order. For the demonstration method to be employed effectively, the learners must be able to clearly see and hear the steps being taught. Therefore, the demonstration method is best suited to teaching individuals or small groups. The use of a big screen or multiple screens for video presentations of demonstrations can allow larger groups to more easily visualize detail. Watching a demonstration can be a passive activity for learners, whose role is to observe the

teacher presenting an exact performance of the required skill. The demonstration can be enhanced by the teacher slowing the actual timing of the demonstration and exaggerating some of the steps (de Tornyay & Thompson, 1987) or breaking lengthy procedures into a series of shorter steps. In the process of demonstrating a skill, it is important to explain why each step needs to be carried out in a certain manner. The performance should be flawless, but the teacher should take advantage of a mistake to show how errors can be handled. Used correctly, an error may increase rapport with some learners. However, too many mistakes disrupt the mental image that the learner is forming. When demonstrating a psychomotor skill, if possible, work with the exact equipment that the learner will be expected to use. This is particularly important for novice learners. For instance, the novice patient or family member who is learning to administer tube feedings at home will be anxious and frustrated if taught the use of one pump in the hospital when another type is used after discharge. Often the learner is too inexperienced to see the skill pattern and instead will handle each pump as a separate task. The seasoned staff nurse, on the other hand, will find it easier to transfer what is already known about tube feeding pumps if called on to learn to use a newly purchased pump from a different manufacturer.

Return demonstration should be planned close to when the demonstration was given. It may be necessary to do some anxiety reduction prior to the beginning of the learner's performance because the opportunity to return demonstrate may be viewed by the learner as a test and may lead to the expectation of a perfect performance for the first time around. Once a learner recognizes that the teacher is a coach and not an evaluator, the climate will be less tense and the learner will be more comfortable in attempting to practice a new skill. Stress the fact that it is expected that the initial performance will not be perfect. In addition, allowing the learner to manipulate the equipment before being expected to use it may help to reduce anxiety levels. Some patients may experience an increased level of anxiety when faced with learning a new skill because they identify the need to learn a skill in relation to their illness. For example, a young woman learning to care for a venous access device may be very anxious because of the diagnosis of cancer that has necessitated use of the device.

When the learner is giving a return demonstration, the teacher should remain silent except for offering cues when necessary or briefly answering questions. Learners may be prompted by a series of pictures or coached by a partner with a checklist. Casual conversation or asking questions should be avoided because they only serve to interrupt the learner's thought processes and interfere with efforts to focus on mentally imprinting the procedure while performing the actual task. Breaking the steps of the procedure into small increments will give the learner the opportunity to master one sequence before attempting the next. Praising the learner along the way for each step correctly performed will reinforce behavior and give the learner confidence in being able to successfully accomplish the task in its entirety (Haggard, 1989). Emphasis should be on what to do rather than what not to do. Practice needs to be supervised until the learner is competent enough to perform steps accurately. It is important that the initial skill pattern be correct before allowing for independent practice. High-risk skills should be practiced first on a model prior to actual clinical application. Learners will need a varying amount of practice to become competent, but once they have acquired the skill, they can then practice on their own to increase speed and proficiency. A critical care nurse will probably need little practice with a new IV pump that is similar to others already mastered. In contrast, a patient learning to manipulate a pump for home IV therapy may need many practice sessions.

It is very important to plan return demonstration sessions close enough together so that the learner does not lose the benefit of the last practice session. As with demonstration, the equipment for return demonstration needs to be exactly the same as that which was used by the instructor and will be expected to be used by the learner. Learners also will require help in compensating for individual differences. If you as the instructor are right-handed and the learner is left-handed, perhaps sitting across from each other would be more helpful than sitting adjacent to one another. The person with difficulty seeing the increments on an insulin syringe may need a magnifying device to facilitate accurate performance of a skill.

These methods actively engage the learner through multiple stimulation of visual, auditory, and tactile senses. The opportunity afforded for mental rehearsal of procedures being demonstrated prior to actual return demonstration has been associated with increased performance levels (Haggard, 1989). Repetition of movement and constant reinforcement of practice are the mainstays of successful learning in the psychomotor domain. Overlearning through extended practice instills confidence on the part of both the teacher and the learner that the skill will be competently performed and will be retained for a longer period of time.

Although the expression "practice makes perfect" is quite true, demonstration and return demonstration sessions are very time-consuming and require plenty of time to be set aside for teaching as well as learning. These methods are expensive because of the necessity of keeping the size of the group small and the need for individual supervision during follow-up practices. There are ways to reduce the cost of this method. If the audience is a homogeneous group of health professionals who need yearly CPR review, demonstration can be via videotape. Return demonstration can initially be performed with a partner supervising the competency of the skill. However, the final evaluation of staff competency must be carried out by an expert to ensure the accuracy of learning. The cost of obtaining, maintaining, and replacing equipment must also be calculated. Expenses can be reduced by reusing equipment if it will not interfere with the accuracy, safety, or completeness of the demonstration/return demonstration.

Nontraditional Methods

Gaming

Gaming is an instructional method requiring the learner to participate in a competitive activity with preset rules. These activities do not have to reflect reality, but they are designed to accomplish educational objectives. The goal is for the learners to win a game by applying knowledge and rehearsing skills previously learned. Gaming is fun with a purpose. Gaming promotes retention of information by stimulating learner enthusiasm and increasing learner involvement. More complex games require the learner to use problem solving and critical thinking strategies. This method adds variety to the learning experience and is excellent for dull or repetitive content that requires periodic review. Games can be placed anywhere in the sequence of a learning activity (Joos, 1984)—as a device to introduce a topic, check learner progress, or summarize information. This method is primarily effective for improving cognitive functioning but can also be used to enhance skills in the psychomotor domain as well as influence affective behavior through increased social interaction (Robinson et al., 1990).

In gaming, the teacher's role is as facilitator. At the beginning of a game, the group needs to be told the objectives and the rules. Any materials needed to play a game are distributed, and the various teams are assigned. Once the game starts, the teacher needs to keep the flow and interpret the rules. The game should be interrupted as seldom or as briefly as possible so as not to disturb the pace (Joos, 1984). When the game is completed, winners should be rewarded. Prizes do not have to be expensive because their main purpose is to acknowledge achievement of learners in a public manner (Robinson et al., 1990).

At the finish of the game, the teacher should conduct a debriefing session focusing on educational content and evaluating the gaming experience. Learners should be given a chance to discuss what they learned, ask questions, receive feedback regarding the outcome of the game, and offer suggestions for improving the process.

Games may be either purchased or designed. Well-known commercial games such as "Trivial Pursuit," "Bingo," "Monopoly," or "Jeopardy" have the advantage in that their formats can be modified, the equipment is reusable for many topics, and many players already have familiarity with the rules of play. Word searches, crossword puzzles, treasure hunts, and card and board games are also flexible in format and can be developed inexpensively and with relative ease. Be sure to pilot games prior to widespread use. Computer games, although much more expensive, are becoming increasingly available and are a popular option for many learners. Gaming is a method particularly attractive to children, who enjoy the challenge of learning through playlike activity. Games can be devised or modified for individual or group learning.

An example of a game is a word search for foods that are known to elevate serum potassium used with patients with end-stage renal disease (Robinson et al., 1990) (Figure 11–1). Another game

called "Emergency Pursuit" has content that is related to emergency situations that might occur on a medical-surgical unit. It uses a question and answer format, with two teams of staff nurses competing against each other (Schmitz et al.,1991).

It is particularly important to remember that games, whether purchased or self-developed, must serve the purpose of helping the learner accomplish the predetermined behavioral objectives. To participate, learners must have the ability and background knowledge sufficient to play the game. Games should be exciting and challenging enough to stimulate learner interest but not so difficult or competitive as to result in frustration, inability to succeed, or the avoidance altogether of this learning opportunity (Walts, 1982).

Along with the advantages, this method also has its limitations. Gaming can create a competitive environment that may be threatening to some learners. The group size has to be kept small for all members to be able to participate. The room must be more flexible than a traditional conference room or classroom to be set up in different clusters for teamwork. The noise level may be higher and the requirements more physically demanding than many other methods. Not all learners may be able to participate if they are restricted by a disability. Lewis et al. (1989) designed a game suitability checklist that is helpful in determining if gaming is a viable alternative to meet the objectives for learning (Figure 11–2).

Economic considerations include the cost for purchasing the game or the time taken by the instructor to design, pilot, and update the material. Some types of gaming also require the instructor to be present each time that the game is played.

Simulation

Simulation is a method whereby an artificial or hypothetical experience is created that engages the learner in an activity that reflects real-life conditions but without the risk-taking consequences of an actual situation. Participants can trial their problem-solving, interactive, and psychomotor skills. Clinical judgment and technical proficiency can also be practiced in a safe environment (Weston & Cranton, 1986). Simulations are effective for teaching higher-level learning in the cognitive domain, as well as promoting the attainment of psycho-

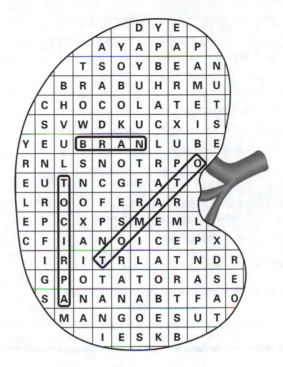

FIGURE 11–1.   Sample Word Search Game for Patients

SOURCE: Reprinted with permission of the American Nephrology Association, publisher, *ANNA Journal*, Volume 17/Number 4 (August 1990), page 307.

motor and affective skills. In actual use, there is overlapping between games, simulations, and role-playing because these three teaching methods all require active participation on the part of the learner in dealing with concrete, realistic learning experiences. All are experiential learning methods that call for the learner to choose an action and see the consequences. They are effective in facilitating problem solving, attitude change, and preparation for anticipated events (Rorden, 1987). It is important to have a discussion with learners after use of these experiential methods to facilitate analysis of the experience.

When planning a simulation, it is most effective if the learning experience is made to resemble real life as much as possible but in a nonthreatening way. The activity should challenge the decision-making ability of the learner. This can be done by imposing time constraints, realistic levels of tension, and the use of actual equipment or other important features of the environment in which the

specific skill will be performed. For example, a scenario could be developed to help parents of a baby with sudden infant death syndrome work through how to handle a situation when the monitor signals respiratory difficulty of their infant. Another example would be when a staff nurse is learning to respond to a chest trauma victim in an emergency room setting and is expected to gather an assessment rapidly and set up a chest tube drainage system with accuracy and speed. All these actions will take place while the nurse is pretending to interact with other team members and a very frightened patient. An effective use of simulation would need to include as many aspects of these complex processes as possible to determine if the learner has the necessary skills to do the activity correctly. Simulation should be followed by a debriefing session (de Tornyay & Thompson, 1987). It should include discussion of what happened during the experience, the decisions made, the actions taken, the consequences of the

GAME SUITABILITY CHECKLIST

Criteria	Yes	No
• Does the game meet the program objectives?	_____	_____
• Can the game be completed within the time allotted?	_____	_____
• Is the size and layout of the room conducive to the game?	_____	_____
• Will the available participants meet the minimum number required for the game?	_____	_____
• Do staff members have the time and interest to design or adapt games? If not, are funds available to purchase games?	_____	_____
• If the game requires equipment or supplies, are they readily available?	_____	_____
a. Are resources or funds available to design or purchase needed materials?	_____	_____
b. Does the game require replacement of materials following each use?	_____	_____
• Does the game require preparation or cleanup time?	_____	_____

FIGURE 11–2. Game Suitability Checklist

SOURCE: Lewis et al. (1989). Reprinted with permission from *The Journal of Continuing Education in Nursing*.

choices, the possible alternatives, and suggestions for improvement in skill performance. Simulation provides the opportunity for anticipatory learning.

There are various types of simulations. A written simulation is the use of a case study to which the learner responds. Staff nurses may be asked to respond by stating how they would handle a staff communication problem or manage a physiologically complex patient in the critical care environment. Models are frequently used in simulation to teach both patients and nurses. For instance, a patient or a nurse may be taught to change a venous access device dressing on a torso model. A peer, instructor, or trained individual may act in the role of a patient as an effective and economical method to teach certain noninvasive skills. Computers can be used to present simulated situations whereby information as well as feedback is given to learners in helping them to develop decision-making skills. Simulation gaming incorporates aspects of both methods (de Tornyay & Thompson, 1987).

A growing phenomenon for use of simulation is the learning laboratory. This is an environment where staff and patients can easily access models, computers, tapes, videos, and other equipment for use in practicing various skills. For example, a staff member may request an audiotape with heart sounds to practice this assessment. The role of the instructor is that of facilitator. Nursing staff report that this is a nonthreatening environment in which to learn (Jeska & Cosgrove, 1992). This type of laboratory has also been used on college campuses for nurses reentering the workforce. These returning students claim the learning laboratory is a stimulating and helpful approach to updating their skills. Following this simulated experience, they have an increase in self-confidence when returning to the workforce (Wood, 1994). Many of the same models and equipment for simulation in the laboratory setting can also be used to train patients or family providers in such skills as transfer techniques, sterile procedures, and urinary catheter care. Even though the equipment for simulation is permanently assigned to the learning center, efforts should be made to make the equipment portable so that it may be used on hospital units, in outpatient clinic settings, or in home settings. Simulated experiences should be followed with the actual experience as soon as possible. The simulation is never exactly the same as the real experience for which one is preparing, and therefore, the learner will need help with the transfer of skills learned in a simulated experience to the actual situation. In the future, virtual reality has the potential to narrow the distance between simulation and real life.

Limitations of this method are that it can be expensive and very labor intensive in many cases. Simulation can be made more cost-effective by reuse of supplies and by teaching a higher volume and a more diverse population of learners (Jeska & Cosgrove, 1992). Findings suggest that the modern learning laboratory in particular is an approach that will help nursing education to function both more efficiently and more effectively in the future (Kleinknecht & Hefferin, 1990).

Role-Playing

Role-playing is a method by which learners participate in an unrehearsed dramatization. They are asked to play assigned parts of a character as they think the character would act in reality. This method is a technique to arouse feelings and elicit emotional responses in the learner. It is used primarily to achieve behavioral objectives in the affective domain. This method is different from simulation, where learners are rehearsing behaviors or roles that they will need to master and apply in real life. For example, the patients in a diabetes self-management education program will need to practice behaviors such as selecting foods from a restaurant menu and setting their insulin pumps for the correct bolus of insulin because these are self-management skills that they are trying to master. In role-playing, on the other hand, the learner is not mastering a role in order to use it but rather to develop understanding of other people. The nurse attending an education program, for instance, may wear an insulin pump containing saline and select the appropriate foods to "see how it feels" to have to be aware of these issues rather than for the purpose of mastering the techniques.

The responsibility of the teacher is to design a situation with enough information for learners to be able to assume character roles without actually giving them a script to follow. Occasionally, people are assigned to play themselves to rehearse desired behavior, or the instructor takes a part to act as a positive role model for the learners. Most often, however, the teacher designates members in a group to play the part of someone else, and then they pretend to be that person for the duration of the exercise. Participants do and say things that they perceive the actual person would do, say, and feel. The purpose is to help learners see and understand a problem through the eyes of others. In other words, it gives them a chance to "walk in someone else's shoes." For example, children may use role-playing with puppets to explore their responses to such illnesses as asthma (Ramsey & Siroky, 1988). When professional caregivers take the place of patients, this role reversal helps to sensitize staff to the care they deliver to their patients.

For role-playing to be employed effectively, the teacher must be sure that the group has attained a comfort level that allows each member to feel secure enough to participate in a dramatization. This method should never be used with learners in the beginning of a group session encounter. Members need time to establish a rapport with one another as well as with the instructor, or else learners may feel embarrassed or self-conscious about playing a part. All learners should be given an assignment. Those who are actual participants need to be informed about the role they are to portray so they can effectively develop the appropriate actions. Those who are designated as observers require specific instructions about what to attend to during the role-playing session. Role-playing is best done in small groups so that all learners can actively take part as players or as observers. Active participation by learners is particularly important during the postactivity discussion or debriefing session. Because this method is most effective for learning in the affective domain, all participants need to discuss how they felt and share what they observed to gain insight into their understanding of interpersonal relationships and their reactions to role expectations or conflicts.

Role-playing can be used in conjunction with other instructional methods, but this requires careful planning as to the sequential placement of this strategy and the important points to be captured during the dramatization period. This method is an opportunity for the learner to explore feelings and attitudes. Role-playing has the potential for bridging the gap between understanding and feeling, thus reducing the role distance between and among clients and professionals (Redman, 1993). One major drawback in using this instructional method is the tendency by some participants to overly exaggerate the roles to which they have been assigned. They become too dramatic, and then the part loses its realism and credibility. This approach also has limitations when participants are uncomfortable in their role and therefore are unable to develop the role sufficiently. Despite these disadvantages, when role-playing is planned and carried out well, it is an effective technique to help learners change feelings or attitudes.

Role-Modeling

The use of self as a role model is often overlooked as a method. Learning from role-modeling is called identification and emanates from socialization theories that explain how people acquire new behaviors and social roles. Nurse educators have many opportunities to demonstrate behaviors they would like to instill in learners, whether they be patients, family members, nursing staff, or students. The competency with which you perform a skill, the way you interact with others, the personal example you set, and the enthusiasm and interest you convey about a subject or problem influence learners' motivation levels and the extent to which they perform a desired behavior. Role-modeling does influence attitudes and is a significant factor in achieving behavior change in the affective domain. "Actions speak louder than words" is a popular saying relevant to the use of self as a role model (de Tornyay & Thompson, 1987).

Self-Instruction Activities

Self-instruction is a method used by the teacher to provide or design instructional activities that guide the learner in independently achieving the objectives of learning. Each self-study module is usually focused on one topic, and the hallmark of this format is independent study. The self-instruction method is effective for learning in the cognitive and psychomotor domains where the goal is to master information and apply it to practice. Self-study can also be an effective adjunct for introducing principles and step-by-step guidelines prior to demonstration of a psychomotor skill. This method

is sometimes difficult to identify as a singular entity because of the variety of terms used to describe it such as mini course, self-instructional package, individualized learning activities, and programmed instruction (de Tornyay & Thompson, 1987). For the purposes of this discussion, the term *self-instruction* will be used and is defined as a self-contained instructional activity that allows learners to progress by themselves at their own pace (Abruzzese, 1992).

Self-instruction modules, which come in the form of workbooks, study guides, videotapes, or computer programs, are specifically designed to be used independently. The teacher serves as a facilitator–resource person to provide motivation and reinforcement for learning. This method requires less teacher time to "give" information, and each session with the learner is for the purpose of meeting individual needs. Some learners and teachers resist the self-instructional method because it appears to depersonalize the teaching-learning process (de Tornyay & Thompson, 1987). This is not necessarily true. There can still be communication between the teacher and the learner, but the focus of instruction is different. The amount of time for direct interaction is more limited than with other so-called traditional methods of teaching. This method adheres to the principles of adult education whereby the learner assumes responsibility and is self-directed.

A self-instruction module is carefully designed to achieve preset objectives by bringing learners from diverse knowledge and skill backgrounds to a similar level of achievement prior to the next step in a series of learning activities. For example, during orientation to an agency, there may be a self-study module on pharmacology prior to staff nurses' attending mandatory medication administration classes. A self-instructional activity can be made available to educate all staff on new infection control practices in an agency. Patients can learn breast self-examination or cardiopulmonary resuscitation techniques by using specifically prepared self-study materials.

Each self-instruction module needs to contain certain elements:

1. *An introduction and statement of purpose,* which generally include a table of contents, the terminal objectives, the intent of the module, and directions for its use.

2. *A list of prerequisite skills* that the learner needs to have to use the module.

3. *A list of behavioral objectives,* which are clear and measurable statements of what skills the learner is expected to acquire on completion of the unit.

4. *A pretest* to diagnostically determine if the learner needs to proceed with the module. Some learners may demonstrate mastery in the pretest and can move on to the next module. Other learners will get a sharper focus on their areas of weakness and may decide to seek additional preparation prior to beginning the module.

5. *An identification of resources and learning activities,* which specifies the equipment needed such as videotapes, slides, or written materials and outlines the actual learning activities that will be presented. Objectives are given to direct the learner, followed by material presented in small units of discrete information called a frame. The total length of a well-designed module is kept relatively short so as not to dampen the motivation to learn. How the material is presented will vary with the objectives and the resources available. For example, information may be given via programmed instruction or through a series of readings on the principles of conflict resolution. This is followed by a video presentation of a relevant case with the requirement that the learner write a response to what has been read and observed.

6. *Periodic self-assessments,* which provide feedback to the learner throughout the module. The user is frequently able to do periodic self-assessments prior to moving on to the next unit. This allows the learner to decide if the previous information has been processed sufficiently enough to progress further.

7. *A posttest* to evaluate the learner's level of mastery in achieving the objectives. If the learner is aware that a posttest needs to be completed, this requirement encourages attention to the information. Keeping a record of final outcomes is helpful in both staff and patient education as documentation of competency, as proof that standards were met, and for the purpose of planning for continuing education.

Self-instruction modules should be piloted with a small group before use with larger groups to determine suitability for the intended learners (Schmidt & Fisher, 1992). Modules can be made readily accessible to learners along with any resources that are needed to complete the self-study program. Inherent in this method of teaching are the advantages of self-pacing, active learning, the chance to review and reflect on information, the ability to get frequent feedback, and a mechanism to prove mastery of material accomplished in a particular time frame. Self-instruction modules have been found to be cost-effective because they are designed to be used by large numbers of individuals with minimal and infrequent revisions. It may be less time-consuming and efficient to purchase rather than produce a self-instruction module if the information presented in a commercial product is appropriate for the target audience. An example of the method's effectiveness in helping learners achieve objectives is a study that compared the use of programmed instruction and traditional classroom methods to teach nurses about how to protect themselves from occupational exposure to hepatitis B virus and human immunodeficiency virus (HIV) (Goldrick, 1989). Self-instruction was found to be efficient because it took half the time to present the information than via classroom instruction. It was also effective because the nurses who learned through programmed instruction scored higher on the posttest than those who attended a lecture, regardless of their pretest scores, experiential backgrounds, or educational levels.

The use of self-instruction is limited with learners who have low literacy skills, which would impede their ability to read or comprehend information as presented. Also, learners with visual and hearing impairments, low levels of motivation, a tendency to procrastinate, or little experience with learning by self-pacing will have difficulty with this method (de Tornyay & Thompson, 1987). Self-study also may be boring if this method is overused with the same population with no variation in the activity design.

Computer-Assisted Instruction

Computer-assisted instruction (CAI) is an individualized method of self-study using the high technology of the computer to deliver an educational activity. CAI allows learners to proceed at their own pace with immediate and continuous feedback on their progress as they respond to a software program. Most computer programs assist the learner to achieve cognitive domain skills but can also be used to master psychomotor behaviors and to change attitudes. Computers integrated with color, sound, and video motion are a type of CAI known as interactive video disc (IAVD) or computer-assisted video instruction (CAVI). This type of instruction is more expensive because of the multimedia applications.

CAI software include a variety of approaches such as drill and practice, tutorial, simulation, and basic problem solving (Anderson, 1992). An example of drill and practice type of application would be a program on drug calculations that teaches by continued repetition of exercises. Tutorials, on the other hand, usually present new information to the learner such as instruction on basic or advanced anatomy and physiology principles. Clinical simulations hold great promise for teaching because learners with background knowledge and experiences are exposed to the requirements of data collection and decision making to test their skills in artificial but realistic clinical situations under very low-risk conditions. An example would be a simulation program challenging the clinical responses of nursing staff to cardiac dysrhythmias. Problem-solving software allows the learner to develop the process of seeking solutions to situations presented.

Computer games, also referred to as *edutainment* (educational software disguised in a game format), introduce content or involve the process of competition in the application of strategies for decision making toward attaining a goal. They are an enjoyable and effective way to teach specific cognitive, psychomotor, and affective skills (Green & Brightman, 1990).

Computer programs can also evaluate learning. One complex type of testing is known as computerized adaptive testing (CAT). CAT presents test items and scores each response made, and then the computer decides what the next item will be based on the previous response by the learner (Halkitis & Leahy, 1993). Nursing students are using this type of testing to take their state nursing licensing examination.

The most valuable aspect of CAI is that it actively involves the learner in the learning process

and instruction is individualized to meet learner needs. The student can set the pace, spend as much time on a subject as needed for mastery, and will do so in a private, nonjudgmental environment (Anderson, 1992). Computer programs have enormous possibilities for teaching fundamental as well as advanced skills. The computer is a reliable, attentive, and tolerant drill and practice partner (Green & Brightman, 1990). CAIs offer consistent presentation of material and round-the-clock accessibility. They are a time-efficient and effective instructional method that reduces student-teacher ratios (McAlindon & Smith, 1994). It has been demonstrated that CAI assists the learner in the achievement of educational objectives in about one-third the time required by traditional methodologies. CAI not only saves time but can accommodate various types of learners. With its extensive branching capacity, CAI provides multiple self-assessment opportunities to allow slow learners to repeat lessons as many times as necessary, while quick-to-grasp users can advance more rapidly or test out of a program (Armstrong, 1989).

The limitations of CAI are that it is labor intensive if self-composed, and this type of instructional design is not a widespread skill among nurse educators (Whiteside et al., 1990). In addition, selection of CAI materials may present difficulty to the educator who is not experienced with this type of technology. Consultation with a nursing informatics specialist is suggested for educators who need to be updated on the use of and possibilities for CAI application to patient and staff education. Nursing informatics is an area of specialization that weds nursing education and practice with information and computer sciences. Postel (1993) suggests review criteria for educators to make the best use of limited informatics personnel and to employ the instructional and clinical expertise of other staff members. There are authoring software systems to assist instructors with designing CAIs.

There is also concern that computer instruction depersonalizes the learning process. Nontraditional methods should not be taken to mean that the teacher is unavailable for guidance in learning. What this technology does is deliver content, which allows more time for the nurse educator to concentrate on the personal aspects of individual reinforcement and ongoing assessments of learning. Because CAI requires self-motivation, this method may not be adequate for learners who have an external locus of control and who need human interaction to learn best (Poston, 1993).

Evidence suggests that nurses have a slightly positive attitude toward computers (McAlindon & Smith, 1994; Scarpa et al., 1992), and this will surely increase as nurses as well as the general public accommodate to this new technology. An effective approach for introducing this type of instruction would be to mix it with other methods of instruction.

Economic considerations remain a real concern because both the hardware and the software for computer instruction are very expensive. The future, however, portends enormous possibilities for widespread use of this method in institutions and agencies for purposes of patient and staff education. For example, CAIs have been used with good patient acceptance for both pre- and postoperative instruction on joint replacement (Tibbles et al., 1992). This instructional method has also been useful in teaching hospital staff nurses the concepts of quality improvement (McAlindon & Smith, 1994). The prediction is that someday soon multimedia systems for learning will be commonplace in educational settings around the globe (Green & Brightman, 1990).

Distance Learning

Distance learning is a telecommunications approach to instruction using video technology to transmit live or taped messages directly from the instructor to the viewer. It is becoming more popular as an instructional technique for staff development and continuing education programs and for student learning in academic settings. Teleconferencing allows for video and audio information to be sent via satellite, microwave, or ground telephone line from one place to another. Distance learning is made possible by network technology and is particularly advantageous for getting information to a wide variety of people located at great distances from each other. It is an ideal way to transmit current information without the cost and time in traveling to meet face to face with the expert delivering the instruction (Kaihoi, 1987). It can be interactive for the learner when teleconferencing is set up to allow for call-in questions via regular telephone. Because this method can reach large audiences, it is a relatively inexpensive approach to teaching. The drawback to this method

of instruction is that the teacher and learner are physically removed from one another, and it can become a lecture-type, one-way interaction session if no telephone hookup is available for interactive question and answer periods. As large health-care networks develop, this method may be useful for staff development and for patient education in a multicenter network.

Distance has also been eliminated as a barrier through access to the Internet. This network provides the learner access to a vast array of resources such as databases and human expertise in a variety of fields. This is a global resource and is limited only by the learner's inquiry skills and energy.

Table 11–1 summarizes the general characteristics of instructional methods.

SELECTION OF INSTRUCTIONAL METHODS

The process of selecting an instructional method requires a prior determination of the behavioral objectives to be accomplished and an assessment of the learners who will be involved in achieving the objectives. Also, consideration must be given to available resources such as time, money, space, and materials to support learning activities. The teacher is also an important variable in the selection and effectiveness of a method.

Teachers are at different levels on the novice to expert continuum, and how seasoned they are influences their choices of instructional methods. An expert skilled at facilitating small-group discussion may be a novice in the design and selection of CAI. A nurse may be an expert clinician but have only limited experience and effectiveness in the teaching role. Nurses are expected to teach but may not have adequate time, inclination, energy, or capability for developing the quality and variety of instruction necessary. Teaching is a skill that can be gained in formal academic settings, in continuing education programs, or through guidance by an expert peer mentor.

Teachers are likely to focus on a particular method because it is the one they feel most comfortable using without considering all the criteria for selection. There is no one right method because the approach is dependent on many variables such as who your audience is, the content to

TABLE 11–1. General characteristics of instructional methods

Methods	Domain	Learner Role	Teacher Role	Advantages	Limitations
Lecture	Cognitive	Passive	Presents information	Cost-effective Targets large groups	Not individualized
Group discussion	Affective Cognitive	Active—if learner participates	Guides and focuses discussion	Stimulates sharing ideas and emotions	Shy or dominant member High levels of diversity
One-to-one instruction	Cognitive Affective Psychomotor	Active	Presents information and facilitates individualized learning	Tailored to individual's needs and goals	Labor intensive Isolates learner
Demonstration	Cognitive	Passive	Models skill or behavior	Preview of "exact" skill/behavior	Small groups needed to facilitate visualization
Return demonstration	Psychomotor	Active	Individualizes feedback to refine performance	Immediate individual guidance	Labor intensive to view individual performance
Gaming	Cognitive Affective	Active—if learner participates	Oversees pacing Referees Debriefs	Captures learner enthusiasm	Environment too competitive for some learners
Simulation	Cognitive Psychomotor	Active	Designs environment Facilitates process Debriefs	Practice "reality" in safe setting	Labor intensive Equipment costs
Role-playing	Affective	Active	Designs format Debriefs	Develops understanding of others	Exaggeration or under-development of role
Role-modeling	Affective Cognitive	Passive	Models skill or behavior	Helps with socialization to role	Requires rapport
Self-instruction	Cognitive Psychomotor	Active	Designs package Gives individual feedback	Self-paced Cost-effective Consistent	Procrastination Requires literacy
Computer-assisted instruction	Cognitive	Active	Purchases or designs program Provides individual feedback	Immediate and continuous feedback Private Individualized	Costly to design or purchase Must have hardware
Distance learning	Cognitive	Passive	Presents information Answers questions	Targets learners who are at varying distances from expert	Lack of personal contact Accessibility

be taught, the setting in which teaching-learning is to take place, and the resources at your disposal. But the ideal method for any given situation is the one that best suits the learner's needs, not your own. If you are a novice, begin instruction with very familiar content so that you can focus on the teaching process itself and feel more confident in trying out different techniques and instructional materials. Ask questions of learners and peers in the evaluation process to ascertain if the method chosen was appropriate for accomplishing the behavioral objectives and meeting the needs of different learners in terms of their learning styles and readiness to learn.

Narrow (1979) emphasized the importance of periodically examining your role as a teacher and assessing the factors of energy, attitudes, knowledge, and skills, which influence the priority you assign to teaching and the ability to teach effectively. The following is a summary of her suggestions.

At any given point in time, your energy level will be influenced by both psychological and physical factors such as the amount of satisfaction you derive from your work, the demands and responsibilities of your professional and personal life, and the state of your health. Your feelings toward the learner also influence the enthusiasm you bring to the teaching-learning situation. If you feel drawn to the learners because you find them interesting or you are concerned or anxious about their situation, then teaching will most likely be a satisfying experience. If, on the other hand, the learners are demanding or display inappropriate behavior, you may feel negatively toward them and find the teaching-learning encounter more difficult and less fulfilling. You can develop the ability to accept individuals without necessarily approving of their behavior. Another factor to consider is your comfort with and confidence in the nature of the subject matter to be taught. If you find certain content to be stressful to teach because you lack relevant knowledge or skills, then additional study and practice to increase understanding of the subject will likely relieve your stress and apprehension so you can function more effectively in the teaching role. If you have difficulty communicating with learners about what you may consider sensitive material such as sexual behavior, mental illness, abortion, birth defects, disfigurement, terminal illness, and the like, it would be important

for you to examine your own feelings, seek support from colleagues, and use resources to help create an effective teaching approach. If the process of teaching-learning is to be a partnership, not only is it crucial to assess the learner but also it is equally important to assess yourself as the teacher. Often teachers fail to take into account their own circumstances and needs.

EVALUATION OF INSTRUCTIONAL METHODS

An important aspect of evaluating any instructional program is to assess the effectiveness of the method. Was the choice selected as effective, efficient, and appropriate as possible? There are five major questions to ask yourself that will help you to decide which method to choose or if the method selected should be revised or rejected:

1. *Does the method help the learners to achieve the stated objectives?* This question is the most important criteria for evaluation because if the method does not facilitate accomplishing the objectives, then all the other criteria are unimportant. Examine how well matched the method is to the learning domain of the predetermined objectives. Will the method expose learners to the necessary information and training to learn the desired behaviors?

2. *Is the learning activity accessible to the learners you have targeted?* Accessibility includes such issues as when information is presented, the location and setting in which teaching takes place, and the availability of resources and equipment to deliver your message. Patients and family members need programs to be offered at suitable times and accessible locations. For example, childbirth preparation classes scheduled during the daytime hours likely would not be convenient for expectant couples who are working.

3. *Is the method efficient given the time, energy, and resources available in relation to the number of learners you are trying to reach?* To teach large numbers of learners, you will have to choose a method that can accommodate groups, such as lecture, discussion sessions, or role-playing, or a method that can reach many individuals at one time, such as the use of various self-instructional formats or CAI.

4. *To what extent does the method allow for active participation to accommodate the needs, abilities, and style of the learner?* Active participation has been well documented as a way to increase interest in learning and the retention of information. Evaluate how active learners want to be or are able to be in the process of gaining knowledge and skills. No one method will satisfy all learners, but adhering to one method will exclusively address the preferred style of only a segment of your audience.

5. *Is the method cost-effective?* It is vital to examine the cost of educational programs to determine if similar outcomes can be achieved by using less costly methodologies. In this era of cost containment, insurers want their monies invested in patient programs that yield the best possible outcomes at the lowest price in terms of preventing illness and injury, minimizing the severity and extent of illness, and reducing the length of hospital stays and readmissions. Health-care agencies want the best staff nurse performance with the most reasonable use of resources and the least amount of time taken away from actual practice.

INCREASING EFFECTIVENESS OF TEACHING

Excellent teachers have one thing in common—a passion to keep improving their abilities. One does not "arrive" at being an expert teacher. The drive toward excellence is an ongoing process that continues throughout the teacher's entire professional life. What constitutes creative teaching? What personal attributes does the creative teacher possess? The following are techniques, not in any priority, that creative teachers use to enhance the effectiveness of teaching. In addition, some general principles for teaching are also put forth that can be used by all teachers.

Present information enthusiastically: The teacher who comes across as invested in the material excites the learner to identify with the subject at hand. No matter how well a lesson is planned or how clearly it is presented,

if it is delivered in a dry and dull monotone, it will likely fall on deaf ears (Cunningham & Baker, 1986). Try to vary the quality and pitch of voice, use a variety of gestures and facial expressions, change position if necessary to make direct and frequent eye contact with everyone in the group, and demonstrate an ardent interest in the topic to attract and fascinate an audience. The enthusiastic teacher is aware that an energetic attitude is contagious and enticing. However, one must exercise caution in overusing body language and overt actions because mannerisms can be distracting and can adversely affect learning.

Include humor: Many creative teachers use humor as a technique to grab, arouse, and maintain the attention of the learner. Appropriate humor can help establish a rapport with learners by humanizing the teacher. Humor does not necessarily require the teacher to tell jokes, and joke telling should not be attempted if this is not a skill one possesses. Furthermore, the teacher should avoid making someone the object of humor if it results in a "put-down." Humor establishes an atmosphere that allows for human error without embarrassment and encourages freedom and comfort to explore alternatives in the learning situations. Humor is a means to reduce anxiety when dealing with sensitive material, to provide poignant examples of everyday life experiences, and to reinforce traditional teaching methods (Freitas et al., 1991).

Exhibit risk-taking behavior: Creative teachers are willing to develop exercises in which many variables can lead to any number of possible outcomes. They use this technique to encourage learners to reach their own conclusions about controversial issues. Regardless of the outcome, creative teachers are prepared to deal with uncertainty. Exercises that allow learners freedom to experiment and express their ideas focus more on the process than on the result (Freitas et al., 1991).

Deliver material dramatically: Creative teachers seek ways to engage the learner emotionally by using surprise, controlled tension, or ploys. The teacher uses strategies that connect the educational material directly to the learner's life experiences so that information is made more understandable and relevant. Learners may be asked to participate in simulations, games, or role-playing to act out a part, live an experience, or test their capacities. These activities involve the learner and can leave a profound, lasting impression that can be recalled vividly and can be drawn upon when faced with a real situation. This technique engages learners by arousing their emotions (Freitas et al., 1991).

Use methods that match the topic rather than the teacher's personality: Most teachers have a preferred style of teaching and tend to rely on this approach regardless of the content to be taught. The effectiveness of teaching will be severely limited when the choice of method is based on the interest and comfort level of the teacher and not on the assessed needs of the learner (Freitas et al., 1991). Creative teachers adapt themselves to a teaching style appropriate to the subject matter, setting, and the various styles of the learners. Flexibility is their hallmark in tailoring instructional design to the unique needs of each population of learners. They are willing to use a variety of teaching methods to provide the best possible experience for achievement of objectives.

Choose problem-solving activities: Whether the learners are staff members or patients, the creative teacher recognizes that learners need to be immersed in activities to help them develop problem-solving skills. In today's world, professionals must have the ability to identify both patient and system problems by searching and sorting data, uncovering problems, and finding solutions. Increasingly, they are expected to work with interdisciplinary teams to determine and implement solutions to health-care problems. Learning activities must be designed to help these nursing staff and students to develop critical thinking and collaborative skills. Patients, especially those with chronic conditions, need problem-solving skills in order to know how to respond to changes demanded by their condition. What should they do differently on a "sick day," or what constitutes an emergency? Patients and families need more than just low-level cognitive information to make adjustments in their lives. The teacher will need to devise and orchestrate opportunities that challenge learners to critically analyze situations as well as support the learner in exploring possible alternative situations. The creative teacher encourages brainstorming sessions and supports the testing out of possible answers by the more nontraditional methods of teaching.

Serve as a role model: The creative teacher constantly seeks new information by keeping abreast of current research, theories, and issues in clinical practice for application relevant to the teaching situation. Expanding one's own knowledge base gives credence to what is taught and gains the confidence of learners in the teacher's expertise. A commitment to lifelong learning transmits an important value to others of their need for continuous personal or professional development. As part of the creative teacher's repertoire of behavior, role-modeling is an effective way to facilitate learning. Teachers are seen as credible role models when they are actively engaged in scholarly activities, are experienced in the field, and have advanced credentials to teach complex skills. The believability of a role model is greatly affected by the values displayed and the congruence demonstrated between what the teacher says and does (Babcock & Miller, 1994). If the learners regard the behavior of the creative teacher as desirable, they will likely imitate that behavior, which they perceive as eliciting positive effects (Narrow, 1979).

Use anecdotes and examples: The creative teacher uses stories, tales, and examples of incidences and episodes to illustrate points. Anecdotes, whether amusing, alarming, sad, or anger provoking, are valuable in driving a point home, clarifying a topic under discussion, or helping someone better relate to an issue. Use examples to reinforce the learning principle that simple representations can assist the learner to grasp complex ideas. Using examples relevant to past experiences and the knowledge base of learners helps them identify and connect in a concrete way with the material being taught.

Use technology: Creative teachers use technology to broaden and add variety to the opportunities for teaching and learning. They continue to increase the level of their own skills by taking advantage of the advances in technology to introduce and coach others in new ways of learning. They recognize that the sophisticated use of technology is a primary skill that will be needed for educational programs of the future. The use of different types of technology assists the teacher in helping learners meet their individual needs and styles of learning. Technology has the potential for making the teaching-learning process more convenient, accessible, and stimulating. Creative teachers are future oriented. A mastery of technological skills assures their ability to teach in innovative and eclectic ways to prepare students for learning into the twenty-first century.

Give positive reinforcement: Educational research is replete with examples of the effects of positive reinforcement on learning. Acknowledging ideas, actions, and opinions of others by using words of praise or approval, such as "That's a good answer," "I agree with you," and "You have a very good point," or using nonverbal expressions of acceptance, such as smiling, nodding, or a reassuring pat on the back, will encourage learners to participate more readily or try harder to improve their performance. Rewarding even a small success can instill satisfaction in the learner. Reproval, on the other hand, will dampen motivation and cause learners to withdraw. A powerful incentive is to ask learners to share their experiences with others. In a group, it is important to recognize the contributions of each member rather than focus primarily on the more aggressive learner or high achiever. What constitutes positive reinforcement for one individual may not suffice for another. Rewards are closely tied to value systems. The quantity of reinforcement varies in its effectiveness from one individual to another. A small amount of praise can have a strong affect for the learner who is not used to succeeding, whereas significant praise may be relatively ineffective for a consistently high achiever. The effects of reinforcement are also transitory. An incentive that works for a learner at one time may not work well at another time. Positive reinforcers, in the form of recognition, tangible rewards, or opportunities, should closely follow the desired behavior (de Tornyay & Thompson, 1987). The clearer the correlation between the desired behavior (cause) and the reward (effect), the more meaningful the reinforcement will be.

Project an attitude of acceptance and sensitivity: The ease with which teachers conduct themselves, the willingness to receive and answer questions, the simple courtesies extended, and the responsiveness demonstrated toward an audience set the tone for a friendly, warm, and receptive atmosphere for learning. If you exhibit self-confidence and self-respect, the learner in turn will feel comfortable, confident, and secure in the learning environment. If you come across as believable, trustworthy, considerate, and competent, you help to put your audience at ease, which serves as an invitation for them to learn. When you exercise patience and sensitivity with respect to race, culture, and gender, this projects an acceptance of others, which serves to establish a rapport and opens up the avenues of communication for the sharing of ideas and concerns. People will learn better in a comfortable and supportive environment. Not only is it important that the physical environment be conducive to learning, but also the psychological climate should be respectful of learners and focused on their need for an atmosphere of support and acceptance. Teachers must have a clear view of their role as facilitators and expert coaches and not as controlling disseminators of information.

Be organized and give direction: Excellent discussions, meaningful experiences in role-playing, or successful attempts at self-study are examples of teaching that do not happen by accident. They are the result of hours of skilled preparation, careful planning, and organization, which allow the learner to stay focused on the objectives. Material should be logically organized, objectives clearly defined and presented up front, and directions given in a straightforward, specific, and easily understood manner. Instructional sessions should be relatively brief so as not to overload the learner with too much detail and extraneous content. "Need to know" information should take precedence over the "nice to know" information to ensure there is enough time for the essentials. Regardless of the method of instruction used, the attention span of the learner waxes and wanes over time, and what is learned first and last is retained the most (Ley, 1972). Audiovisual materials selected to supplement various methods of teaching should clarify or enhance a message. Advance organizers should be used to structure information and assist the learner in identifying the subject to be presented and in what order.

Elicit and give feedback: Feedback should be a reciprocal process. It is a strategy to give information to the learner as well as to receive information from the learner. Both the teacher and the learner need to seek information about the quality of their performance. Feedback should be encouraged during and at the end of each teaching-learning encounter as well as at the completion of an educational program. Feedback can come from verbal as well as nonverbal responses to a situation. Feedback that learners receive can be subjective or objective. Subjective data, physiological or psychological, come from within the learners themselves. People sense how they are reacting to a situation. Internally, they usually know how well they performed or how they feel by their own responses, such as fatigue, anxiety, disinterest, or satisfaction. Learners are able to compare their own performance to what they expect of themselves or what they think others expect of them. Objective data come to the learners from the teacher, who measures their behavior based on a set of standards or criteria and who gives them an opinion on the progress they have made. To get feedback, the learner might ask, "How well did I do?", "Am I on track?", "Did I do all right?", or "What do you think?"

Feedback to the teacher is equally important because the effectiveness of teaching depends to a great extent on the learners' reactions. Whether positive or negative, verbal or nonverbal, feedback enables you to determine if you should maintain or modify your approach to teaching. Feedback indicates whether to proceed, take time to review or explain, or cease instruction altogether for the moment. The teacher should be direct in eliciting feedback from the learners by asking questions such as "Did I answer your questions?", "Is this clear?", "Do you need me to explain it further?", or "What more can I help you with?" The teacher should also be sensitive to nonverbal expressions such as a nod, a smile, a look of bewilderment, or a frown indicating an understanding or lack thereof.

Feedback is neutral unless it is compared with established norms, preset criteria, or past behavior. How much someone learned, for example, is meaningless unless compared to what the person knew previously or how the person stacks up against other learners under similar conditions. Feedback, either positive or negative, is needed by both the learner and the teacher. Praise reinforces behavior and increases the likelihood the behavior will continue. Constructive criticism tends to redirect behavior to conform with expected norms. Labeling someone's personality, such as cooperative, smart, stubborn, unmotivated, or uncaring, is harmful, but it is helpful to label someone's performance to give that person specific information for improving, correcting, or continuing the behavior (Narrow, 1979).

Use questions: Questioning is one of the means for both the teacher and the learner to elicit feedback about performance. If the teacher is skillful in the use of questioning, it serves a multipurpose approach in the teaching-learning process. Questions help to clarify or substantiate concepts, assess what the learner already knows about the topic, stimulate interest in a new subject, or evaluate the learner in mastery of the predetermined objectives.

Babcock and Miller (1994) identified three types of questions that can be used to elicit different types of answers. The first type of question is known as a factual or descriptive question. It begins with words such as *who, what, where,* or *when* and asks for recall-type responses from the learner. Factual questions such as "What foods are high in fat?" or "Whom should you call if you run out of medication?" elicit straightforward facts. Descriptive questions take a more open-ended approach, such as "What kinds of exercise do you get daily?", "Tell me what problems you have with activities of daily living?", or "What are the signs and symptoms of infection?", which require a more detailed and organized response from the learner. The second type of questioning involves using clarifying questions that ask for more information and help the learner to convey thoughts and feelings, such as "What do you mean when you say. . . . ?" or "I'm not sure I understand exactly what you are expressing."

The third type of question is known as a high-order question, and it requires more than memory or perception to answer by asking the learner to make inferences, establish cause and effect, or compare and contrast concepts, such as "Why does a low-salt diet help to control blood pressure?" or "What do you think will happen if you don't take your medication?" or " What do you see as the advantages and disadvantages in following the treatment plan?" After asking questions, a period of silence may occur, which can be uncomfortable for both the teacher and the learner. Anxiety over silence may be reduced by encouraging the learner to think about the answer before responding. In a group, this strategy also allows all participants to have a chance to think through their responses to the questions, which gives them the opportunity for a more thoughtful and deliberate response. Questioning helps the teacher appropriately pace the material being presented and arrive at an evaluative judgment as to the progress the learner is making in the achievement of the behavioral objectives.

Use repetition and pacing: Repetition, if used with discretion, is a technique that strengthens learning. Repetition reinforces learning by aiding in the retention of information. If overused, it can lead to boredom and frustration because you are repeating what is already understood and remembered. If used deliberately, repetition assists the learner in focusing on important points and keeps the learner on track. Repetition is especially important when presenting new or difficult material. The opportunity for repeated practice of behavioral tasks is called skill inoculation. Repetition can take the form of a simple reminder, a review of previously learned material, or the continued practice of a skill. Assessing where the learner is will help you to use repetition effectively. Pacing refers to the speed at which information is presented.

Some self-instruction methods of teaching, such as programmed instruction, allow for individualized pacing so that learners can proceed at their own speed, depending on abilities and style of learning. Other methods of group learning require the teacher to take command of the rapidity at which information is presented and processed. Many factors determine the optimal rate of teaching such as previous history with learning, attention span, the domain in which learning is to take place, how eager and determined the learner is to obtain a reward or attain a goal, the degree of progress in learning, and the learner's ability to cope with frustration and discomfort. Keeping in touch with your audience will help you to pace your teaching so that it is slow enough for assimilation of information, yet fast enough to maintain interest and enthusiasm (Narrow, 1979).

Summarize important points: Summarizing of information at the completion of the teaching-learning encounter gives a perspective on what has been covered, how it relates to the objectives, and what you expect the learner to have achieved. Summarizing also reviews key ideas to instill information in the mind and helps the learner to see the parts of a whole. Closure should be used at the end of one lesson before proceeding on to a new topic. Summary reinforces retention of information. It provides feedback as to the progress made, thereby leaving the learner with a feeling of satisfaction with what has been accomplished.

SUMMARY

In this chapter, all the major traditional and nontraditional methods of instruction have been presented. An in-depth review of the various instructional methods highlights the means for effective use, addresses the specific domains for learning, and compares the advantages and limitations relative to each approach. Emphasis was given to the importance of taking into account the learner characteristics, behavioral objectives, teacher characteristics, and available resources prior to selecting or designing any of the vast array of methods at the teacher's disposal. In many instances, guidelines were put forth to assist nurse educators in planning and developing their own instructional activities. In addition, the major questions to be considered when evaluating the effectiveness of instructional methods were assessed in detail. Lastly, but equally as important as selecting the right method, are the strategies a creative teacher uses as well as the general principles all teachers should use to effectively communicate with learners. What must be stressed are the inherent qualities of each method and that no one method is better than another. The effectiveness of any method depends on the purpose for and the circumstances under which it is used. Nurses in the role of educators are urged to take an eclectic approach to teaching by avoiding reliance on any one particular method and by using a combination of teaching methods to accomplish the objectives for learning while at the same time meeting the different needs and styles of each and every learner. Multisensory stimulation is best for increasing the acquisition of skills and the retention of information.

References

Abruzzese, R.S. (1992). *Nursing staff development: Strategies for success.* St. Louis: Mosby–Year Book.

Anderson, J.M. (1990). Health care across cultures. *Nursing Outlook, 38,* 136-139.

Anderson, S.K. (1992). *Computer literacy for health care professionals.* Albany, NY: Delmar.

Armstrong, M.L. (1989). Orchestrating the process of patient education. *Nursing Clinics of North America 24,* 597-604.

Arnold, E., & Boggs, K. (1989). *Interpersonal relationships.* Philadelphia: Saunders.

Babcock, D.E., & Miller, M.A. (1994). *Client education: Theory and practice.* St. Louis: Mosby–Year Book.

Cunningham, M.A., & Baker, D. (1986). How to teach patients better and faster. *RN, 49*(9), 50-52.

del Bueno, D.J., Griffin, L.R., Burke, S.M., & Foley, M.A. (1990). The clinical teacher as a critical link in competence development. *Journal of Nursing Staff Development, 6,* 135-138.

de Tornyay, R., & Thompson, M.A. (1987). *Strategies for teaching nursing,* 3rd ed. New York: Wiley.

Fredette, S.L. (1990). A model for improving cancer patient education. *Cancer Nursing, 13,* 207-215.

Freitas, L., Lantz, J., & Reed, R. (1991). The creative teacher. *Nurse Educator, 16*(1), 5-7.

Goldrick, B.A. (1989). Programmed instruction revisited: A solution to infection control inservice education. *Journal of Continuing Education in Nursing, 20,* 222-227.

Green, P., & Brightman, A.J. (1990). *Independence day: Designing computer solutions for individuals with disabilities.* Olm Park, Allen, TX: Apple Computer.

Haggard, A. (1989). *Handbook of patient education.* Rockville, MD: Aspen.

Halkitis, P.N., & Leahy, J.M. (1993). Computer adaptive testing: The future is upon us. *Nursing & Health Care, 14,* 378-384.

House, B.M., Chassie, M.B., & Spohn, B.B. (1990). Questioning: An essential ingredient in effective teaching. *Journal of Continuing Education in Nursing, 21,* 196-201.

Jeska, S.B., & Cosgrove, K. (1992). Education centers: Which features are best? *Journal of Nursing Staff Development, 8,* 109-113.

Joos, I.R.M. (1984). A teacher's guide for using games and simulation. *Nurse Educator, 9*(3), 25-29.

Kaihoi, B.H. (1987). Implementing use of learning resources in our technical age. In C.E. Smith (Ed.), *Patient education: Nurses in partnership with other health professionals* (pp. 189-232). Philadelphia: Saunders.

Kaplan, S.H., Greenfield, S., & Ware, J.E., Jr. (1989). Assessing the effects of physician-patient interactions on the outcomes of chronic disease. *Medical Care, 27* (Suppl. 3), S110-S127.

Kleinknecht, M.K., & Hefferin, E.A. (1990). Maximizing nursing staff development: The learning laboratory. *Journal of Nursing Staff Development, 6,* 219-224.

Lewis, D.J., Saydak, S.J., Mierzwa, I.P., & Robinson, J.A. (1989). Gaming: A teaching strategy for adult learners. *Journal of Continuing Education in Nursing, 20,* 80-84.

Ley, P. (1972). Primacy, rated importance, and recall of medical statements. *Journal of Health and Social Behavior 13,* 311-317.

Lorig, K., & Gonzalez, V.M. (1993). Using self efficacy theory in patient education. In B. Gilroth (Ed.), *Managing hospital-based patient education* (pp. 327-337). Chicago, IL: American Hospital Publishing.

Magenty, J., & Magenty, J. (1982). *Patient teaching.* Bowie, MD: Brady.

McAlindon, M.N., & Smith, G.R. (1994). Repurposing videodiscs for interactive video instruction: Teaching concepts of quality improvement. *Computers in Nursing, 12,* 46-56.

Narrow, B. (1979). *Patient teaching in nursing practice: A patient and family centered approach.* New York: Wiley.

Peters, F.L., & Connell, K.M. (1991). Incorporating the affective component into an AIDS workshop. *Journal of Continuing Education in Nursing, 22,* 95-99.

Postel, N. (1993). Guidelines for the evaluation of instructional software by hospital nursing departments. *Computers in Nursing, 11*(6), 273-276.

Poston, I. (1993). How to develop computer assisted instruction programs. *Nursing & Health Care, 14,* 344-349.

Ramsey, A.M., & Siroky, A.S. (1988). The use of puppets to teach school age children with asthma. *Pediatric Nursing, 14,* 187-190.

Redman, B.K. (1993). *The process of patient education,* 7th ed. St. Louis: Mosby–Year Book.

Robinson, K.J., Lewis, D.J., & Robinson, J.A. (1990). Games: A way to give laboratory values meaning. *American Nephrology Nurses Association Journal, 17,* 306-308.

Rorden, J.W. (1987). *Nurses as health teachers: A practical guide.* Philadelphia: Saunders.

Rothwell, W.J., & Kazanas, H.C. (1992). *Mastering the instructional design process: A systematic approach.* San Francisco: Jossey-Bass.

Scarpa, R., Smeltzer, S.C., & Jasion, B. (1992). Attitudes of nurses toward computerization: A replication. *Computers in Nursing, 10,* 72-79.

Schmidt, K.L., & Fisher, J.C. (1992). Effective development and utilization of self-learning modules. *Journal of Continuing Education in Nursing, 23,* 54-59.

Schmitz, B.D., MacLean, S.L., & Shidler, H.M. (1991). An emergency pursuit game: A method for teaching emergency decision making skills. *Journal of Continuing Education in Nursing, 22,* 152-158.

Tibbles, L., Lewis, C., Reisine, S., Rippey, R., & Donald, M. (1992). Computer assisted instruction for preoperative and postoperative patient education in joint replacement surgery. *Computers in Nursing, 10,* 208-211.

Walts, N.S. (1982). Games and simulations. *Nursing Management, 13*(2), 28-29.

Weston, C., & Cranton, P.A. (1986). Selecting instructional strategies. *Journal of Higher Education, 57*(3), 259-288.

Whiteside, M.F., McCulloch, J., & Whiteside, J.A. (1990). Helping hospital educators and clinical nurse specialists learn to use and develop computer assisted instruction. *Journal of Continuing Education in Nursing, 21,* 113-117.

Whitman, N.I., Graham, B.A., Gleit, C.J., & Boyd, M.D. (1992). *Teaching in nursing practice: A professional model,* 2nd ed. Norwalk, CT: Appleton and Lange.

Wood, R.Y. (1994). Use of the nursing simulation laboratory in reentry programs: An innovative setting for updating clinical skills. *Journal of Continuing Education in Nursing, 25,* 28-31.

CHAPTER 12

Instructional Materials

Diane S. Hainsworth

CHAPTER HIGHLIGHTS

KEY TERMS

audiovisual materials
instructional materials
aids/tools
realia
illusionary representations

delivery system
media and task characteristics
learner characteristics
replica, analogue, and symbolic models

OBJECTIVES

After completing this chapter, the reader will be able to

1. Differentiate between instructional materials and methods of instruction.
2. Identify the three major variables (learner, task, and media characteristics) to be considered when selecting, developing, and evaluating instructional materials.
3. Cite the three components of instructional materials required to effectively communicate educational messages.
4. Discuss general principles applicable to all types of media.
5. Identify the multitude of audiovisual tools, both print and nonprint materials, available for patient and professional education.
6. Describe guidelines for development of printed materials.
7. Analyze the advantages and disadvantages specific to each type of instructional medium.
8. Evaluate the type of media suitable for use depending on the characteristics of the audience, seating, preference, resources available, nature of the subject, and characteristics of the learner, such as age, literacy level, and sensory deficits.
9. Identify where educational tools can be found.
10. Critique tools for value and appropriateness.
11. Recognize the supplemental nature of media's role in patient education.

Just as the *instructional methods* are the approaches or processes used for instructor-client communications, the *instructional materials* are the resources and tools used as vehicles to help communicate the information. Often the terms *instructional strategy* and *teaching technique* serve to describe both the methods and the materials used in teaching (Weston & Cranston, 1986). Instructional materials are tangible substances and real objects that provide the audio and/or visual component necessary for learning. Many of them can be manipulated. They stimulate a learner's senses and may have the power to arouse emotions. They help the teacher make sense of abstractions and simplify complex messages (Babcock & Miller, 1994). In this chapter, the term *instructional materials,* also referred to as *tools* and *aids,* includes both print and nonprint media that are intended to supplement, not replace, actual teaching.

The selection and development of teaching materials are a complex component of the educational process, yet the means by which information is communicated to the learner is often not considered in depth (Weston & Cranston, 1986). Thus, a discussion of media goes hand in hand with methods because of the need to expand the teacher's understanding of the full potential that broad knowledge of media brings to instructional methods.

The purpose of instructional media is to help the nurse educator deliver a message creatively and clearly. The advantage of a multimedia approach for teaching is to assist learners in gaining increased awareness and skills and in retaining more effectively what they learn (Rankin & Stallings, 1990). In addition, teaching materials stimulate the learners' bodily senses, help clarify abstract or complex concepts, add variety to the teaching-learning experience (Babcock & Miller, 1994), reinforce learning, and potentially bring realism to the experience as well, saving time and energy on the part of both the teacher and learner. Research indicates that the use of audiovisual aids facilitates learning (Haggard, 1989; Rankin & Stallings, 1990).

Considering such factors as the time constraints on health-care professionals as a result of increased workloads, the decreasing length of patient hospital stays, the increase in patient acuity, the alternative health-care settings in which education is now delivered, and shrinking resources for educational services, to name a few, the nurse educator must look to ways to supplement teaching and provide alternative approaches to educating learners.

This chapter provides an overview of the process for selecting, developing, and evaluating instructional materials. A systematic approach is used to examine various types of instructional media with an eye to matching their use to particular kinds of learners and to particular kinds of topics and situations. The advantages and disadvantages of media types will be discussed. Although the choice of what instructional materials to use often depends on availability or cost, whatever materials are selected should enhance the intended learning. The purpose of this chapter is to inform nurses about various media options and allow them to make informed choices regarding appropriate instructional materials that fit the learner, that will accomplish the learning task, and that will have impact on the motivation of the learner. Whether nurses educate patients and families or other health-care professionals, the same principles apply in making selection decisions about the type of instructional materials to use for teaching.

GENERAL PRINCIPLES: AUDIOVISUAL MATERIALS

Before selecting or developing media from the multitude of available options, you should be aware of the following general principles regarding the effectiveness of audiovisual tools:

- Print and nonprint materials do change behavior by influencing a gain in cognitive, affective, or psychomotor skills.
- No one tool is better than another in enhancing learning. The suitability of a medium depends on many variables.
- The tools should complement the instructional methods.
- The choice of media should be consistent with course content and match the tasks to be learned to assist the learner in accomplishing predetermined behavioral objectives.
- The instructional materials should reinforce and supplement, not substitute for, the educator's teaching efforts.
- Media should match the available financial resources.
- Instructional aids should be appropriate for the physical considerations and the learning environment, such as the size and seating of the audience, acoustics, space, lighting, and display hardware (delivery mechanisms) available.
- Media should complement the sensory abilities, developmental stages, and educational level of the intended audience.
- The message imparted by instructional materials must be accurate, valid, authoritative, up-to-date, state-of-the-art, appropriate, unbiased, and free of any unintended messages.
- The media should contribute meaningfully to the learning situation by adding diversity and additional information.

CHOOSING INSTRUCTIONAL MATERIALS

There are many important variables to consider when choosing instructional materials. The role of the nurse educator goes beyond the dispensing of information only. It also involves skill in the designing of and planning for instruction. Learning can be made more enjoyable for both the learner and the teacher if the educator knows what instructional materials are available, as well as how to select and use them to enhance the teaching-learning experience. Knowledge of the diversity of instructional tools and their appropriate use will enable the teacher to make education more interesting, challenging, and effective for all types of learners. With current trends in health-care reform, educational strategies to teach patients will need to include instructional materials for health promotion and illness prevention among well persons, as well as for health maintenance and restoration for ill persons. Making appropriate choices of instructional materials depends on a broad understanding of several major variables: (1) characteristics of the learner, (2) characteristics of the task to be achieved, and (3) characteristics of the media that make them suitable for achieving the objectives of the task (Frantz, 1980).

1. *Characteristics of the learner:* Since variables in the learner are known to have an impact on learning, it is important to "know your audience" in order to choose media that best suit their needs. You must consider the learner's perceptual abilities, reading ability, motivational level (locus of control), developmental stage, and learning style.

2. *Characteristics of the task:* Task characteristics are defined by the predetermined behavioral objectives. The task to be accomplished depends on identification of the learning domain and the complexity of behavior required by the task.

3. *Characteristics of the media:* The nurse educator has the opportunity to choose from a wide variety of media to enhance methods of instruction: *print and nonprint.* Nonprint media include the full range of audio and visual possibilities. An enormous variety of educational materials is available. The tools selected are the *form* through which the information will be communicated. No single medium is most effective. Therefore, the educator must be flexible, sometimes combining a multimedia approach.

THE THREE MAJOR COMPONENTS OF INSTRUCTIONAL MATERIALS

Whatever instructional method is used, decisions will also have to be made regarding the media necessary to help communicate information. The delivery system (Weston & Cranston, 1986), content, and presentation (Frantz, 1980) are the three major components of media that should be kept in mind when evaluating media for potential instruction.

Delivery System

The delivery system is both the physical form of the materials and the hardware used to present the materials. For instance, a person is the delivery system for a lecture. This lecture might be embellished through other delivery systems, such as the use of overhead transparencies or slides (physical form), and a projector (hardware). Videotapes (physical form) in conjunction with VCRs (hardware) and computer programs (physical form) in conjunction with the computer (hardware) are other examples. The delivery system is independent of the content of the message. The choice of the delivery system is influenced by the size of the intended audience, the pacing or flexibility needed for delivery, and the sensory aspects most suitable to the audience.

Content

The content, or message, is the actual information that is communicated to the learner, which might be on any topic from sexuality to educational psychology. When selecting media, the nurse educator must consider several aspects:

- Is the information presented accurately?
- Is the medium chosen appropriate to convey particular content? For example, audiotapes can be a very appropriate tool for teaching content related to the cognitive or affective domain but not a good tool for teaching a psychomotor skill. Content relative to psychomotor behavior might be better served with printed pamphlets, videos, or the use of real equipment through demonstrations.
- Is the readability of the materials appropriate for the audience to accomplish a given task? The more complex the task, the more important it is to write clearly understandable instructions at a level appropriate to the learner. Readability of any printed materials is enhanced through the use of illustrations or the rewriting of instructions in simple, succinct language (see Chapter 7).

Presentation

Frantz (1980) describes presentation as those variables that affect the way in which the content or message to be learned is delivered. Weston and Cranston (1986) state that the *form* of the message is the most important consideration for selecting or developing instructional materials, a consideration that is frequently ignored. They describe the form of the message as occurring along a continuum from concrete (real things) to abstract (symbols).

Realia

Weston and Cranston (1986) term the most concrete form of stimuli that can be used to deliver information as *realia*. For example, an actual woman demonstrating breast self-examination is the most concrete example of realia. Because this form of presentation might be less acceptable for broad teaching situations, the next best choice would be a model, which has many characteristics of reality, including three-dimensionality, without the accompanying embarrassment for the learner. The message is less concrete, yet using a model as an instructional medium allows for an accurate presentation of information with near-maximal use of the learners' perceptual abilities. Further along the continuum of realia is a video presentation of a woman performing breast self-examination. The learner could still learn accurate breast self-examination this way, but the aspect of dimensionality is absent. The message becomes less concrete and more abstract.

Illusionary Representations

Many realistic cues, including dimensionality, are missing from this category of instructional materials. Moving or still photographs and audiotapes projecting live sound are good examples of illusions, as are representations through drawings and graphs (Weston & Cranston, 1986). They are less concrete and more abstract, but the instructional advantages of illusionary media are that these forms can offer learners experiences that they might otherwise not have access to because of such factors as size, location, or expense. Examples, such as pictures of how to stage decubitus ulcers or audiotaping how to discriminate between normal and various abnormal lung sounds, although more abstract in form, still do to some degree resemble realia.

Symbolic Representations

Numbers and words, written and spoken, which are used to convey ideas or represent objects, are the most common instructional materials, yet are the most abstract forms of messages (Weston & Cranston, 1986). Oral presentations, written texts and handouts, and the use of blackboards are just a few examples of messages delivered in symbolic form. The chief disadvantage of symbolic representations stem from their lack of concreteness and a potential need to tailor their form and content to the cognitive abilities and limitations of learners. For that reason, their use is limited with young children, learners from different cultures, learners with low literacy skills, and cognitively and sensory impaired individuals.

When making decisions about how to best accomplish teaching objectives, the nurse educator must carefully consider the three components of instructional materials. The various delivery systems available, the content or message to be conveyed, and the form in which information will be presented are all important considerations. There is a wide range of choices among various media. Remember, no one type of media is known to provide a clear advantage over another in promoting acquisition of knowledge; however, the mere acquisition of knowledge does not guarantee that the learner will learn. It is important to keep in mind the supplemental nature of instructional materials. In other words, nurse educators must know how to select the tools that will best complement and support their teaching efforts for a particular audience and that will emphasize the key points to accomplish the behavioral objectives.

TYPES OF INSTRUCTIONAL MATERIALS

Written Materials

Handouts, leaflets, books, pamphlets, brochures, and instruction sheets are the most widely employed and most accessible type of media used for teaching. Although printed teaching materials have been described as "frozen language" (Redman, 1993), written materials are, nonetheless, the most common form of teaching tool.

There are distinct advantages to the use of printed materials. The greatest virtue of written materials is that they are available to the learner as a reference for information when the nurse educator is not immediately present to answer questions or clarify information. Also, printed materials are widely used at all levels of society, so this type of media is acceptable and familiar to the public. In addition, enormous varieties of materials are available through commercial sources and easily obtainable, usually at relatively low cost, for distribution by educators. They often come in convenient forms, such as pamphlets, which are portable and usually contain concise amounts of information. Their ready availability makes them especially useful for learners who prefer reading as opposed to receiving messages in other formats. The speed at which materials are read may be controlled by the reader, which is an asset for comprehension of complex concepts and relationships. Content may also be altered to target specific audiences.

The disadvantages to printed materials include the fact that they are the most abstract form of reality, possibilities for immediate feedback are limited, and the proper reading level is essential for full usefulness. A large percentage of materials is written at too high a level for comprehension. Learners with low literacy skills or those persons who are visually or cognitively impaired may not be able to take full advantage of written materials, and illiteracy negates the use of printed materials altogether.

Commercially Prepared Materials

A wealth of commercially prepared brochures, posters, pamphlets, and patient-focused texts is currently available. Whether they enhance the quality of learning is an important question for nurse educators to consider when trying to evaluate these products for content and presentation. Examining the factuality of material presented is very important because commercial products may or may not be produced in collaboration with health professionals (Foster, 1987). Attention must also be paid to the cognitive level at which materials are aimed. For example, Foster described a preoperative instruction booklet advertised as appropriate for children of all ages that depicted animal caretakers of a young child. Since young children tend to interpret what they see concretely, very young children

might believe that real animals would be caring for them and could become frightened. For that reason, this particular booklet was clearly inappropriate for such a broad audience.

Several factors must be considered when reviewing commercial materials for possible use (Foster, 1987):

- Who produced the item? Was there any input from health-care professionals?
- Can the item be previewed? The educator should have an opportunity to examine accuracy and appropriateness of content to ensure that the item will provide the target group with the information needed.
- The price of any teaching tool must be consistent with its educational value. Getting across an important message effectively may justify a higher cost outlay, especially if the tool can be used with large numbers of learners, but simple printed sheets may do the job just as well. Another cost consideration is how quickly the information will become outdated.

The advantage of using commercial materials is their availability. Using commercially prepared materials is certainly less time-consuming and often cheaper for educators than designing their own instructional materials. For instance, the American Heart Association produces many fine booklets on cardiac and stroke education for patients and families that cost 50 cents or less when bought in bulk. An educator would need to spend hours researching, writing, and copying materials to create information packets of equal quality.

The disadvantages of using commercial materials may include issues of cost, accuracy and adequacy of content, and readability of the materials. Some educational booklets are expensive to purchase and impractical to give away in large quantities to learners. The American Parkinson's Disease Association produces a number of fine but costly booklets, and an educator might encourage learners to buy their own rather than provide them for free. Also, the actual usability of commercially prepared instructional materials for individual learners must be evaluated on a one-to-one basis because the level of readability might be a problem for some and the content might not completely and accurately cover all the information the learner needs to know.

Self-Composed Materials

Educators may choose to write their own instructional materials for several reasons, which might include cost saving or the need to tailor content to specific audiences.

Advantages to composing your own materials are many. By writing your own materials, you can tailor the information to fit your own institution's policies, procedures, and equipment. You can build in answers to questions asked most frequently by your patients, highlighting points considered especially important to physicians or other health-care professionals. Tailoring your written materials to reinforce specific oral instructions will enhance their efficacy and gives you the opportunity to clarify difficult concepts by using multifaceted approaches that work well for getting the message across (Haggard, 1989). The following example illustrates this point nicely. Using teacher-generated instructional materials, Rice and Johnson (1984) found that groups of patients receiving specific instructions were more likely to follow directions and required less oral teaching time than groups of patients receiving general or nonspecific instructions.

There are, of course, disadvantages to composing your own materials. You need to exercise extra care that materials are well written and well laid out, which can be time-consuming. Many tools written by patient educators are too long, too detailed, and written at too high a level for the target audience (Haggard, 1989). If this is a skill you find difficult to master, it may be easier to use commercially prepared tools or follow the simple guidelines below.

Boyd (1987) points out that accuracy of content is a very important factor in written patient education materials, but another very important factor is that patients must be able to read and understand the materials. Nurse educators are expected to enhance their methods of teaching with audiovisual materials, but few have ever had formal training in the development and application of written materials. Boyd (1987) and Haggard (1989) suggest the following guidelines for writing patient education materials with clarity and completeness:

- Make sure the content is accurate and up to date.
- Organize the content in a logical, step-by-step fashion so learners are being informed adequately but are not being overloaded. Prioritize the content to address what they "need to know" first. Content that is "nice to know" can be addressed with less immediacy or emphasis.
- Make sure the information succinctly discusses the what, how, and when. Do not overwhelm the reader with large amounts of information. Follow the KISS rule: Keep it simple and short. Avoid giving detailed rationales because this may unnecessarily lengthen the written information. Try to integrate information that you think the learner *needs* to know with information they *want* to know. For instance, patients need to know how to turn, cough, and deep breathe after surgery, but they will also want to know when they can eat. This can best be handled by putting the information into a question and answer format or by dividing the information into subheadings according to the nature of the content.
- Regardless of format, avoid medical jargon whenever possible, and define any technical terms in layman's language. Sometimes it is important to expose patients to technical terms because of complicated procedures and ongoing interaction with the medical team, so careful definitions can minimize misunderstandings. Be consistent in words used.
- Find out the average grade in school completed by the targeted patient population, and write the patient education materials two to four grade levels below that level. Follow guidelines for decreasing reading level (see Chapter 7). Readability level appropriate to the audience cannot be emphasized enough.
- Keep words and sentences short and to the point. Write in a conversational style.
- Write in the active voice. For example, "Clean the wound with soap and water" is more directive and effective than "It is important to keep the wound clean."
- Use the second person *you*, instead of the third person.
- Present the most important information first by making the first sentence of a paragraph the topic sentence.
- Use adequate spacing, which is more restful to the eye.
- Do not use all capital letters because words in capitals are much more difficult to read than words printed with lowercase letters.

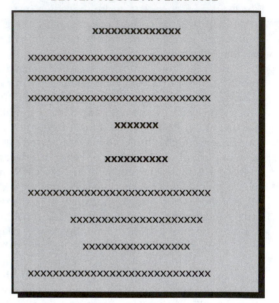

FIGURE 12–1. Inadequate versus Adequate Appearance and Formatting

- Use advance organizers, such as outlines, to set the frame of reference for the learner.
- Build in reviews at the end of written materials to reemphasize key points.

In addition to the guidelines for clarity and completeness in constructing written materials, format and appearance are equally important in motivating learners to read the printed word. If the format and appearance are too detailed, learners will feel overwhelmed, and instead of attracting the learners, you will discourage and repel them (Figure 12-1). To avoid common pitfalls in writing good instructional tools, follow these important tips (Haggard, 1989):

- Allow plenty of white space. This includes double spacing, generous margins, indenting important points, and highlighting or setting off key statements.
- Do not put too much written information on the document.
- Use illustrations to break up blocks of print and to reinforce important information in the text.

- Note that a clear, concrete line drawing may be just as or more effective than a photograph or an elaborate piece of artwork.
- Always state things in positive not negative terms. Never illustrate incorrect messages. For example, depicting a hand holding a metered dose inhaler in the mouth not only incorrectly illustrates a drug delivery technique (Weixler, 1994) but reinforces that message by its visual impact alone (Figure 12-2 illustrates the correct way to use an inhaler).

As a way of evaluating the effectiveness of self-composed materials, Boyd (1987) also suggests interviewing a few patients with different educational levels and asking them for reactions to the materials you write. Computerized readability formulas for writing patient education handouts are also available (see Chapter 7). Baker (1991) offers specific suggestions for writing easily readable handouts, including examples of original and rewritten text.

Evaluating Printed Materials

When evaluating printed materials, the following considerations should be kept in mind.

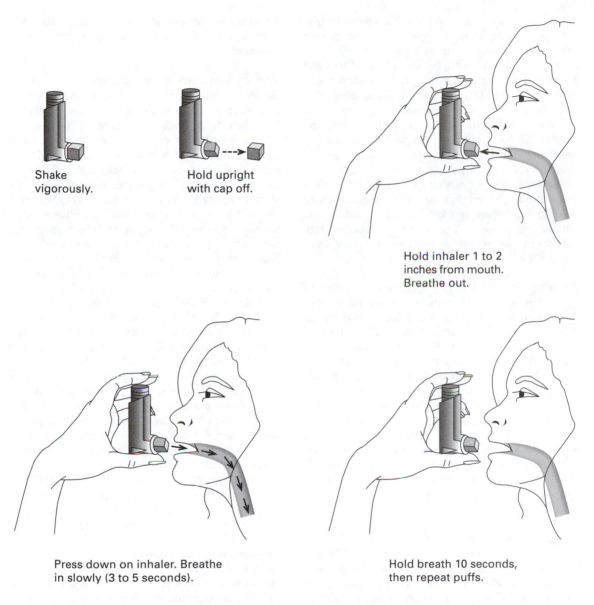

Shake vigorously.

Hold upright with cap off.

Hold inhaler 1 to 2 inches from mouth. Breathe out.

Press down on inhaler. Breathe in slowly (3 to 5 seconds).

Hold breath 10 seconds, then repeat puffs.

FIGURE 12–2.   Diagram Illustrating Proper Technique for Inhaler Use

Nature of the audience   What is the average age of the audience? Certain age groups learn better with one type of media than another. For instance, older adults tend to prefer printed materials they can read at their leisure. Children like printed materials short in length with many illustrations.

What are the preferred learning styles of particular audiences? For example, printed materials with few illustrations are poorly suited to patients who not only have difficulty reading but who do not like to read. Representations of information in the form of graphs and charts can be included with the content of printed materials for those who are visual and conceptual learners.

Older learners, in particular, like handouts. With this group, written materials are most effective when combined with oral presentations, especially on a one-to-one basis. However, vision deficits are common, and short-term memory may be a problem for comprehension. Having materials that can be reread at their own convenience and pace can reinforce earlier learning and minimize confusion over instructions or treatments. Lengthy materials are less problematic for older learners, who frequently have enough time and patience for reading educational materials. Diagrams should be explicit. Examples should relate to activities relevant to the audience's lifestyle. Advice for dealing with problems should be explicit. To accommodate those with vision impairments, use a large typeface and lots of white space in printed materials. Separate one section from another with ample spacing and highlight important points (Haggard, 1989).

Literacy level required   The effectiveness of patient education materials for helping the learner reach instructional objectives can be totally undermined if the materials are written at a level beyond the comprehension of the learner. A study of patients' reading abilities in a public hospital by Glazer-Waldman et al. (1985) found that only 40% of their sample could read at the sixth-grade level. This underscores the importance of screening potential educational tools to be used as adjuncts to various teaching methods. A number of formulas (e.g., Fog, SMOG, Flesch, Fry) are available for determining readability (see Chapter 7 and Appendix A). Boyd's (1987) guidelines, listed previously, are helpful in reducing the reading level of materials you write yourself.

Linguistic variety available   Linguistic variety refers to choices of printed materials in different foreign languages, which may be limited because duplicate materials in more than one language are costly to publish and not likely to be undertaken unless the publisher anticipates a large demand. The growth of the Latino population in the United States has promoted increasing attention to the need for Spanish language teaching materials. Thus, organizations like the American Heart Association, the Parkinson's Disease Association, and the National Institute for Head Trauma have begun providing Spanish and English language versions of their most widely used printed materials. Regional differences exist, so there may be more availability of Asian language materials on the West Coast and more Spanish language materials in the Southwest and Southeast than in other parts of the country.

Brevity and clarity   In education, as in art, the simpler is the better. Remind yourself of the KISS rule: Keep it simple and smart. Address the critical facts only. What does the patient NEED to know? Choose words that explain *how*; the *why* can be filled in by the lecture or the discussion. Including rationales in handouts lengthens materials unnecessarily (Haggard, 1989). Remember, ideally, instructional materials are *supplements* to learning. Figure 12–3 is a good example of a clear, easy-to-follow instructional tool used to teach an asthma patient how to determine when a metered dose inhaler is empty. Using simple graphics and minimal words, it guides the learner through the procedure with very little room for misinterpretation and is suitable for a wide range of audiences.

As another example, Hanafin (1993) described a pamphlet called *The 5-Minute Teaching Series,* which was designed for brief in-service topics at the Minneapolis Veterans Affairs Medical Center. Each topic is printed on a single, brightly colored 8½-by-11-inch paper folded into thirds. On the inside of the pamphlet is information about the topic being covered, while the outside flaps are used for aspects of the topic to be emphasized. Development of content for this teaching series is based on adult learning principles. Topics chosen are problem related and immediately applicable to nursing responsibilities. These pamphlets are easily distributed, are cost-effective, and have been used to meet a variety of learning needs.

Layout and appearance   The appearance of written materials is crucial in attracting learners' attention and getting them to read the information. If the potential tool has too much wording, with inadequate spacing between sentences and paragraphs, small margins, and numerous pages, the intended learner may disregard it under the impression that it is much too difficult and too time-consuming to read. Figure 12–4 illustrates an example of this problem. Figure 12–5 illustrates an improved version of the same material.

Haggard (1989) points out that allowing plenty of white space is the most important step that should be taken to improve the appearance of written materials. This means double-spacing,

How to Tell When Your Metered Dose Inhaler Is Empty

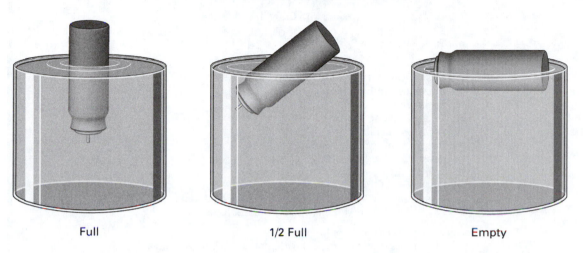

| Full | 1/2 Full | Empty |

FIGURE 12–3. Example of a Clear, Easy-to-Follow Instructional Tool for an Asthma Patient

leaving generous margins, indenting important points, using bold characters, and separating out key statements with extra space. Inserting a graphic in the middle of the text can break up the print and may be visually appealing, as well as providing a mechanism for reinforcing textual information. Redman (1993) states that pictorial learning is better than verbal learning for recognition and recall. For subjects that lend themselves to concrete explanations, this is especially true. An example of this is teaching the psychomotor task of using a metered dose inhaler (see Figure 12–2). More abstract topics, such as teaching communication skills, rely heavily on written information in combination with use of demonstration.

Opportunity for repetition   Written materials can be read later, again and again to reinforce your teaching. This is especially important when you are not there to answer questions. This might be the advantage of materials that are laid out in a question and answer format. If you are writing your own materials, be mindful of the need to keep them current, and update them against changing patient populations.

Concreteness and familiarity   Using the active voice is more immediate and concrete. For example, "Shake the inhaler very well three times" is

more effective than "The inhaler should be shaken thoroughly" (Figure 12–6). Also, the importance of using plain language instead of medical jargon cannot be overstated. Byrne and Edeani (1984) surveyed knowledge of medical terminology among hospital patients and determined that inadequate patient understanding of common medical terms used by health-care providers could be a significant factor in noncompliance with medical regimens by patients. Their own study indicated that patients understood medical terms at a lower rate than health professionals expected.

In summary, self-designed or commercially produced printed teaching materials are widely used for a broad range of audiences. They vary in literacy demand levels and may be found written in several languages. Their major advantages and disadvantages are summarized in Table 12–1.

Demonstration Materials

Demonstration materials include many types of nonprint media such as models and real equipment, as well as displays, which include posters, diagrams, illustrations, charts, bulletin boards, flannel boards, flip charts, chalkboards, photographs, and drawings. All represent unique ways of communicating messages to the learner. These aids

DYSPHAGIA
(Swallowing and Chewing Disorder)

Major Risk: Aspiration Pneumonia

Telltale Clues:
1. Dysarthria (difficulty articulating words)
2. Decreased tongue mobility
3. Facial weakness
4. Decreased gag reflex
5. Weak or hoarse cough
6. Coughing or choking during or after meals
7. Pockets of food in mouth
8. Wet or gurgly voice quality

Diagnosis based on: Modified Barium Swallow or Bedside Evaluation
by qualified speech pathologist

Common Etiologies (causes):
CVA, traumatic brain injury, cerebral palsy, ALS, myasthenia
gravis, multiple sclerosis, muscular dystrophy, Parkinson's,
spinal cord dysfunction, head and neck cancers, COPD, confused
patients, encephalitis.

Nursing Diagnosis: Potential for Injury (Aspiration), related to
impaired swallowing secondary to _____.

Nursing Interventions:
1. HOB up > 30 degrees AAT.
2. Feed in upright position (approx. 90 degrees), neck
   slightly flexed forward (chin tucked).
3. Supraglottic diet, unless otherwise ordered.
4. Suction equipment on standby AAT.
5. Dentures in for meals, when applicable.
6. If unilateral facial weakness, place food on unaffected side.
7. Small bites, chew food well.
8. Patience. Allow plenty of time to eat.
9. No straws, unless individually evaluated.
10. Check mouth for residual food after each swallow.
11. Leave in upright position 30 minutes after meal.

FIGURE 12–4.   Example of a Poorly Formatted Teaching Tool

primarily stimulate the visual senses but can combine the sense of sight with touch and sometimes even smell and taste. From these various forms of demonstration materials, the educator can choose one or more to complement teaching efforts in reaching predetermined objectives. Just as with written tools, these aids must be accurate and appropriate for the intended audience. Ideally, the purpose for using these media forms is to bring the learner closer to reality and actively engage the learner in a visual and sometimes participatory manner. As such, demonstration tools are useful for cognitive and psychomotor skill development. The major forms of demonstration materials—displays and models—will be discussed in detail.

Displays
Displays can be permanently installed or portable. They have been referred to as static instructional

DYSPHAGIA
(Swallowing and Chewing Disorder)

Major Risk: Aspiration Pneumonia

Major Causes in Neuroscience Patients:
Stroke, ALS, Myasthenia Gravis, MS, Parkinson's Disease, Spinal Cord Injury, Confusion

Important Clues:
1. Difficulty articulating words
2. Weak tongue movement
3. Facial droop one side
4. Decreased gag reflex
5. Weak or hoarse cough
6. Coughing or choking during or after meals
7. Wet or gurgly voice quality

Most Important Nursing Interventions:
1. Head of bed up greater than 30 degrees at all times.
2. Feed in upright position with chin tucked in slightly.
3. Suction equipment on standby at all times.
4. Supraglottic diet, unless otherwise ordered.
5. If face weak on one side, place food on unaffected side.
6. Small bites, chew food well.
7. Patience. Allow plenty of time to eat.
8. Check mouth for food after each swallow.
9. Leave in upright position 30 minutes after meal.

FIGURE 12–5.   Example of a Properly Formatted Teaching Tool

STEPS FOR CORRECT INHALER TECHNIQUE

1. Shake the container well.
2. Remove cap and hold inhaler upright.
3. Hold the inhaler 1 to 2 inches from mouth.
4. Tilt head back slightly, and breathe out fully.
5. Press down on the inhaler and start to breathe in slowly.
6. Breathe in slowly (3 to 5 seconds) and deeply to pull medication deeper into the lungs.
7. Hold breath for 10 seconds to hold the medicine in the lungs.
8. Take a few normal breaths.
9. Repeat puffs as directed.

FIGURE 12–6.   Example of Instructions Written in the Active Voice

TABLE 12–1.   Advantages and disadvantages of printed materials

Advantages	Disadvantages
Always available	Impersonal
Rate of reading is controllable by the reader	Limited feedback; absence of instructor lessens opportunity to clear up misinterpretation
Complex concepts can be explained both fully and adequately	Passive tool
Procedural steps can be outlined	Highly complex materials may be overwhelming to the learner
Verbal instruction can be reinforced	Literacy skill of learner may limit effectiveness
Patient is always able to refer back to instructions given in print	

SOURCE: Adapted from Hinkle et al.,1993.

tools because they are usually stationary and unchanging (Haggard, 1989), but that does not imply that they are immovable or unalterable. Some of these demonstration materials, such as posters (discussed later in more detail), are self-explanatory tools, effectively achieving their teaching objectives and vividly representing the essence of relationships between objects without the presence of the teacher (Rankin & Stallings, 1990). However, others, such as chalkboards and flip charts, require an instructor to directly assist in the flow and interpretation of information being depicted. Displays such as chalkboards, white markerboards, flip charts, bulletin boards, and flannel boards are found in almost any educational setting and are useful for a variety of teaching purposes. They can advertise events, convey simple or quick messages about health-care issues, and clarify, reinforce, or summarize important themes.

The proverbial chalkboard and flip charts and the more recent white markerboard are particularly helpful in delivering information. These tools are most useful during brainstorming sessions in formal classes or group discussions. You can use them spontaneously to make drawings or diagrams (with contrasting colored chalk or markers if you wish) or jot down ideas generated from participants while you are in the process of teaching. You can add, correct, or delete information quickly while the learners are actively following what you are doing or saying. These board devices are excellent in promoting participation, keeping the learners' attention on the topic at hand, and reinforcing the contributions of someone else. They are a mode that provides opportunity for the teacher, in

an immediate and direct fashion, to organize data, integrate ideas, perform on-the-spot problem solving, and compare and contrast various points of view. Unlike some other types of visuals, these display tools are unique in that they allow learners to see parts of a whole picture while assisting the teacher in filling in the gaps. Babcock and Miller (1994) list guidelines for use of chalkboards and white markerboards. The most important points include using legible and discernible lettering, being sure to step aside and face the audience after putting notations on the board to maintain contact with the audience and allowing learners to copy the message, and enlisting a good note-taker to capture a creative design or record an idea before the board is erased.

How sophisticated a display is depends on the budget available to produce it, as well as the detail you desire and the creativity you put into getting the message across (Haggard, 1989). On one end of the continuum, you might have a simple illustration with print and line graphics, like Figure 12–3, which can be used to teach asthmatics how to tell when a metered dose inhaler is empty or full. A more sophisticated display might be used to help teach the same content with colored photos, three-dimensional objects, and more sophisticated graphics and print.

Displays can be an effective way of achieving learning outcomes, although they may be time-consuming to use or prepare and sometimes, like models, expensive to purchase (Haggard, 1989). However, computer technology has made it easier to create attractive, up-to-date, and impressive posters as well as to revise ones already made (Bushy, 1991).

ASPIRATION PRECAUTIONS

1. <u>HOB up > 30 degrees AAT.</u>
2. <u>Feed</u> in upright position (approx. <u>90 degrees</u>), neck slightly flexed forward (chin tucked).
3. <u>Supraglottic diet</u>, unless otherwise ordered.
4. <u>Suction</u> equipment on standby AAT.
5. Dentures in for meals, when applicable.
6. If unilateral facial weakness, place food on <u>unaffected</u> side.
7. Small bites, chew food well.
8. Patience. Allow plenty of <u>time</u> to eat.
9. No straws, unless individually evaluated.
10. Check mouth for residual food after each swallow.
11. Leave in upright position 30 minutes after meal.

FIGURE 12–7. Example of a Sign Designed for Display in a Stroke Unit

The following are some advantages of displays as teaching tools:

- A quick way to attract attention and get an idea across.
- Flexible (especially if made for easy modification).
- Portable (Many posters can be folded for storage and unfolded for mounting. Some blackboards and bulletin boards are on rollers.).
- Reusable.
- Stimulate interest or ideas in the observer.
- Can change or influence attitudes.
- Purchasable, and depending on the educator's budget, many can be made. Figure 12–7 shows an example of an "Aspiration Precautions" sign made by an educator to be displayed for use by nurses over patients' beds on a stroke unit.

Some of the *disadvantages* of displays include the following:

- Take up a lot of space
- Time-consuming to have prepared, and for that reason tend to be reused again and again, which increases the risk of their becoming outdated.
- May be overused—they need to be used as *supplements* to learning, not as an end in themselves.
- Unsuitable for large audiences if information is to be viewed simultaneously.

- Cannot present large amounts of information at one time.
- Not good for teaching psychomotor skills when movement needs to be demonstrated.
- Get too cluttered when too much information is placed on them.
- May be ignored if posted too long or poorly arranged.
- If permanently mounted on a large backing, difficult or impossible to transport.
- The symbolic nature of the message may be misunderstood, a problem that underscores their importance as *supplements* to learning.

Some displays, like posters, are essentially hybrids of print and nonprint media because they heavily employ the use of the written word as well as graphic illustration. Because of the increasing use of two-dimensional posters as a legitimate and reasonable alternative to more formal presentations for conveying information (Duchin & Sherwood, 1990), this type of display tool will be discussed in more detail. Posters have become an important educational strategy, particularly as a mode to disseminate information less formally in classrooms and clinical settings to patients and families, as well as at educational seminars and research meetings to educate staff and students.

As a visual aid, posters can be used as an independent source of information or in conjunction with other modalities. Some critics view the poster as a passive instructional medium, but this can easily be disputed because reading and recall require involvement on the part of the learner. Inherent in the design, the message conveyed by a poster is brief, constant, and interactive with the audience (Duchin & Sherwood, 1990). Since the primary mode of the poster is visual stimulation, it must be designed to attract attention. Effective posters leave a mental image long after they are seen. This mental image is a cue to the viewer to recall the message. Much like a bumper sticker you see on a car in front of you while driving, effective poster displays can potentially leave lasting impressions that are easily recalled at some future date.

The advantage of posters is that they can be used as a cognitive reinforcer, as a way to synthesize information, and as an ongoing instructional resource. The value is in the repetition, individual pacing, and availability of the message across various settings (Duchin & Sherwood, 1990). Posters serve as an important teaching tool to help bring about a change of behavior by adding knowledge, reinforcing skill, or appealing to attitudes. By forcing content brevity and utilizing eye-catching imagery, a message can be conveyed quickly and simultaneously to a large audience in a variety of settings. The poster can also be used with individuals and small groups to transmit or reinforce information with or without the teacher present. They are relatively inexpensive to produce. With practice, an educator can become skilled at putting together effective posters in an efficient and timely way.

The disadvantage of posters is that the content is static and, therefore, may become quickly dated. If the same poster is kept around too long, the potential audience begins to disregard its message. The key to a poster's effectiveness lies in its planning and design. Bushy (1991, p. 11) states that ". . . good ideas do not speak for themselves . . . a good poster display cannot rescue a bad idea, but a poor one can easily sink the best idea. . . ." She puts forth important aesthetic considerations when preparing and evaluating poster presentations specifically for research purposes. Duchin and Sherwood (1990) also provide guidelines for developing attractive, simple, yet effective posters that incorporate assessment of content, audience needs, and settings. Both Bushy (1991) and Duchin and Sherwood (1990) refer to the application of design elements such as color, spacing, graphics, lettering, and borders required to create presentations that not only catch the eye but persist in memory. Duchin and Sherwood (1990) further point out that effective imagery can be in the form of graphic designs or photographs. Great artistic skill is not required. Simple pictures, in the form of schematics, outlines, and stick figure drawings, work well and can be illustrated using colored pencils, markers, or construction paper. The ability of a poster to influence behavior or increase awareness can be greatly enhanced by careful consideration of content, audience, and design elements.

Because aesthetic appeal is critical in capturing learners' attention, the following tips, adapted from Bushy (1991), Duchin and Sherwood (1990), and Haggard (1989) should be adhered to when making and critiquing a poster for use as a teaching tool:

- Use complementary (opposite-spectrum) color combinations, taking into consideration the three color aspects of hue (wavelength of the light spectrum), saturation (purity of color), and value (brilliance of color). Two colors clash when they are close to each other in these three elements. See Duchin and Sherwood (1990) for a discussion of the use of color in posters.
- One color should make up 70% of the display. No two colors should be used in equal proportions, and a third color should only be used to accent or highlight the printed components such as titles, subheadings, or credits. Too many colors make the design appear cluttered and complicated.
- Because pictures are worth a thousand words, graphics should be used to break up blocks of script or lettering.
- Use simple, high-quality (but not necessarily sophisticated or ornate) drawings or graphics that can be easily interpreted.
- Balance script with white space (or another background color) and graphics to add variety and contrast.
- Use high-quality photographs with colored borders and different contours, widths, and shapes.
- Convey the message in common, straightforward language, avoiding jargon and unfamiliar abbreviations or symbols.
- Adhere to the "KISS" principle (keep it simple and smart) when using words to decrease

length, detail, and crowding. Simplicity and neatness attract attention.

- Be concise; do not repeat. Include only essential information, but be sure the message is complete.
- Keep objectives in mind for the focus of the display.
- Be sure content is current and free of spelling, grammar, and mathematical errors.
- Add textures by using a variety of paper and fabrics.
- Make titles catchy and crisp, using 10 words or less (no longer than two lines) and lettering large enough to read from a distance of at least 4 to 6 feet.
- Use a title or introductory statement that orients readers to the subject.
- Logically sequence the written and graphic components.
- Use letter-quality script or laser print instead of dot matrix if using computer-generated type.
- Letters should be straight and at least 1 inch in height. Avoid using all capital letters except for very short titles and labels.
- Use arrows, circles, or directional lines to merge the parts to achieve correct focus, flow, sequence, and unity.
- Achieve balance in visual weight on each side by positioning information around an imaginary central axis running vertically and horizontally.
- Handouts can be used to supplement the highlights and reinforce the messages conveyed by the poster.
- If a poster is to be transported, use durable backboards and overlays (styrofoam, heavy cardboard, lamination, or acrylic sprays).

Bushy (1991) also has devised a 30-item poster appraisal tool (R-PAT) to further assist nurses in critiquing posters specifically designed for research. This tool can be modified for use in preparing and evaluating posters as tools for educational purposes.

The ability of a poster to influence behavior or expand awareness can be greatly enhanced by careful consideration of its content, intended audience, and design elements. The poster for AIDS awareness (Figure 12–8) is a stunning example. The interaction of the viewer with the message is the key to a poster's success. This AIDS awareness poster and the World War I poster "Uncle Sam Wants YOU!" are examples of the element of visceral connection between viewer and message that linger in memory.

Computers and printers have opened the door to very professional-looking productions of posters by almost any user. Software programs such as The Print Shop Deluxe and Canvas are frequently used for these purposes.

Models

Models are three-dimensional instructional tools that allow the learner to immediately apply knowledge and psychomotor skills by observing, examining, manipulating, handling, assembling, and disassembling objects while the teacher provides feedback (Rankin & Stallings, 1990). In addition, these demonstration aids encourage learners to think abstractly and give them the opportunity to use many of their senses (Whitman et al., 1992). Whenever possible, the use of real objects and actual equipment is ideal, but a model is the next best thing when the real object is not available, accessible, or feasible, or is too complex to use. The three specific types of models used for teaching and learning are replicas, analogues, and symbols.

A *replica* is a facsimile constructed to scale that resembles the features or substance of the original object. The dimensions of the reproduction may be decreased or enlarged in size to make demonstration easier and more understandable. Replicas can be examined and manipulated by the learner to get an idea of how something works. They are excellent for teaching psychomotor skills by giving the learner an opportunity for active participation through hands-on experience. Not only can the learner assemble and disassemble parts to see how they fit and operate, but also the pace of learning can be controlled by the learner (Babcock & Miller, 1994).

Replicas are used frequently by the nurse educator when teaching anatomy and physiological processes. Models of the heart, kidney, ear, eye, joints, and pelvic organs, for example, allow the learner to get a perspective on parts of the body not readily viewed without these teaching aids (de Tornyay & Thompson, 1987). Resuscitation dolls are a common type of replica used to teach the skills of cardiopulmonary resuscitation. Breast

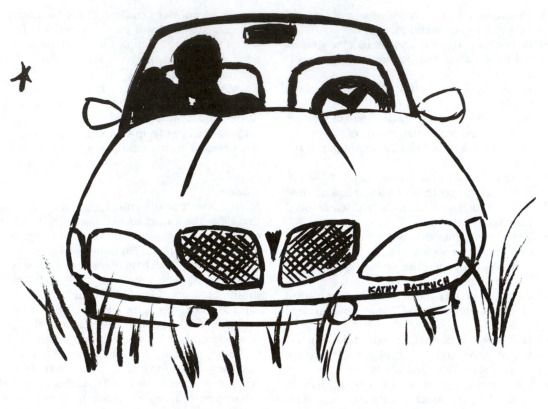

Last night Jennifer had a fatal accident.
She just doesn't know it yet

FIGURE 12–8.   Example of an Effective Poster for AIDS Awareness

self-examination is another topic best taught to wide audiences through the use of a model. Pinto (1993) assessed training and maintenance of breast self-examination skills. The high incidence of deterioration in breast self-examination skills led her to evaluate approaches for improving maintenance. Learners who regularly refreshed their skills using demonstration models as instructional tools were more likely to maintain regular and effective use of the technique than learners who did not participate in these courses.

Using inanimate objects first is a technique educators can use to desensitize learners before doing injections or procedures on themselves or other human beings (Haggard, 1989). Teaching a diabetic how to draw up and inject insulin can best be accomplished by using a combination of real equipment and replicas. Patients first draw up sterile saline in real syringes, then practice injecting oranges, and progress to a model of a person before actually injecting themselves.

For lessons aimed at psychomotor learning, skills checklists can be used as a mechanism for evaluating whether the message has been incorporated by the learner (Grier et al., 1991). These are easily used in observation of return demonstrations. Simulation laboratories use this evaluation method frequently. Sims (1992) describes "Demonstration Day" in a neonatal unit, which had stations for chest tube care, umbilical artery catheter placement, exchange transfusion, metabolic screening and rhythm strips, and code arrest. Using various models, this demonstration day was a way to provide hands-on practice to all new staff nurses, as well as for annual review of seasoned nurses.

The second type of model is known as an *analogue* because it uses analogy to explain something by comparing it to something else. Unlike replicas, an analogue model can be used effectively to explain and represent dynamic systems (de Tornyay & Thompson, 1987). An analogue performs like the real object because it has the same properties as the dynamic system under consideration. Mechanical devices such as extracorporeal and dialysis machines are good examples of analogues. Although they do not look like the actual anatomy of a person, they are artificial equipment that perform similar physiological functions of the heart, lungs, and kidneys. Another popular analogue is the use of a computer model as a comparison to how the human brain functions (Babcock & Miller, 1994).

The third type of model is a *symbol*, which is used more frequently in a teaching situation. Words, mathematical signs and formulas, diagrams, musical notes, cartoons, stick figures, and traffic signs are all examples of symbolic models that convey a message to the receiver through imaging, convention, or association. As Babcock and Miller (1994) further point out, the meaning of words as symbols to convey concepts and ideas can vary depending on the language familiar to the one giving the message or the one receiving it. Symbols, such as the international signs, are increasingly being used in multilingual or multicultural areas. However, abbreviations common to health-care personnel, such as NPO, PRN, GTTS, and PO, should be avoided when interacting with consumers because they may not be familiar with these acronyms. To differentiate the three types of models, Babcock and Miller (1994) suggest associating a *r*eplica with the word *resemble*, an *a*nalogue with the term *act like*, and a *s*ymbol with the words *stands for*.

The advantage of models is their usefulness when the real object is too small, too large, too expensive, too complex, unavailable, or a potential source of difficulty for learners. Models also allow learners to practice acquiring new skills without compromising themselves in practicing self-care activities or in risking damage to valuable equip-

ment (Haggard, 1989). Learners become more actively involved, and the application of knowledge and skills is immediate, as is the feedback from the instructor. These tools are especially attractive and useful for the kinesthetic learner who prefers the hands-on approach to learning. A whole array of models can be purchased from commercial vendors at varying prices (some for free) or improvised by the teacher. Models do not need to be expensive or elaborate to get concepts and ideas across (Rankin & Stallings, 1990).

Considering the disadvantages, some models may not be suitable for the learner with poor abstraction abilities or for visually impaired audiences, unless each individual is given the chance to tangibly appraise the object using other senses. Also, some models can be fragile and others very expensive, like Resusci-Annie used to teach cardiopulmonary resuscitation. Many are bulky to store and difficult to transport. Unless models are very large, they cannot be observed and manipulated by more than a few learners at any one time. This can be overcome by using team teaching and by creating different "stations" at which to arrange the replica for demonstration purposes (Babcock & Miller, 1994).

Table 12–2 summarizes the advantages and disadvantages of demonstration materials.

Audiovisual Materials

Technology has changed the traditional approach to teaching. Nowhere is this more evident than in the audiovisual arena. Audiovisual tools support and enrich the educational process by stimulating the learner's visual and auditory senses, adding variety to the teaching-learning experience, and instilling visual memories, which have been found to be more permanent than auditory memories (de Tornyay & Thompson, 1987). Some visual aids, such as pictures and diagrams as demonstration materials, have been around since antiquity. But it is only relatively recently that technology has allowed for application of audiovisual tools for purposes of instructing and learning. They are exceptional aids because many can influence all three domains of learning by promoting cognitive development, effecting attitude change, and helping to build psychomotor skills. Audiovisuals have been known to increase retention of information by combining what we hear with what we see.

TABLE 12–2.   Advantages and disadvantages of demonstration materials

Advantages	*Disadvantages*
Brings the learner closer to reality through active engagement	Content may be static, easily dated.
Useful for cognitive reinforcement and psychomotor skill development	Can be time-consuming to make
Effective use of imagery may impact affective domain	Potential for overuse
Many forms are relatively inexpensive	Not suitable for simultaneous use with large audiences or for presenting large amounts of information.
Opportunity for repetition	Not suitable for visually impaired learners or for learners with poor abstraction abilities

Because we live in an increasingly technological age, educators have to be aware of what audiovisual tools are available, how tools potentially and actually impact on the ability to learn, and how to effectively and efficiently implement the various tools at our disposal. When and to what extent we should use them to augment teaching depend on many variables, not the least of which is the educator's comfort level and expertise in operating these technological devices. We assume that all educators are oriented to the use of audiovisual aids. However, this is not necessarily true, especially in light of the newness of some of the technology, such as computer-assisted instruction. Also, it should not be forgotten that the learner may have difficulty orienting to the newer modes of learning, as well as have physical or cognitive limitations that may preclude the use of some types of audiovisual tools.

As with any teaching aids, audiovisuals must be carefully previewed for accuracy and appropriateness of content. Another major concern affecting which media you choose will depend on budgetary resources available for the purchase or rental of hardware equipment and software programs. It is extremely costly, in terms of time and money, as well as technologically demanding to self-produce audiovisual instructional materials. Thus, the three issues (Smith, 1987) that must be addressed are

1. *Technical feasibility:* technical expertise, professional and repair service support, equipment fit and replacement.
2. *Economic feasibility:* budgetary allowance and justification of cost.

3. *Social/political acceptability:* learner's willingness to use, impersonality of machines, acceptance by institutional administrations.

There are many nonprint media whose primary mode of presentation is visual or audio or a blend of these two forms. Audiovisual materials can be categorized into five major types: projected, audio, video, telecommunications, and computer formats. Most of these learning resources are popular devices common to the general public. Others, like the computer, have only recently been applied to education, and therefore, learners are not as accustomed to receiving information via this type of media. Kaihoi (1987) has conducted a thorough review of these learning resources for implementation into health education in our technological age. The following is a summary of the various types of audiovisual tools available for teaching based largely on Kaihoi's findings.

Projected Learning Resources

The category of projected media, the best known of all audiovisual formats, includes movies, filmstrips, slides, overhead transparencies, computer outputs and video that can be projected on a screen. These media types are most frequently used with audiences of various sizes but can be an effective tool for teaching individuals, as well.

Movies and filmstrips   Sixteen-millimeter movies and filmstrips have been to date some of the most common health education aids. A large selection of commercially prepared films is available, and the picture quality is usually very good.

They have the advantage over videotapes in that different sized screens can be used for variable sizes of audiences. Images often can be seen even by visually impaired persons because the picture size can be adjusted by placing the projector closer or farther away from the screen (Haggard, 1989). Also, films with closed captions can accommodate the hearing impaired. Illiterates or persons with low literacy skills benefit, as well, from this form of visual stimulation (Boyd, 1983). Because films can depict real-life situations, this method is useful in encouraging attitude changes and cognitive learning. In addition, films are useful for teaching step-by-step demonstration of psychomotor skills.

The lack of flexibility is the biggest disadvantage, because the content is not alterable once the film is made. For this reason, videotapes are fast replacing this medium for educational purposes. Films should be reviewed periodically because information may become outdated and no longer be accurate or appropriate for use in teaching. A film that is outmoded can be very distracting to the audience and cause them to lose interest in the main concept being presented. The second major drawback is the expense. Unlike relatively inexpensive videotapes, 16-mm films, as well as movie projectors for showing them, frequently cost hundreds of dollars. For small audiences, this is not cost-effective. Film is fragile and can break easily. The instructor also must have the facility and dexterity to thread and rewind the film, not necessarily an easy task. In addition, lack of portability is a drawback. The projector is bulky, and the film requires a screen and a dark room for viewing. Films are less flexible as well because they are unlikely to be played independent of an instructor.

Slides   There exist both the conventional slide shows that appear static as slides are advanced one by one manually and the newer slide/sound programs that change slides automatically in a rapid, synchronous manner to simulate motion. Slides have many advantages. They offer the instructor a great deal of flexibility. They are inexpensive both to purchase and to make. Out-of-date material can readily be redone and replaced. Slides also can be easily rearranged and added to the original sequence. Close-ups can be made for a look at important details. During a slide presenta-

tion, it is easy to go backwards to review information for purposes of reinforcing or clarifying a point (Haggard, 1989). They can enhance an oral presentation by adding visual dimensions to the narration. Slide cassettes and projectors are portable, can fit into small rooms for viewing, and are easily stored. Most importantly, learners can start and stop equipment by themselves. Slides are excellent for conveying a message because they are an attractive mode for learning at all ages and facilitate retention and recall. Slides can capture real situations and can be personalized or tailored to meet specific audience needs.

The biggest disadvantage is that slides must be shown in darkness for best visibility. With the lights lowered, the teacher can lose eye contact with the audience, and learners are less likely to ask questions or raise concerns when in the dark. A screen and projector setup must be available. Because slide equipment is manufactured by so many companies, you must be sure the carousel and projector being used are compatible. Careful composition of the slides is needed to avoid clutter or complex visuals that are too boring or too difficult for the viewer to assimilate. In addition, slide programs take time to prepare and may not be appropriate for those with vision impairment.

Haggard (1989) suggests the following special considerations when preparing slides:

- Illustrate one idea per slide.
- Keep images simple by using clear pictures, symbols, or diagrams. Put long lists of words or complex figures on handouts that supplement the slides.
- Avoid distorted images by keeping the proportion of height to width at 2:3.
- Use large, easily readable, and professional-looking lettering.
- Use a 35-mm camera and slide film for photographing.

Overhead transparencies   This medium is frequently used for teaching in a variety of settings, both in the classroom and for large conference presentations. Its advantages are many. Large numbers of people can see the projected images at one time while information is being explained. It is a particularly useful tool to stimulate group discussion. Overheads share some of the same qualities of slides, such as the ability to isolate single facts, ideas, or themes. They also can be used to enlarge images. The biggest advantage from a teaching standpoint is that they can be shown in lighted rooms. They are also inexpensive to produce or purchase. Diagrams and figures can readily be photocopied and made into transparencies. Multiple transparencies can be overlaid to illustrate changes in the content of teaching material. Transparencies can be black and white or color. Use of colored acetates or colored felt pens provides contrast to images and lettering to enhance important teaching points. Color is known to attract attention and help differentiate information for better retention and recall (Cooper, 1990).

Among the disadvantages of overhead transparencies are the need for both equipment for projection and the support of verbal feedback. For this reason, they are more conducive for use in a classroom than for purposes of individual self-instruction. The projector itself is awkward to transport, and the noise given off by the fan of the machine can be distracting in a small room. It is essential that finished transparencies be viewed ahead of time for an assessment of readability specifically related to the size of the lettering. Usually letters ¼-inch high or letters that can be read at a distance of 10 feet before projection are sufficient for easy reading (Haggard, 1989). Too much content on an overhead transparency will also decrease its efficacy as a teaching tool.

Babcock and Miller (1994) recommend helpful guidelines in the use of overhead projectors and transparencies. These are summarized as follows:

- Do not block the audience's view of the screen by standing in front of the machine. This is a common error that can best be solved by making a habit of sitting or standing to the side to avoid interference with the projected image.
- Turn the projector off when finished referring to the transparency to keep the learners' attention on you and away from what is being projected. Constant use of the machine is also distracting because of the fan noise.
- Keep the message on the transparency simple. Use handouts to cover complex information as a supplement to your message.
- Display only one point at a time by masking the rest with a piece of paper if you have listed several ideas on one transparency. This allows the listener to focus on what you are saying and gives them time for note taking.
- Use a screen large enough for the audience to read the information projected.
- Use a light-colored blank wall if a screen is unavailable or too small.
- Pull the projector closer or farther away from the screen to change the size of the projection.
- Use tinted film to reduce glare of light.
- Use colored pens to help organize information or make specific points.
- Use overlays to help illustrate complex or sequential ideas. However, too many can make the picture fuzzy.

Table 12–3 summarizes the advantages and disadvantages of projected learning resources.

Audio Learning Resources

Audio technology, although it has existed for a long time, has not been used to any great extent for educational purposes until recently. For years, it has been a useful tool for the blind or for those with serious visual or motor impairment. But with significant advances in audio hardware and soft-

TABLE 12–3.   Advantages and disadvantages of projected learning resources

Advantages	Disadvantages
Most effectively used with groups	Lack of flexibility due to static content for some forms
May be especially beneficial to hearing-impaired, low-literate patients	Some forms may be expensive
	Requires darkened room for some forms
Excellent media for use in teaching psychomotor skills	Requires special equipment for use

ware and a turn away from the purely commercial use of this technology, audiotapes, compact discs (CDs), and radio have become more popular tools for teaching and learning. They can be used to relay many different types of messages, can help learners who benefit from repetition and reinforcement, and are well suited for those who enjoy or prefer auditory learning. They are also useful adjuncts for teaching illiterate persons.

Audiotapes   The most popular format today is the cassette tape. This medium has been growing in use by educators. The biggest advantage of cassettes is their practicality. They are small, portable, inexpensive, simple to operate, and easy to prepare or duplicate, and the required recorders also are of minimal expense. The audiotape recorder can be a powerful tool to augment other teaching methods by providing the listener with the opportunity to review previously heard information, to receive taped feedback from instructors, or to hear information available from no other source (Haggard, 1989). A good example of the latter is recorded lung sounds, which allow comparison between normal and abnormal breathing.

Cassettes are now available on a variety of health topics, from stress reduction to how to stop smoking, and can be prepared specifically to meet the needs of a learner by reinforcing facts, giving directions, or providing support. If the tapes are self-made, the learner derives much comfort from hearing your familiar voice and reassuring words. This tool is used extensively by the Regents College, a nursing external degree program of independent study, to provide direct feedback to students on the results of their examinations. Fredette (1984) described the use of audiotapes for process recordings as a way to individualize clinical instruction for nursing students. Information can be listened to at the leisure of the learner and reviewed as often as necessary. They can be used almost anywhere, such as the home, office, clinic, or hospital setting, and can be listened to while simultaneously driving a car or fixing a meal, thus filling in what normally would be considered wasted time. Developing a sizable library of tapes is well within the capability of most instructors because of the low cost and easy storage of this medium. Pictures, diagrams, and printed handouts can accompany these instructional tools to fit the needs of a variety of learners.

The disadvantages of using audiotapes are few. The biggest drawback is that since audiotapes address only the one sense of hearing, they cannot be used for the hearing impaired, and some learners can be easily distracted from the information being presented unless they have visuals to accompany the tapes. There is also no opportunity for interactive feedback between the listener and the speaker. As with any medium, audiotapes should be used only as supplements to the various methods of instruction.

Radio   The radio has impacted tremendously on all of our lives for many years and is the oldest form of audiotechnology. However, due to its commercial nature and appeal to mass audiences, it has been used more for pleasure than for education. More recently this major advantage of radio has been exploited by both public and private radio stations, which have turned more and more to airing community service and medical talk shows for public education on health issues. These programs are helpful in delivering a message, and because of the convenience and popularity of radio as a communication tool, it could become more useful as a vehicle in teaching and learning. The disadvantage lies with the difficulty of consistently delivering information on major topics to general as well as specific populations. The nurse educator has little control over the variety and depth of topics discussed or how regularly one listens to a program, and the general nature of radio programs is not tailored to meet individual needs. Unlike audiotapes, radio does not allow the opportunity for repetition of information. However, because of its widespread use and versatility, it has the potential for becoming a major source for broadcasting important and useful healthcare information, especially if air time is funded by private foundations or sponsored by special groups or agencies dedicated to health teaching.

Compact discs   This modern form of media has replaced the traditional vinyl record albums. The major advantage of CDs is their superior fidelity, which does not deteriorate over time. Other advantages and disadvantages of CDs are similar to those of audiotapes except for the fact that they are still relatively expensive. In addition, not as many people or institutions have the recording hardware or the computer capability to accommodate the use of this tool. Thus, its versatility for application to education is currently limited, but as with all new technological advances, its cost will eventually go down, and the hardware availability will increase in the near future.

Table 12–4 summarizes the advantages and disadvantages of audio learning resources.

Video Learning Resources

Videotapes, along with the videotape recorders and television sets as the electronic devices to view the tapes, have become commonplace in homes and health-care settings. Camcorders and video cameras to make tapes are also owned by a growing number of people and institutions. People are becoming more accustomed to receiving information via this medium, and health educators are using it extensively for teaching in a variety of settings. Videotapes are becoming one of the major nonprint media tools for enhancing patient/family, staff, and student education because tapes can be both entertaining and educational at the same time. However, the major disadvantage of this medium is that videotapes and video recorders come in two major formats, Beta and VHS, which are not interchangeable, and therefore, the type of tape and machine used must be compatible with one another. In addition, videotapes are found in varying sizes, the most common of which are the ½-inch and ¾-inch sizes. You probably have found yourself more than once with a ½-inch or ¾-inch tape in hand but not the right size machine on which to play it. As technology advances, most hospitals and other health-care agencies and educational institutions will convert to the less costly (but not less quality) ½-inch size videotapes.

Over the last few years, health-care facilities have begun to use videotapes to develop patient education materials and broadcast them over in-house televisions. Convenience and flexibility allow an educator to use the VCR for individual patient teaching situations, as well as for large groups. Role modeling of particular behaviors, attitudes, and values may be demonstrated powerfully through this medium. Videotapes are a good means to promote discussion because they can capture real-life situations. Videotaping may be used as a teaching tool for nurse educators because its use as a critiquing instrument may provide direct feedback regarding learners' performances of complex interpersonal and psychomotor skills (Nielsen & Sheppard, 1988). Minnick et al. (1988) described such use of audiovisual modeling to improve teaching skills of baccalaureate nursing students. This has been especially beneficial for students with high performance anxiety and to convey teaching-learning principles to large groups in nonclinical settings.

The usefulness of videotape is in its flexibility as a tool for instruction. The advantages of color and motion and different angles, as well as sound, enhance learning through visual as well as auditory senses. Videotaping has become extremely inexpensive, although whether the recorder is rented or owned by the user is a cost factor. Portability of recorders allows access to learning situations unavailable elsewhere.

The disadvantage of purchased tapes is that they may be beyond the viewers' level of understanding, inappropriate for learner needs, or too long. The attention span of the learner is variable, and the ideal length of tapes in most instances should be limited to 15 to 20 minutes. To avoid the possibility of creating a "talking head" effect, the operator of the recorder needs to be knowledgeable in the use of motion picture technology. Use of close-ups, dramatization of situations, and angle effects are not in the usual repertoire of many nurse educators. Scheduling for videotape viewing

TABLE 12–4.   Advantages and disadvantages of audio learning resources

Advantages	Disadvantages
Widely available	Relies only on sense of hearing
May be especially beneficial to visually impaired, low-literate patients	Some forms may be expensive
May be listened to repeatedly	Lack of opportunity for interaction between instructor and learner
Most forms very practical, cheap, small, and portable	

must take into account unit routines and the importance of repeat viewing opportunities (Nielsen & Sheppard, 1988). If you are planning to do your own videotapes, Haggard (1989) suggests striving for network-quality production by using the following guidelines:

- Write a script for the program. Rehearse thoroughly.
- Consider hiring a video technician on a per diem basis. This may be time- and cost-effective.
- For a small budget, a single camera with zoom capacity should be used. A larger budget may allow hiring a professional to edit the final product.
- Always be mindful of the program's objectives to avoid being seduced by the glamour of the process.
- Keep the program short. The longer the video, the more risk of losing viewer interest. Five to 15 minutes is ideal.

Table 12–5 summarizes the advantages and disadvantages of video learning resources.

Telecommunications Learning Resources

Telecommunications is a means by which information can be transmitted via electrical energy from one place to another in a sense that is meaningful for the person receiving it. This form of media includes television and telephone and its related modes of audio and video teleconferencing and closed-circuit, cable, and satellite broadcasting. Telecommunication devices have allowed messages to be sent to many people at the same time in a variety of places at great distances.

Television   The television, ubiquitous in American homes, has been used for many years as an entertainment tool. Today, there are more televisions than telephones in private residences. The TV is also well suited for educational purposes and has become a popular teaching-learning tool in homes, as well as schools, businesses, and health-care settings. The power to influence cognitive, affective, and psychomotor behavior is well demonstrated by the television commercials whose messages are simple, direct, and variously repetitive to effectively impact on intended audiences. Cable TV under the law must provide public access programming by offering channels for community members to air their own programs. Health education, if placed on the cable system, can be seen in any home hooked up to cable. The advantage of this option is that distribution of programs is relatively inexpensive. The disadvantage is that one cannot control who is watching, and this medium cannot serve as an interactive question and answer experience unless call-in phone lines are provided.

Closed-circuit TV allows for education programs to be sent to specific locations, such as patient rooms or staff units. The learner can request a particular program at any given time, much like a guest in a hotel can choose from a variety of movies day and night. This telecommunications technology requires programs to be played intermittently or continuously, with program availability clearly advertised. Because the learner controls program viewing, the nurse educator must follow up to answer questions and determine if learning has, in fact, occurred. Satellite broadcasting, a newer form of telecommunications, can reach far more distant locations, and a number of programs can be carried at any one time. Because of its

TABLE 12–5.   Advantages and disadvantages of video learning resources

Advantages	*Disadvantages*
Widely used educational tool	Viewing formats limited depending on use of Beta or VHS and size of tape
Inexpensive, for the most part	
Uses visual and auditory senses	Some commercial products may be expensive
Flexible for use with different audiences	Some purchased materials may be too long or inappropriate for audience
Powerful tool for role-modeling, demonstration, teaching psychomotor skills	

expense, not many institutions send health information via this mode, but many receive it. There are several health networks, such as Lifetime, that broadcast to cable companies and hospitals. New types of satellite systems are being developed such that this form of communication for educational purposes will become possible in the near future on a worldwide basis.

Telephones   It is almost impossible to imagine being without the telephone as a daily tool. Americans have come to depend on it as a fundamental means of communication. It is not surprising, therefore, that the telephone can be used effectively for education. In recognition of this, many health-care associations have begun to provide telephone services with messages about disease treatment and prevention. The American Cancer Society, as one example, has established a toll-free number for the public to obtain short taped messages about various types of cancer. Hospitals, too, have set up call-in services about a variety of health-related topics and sources for referral. The advantage is that these services are relatively inexpensive and can be operated by someone with minimal medical knowledge because the taped message contains the substance of the content. Another advantage is that this type of service is available in most cases around the clock. The disadvantage is that there is no opportunity for questions to be answered directly.

Telecommunications as an instructional tool is becoming increasingly popular and sophisticated. Many hospitals and health-care agencies are now establishing hot-line consumer information centers, which are manned by knowledgeable health-care personnel so that information can be personalized and appropriate feedback can be given on the spot. The Poison Control hot line is a good example of the use of this medium.

Table 12–6 summarizes the advantages and disadvantages of telecommunications learning resources.

Computer Learning Resources

In our technological society, the computer has changed our lives dramatically and has had widespread application in industry, businesses, schools, and homes. The computer can store large amounts of information, it is designed to display pictures and graphics, as well as text, and the presentation of information can be changed depending on user input.

Although computer technology is fairly recent on the educational scene, it is becoming more common, especially with the rapid increase of computer literacy among students, professionals, and the general public. There is a great deal of evidence that computer-assisted instruction (CAI) promotes learning in primarily the cognitive domain. More research needs to be done to establish its usefulness to change attitudes and behaviors or promote psychomotor skill development. Retention is improved by an interactive exchange between learner and instructor, regardless of whether the instructor lives and breathes! CAI simulates the feedback of a face-to-face exchange between individuals. For instance, the computer game "NumberMaze," developed by Great Wave Software for the Macintosh, was designed to teach math at a variety of skill levels. Instructions can be selected that will present more word problems or more numerical problems to learners at a pace of their own choosing. Its changeability makes it endlessly challenging and new to the user.

More recently, the growth of the computer Internet has opened new doors for learners to gain access to libraries and to direct learning experiences, which can include on-line discussions with educators at great distances from the learner. Use

TABLE 12–6.   Advantages and disadvantages of telecommunications learning resources

Advantages	Disadvantages
TV program distribution relatively inexpensive to wide audiences	Complicated to set up interactive capability
Telephone relatively inexpensive, widely available	Expensive to broadcast via satellite

of the Internet is not restricted to any age group. Anyone with a computer and access to on-line technology can make use of this tremendous resource.

CAI has many advantages. The ability to individualize instruction to the learner on a moment by moment basis is a unique feature of CAI. Lessons can be varied readily, and the learner controls the pace. With no time constraints, the learner can move as quickly or as slowly as desired to master content without penalty for mistakes or performance speed. An instructor can easily track the level of understanding of the learner. Because the computer has the ability to ask questions and analyze responses, it can perform ongoing assessment of the learner and alter the content, pace, and examples presented. Computers can be programmed to provide feedback to the educator regarding the learner's grasp of concepts, the speed of learning, and what aspects of learning need reinforcement.

The interactive features of this medium also provide for immediate feedback to the learner. Many software packages are available from a wide variety of sources. Even costly packages may be cost-effective if the potential audience is large (Gillespie & Ellis, 1993). Time efficiency is a major advantage of CAI in that the teacher has more time to devote to teaching other tasks not taught via computer, such as affective and psychomotor skills. In addition, the content of CAI programs is consistent for all learners because they are exposed to the exact same information. Computers are also valuable tools for those with aphasia, hearing impairment, or learning disabilities.

The major disadvantage of CAI is that both hardware and some software can be substantially expensive, making it unattainable for some learning situations. In most cases, programs must be purchased because they are too time-consuming and too complex for the educator to develop. Even if someone has programming skills, it can take up to 500 hours to produce 1 hour of instructional material (Whitman et al., 1992). Lack of computer literacy or a comfort level with computers may be a barrier to some learners and even some nurse educators. As Whitman further points out, many older adults are computer shy or computer illiterate. Also, those people with reading problems will likely have major difficulty making sense of the information on the screen. In addition, learners with physical limitations, such as arthritis, neuromuscular disorders, pain, fatigue, paralysis, or vision impairment, find computer use difficult if not impossible. Moreover, it should not be forgotten that the computer is a machine, and therefore, the learner is deprived of the personal, compassionate, one-to-one interaction that only a teacher can provide to facilitate learning. Because of the independent nature of the computer learning experience, it is not very suitable for nondirected or poorly motivated learners. Lack of access to computers may be a barrier, even for the computer literate. Although the market for computer software has skyrocketed, only a small percent to date have dealt with patient education, and the quality of the product is uneven (Gillespie & Ellis, 1993).

Table 12–7 summarizes the advantages and disadvantages of computer learning resources.

TABLE 12–7. Advantages and disadvantages of computer learning resources

Advantages	*Disadvantages*
Interactive potential promotes quick feedback, retention of learning	Primarily promotes learning in cognitive domain; less useful in changing attitudes and behaviors or promoting psychomotor skill development
Potential database enormous	Both software and hardware expensive, therefore less accessible to wide audience
Instruction can be individualized to suit different types of learners or different pace for learning	Must be purchased—too complex and time-consuming for most educators to prepare
Time-efficient	Limited use for many elderly, low-literate learners, and those with physical limitations

EVALUATION CRITERIA FOR SELECTING MATERIALS

Choosing the right tools for patient education calls for judgment on the part of the nurse educator, who must take into consideration the learner, the task, and the media available to help achieve the task. Decisions may need to be made on an individual basis or for large groups, depending on the size and characteristics of the audience. There may be multiple objectives. Not only must the educator consider the media available in general, but different objectives may best be reached with different teaching materials.

Both the learning objectives and the domains of learning in which instruction must occur will dictate the most appropriate materials. Discenza (1993) states that the method for selection of instructional materials is the same, regardless of the domain of learning. Selection is based on the ability of materials to help with the instruction of a given behavioral objective. Materials should not be selected before the objectives are set. He also states that evaluation of media involves evaluating the content, the instructional design, the technical production of the instructional material, and the packaging. Figure 12–9 is Discenza's check-list for selecting and evaluating instructional materials:

	Yes	No
A. Content		
Is the content valid?		
Relevant?		
Current?		
Is the purpose of the program stated?	___	___
Are instructional objectives given?	___	___
B. Instructional Design	___	___
Are the ideas and information presented logically?	___	___
Is the format of the program appropriate for the audience?		
Does the instructor actively engage the learner?	___	___
Is there evidence of formative evaluation?	___	___
Is summative evaluation material provided?	___	___
C. Technical Production	___	___
Is the visual material sharply focussed and clear?		
Is the image composition clear and uncluttered?		
Is the text legible at the maximum viewing distance?	___	___
Is the audio clear and intelligible?	___	___
Is there any distracting background noise?	___	___
Is the pace of the narration appropriate for the audience?	___	___
D. Packaging	___	___
Is the material available in a format for which equipment is available?		
Is descriptive information provided?	___	___
Is a User's Guide provided?	___	___
Has the instructional material won any awards?	___	___

FIGURE 12–9. A Checklist for Selecting and Evaluating Instructional Materials

SOURCE: David J. Discenza (1993). A systematic approach to selecting and evaluating instructional material. *Journal of Nursing Staff Development, 9*(4), p. 198. Reprinted by permission of J.B. Lippincott Company.

TABLE 12–8.   Effectiveness of teaching tools and methods

Mode of Learning	*Retention*	*Media*	*Methods*
Reading	Learners retain 10% of what they read.	Leaflets, books, brochures, flip charts, chalkboards, instruction sheets	Self-instruction
Hearing	Learners retain 20% of what they hear.	Audiotapes, telephones	Lectures, discussion
Watching	Learners retain 30% of what they see.	Silent films, displays, photos, pictures, posters, cartoons, drawings	Demonstration, self-instruction
Watching and hearing	Learners retain 50% of what they see and hear.	Movies (films), TV, video-tapes, slides, overheads, models	Lecture or demonstration
Watching and speaking	Learners retain 70% of what they see and talk about.	Audiovisual media	Group discussion, 1:1 verbal interactions, demonstrations
Speaking and doing	Learners retain 90% of what they talk about and do.	Interactive media	Demonstration, return demonstration, gaming, role-playing

SOURCE: Adapted from Heinich et al. (1992).

Written materials are one of the most important tools available in comprehensive patient education. They are available for direct learning and as reinforcement for oral and audiovisual presentations. An evaluation of readability is essential when selecting print media that will best enhance a given audience's learning. Pastore and Berg (1987) offer a practical guide for developing and evaluating written patient education materials, especially pamphlets. It focuses on needs assessment of audience, consideration of readability including formatting and readability formulas, patient and staff reviews of materials, and agency approval.

Remember to consider the predetermined behavioral objectives. Ask yourself what *materials* will best support the teaching to meet *these objectives* with *this audience*? Also, remember that *active* is best, *real* is best, and instructional materials should be used only to *support* the learning.

Finally, Table 12–8 may be helpful as an easy-to-use reference for selection of media.

SUMMARY

This chapter was designed to address the major categories of instructional materials and to answer questions about how to select media from a range of possible options and how to evaluate their effectiveness. Nurse educators are expected to be able to make these choices every day, whether it be to meet the needs of an individual learner or design a large educational program to satisfy a broader, more diverse group. In this chapter, the importance of considering characteristics of the learner, the task, and the media when choosing instructional materials was emphasized. The supplemental nature of teaching materials has been stressed, as well as the need to keep the teaching objectives and behavioral objectives in focus when selecting these materials as adjuncts to instruction.

When using print and nonprint media, it is crucial that nurses alert patients to watch for specific points of information. This individualizes content by helping patients focus on what is particularly important to them. After viewing any program, make yourself available (be there) to answer questions or provide opportunity for cognitive practice on what they have seen or read. Audiovisual programs that have accompanying reference materials on which patients can jot notes and write questions and that they can take home can be effective in engendering patient involvement and retention.

The major categories of print and nonprint media were reviewed in full. Where appropriate, examples of effective teaching tools were contrasted with examples of less effective instructional aids. Finally, comprehensive evaluation criteria were presented to assist the educator in selecting appropriate tools for purposes of teaching and learning.

Print media include both commercially prepared and self-composed materials. The problem of matching literacy level and cognitive level of learners to instructional tools is relevant to both types of media. The major advantages of printed tools are their wide availability, that patients are able to refer back to these materials for review at any time and at their own pace, and that they have potential for reinforcing explanations of complex concepts. Disadvantages include the limited opportunity for learner-educator feedback. For some learners, literacy level and complexity of information may be significant barriers to full utilization of printed tools. This chapter contains several guidelines that should be useful to educators in selecting or developing printed materials appropriate to both the audience and the task.

Demonstration materials include many types of nonprint media, such as models, real equipment, diagrams, charts, flip charts, posters, photographs, and drawings. They may exploit the senses of sight, touch, smell, and even taste. They are especially useful for cognitive and psychomotor skill development and may even impact the affective domain through creative imagery. Other advantages include bringing the learner closer to reality through active engagement and the opportunity for repetition. The major disadvantage of demonstrations is the potential for static content or overuse, as demonstrations are often time-consuming to prepare and the educator may be reluctant or unable to revise these materials frequently. In addition, these materials are not suitable for large audiences, visually impaired learners, or those with poor abstraction abilities. Guidelines for selecting demonstration media are contained in this chapter.

Audiovisual materials are the fastest growing category of instructional tools. Their ability to stimulate learners' visual and auditory senses enhances their power to actively engage the learner and increase retention of information. Many audiovisual tools can influence all three domains of learning by promoting cognitive development, effecting attitude change, and helping to build psychomotor skills.

This chapter examined the five major categories of audiovisual tools: projected, audio, video, telecommunications, and computer formats. Discussion included audience appropriateness, expense, and convenience of use. Comprehensive guidelines for selecting and developing audiovisual materials were discussed. The principal advantages and disadvantages of the five categories were also described. Learners with low literacy skills may benefit from most categories of these media except computer formats. Visually impaired learners may be limited to audio materials, while hearing-impaired learners may do well with projected, video, computer, and some forms of telecommunications.

References

Babcock, D.E., & Miller, M.A. (1994). *Client education: Theory and practice*. St. Louis: Mosby–Year Book.

Baker, G.C. (1991). Writing easily read patient education handouts: A computerized approach (review). *Seminars in Dermatology, 10*(2), 102-106.

Boyd, M.D. (1983). An emergency room teacher's guide. *Nursing Management, 14*(2), 65-67.

Boyd, M.D. (1987). A guide to writing effective patient education materials. *Nursing Management, 18*, 56-57.

Bushy, A. (1991). A rating scale to evaluate research posters. *Nurse Educator, 16*(1), 11-15.

Byrne, T. J., & Edeani, D. (1984). Knowledge of medical terminology among hospital patients. *Nursing Research, 33*(3), 178-181.

Cooper, S.S. (1990). Teaching tips, one more time: The overhead projector. *Journal of Continuing Education in Nursing, 21*(3), 141-142.

de Tornyay, R., & Thompson, M.A. (1987). *Strategies for teaching nursing*, 3rd ed. Albany, NY: Delmar.

Discenza, D.J. (1993). A systematic approach to selecting and evaluating instructional materials. *Journal of Nursing Staff Development, 9*(4), 196-198.

Duchin, S., & Sherwood, G. (1990). Posters as an educational strategy. *Journal of Continuing Education in Nursing, 21*(5), 205-208.

Foster, S.D. (1987). Are commercial patient education materials right for you? *MCN: American Journal of Maternal Child Nursing, 12*(4), 287.

Frantz, R. A. (1980). Selecting media for patient education. *TCN/education for self-care*. Rockville, MD: Aspen.

Fredette, S. L. (1984). Individualized clinical teaching via the tape recorder. *Image, 16*(3), 80-83.

Gilliespie, M.O., & Ellis, L.B. (1993). Computer-based patient education revisited (review). *Journal of Medical Systems, 17*(3-4), 119-125.

Glazer-Waldman, H., Hall, K., & Weiner, M.F. (1985). Patient education in a public hospital. *Nursing Research, 34*(3), 184-185.

Grier, E.C., Owens, C., Peavy, B.A., & Pelt, F. (1991). Use of a checklist to teach advanced technical skills. *Nurse Educator, 16*(5), 37-38.

Haggard, A. (1989). *Handbook of patient education*. Rockville, MD: Aspen.

Hanafin, L.F. (1993). The 5-minute teaching series: Pamphlet designed for brief inservice topics. *Journal of Nursing Staff Development, 9*(4), 199-220.

Heinich, R., Malenda, M., & Russell, J.D. (1992). *Instructional media and the new technologies of instruction*, 4th ed. New York: Macmillan.

Hinkle, J.L., Albanese, M., & McGinty, L. (1993). Development of printed teaching materials for neuroscience patients. *American Association of Neuroscience Nurses, 25*(2), 125-129.

Howell, J.H., Flaim, T., & Lung, C.L. (1992). Patient education (review). *Pediatric Clinics of North America, 39*(6), 1343-1361.

Kaihoi, B.H. (1987). Implementing use of learning resources in our technological age, Chapter 7 in C.E. Smith, *Patient education: nurses in partnership with other health professionals.* Philadelphia: Saunders.

Minnick, A., Peterson, L.M., & Krawczak, J. (1988). The effects of audiovisual modeling and reading on baccalaureate students' patient teaching. *Western Journal of Nursing Research, 10*(6): 766-777.

Nielsen, E., & Sheppard, M.A. (1988). Television as a patient education tool: A review of its effectiveness. *Patient Education and Counseling, 11*, 3-16.

Pastore, P.O., & Berg, B.K. (1987). The evaluation of patient education materials: Focus on readability. *Patient Education and Counseling, 9*(2), 216-219.

Pinto, B.M. (1993). Training and maintenance of breast self-examination skills. *American Journal of Preventive Medicine, 9*(6), 353-358.

Rankin, S.H., & Stallings, K.D. (1990). *Patient education: issues, principles, and practices*, 2nd ed. Philadelphia: Lippincott.

Redman, B.K. (1993). *The process of patient education*, 7th ed. St. Louis: Mosby–Year Book.

Rice, V.H., & Johnson, J.E. (1984). Preadmission self-instruction booklets, postadmission exercise performance, and teaching time. *Nursing Research, 33*(3), 147-151.

Sims, S. (1992). Demonstration day: A unique way to learn. *Neonatal Network—Journal of Neonatal Nursing, 11*(1), 41-44.

Smith, C.E. (1987). *Patient education: Nurses in partnership with other health professionals*. Philadelphia: Saunders.

Weixler, D. (July 1994). Correcting metered-dose inhaler misuse. *Nursing, '94, 24*(7), 62-65.

Weston, C., & Cranston, P.A. (1986). Selecting instructional strategies. *Journal of Higher Education, 57*(3), 259-288.

Whitman, N.I., Graham, B.A., Gleit, C.J., & Boyd, M.D. (1992). *Teaching in nursing practice*, 2nd ed. Norwalk, CT: Appleton & Lange.

CHAPTER 13

Instructional Settings

Virginia E. O'Halloran

CHAPTER HIGHLIGHTS

Emerging Trends in Health Care

Classification of Instructional Settings

Factors Impacting on Instructional Settings
 Organizational Factors
 Environmental Factors
 Clientele Factors

Health-Care Setting
 Hospitals
  Organizational Factors
  Environmental Factors
  Clientele
 Home Care
  Organizational Factors
  Environmental Factors
  Clientele

Health-Care-Related Setting

Non-Health-Care Setting
 Occupational Health
  Organizational Factors
  Environmental Factors
  Clientele

Sharing Resources Among Settings

KEY TERMS

instructional setting   health-care setting
health-care-related setting   non-health-care setting

OBJECTIVES

After completing this chapter, the reader will be able to

1. Classify the instructional setting in which the role of nurse as educator occurs.
2. Recognize the trends in health care that are expanding opportunities and expectations of the nurse in the role of educator.
3. Describe the factors that impact on the nurse in the role of educator in each setting.
4. Select the preferred teaching strategies for each instructional setting.

Traditionally, the primary focus of nursing practice has been on the delivery of acute care in hospital settings. Within recent years, the practice of nursing in community-based settings has experienced tremendous growth. The reasons for the shift in orientation of nursing practice from inpatient care sites to outpatient sites relate to the trends affecting the nation's health-care system such as cost-containment measures, regulatory mandates, public and private reimbursement policies, changing population demographics, advances in health-care technology, an emphasis on wellness care, and increased consumer interest in health accompanied by demands for care options. In response to these trends, the domains of nursing practice have broadened to include a greater emphasis on the delivery of care in community settings such as homes, clinics, health maintenance organizations (HMOs), physicians' offices, public schools, and the workplace.

Since health education is an integral component of nursing practice and has become an increasingly important responsibility of nurses in all practice environments, it is imperative to examine the factors influencing the teaching-learning process in various settings where clients, well or ill, are consumers of health care. The chief difference in the delivery of nursing care in acute-care and long-term care facilities versus community-based environments is not only in the health status of the client but also in the length of time and resources available for educational activities. This chapter will

- Examine the trends in health care impacting on the delivery of instruction in various settings.
- Classify instructional settings in which health teaching takes place.
- Present a comparative analysis of the variables affecting educational efforts within different practice environments.
- Recommend teaching strategies best suited for specific settings in which teaching and learning take place.

EMERGING TRENDS IN HEALTH CARE

The major trends impacting on the nation's health-care system come from health-care economics coupled with advances in medical technology, resulting in patients being discharged "quicker" and "sicker," with many of them receiving sophisticated treatment modalities outside the acute-care environment. This has forced providers to cope with delivering high-tech, complex care in less structured and at times less supportive community environments and with clients and their families having to assume increasingly more responsibility for the ongoing management of the medical regimen within their homes. Managed care, as part of the health-care reform movement sweeping the country, has become a reality and is influencing the practice of nurses everywhere. Bridging the gap between inpatient services and community-based services has required all nurses to have greater involvement in client teaching for self-care management, discharge planning, and providing for continuing care (Zarle, 1989).

With the increased focus on prevention, promotion, and independence in self-care activities, today's newly emerging health-care system mandates the education of consumers to a greater extent than ever before. Opportunities for client teaching have become increasingly more varied in terms of the types of clients encountered, their particular learning needs, and the settings in which health teaching occurs. For health education to have a meaningful impact on the lives of others, nurse educators must have a sound understanding of the teaching-learning process to take advantage of the multitude of opportunities to educate consumers. They are also expected to be increasingly adept at identifying the type of content and instructional methodologies that most effectively and efficiently deliver the intended health messages.

CLASSIFICATION OF INSTRUCTIONAL SETTINGS

Although the professional literature contains a significant number of articles related to the practice of nursing in home health care, ambulatory care, school and occupational health care, and institutional care for the acutely and chronically ill, little attempt has been made by authors to comprehensively categorize settings specifically with respect to the nurse's role in patient/client education. Most of the major textbooks on patient education do not present a clear definition of instructional settings. Various authors refer to education taking place in a hospital, a client's home, a physician's office, or unit-based environments for cardiac care, kidney dialysis, or intensive care (Haggard, 1989; Rankin & Stallings, 1990; Redman, 1993). Others identify location of practice by the level of service given such as acute, episodic, rehabilitation, or long-term care. The implication is that these identified "areas" for practice serve a variety of clients with different educational needs requiring different teaching approaches (Cupples, 1991).

Graham and Gleit (1992) describe the teaching role of nurses from the perspective of community versus inpatient, labeling these various practice areas as service settings. Redman (1993) refers to the larger organizations or agencies where health or patient education is provided as health-care delivery systems and presents client teaching situations within the context of a system to describe the tools needed for organizing, evaluating, and documenting teaching content. Cupples (1991) and Leckrone (1991) present data from various studies on the effectiveness of teaching in a variety of "situations," which they identify as settings. The consensus is that a "setting" is generally implied to be that place where health teaching occurs.

The setting for client and patient education is being viewed by this author in a different manner than presented by nurse educators in the past. An instructional setting is conceptualized on the basis of what relationship health education has to the primary function of the organization, agency, or institution within which it occurs. This approach is derived from the method used by Knowles (1964) and Schroeder (1980) to classify settings for adult education. Both of these experts in the field of adult education categorized instructional settings according to the extent to which education is a primary or secondary function of an agency, institution, or organization. For example, they term an academic institution as clearly a setting whose primary purpose is education.

In this chapter, instructional settings are classified according to the primary purpose of the organization or agency that sponsors health education encounters. An *instructional setting* is an entity whose fundamental mission is to provide health care, to engage in activities related to health care, or to be involved primarily in activities unrelated to health care (Figure 13–1). Based on this perspective, three types of settings for the education of clients have been identified:

1. *A health-care setting* is one in which the delivery of health care is the primary or sole function of the institution, organization, or agency. Hospitals, visiting nurse associations, public health departments, outpatient clinics, extended-care facilities, health maintenance organizations, physician offices, and nurse managed centers are examples of organizations whose primary purpose is to deliver health care, for which health education is

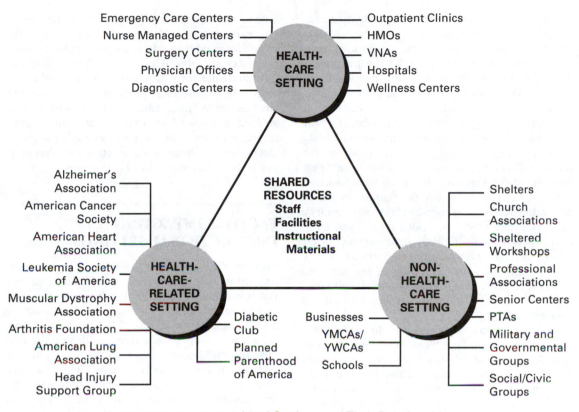

FIGURE 13–1. Instructional Settings and Their Relationships

an integral aspect of the overall care delivered within these settings. Nurses function to provide direct patient care, and their role encompasses the teaching of clients as part of that care.

2. *A health-care-related setting* is one in which health-care-related services are offered as a complementary function of a quasi–health agency. Examples of this type of setting are the American Heart Association, the American Cancer Society, and the Muscular Dystrophy Association. They provide client advocacy, conduct health screenings and self-help groups, disseminate health education information and materials, and support research on disease and lifestyle issues for the benefit of consumers within the community. Education on health promotion, disease prevention, and improving the quality of life for those who live with a particular illness is the key function of nurses within these agencies.

3. *A non-health-care setting* is one in which health care is an incidental or supportive function of an organization. Examples of organizations found within this type of setting are businesses, industries, schools, and military and penal institutions. The primary purpose of these organizations is to produce a manufactured product or offer a non-health-related service to the public. Industries, for example, are involved in health care only to the extent of providing health screenings and nonemergent health coverage to their employees through a health office within their place of employment, making available instruction in job-related health and safety issues to meet Occupational Safety and Health Administration (OSHA) regulations or providing opportunities for health education through wellness programs to reduce absenteeism or improve employee morale.

Thus, an *instructional setting* is defined as an environment in which health education takes place to provide individuals the opportunity to engage in learning experiences for the purpose of improving their health or reducing their risk for illness. It is best to select a broad definition of an instructional setting to enable nurses to consciously recognize the opportunities available for the teaching of those who are currently or potentially consumers of health care. Given that teaching is an important aspect of health-care delivery, nurses engage clients of various ages and at various stages along the wellness-illness continuum in health education activities, which can take place under a variety of circumstances, both formal and informal. Wherever and whenever teaching takes place, nurses need to recognize the importance of consciously applying the principles of teaching and learning to these encounters for maximum effectiveness in helping clients to attain and maintain optimal health.

Health teaching can occur during any encounter between a health-care professional, in this case the nurse in the role of educator, and another person or group seeking health-related information, regardless of the setting in which the information is shared. The client who is the recipient of formal health teaching can be the patient who is ill, the patient's family members or significant others, or individuals or groups in the community who are presently well. Health teaching can also occur during impromptu or informal encounters between the nurse and anyone seeking health information.

Classifying instructional settings in which the nurse functions as educator provides a frame of reference to better understand the interrelationship between the components of the organizational climate, the target audience, and the resources within the environment influencing the educational tasks to be accomplished. The role and functioning of the nurse as client educator are impacted differently by these components in each of the identified settings.

Approaching instructional settings from the perspective of these three components will assist the professional nurse responsible for teaching to gain insight into the common elements to be considered across settings as well as the unique factors associated with particular settings. According to this classification, the nurse educator then is able to more accurately determine who the potential learner is, consider the circumstances under which learning is to take place, and understand the resources available, which can limit or dictate specific strategies for teaching or conversely allow for a diversity of teaching options for maximum effectiveness in learning. Each setting should be considered in terms of what factors have the greatest impact on it and how these factors affect the client, the nurse educator, and the teaching-learning process in the selected practice environment.

FACTORS IMPACTING ON INSTRUCTIONAL SETTINGS

Prior to a discussion of the specific types of settings in which health-care teaching can be carried out, it is necessary to acknowledge those common factors that can have a major impact on teaching and learning across settings. These general factors, which positively or negatively influence the success of teaching strategies and the outcomes of learning in any particular situation, fall into three main categories: organizational, environmental, and clientele variables. If any elements within these categories are insufficient or not conducive to the support of the teaching-learning process, they may act as barriers that reduce the effectiveness of health education interventions by interfering with either the teacher's or the client's level of participation.

The following questions in relation to these factors must be taken into account when planning for the delivery of education programs in the various settings in which the nurse functions (Table 13–1). These elements will be specifically addressed later in the chapter as they apply to the discussion of selected settings.

Organizational Factors

1. What is the administrative perspective regarding health education? The philosophy of the organization emanates from those who are in control of operations. The attitude of administration about the teaching of health information is of utmost importance to the success of educational endeavors. Administrative support influences the amount and types of resources available for education.

TABLE 13–1. Instructional settings, impacting factors, and teaching strategies

Instructional Settings	Impacting Factors and Elements	Teaching Strategies
Health-care	Organizational	One-to-one instruction
Health-care-related	Administrative perspective	Lecture
Non-health-care	Time constraints	Group discussion
	Resources	Printed material
	Teaching expertise	Audiovisual materials
	Collegial support	Interactive media
	Environmental	Individual and group sessions
	External resources	Role-playing
	Structural characteristics	Simulated games
	Clientele	Situational problem solving
	Health status	Demonstration and return
	Nature of contact	demonstration
	Characteristics	
	Self-directedness	
	Educational need	
	Resources	

Within health-care organizations and agencies, patient education carries an economic benefit because it is considered skilled care and is reimbursable by third-party payers in most instances. When patient education is a non-revenue-generating activity, the cost of educational interventions is balanced by a reduction in the incidence of illness, an improved quality of life, and decreased rehospitalization, or overutilization of other services within the health-care system (Shendell-Falik, 1990).

Within non-health-care organizations, such as in occupational settings, employers can reduce their indirect health-care costs by sponsoring health education programs that can decrease absenteeism and increase safety and well-being of workers. Because health insurance premiums paid by employers are often determined by the health-risk level of their employees, these programs can offer employers an immediate, tangible financial reward for their efforts (Graham & Gleit, 1992). Thus, the value given by administrators to health education as a service to their clientele or employees, relative to the emphasis placed on other aspects of their operations, influences the development and provision of health education programs within an organization.

2. How much time is allocated to the teaching of health information? Regardless of the instructional setting, time is a valuable resource that exerts a major influence on the delivery of education to clients. The length of time a client has contact with the health-care system for receipt of services is shrinking as a result of economic factors. Time for educational activities is often a scarce commodity within any organization, but particularly in health-care agencies where the amount of contact time with patients is being further limited by organizational responses to external health-care reforms, resulting in fewer nurses for the same or more clients.

In addition, although advances in technology have generally improved care, they also have reduced contact time by allowing patients to be discharged earlier from inpatient facilities to care for themselves at home. Early discharge requires patients to learn how to operate high-tech equipment within time constraints imposed by the managed-care mandates of most HMOs and insurance providers. Time constraints will force nurses in the role of educators to become more proficient when providing health education. Their focus must be on providing only essential information and skill development needed by the client during the recovery or convalescence period, prioritizing content that can be taught in shorter time frames, and selecting instructional methodologies that allow for more self-directed client involvement with less direct educator presence. A concentrated effort must be made to use every available opportunity, no matter how brief, for client teaching and reinforcement of information across all levels of prevention including health promotion.

3. To what extent are resources available to carry out educational endeavors? Sufficient financial support is required to ensure adequacy of nursing staff, the purchase of needed audiovisual materials and instructional equipment, time to develop content-specific materials, and the provision of space for teaching. Adequate resources make possible the implementation of efficient and effective educational interventions. Without the required resources, information fails to be consistently provided, and the specific needs of clients go unaddressed. Teaching time can be decreased with the use of more standardized teaching materials along with the sharing of resources among health-care settings, thereby reducing bottom-line costs.

4. Is the staff within the organization expert in the teaching role? Although undergraduate nursing education includes principles of teaching and learning in patient education, a basic understanding is generally insufficient to prepare nurses to creatively integrate teaching into their demanding work schedules in a health-care environment where the informal reward system often recognizes physical care as more important than the teaching of self-care. Patient care is frequently viewed by nurses as a series of tasks rather than as an interactive process to support the development of new skills by the client. Furthermore, when staff nurses do teach, they often concentrate on presenting large amounts of didactic information rather than incorporating educational strategies that allow for skills training, family involvement, and the provision of opportunities to practice new skills in realistic situations.

The emphasis on improving cognitive skill levels rather than changing attitudinal or psychomotor behaviors is due to the fact that teaching efforts to meet cognitive needs are easier to deliver, are less time-consuming, and tend to be a less threatening role for nurses (Zarle, 1989). The perspectives of nurses toward client education as well as their competencies with respect to their preparation for and experience with teaching must be evaluated in each environment. As more nurses become prepared at the baccalaureate level, with teaching, health promotion, and community experiences as an integral part of their learning, future nurses will be better prepared for the client teaching role, whether it be in the acute-care or community situation.

5. What is the level of support from physicians and other colleagues? Although a growing number of nurse educators are quite capable of identifying clients' learning needs and providing for the education to meet those needs, in health-care settings physician support is imperative in providing for that education. Presently, Medicare and other third-party reimbursement payments will not be received if the service is not a direct order by a physician. Within health-care organizations, instituting innovative client education approaches is facilitated when the support of physicians and other professional colleagues is present (Shendell-Falik, 1990). Good communication and positive relationships among colleagues are necessary to provide continuity of care, which includes patient education as one very important aspect of overall treatment.

Environmental Factors

1. What external resources are available within the environment to support and promote the educational process? The services of consultants and specialists from other health-care disciplines such as dieticians, occupational therapists, physicians, physical therapists, speech therapists, and social workers must be available to complement the efforts by nurse educators in helping clients to acquire skills needed to attain or maintain optimum wellness. Members of the clergy and self-help groups may play a key role in assisting the client to adjust emotionally and socially to a difficult situation. Community-based organizations often are an excellent vehicle for disseminating information and providing a source of funding for client education services. The nurse's role is to facilitate and coordinate the interactions among these resources.

2. What structural characteristics may stimulate or impede the development and use of educational programs? Consideration must be given to location, travel time, space availability, costs, scheduling, and accessibility when designing a new program or continuing with an existing one. The physical layout of a given area needs to be evaluated with attention paid to determining its adequacy for client privacy, low distraction potential, roominess, comfort, and the ability to easily accommodate equipment related to the topics and skills being taught.

Clientele Factors

1. What is the health status of the client? The client who is well most likely has a low or moderate state of anxiety and is therefore likely to be receptive to teaching and learning. For the patient who is acutely or chronically ill, symptom distress such as fatigue, discomfort, and anxiety, along with the client's and family's perceptions of the illness and support systems available, may adversely affect the person's ability to learn. For those who are hospitalized, the loss of personal control, lack of privacy, and social isolation can have a negative impact on their ability to actively participate in acquiring needed skills for self-care.

2. What is the nature of the contact with the client over time? Contact with the client is highly variable, depending on the situation. If the patient is hospitalized, the opportunity for frequent contact may be more concentrated, over a week or just a few days or even hours in the case of same-day surgery units. The trend toward decreased lengths of stay means that there is less contact time for nurses to do the required teaching and patients are likely to be sicker and less likely to be receptive to educational interventions.

If care is being given in the home setting, the nurse's visits may be limited to only a half hour or so because of fee-for-service or insurance reimbursement regulations or the number of clients to be seen that day by the nurse, but repeated visits may be scheduled over a period of weeks or months, allowing opportunity for the nurse to establish an ongoing relationship with the patient and family and to pace the learning to the individual client situation. Ambulatory care provides for short and intermittent contacts, and the client may not consistently be cared for by the same nurse at every visit.

Rehabilitation settings, on the other hand, allow for extended contact in which to build rapport with the client and provide practice opportunities to learn self-care skills. In today's managed-care climate, clients receive instruction across a continuum of care settings, requiring that attention be given to the coordination of teaching to guarantee that information is complete and the content presented and reinforced is similar.

3. What are the developmental levels, language skills, age, literacy levels, disabilities and cultural beliefs of the client? For settings that serve special populations or multilingual, low-literate, or diverse cultural groups, education methods and materials must be specifically designed to meet the needs of these clientele (see Chapters 5, 7, 8 and 9). The nurse educator must determine the homogeneity and heterogeneity of the populations in different settings when planning educational strategies.

4. How self-directed is the client in seeking information? A major goal of education is to gain the compliance of the learner in carrying out treatment regimens and self-care activities. Research on locus of control suggests that internally oriented individuals prefer to maintain self-control and are likely to be health oriented, compliant with treatment regimens, and receptive to health teaching. Those with an external locus of control, on the contrary, prefer to relinquish control to health-care providers and present a challenge for the nurse educator in motivating them to attend educational sessions and actively participate in learning activities. This can become an even greater challenge to the health educator as the health-care system demands more self-care responsibility from the client.

5. How critical to the health and well-being of the learner is the educational content being presented? If what is being taught is viewed as important information that can be used to help attain or maintain optimal health or reduce the likelihood of an emergency situation, then the clients' attention will be oriented to learning. If the learners do not see the relevance of the information to improving their lifestyle and health status, it is unlikely they will have much motivation for learning or participating in self-care (see Chapter 6).

6. What resources are available to assist clients in achieving educational outcomes? The clients' financial resources must be taken into account because they cannot be expected to follow a specific regimen of care if money to obtain the necessary equipment, medications, foods, or services prescribed is not available. Even healthy individuals who attend programs for promotion of health and disease prevention may not have the financial resources to carry through with suggested lifestyle changes. Psychosocial resources, such as the presence of supportive family members or significant others is most beneficial to the learning experience because they can reinforce the teaching-learning process and provide assistance with self-care activities for those less able for whatever reason.

HEALTH-CARE SETTING

Within the health-care setting are many types of institutions, organizations, and agencies, large and small, whose main focus is the delivery of patient care, with clients receiving patient education as a mandated part of their overall care. Some of these settings provide care on an inpatient basis, such as hospitals, nursing homes, and other extended- or skilled-care facilities, while others provide outpatient care in the home and community, such as visiting nurse associations (VNAs), health maintenance organizations, neighborhood health clinics, physicians' offices, and nurse managed centers. In addition, individual hospitals and large health-care management networks own and operate smaller general or specialty-based units such as one-day surgery centers, outpatient clinics, and diagnostic and rehabilitation centers. Some of these units are located within hospitals, while others are physically located outside the organization as an extension of its services. They are commonly referred to as ambulatory and community outreach centers (Figure 13–1).

This broad spectrum of patient care services provides a wide range of sites in which nurses provide care and client education. In addition to providing patient care, these organizations or institutions are employing agencies as well. In this respect, they are like any other business entity in that they must conform to OSHA regulations and the required standards of various accrediting bodies and state licensing departments to provide workplace safety and health promotion instruction for all of their employees. They must also provide inservice education or staff development programs to maintain the practice competencies of their professional caregivers. Therefore, the re-

sponsibility of nurse educators in these health-care settings is not only to teach patients but to instruct nursing staff and other personnel as well.

Teaching strategies incorporate a wide variety of instructional methods and tools to deliver content. They enhance the capacity of the learner to obtain, retain, and apply knowledge and skills. These techniques include such teaching methods as traditional lectures, group discussions, and simulated games as well as audiovisual materials (Table 13–1). Today's learners are most responsive to teaching strategies that employ stimulation of several senses and participatory learning exercises whenever possible (Rankin & Stallings, 1990; Stulginsky, 1993a). Knowles (1983) predicts that by the end of the twentieth century, most educational services will be delivered electronically.

Nurses will need to be prepared to utilize this new technology in delivering health education. Computer-assisted instruction (CAI), interactive video programming, and virtual reality will soon be readily accessible in all settings. These strategies reduce the amount of direct contact time a nurse needs to spend providing education, allows for diverse learner needs, and provides for pacing, repetition, and flexibility of learning (Blackwood & White, 1991). The general content available in multimedia format can be used for initial instruction and repetitive learning for one or several learners at a time. It allows the nurse to use the limited time with the client to individualize instruction when needed. (For more details related to instructional methods and materials, see Chapters 11 and 12.)

Within the health-care setting, there is a range of teaching situations that require different strategies based on the characteristics of the clientele, their health-care problems, and the type and extent of services they are receiving. A client on the inpatient unit and one in the outpatient clinic can be presented with some similar and some different strategies. Teaching strategies should be selected based on responses to the following four concerns:

- How much does the client need to know now and later?
- Is the information to be learned life sustaining or general content that the client ought to know?
- To what degree will the client's physical and psychological condition interfere with knowledge acquisition and retention?

- How much teaching time and client contact over time are possible?

General care units, specialty units, outpatient units, community medical care centers, and physician offices all require teaching of clients. The strategies include one-to-one, lecture, and group discussions; brief, concise, printed instructions; and demonstration with return demonstration when necessary. The client situation will dictate whether teaching sessions need to be individual or group presentations, recognizing that teaching clients in a group should be selected whenever possible because this approach uses staff time more effectively, is less costly, and affords the client an opportunity to have a shared experience. However, when the client situation is more individualized, such as on a same-day surgery unit, individual one-to-one teaching strategies need to be emphasized, along with the other modalities.

When contact with the client is expected to include revisits over time, such as in home-care visits, outpatient clinics, HMO centers, and physician offices, then a multisensory approach is used, with films, videos, and take-home printed material, with staff accessible and actively engaging the clients in individualized discussions, clarification, and reinforcement of content after they have had the opportunity to view or read the materials or interact with the learning modules.

When more time is available and the health education involves more general care or ought-to-know content related to chronic conditions or lifestyle changes, then participatory learning strategies such as problem-solving situations, simulated games, and role-playing can be employed, with video films added for more varied sensory input and for repetition, to enhance understanding and retention of content. Charts or diagrams are a particularly helpful strategy to review content, to emphasize steps in a procedure, or to help clients learn the sequencing in an event (Breckon et al., 1985). Providing small increments of information over time is a better strategy when attention span is short. This is the case when the client is a child, mentally disabled, an older adult, or very anxious. A follow-up contact by phone should be included if discharge is immediate after the teaching session or contact with the client is brief such as in an emergency-care or same-day surgery center. The phone contact is used to evaluate the learning and

to reinforce teaching as well as to assess physical status. A follow-up phone contact would also be used if the problems the client may encounter are likely to occur between the discharge time and the follow-up visit (Rankin & Stallings, 1990).

The instructional category of health-care setting provides a wide variety of practice environments for the nurse educator, and a few will be described. In reviewing the factors that impact on the role of the nurse educator in large and small practice environments, an understanding will be gained regarding the clientele, environmental resources, and organizational characteristics of other similar but somewhat different practice environments not described, yet part of the instructional category of health-care setting (Figure 13–1).

Hospitals

Since the 1970s, patient education has been an integral part of hospitals. Organizational support and commitment of staff, resources, and time exist in hospitals for client health education and for the nurse as the primary provider of that education because mandates from accreditation and licensing bodies require it (Simonds, 1973). The shortened hospital stay and the expansion of services into areas like same-day surgery centers, hospital-based home-care departments, cardiac rehabilitation centers, and hemodialysis centers are already increasing the emphasis on health education as part of the continuum of care. Continuity of care ensures that from admission through posthospital care, the patients have what they need in treatment, medical equipment, knowledge, and skills to carry them to the end point of service, bridging the gap between acute inpatient service and less acute community service needed after rapid discharge, especially for older adults and those with chronic illnesses (Zarle, 1989). Patient teaching and the role of the nurse educator must become a more integral part of this system to identify and implement teaching plans needed to prepare clients for each phase of recovery.

Organizational Factors
Hospitals, like other large health-care delivery systems or networks, are complex organizations that have a variety of organizational structures, with specialty units within the hospital or situated

offsite in community centers. Although the nurse educator has organizational support, large organizational systems require formal, hierarchical communication among units, whether on or off premises, resulting in cumbersome negotiations when planning to establish an innovative patient education program or make changes in existing ones. It requires knowledge and application of change theory and involvement of multidisciplinary planning teams to ensure success (Rifas et al., 1994; Shendell-Falik, 1990). Regardless of the size of the health-care organization or the mandated regulations, it is often difficult to garner support of our medical colleagues for client education programs, and it is often achieved only through persistent, lengthy, one-to-one discussions with key medical staff. Although difficult to obtain, their support is essential to comply with present insurance payment requirements. However, as consumers demand more information and health-care systems require more self-care from clients, the client education component will become a more important part of the entire package of care delivered, with nurses providing it without specific medical orders.

The health-care setting does not separate out the cost of patient teaching activities because many third-party payers at present do not pay for teaching, whether provided in the inpatient or outpatient unit. The future may see health-care organizations being required to itemize separately patient or health education as well as many other items for the sole purpose of insurance reimbursement. The current state of financial reimbursement impacts on the setting in that no monies are specifically marked for this purpose and monies needed for patient education must come from the "common pot." The value placed by the organization on health education will determine the percentage of financial support provided to such programs.

Nurse educators in these practice environments are restricted by many constraints imposed by organizational factors and are more traditionally bound by the established criteria to be met or required content to be taught. They may be limited by monies or technical resources available to obtain or develop teaching materials or by the staff time allowed to prepare and deliver content. This is especially true for outreach centers, which often operate on grant funds or time-limited financial support.

However, these detached services or specialty units often allow for a closer relationship to develop between physicians and nurses who provide care to clients, enhancing a collegial, collaborative relationship in joint efforts to meet patient education needs with less physician resistance evident. Teaching is still a less quantifiable, non-revenue-generating function, hampering its general acceptance and implementation in all ambulatory care situations. This is especially true for physician offices, where the nurse educator role is far less defined or developed and time for teaching underutilized (Hiss et al., 1986).

The attitudes and value placed on client education by all involved, from administrators to staff-level nurses, can affect the quantity and quality of client education (DeMuth, 1989). The focus of care is still tasks and procedures, with seeing a high number of both scheduled and emergency clients within posted hours of operation taking priority and leaving little time for the nurse educator to engage in creative thinking to prepare or evaluate teaching plans, materials, or strategies. Client education must be a well-integrated activity with well-designed strategies and tools if it is to be a meaningful, worthwhile intervention. Planning ahead is essential, with input into yearly budgets to ensure that monies for client education activities and equipment are there, making what is needed a reality in the year ahead.

Hospitals and their associated specialty units are more likely to have on staff nurse educators who oversee client education programs or who support less-prepared unit-level nurses in their teaching efforts. Unfortunately, these resources are not fully utilized, and there remain a significant number of unit-level nurses who are inadequately prepared in application of teaching-learning principles. They do not discriminate the "need to know" from "nice to know" content to be taught, fail to assess what the clients perceive as important for them to learn about self-care, or lack sufficient knowledge regarding the aftercare situation for which the nurse needs to prepare the client (Bubela et al., 1990; Naylor & Shaid, 1991).

In general, these environments provide an opportunity for nurse educators to prepare extensively to meet the educational needs of the learners because they know the composition of the learning group, can anticipate their needs, and can individualize the educational plan using appropriate teaching strategies. Anticipated problems such as staff schedules and language or sensory disabilities of the learners can be discussed and solutions proposed ahead of time to make for a more successful learning situation, with fewer unanticipated difficulties arising in this type of setting.

For a variety of reasons, what clients learn in the hospital is not well recalled after discharge, necessitating reteaching by home-care nurses. The patient education component of the system could be better organized, more efficient, and more effective if there was greater involvement and closer coordination among hospital-based patient educators, discharge-planning nurses, and home-care nurses. It is essential to increase standardization of content and teaching materials across units of patient care and to facilitate the development and implementation of teaching protocols for the more common acute and chronic health problems from the moment of admission through to discharge to home-care, focusing on education for self-care as a major component to be addressed when planning for discharge. This would make possible cost-effective use of the nurse's teaching time and patient learning time, smooth the transition from acute to home care, from dependent to more independent client functioning, and include client education to ensure the quality of continuity of care and discharge planning.

Documentation in a health-care setting is an important and integral component of the patient education activity because it provides the basis for financial reimbursement of that portion of care. On one large metropolitan hospital's postpartum unit, a checklist is used to document standard teaching content for self and baby care. Every client is provided with the same content, which is documented on the checklist by the nurse who does the teaching. When home-care nurses make the follow-up visit after discharge, they know what the clients have been taught, they can assess retention of that knowledge, reinforce if necessary, and move on to other mutually agreed on client education topics best taught in the home setting. Between the two experiences, the new mother will have had a total educational packet begun in the hospital and completed after discharge in the home (Smith, 1986).

For a number of years, both major and smaller community hospitals have utilized their nursing education departments creatively and fully by providing health promotion programs to the general community and many area businesses, such as offering free or fee-for-service cholesterol screening and weight management programs supported by small grants, or for a break-even cost. In the future, this area of practice for the nurse educator will expand and become a more profitable, revenue-generating endeavor in this health-care setting, offering opportunity for collaboration and sharing of expertise among staff, of facility space, and of instructional materials as well as meeting the general community's need for health promotion education provided by nurse educators.

Environmental Factors

The resources including consultants and specialists from all health-care disciplines are extensive and easily accessed in the hospital or large network practice environments. Even when the care delivery sites are off premises, the resources of the parent facility are present, with time and distance as the major barriers.

Specific teaching materials, such as pamphlets and films, on standardized topics are often provided free through vendors who service health-care settings. Closed-circuit TV and freestanding TV/VCR units are commonly provided to any patient-occupied area. Classrooms or conference rooms are likely available but may need to be scheduled in advance if not dedicated for the sole use of patient education departments. Patient waiting areas, lounges, and patients' rooms are often used for small group or individualized client education sessions, providing an attractively furnished, comfortable environment and fostering inclusion of family or support persons in the sessions.

Even when space is available, the client's other medical-care-related activities may take priority over scheduled patient education time because patient education is not viewed as having the same importance as other higher-cost interventions. The organization may not place as much value on the teaching component needed but focus more on the need to discharge the client as rapidly as possible, regardless of the client's psychological preparedness. In this instance, knowledge and skills for aftercare may be compromised.

Ambulatory care units such as same-day surgery, outpatient clinics, or emergency rooms process a high volume of clients in a brief time period, with major space and time constraints for care delivery including much needed client education presentations. A greater reliance on audiovisual and take-home printed materials coupled with follow-up phone calls to evaluate client status and teaching effectiveness can provide for client learning needs in those situations.

SCENARIO

This is a same-day surgery unit of an ambulatory care center. Clients A and B are admitted for a diagnostic procedure. Client A is a schoolteacher, and Client B is a housewife with a limited understanding of English. The unit is fast paced and dictated by schedules. Most clients have a mild to moderate anxiety level. The nursing staff must relate to many physicians and adhere to many protocols. The nurse-client encounters are brief, and the total length of stay for the client is less than 12 hours. Instructional encounters within this health-care setting require brief, concise teaching of only key points. An explanation of the client's recovery process is done through use of a video individually viewed over a bedside TV. Staff are available to respond to client questions, to provide discharge instructions, both verbal and written, and for follow-up phone calls the next day to assess client status, evaluate learning, and provide additional teaching interventions. If the client has a vision problem or a language barrier, an audiocassette of instructions is provided for listening, with the audio and written instructions available in the more common languages.

This setting dictates individual teaching strategies as a primary mode augmented with group presentations and multimedia materials whenever possible.

The type and range of teaching strategies used in any instructional setting will be influenced by the value the organization places on client education, resources available to support the development and delivery of educational programs, and the characteristics of the clients to be served.

In most health-care settings, the learning need is responded to more from the health provider's perspective and less from the client's. For example, if it is decided that a newly diagnosed diabetic client needs to know how to test for blood sugar regularly and what the readings indicate, although the patient may not desire to learn that part of self-care first, the patient will be taught despite the probable lack of readiness to learn because discharge may be only a day away.

Clientele

The characteristics and needs of the clients serviced by large or smaller health-care organizations and their specialty units dictate the specific content to be taught, the time and the amount of client teaching undertaken, and the most appropriate teaching strategies to be used. Clients admitted to these facilities are sicker and have higher anxiety levels due to the acute nature of their health problems at the time of contact with the setting, making them less receptive to learning. They may have one or more chronic illnesses, have a variety of compounding socially related issues such as homelessness or poverty, be newly diagnosed, or be at advanced stages of an illness.

Ambulatory care units such as outpatient clinics and emergency care centers see and treat clients for episodic conditions with decreased opportunities for future encounters for more individualized health promotion and disease prevention focused teaching. If clients return at a later point to one of the large or high-volume care areas, they will probably see a different nurse each time, reducing the possibility of continuity in client teaching. Therefore, most teaching content should focus on the common concerns for the clients at whatever stage on the illness continuum they are, providing verbal and written information on signs and symptoms to report, medication or treatment regimens, and safety in self-care management (DeMuth, 1989).

Clients are oriented to receiving diagnostic procedures and treatments but not necessarily health education as an integral part of a visit to an ambulatory care facility. For clients to participate in teaching-learning as a part of their experience in ambulatory care, they must know ahead of time to expect health teaching as a component of their care, facilitating their readiness to learn at each visit.

The limited contact the nurse has with the client, for whatever reason, will require that it be utilized to the fullest, with the nurse providing teaching sessions and reinforcement of information woven into every patient contact. Hospitalized clients' acuity level makes them less receptive to learning, and not being provided with an opportunity to apply the learning to their present condition makes retention difficult. They are not asked to self-medicate or do their own dressings while hospitalized and therefore are less likely to be skilled in these areas when discharged, unless the facility and the nurse educator have provided some realistic opportunities for application of self-care skills.

Although the ideal is to set up self-care units such as exist in New York University's Cooperative Care Model or the one at Newark Beth Israel Medical Center, that may not be financially possible for many hospitals. A smaller model like the Recuperative Skills Training Center at Sacramento's Kaiser Permanente Medical Center, where patients go to practice needed self-care skills, may be more feasible (Rifas et al., 1994). It is also possible to reorient staff nurses to "do less" and "teach more" by allowing able patients to do their own dressings with staff supervision or provide group teaching sessions where patients on restricted diets select their daily menus with the teaching and guidance of the nurse educator and dietician. This approach is facilitated by the fact that the client in the hospital situation is narrowly focused toward the disease condition with interest in treatments, side effects, medications, impact on lifestyle, and activities of daily living, with little concern related to the general aspects of the disease or primary prevention components (Naylor & Shaid, 1991). Including the family or significant other in teaching sessions whenever possible will improve retention of content, increase support for the client, and enhance compliance with treatment regimens. Triad communication involves a third person who is assisting with daily care management decisions (Davidhizar & Rexroth, 1994).

There is a wide range of demographic characteristics of today's client, and that is true in this setting as in all others, requiring the nurse's rapid, comprehensive assessment of the client's developmental level, language skill, literacy level, cultural and religious orientation, self-directedness, readiness to learn, and available support system. Regardless of the psychosocial readiness factors, the system mandates that the client be taught self-care with referral to home care for follow-up. Because this is the case, the nurse educator must select and prioritize the "must knows" from the "ought to knows" to accomplish the minimum

teaching requirements. Many of the client characteristics and limited time frames for teaching are the same in most health-care environments. However, it is the acuity of the clients, their anxiety level, and the number of contacts with the clients over time that vary in each setting. To meet the learning needs in complex situations, clients with multiple health problems, life-threatening illnesses or complications, conditions requiring complex technical treatments, or multiple medication regimens should be identified as requiring more intense teaching begun as early as possible (Bubela et al., 1990).

Although large health-care settings such as hospitals and their community-based units can more easily obtain reimbursable medical supplies and equipment or other support services, some items require out-of-pocket funds by the client with or without future reimbursement, which may be an issue for the aged or others on fixed or limited income. Financial constraints may prevent compliance with health teaching.

Nurse educators need to be prepared for the wide variety of client characteristics and health-related elements encountered in the hospital setting that dictate learning needs. Nurses must revise the expectations of themselves, refrain from attempting to "teach it all," and adopt an abbreviated, efficient, and expeditious form of client education that meets the client's basic self-care needs (Ruzicki, 1989).

Home Care

Home health care is one of the most rapidly growing practice settings, driven by early discharge and the need to provide acute and high-tech care as the client is shifted from hospital to home (Humphrey, 1988). The home of today is the hospital of yesterday, with clients being maintained at home with skilled care until their next life-threatening episode brings them back to the hospital. Hospital administrators recognize that the home-care clientele is fast replacing their shrinking hospital bed clients and welcome the opportunity to be involved in this area of community care through hospital-based home-care units. At present, home care can be situated within a variety of large or small health-care organizations such as VNAs, hospice associations, extended care facilities, and large or small for-profit home-care organizations. Some agencies provide home care for their own parent institutions as well as for other facilities that are not able to provide the home care directly but whose clients require these services, such as institutions outside the geographical area. If the parent organization is the more traditional hospital, for example, then teaching is impacted by the factors of that organization, its environmental resources, and its clientele.

Organizational Factors

When home care is a unit within a larger organization, it is committed to health education and will vary only somewhat based on individual philosophies or values of the facility. When the home-care agency is a smaller independent agency or one for profit, the organizational philosophy, value placed on client health education, scope of services provided, organizational structure, and legislative regulations will vary much more from agency to agency and impact to a greater extent on how much patient education is provided, especially in today's money-driven system. For example, if the nurse's primary purpose for the visit is to oversee care and supervise home health aides in a long-term care program or a for-profit home-care agency, then the nurse educator role is focused more on staff learning needs related to their care of the client and less on client-based learning needs regarding medications and treatments. Third-party payers, such as Medicare, in these instances will pay only for a nursing visit to reassess ongoing care needs and aide supervision once every few weeks in what is considered to be a more stable chronic-care situation. Thus, the type of home-care agency and services rendered will directly impact on the nurse educator in terms of who is the learner, the nature of the content, and the time allocated.

Documentation for client teaching in the home setting is essential in all instances regardless of the size of the organization because many insurance payers, such as Medicare, specifically look for teaching related to treatments and medications in nursing notes to support their reimbursement. Time allotted for client visits including client education activities is becoming more limited by the increasing workload, with more cases to be seen each day as a result of reduced staffing and insurance reimbursement pressures.

The home-care nurse is truly alone in the home environment, without colleagues to verify assessments or give assistance. Instead, home-care nurses must rely on theoretical knowledge, past experience, creativity, and often intuition to provide for the health education needs of clients, where every home presents a different scenario. The positive side of this very different and solitary practice environment is that there are less turf issues than in other health-care disciplines. Health-care teaching for self-care management is an expected component of care not in every instance requiring a physician order for implementation or reimbursement. If a client requires a dressing change daily, that activity is ordered by the physician, and the nurse is expected to teach the signs and symptoms of infection to be reported to the physician and teach the client or caregiver to do the dressing change, if possible, even though it was not specified by the physician's order. The home-care nurse must be adept at rapid and comprehensive assessment of client learning needs for self-care management, prioritizing learning goals that meet both the nurse's and client's perceived needs. The nurse must be able to switch from the planned content of a teaching session to what the client wants or needs to learn, perhaps delaying intended objectives for learning until the next visit.

Because home care is one of the few practice areas less impacted on by restructuring, nurses are seeking such positions with little or no realization of the knowledge and skills required. While most hospital-based home-care agencies and VNAs hire baccalaureate-prepared nurses, the smaller or for-profit agencies may not. Despite the educational preparation of the baccalaureate-prepared nurse, few nurses are adequately prepared when it comes to patient education in complex client situations in the home. This has been recognized as a problem, and an innovative partnership between the New York State Nurses Association and Pace University's Department of Continuing Education in Nursing has developed a program of classroom and clinical experiences to help transition nurses from shrinking acute-care positions to home-care nursing, enhancing their level of competency and feelings of comfort working within such a different practice environment (Opening the door to home care, 1995).

Environmental Factors

Home-care nurses are permitted into clients' homes, as guests, interacting collaboratively with clients and caregivers, who are the primary decision makers in all aspects of their care. Home care provides an opportunity to see clients in their familiar surroundings, observe behavior that is more natural, determine the problems encountered in the home, and assess clients' perspective of their illness and limitations now that they are in their own environment. The learning goals established must be mutually acceptable, and there is joint nurse/client responsibility and negotiation as part of the caregiving process (Pesznecker et al., 1989). For example, if the client does not wish to take narcotics for pain as prescribed, then through teaching and negotiation by the nurse, the client may agree to take the narcotic at bedtime and a non-narcotic analgesic with use of relaxation techniques taught by the nurse for daytime relief. The client has more freedom of choice in this setting. Health education needs must be prioritized based on the potential threats to health, the degree of client concern about a problem, and the ease of solution (Stulginsky, 1993b).

The home can pose distractions that are not under the nurse's control and that are different for each home and client situation, unlike the hospital, where the environment of a patient unit or clinic is essentially the same. Disruptive family members, visitors, environmental noise, household pets, confined quarters, and inadequate or unfamiliar medical supplies and equipment are some of the distractions or impediments for the client and the challenges the nurse may encounter in the provision of health care in the home setting. (Pruitt et al., 1987). A client might have believed they could do the dressing or injection taught in the hospital before discharge, but once home, reality sets in, and barriers within the home may interfere with the patient's ability to apply what had been learned.

Most homes have TVs, and many have VCRs or cassette players as potential instructional tools to present, support, or reinforce teaching content. Many teaching materials can be obtained from the parent facility, borrowed from other health facilities in the community, or provided from the nurse's own supplies to be brought into the home. The home-care nurse has access to many of the same health-care educational materials provided by health-care vendors, much of which is free to health-care professionals. With creativity and imagination, the nurse educator working in home care can develop a small library of teaching tools that address many of the common chronic illnesses or health problems, such as diabetes, cardiovascular disease, hypertension, chronic obstructive pulmonary disease, hip fractures, and cancer.

The nurse focuses on health education related to self-care management and can enlist the assistance of such professionals as dieticians, physical therapists, or speech therapists for their expertise while reinforcing the specialized content they provide at subsequent visits. Knowledge regarding area community agencies, self-help groups, and church-affiliated programs is essential to assist in providing specialized teaching materials, equipment, or financial and psychosocial support for the learning needs of clients, facilitating client compliance with the prescribed regimen.

Clientele

The clients in home care have the same requirements for needs assessment as those described for clients in hospital teaching situations. Clients in the home are less acutely ill. Most are chronically ill with multiple diseases and although less anxious than hospitalized patients, they are still fearful that the next symptoms might send them back to the acute-care setting or that their lifestyle, quality of life, and level of independence will deteriorate as a result of their last acute-care episode. Focusing on their educational needs that reflect these concerns will facilitate the teaching-learning process and ultimately achieve self-care goals desired by the nurse and the client.

Client teaching in the home situation often needs to involve not only the client but also the primary caregiver or any other concerned family members who need health education information related to the client's care needs and condition (Johnson & Jackson, 1989). The home-care situation offers the opportunity for extended contact with the client and caregiver over time and an ability to evaluate the effectiveness of the teaching-learning process, enabling adjustments to be made as adaptation to levels of wellness occur. The degree of self-directedness in learning is dependent on each individual client and varies according to clients' views of their wants and needs. Since the home is their "turf," clients feel freer to question advice or teaching they receive, do things their way, and establish their own time schedules and priorities, all of which may prove challenging from the perspective of the nurse's teaching efforts. The nurse must be flexible and prepared for the unexpected, a hallmark of home-care delivery. The goal is to maintain the client within the home and out of the acute- or chronic-care institutions for as long as possible through teaching self-care management skills. The focus of health teaching tends to be less on primary prevention or health promotion and more on secondary or tertiary levels of intervention. Teaching needs to be individualized, holistic, short-term, and often chronic care oriented. Client education is increasingly challenging because more high-tech equipment and greater acute-care needs are being met in the home-care situation than ever before, with increased responsibility for management left to clients, family, neighbors, or unlicensed assistive personnel (Stulginsky, 1993b).

Home-care services including health education are paid for by Medicare and most third-party payers, who recognize that these services are appropriate, cost-effective approaches to handling acute- and chronic-care needs (Johnson & Jackson, 1989). Although the home situation allows for contact with clients over several visits, insurance payers are beginning to circumscribe the number of visits for teaching clients, as they already have done for the newly diagnosed diabetic. Nurses will need to be creative in providing for the variety of teaching needs of clients, including aspects that may not be reimbursed, to meet client learning needs in a holistic, individualized manner.

Teaching strategies need to focus on priority content with brief explanations and easy to identify instructional guidelines, offering more detailed information and instructional materials at later visits. A multisensory approach to presenting content is a helpful strategy for reinforcement and retention in the home situation, as it is in all other situations. The use of more sophisticated interactive media in the home teaching situation is rapidly becoming more popular and should be applied to the fullest extent possible. An educational video may be made available for the nurse to take to the home for viewing with the client and family members during a teaching session, or a copy sent ahead to be viewed by the client in preparation for the visit and teaching session. Videotapes can be left in the home until the next visit for the client and family members to review for reinforcement of learning.

The teaching strategies that can be used with clients in health-care settings are many. Whenever hardware for audiovisual materials is unavailable, printed materials to supplement various methods of teaching may be likely substitutes. The selection of instructional strategies in the health-care setting is dictated more by the client factors than available resources and organizational factors because health education and patient teaching are recognized and expected responsibilities of the nurse in these settings.

HEALTH-CARE-RELATED SETTING

Within health-care-related settings are voluntary, nonprofit agencies, organizations, and institutions, such as the American Lung Association, the American Heart Association, the American Cancer Society, and the Muscular Dystrophy Association (Figure 13-1), whose major purpose is client advocacy, education, and/or research (Breckon et al., 1985). Health education may be the primary purpose of the organization, or it may have a secondary or equally valued advocacy or research goal. The educational services offered to the consumer by these agencies are directed toward emphasis on health promotion and disease prevention for the well public as well as maintenance and rehabilitation efforts to improve the quality of life for those who are living with a particular health problem.

In addition to responding to the needs of the general community, these organizations also serve health professionals who are seeking up-to-date, reliable information either for the benefit of their patients or to enhance their own knowledge base. Relative to the primary concern of each of these organizations, they provide information on the latest research, treatments, or techniques available in their field of interest. Health education is viewed by these health-care-related entities as a vehicle to further the general public's and the professional's knowledge regarding the magnitude and impact that a particular health problem or issue has on society as a whole.

The information provided by these various organizations and agencies is narrowly focused on one topic area, which is the primary reason for their existence, and their clientele have similar learning needs driven by the motivation for a healthier heart or improved breathing, for example. Contact with these agencies is often initiated by the clients, but they can be referred by a provider for the desired information or support services. The clients using their services tend to be less anxious than clients found in health-care settings, are more self-directed in meeting learning needs, and seek information that is disease specific or involved with lifestyle changes such as smoking cessation.

Characteristic of these agencies is their single-minded focus on one specific health problem or issue, often with a fervor that can be all-consuming for their supporters. This narrow perspective influences their educational offerings, research initiatives, and client advocacy efforts. With a serious commitment to education about a specific identified health problem or issue, these associations are heavily involved in the development and dissemination of printed materials and audiovisual tools for purposes of teaching and learning.

As nonprofit organizations with limited funding sources, these organizations are primarily supported through individual charitable contributions and public or private grants. Some receive monetary allocations from community fundraising efforts, such as the United Way, while others are dependent solely on direct public donations, potentially causing their resources and programs to wax and wane based on their current financial status. Many of the services provided are free of charge, although nominal fees are usually established for multiple copies of their printed materials because this offers them partial financial return to offset production costs. Because printed materials are heavily relied on by these associations as a medium through which to widely disseminate health information, the nurse as educator must be responsible for evaluating the literacy level and content of these various materials to determine whether they are suitable for the intended audiences.

Many of the larger, well-supported organizations such as the American Cancer Society and the American Heart Association have professional nurses on staff as paid employees or as voluntary members to develop health education materials, to plan and participate in programs such as conferences or health screenings, or to lead support groups. Teaching is a major responsibility of nurses functioning within agencies that operate in the health-care-related setting. As referral sources, these agencies also exist to share informational materials and deliver educational services to augment and complement resources of institutions and organizations belonging to the other health-care or non-health-care settings (Figure 13–1).

The teaching strategies used by nurses in the role of educators in this type of setting depend on the nature and size of the prospective audience as well as the learning situation. Instructional methods often involve group activities that stimulate active participation of the learner, such as discussion sessions, role-playing, and simulations augmented with audiovisual tools as effective means to involve the consumer. Health-screening encounters and telephone inquiries provide the opportunity for individual one-to-one teaching possibilities with a client. Although the emphasis for teaching is on health promotion and disease prevention with healthy individuals and groups, the nurse must also deal with ill clients who present themselves looking for information that can assist them in reaching optimal levels of functioning. Thus, the nurse functioning in this setting must demonstrate versatility and flexibility in the role as educator, employing a variety of teaching strategies to meet the needs and satisfy the demands of the various clients served by these community-based health-care-related agencies.

NON-HEALTH-CARE SETTING

Included within the non-health-care setting are organizations, institutions, or agencies whose primary purpose is anything other than health care and who voluntarily seek to provide health education or health care to its membership as a benefit or service. Of the three types of instructional settings under discussion, this type of setting includes the most varied kinds of organizations. Examples are industries; businesses; schools; YMCA/YWCAs; community civic, social, and religious associations; senior centers; shelters for the homeless or abused; and others (Figure 13-1). Non-health-care settings have clientele who vary widely in their educational needs and desires because they can be employees in industry or business, schoolchildren of various ages, parents in a parent-teacher organization, or members of all ages in civic or church groups. Some generalities can be applied to the members of these varied facilities in that most are an adult working population in need of educational programs covering a wide variety of topics—safety in the work environment, stress reduction, the importance of health screening for elevated blood pressure, lowering cholesterol or glucose levels, or health problems for which members are at risk, including controversial topics such as HIV.

Most institutions and organizations in the non-health-care setting view health education as a service to its members or a benefit for employees in the work environment. Employers see health education as a method for reducing health-care costs associated with unhealthy lifestyles or keeping absenteeism at a minimum. Nonwork settings that include civic, religious, or social organizations frequently view health education as meeting either the expressed need of its membership or the needs of the community as a whole. Those agencies and institutions that embrace a community perspective believe that improving the health of the public is everyone's responsibility. Health-related education in these organizations can range from a substantial commitment to only a minimal interest on the part of the leadership in the health and well-being of their membership. Agencies and institutions within this setting will usually identify the topic that is to be provided, without detailing content, and provide the resources to accomplish the desired outcome by bringing in a nurse educator or other health professional to present the material to their members or employees. The nurse's responsibility for the health education encounter may be a brief one-session experience to meet a specific health need of a population of clients, or it can be a series of sessions occurring over an extended period of time.

Because this instructional setting comprises a kaleidoscope of practice environments and populations, attention will focus on occupational health as one illustration of how the three factors of organization, resources, and clientele interact and impact on the client education role of the nurse.

Occupational Health

Occupational health nurses compose the largest health specialty group employed in industry. They can be found in most large companies, providing for the health-care needs of employees and working closely with management to expand their view of what constitutes health care in the workplace. In other instances, companies contract with hospitals or ambulatory care centers to provide services to meet their employees' health-care needs, usually at a secondary level of prevention, such as yearly health screenings, with little emphasis on activities promoting health or preventing disease. However, most industries are mandated by governmental regulations from OSHA to provide some level of safety or injury prevention programs, which may be presented by occupational health nurses. Occupational nurses in the role of educator have an opportunity to teach employers, to go beyond physical care of the ill or injured worker, to broaden their view of what encompasses the role of the nurse, and to include health education for health promotion and disease prevention for the benefit of workplace wellness in providing health services to employees.

Organizational Factors

The attitude and perspective of company chief executive officers are a major influence on what is made available to employees through their health programs. Management's understanding of their decision-making responsibility in providing health-care services to employees, the scope of those services, and how the health of their employees impacts on meeting the company production goals will determine the organizational commitment of resources to the health education component of the occupational nurse's role. The size of the business or industry may impact on the resources available to provide health-related education, but a positive view of health education by management will mean more programming even with limited resources. Here is where creative thinking and resource networking on the part of the nurse educator can make a real difference by designing programs to provide health education at no cost, at a minimal fee for service, or with cost sharing by the employers and employees.

Contracting with local hospitals or the American Lung Association for specific programs at a reduced or group rate for employees of area businesses provides the expertise in a particular content area of health education that the occupational nurse is necessarily not prepared to offer. Networking, sharing expertise with nursing colleagues, and attending continuing education programs in worksite wellness programming can help the less prepared occupational nurse acquire the knowledge necessary to plan, implement, and evaluate health education programs at the workplace. Financial reimbursement from third party payors for health education programs in non-health-related settings is indirect and minimal or nonexistent in most cases. However, some health insurance companies will provide free on-site wellness programs such as cholesterol screening, weight management, stress reduction, or healthy back programs for their subscribers. Others will give financial rebates in the form of reduced premiums to employers or employees based on lower employee illness risk or employee participation in weight management or exercise programs, which foster healthy lifestyle behaviors. This commitment by insurers, although minimal at best, provides employers and employees with some tangible return for their investment in wellness programs. The occupational nurse's activities are quite similar to those of the nurse in a physician's office. Episodic care is provided for minor on-the-job injuries or illnesses, with client education information regarding signs and symptoms of complications or safety precautions delivered via verbal or written format and specific to the problem presented. Some organizations may or may not provide the nurse with time during the workday for assessing the health education needs of management and employees or with planning, implementing, and evaluating programs focused on health promotion and disease prevention in the workplace.

Environmental Factors

The occupational health nurse has access to a variety of resources, usually within the limitations of the geographical area, such as consultation with other health-care professionals and health-care-related organizations such as the American Cancer Society, who can assist in providing health promotion materials or programming on or off premises. The health office, cafeteria, conference room, and reception area space can be creatively utilized to provide attractive, eye-catching health promotion literature at designated times during the year, such as during Diabetes Awareness Month, or throughout the year with changing monthly themes. Conference rooms or other suitable presentation areas are usually available within employing facilities and suitable for health program presentations to small or large groups, but programming may need to be planned in advance to fit room availability. Standardized printed and audiovisual health education materials are available in limited or bulk quantity for free or for a nominal fee through health-care product vendors, the Department of Health, or organizations like the American Heart Association.

Clientele

The clients serviced by occupational health nurses are both management and employees, who are mostly a well adult population. Although they are well adults, some of them have lifestyle behaviors that put them at risk for diseases, have episodes of acute and chronic illness, could benefit from health promotion programs to reduce their risk factors, and need screening programs to detect the early stages of disease. The clients in this type of environment, as adult learners, are self-directed in seeking health education information. High anxiety levels are usually not present to interfere with the teaching-learning process. Often health education and promotion programs are offered at no charge to employee participants, who are then free to choose to attend or not attend. Motivating those less interested is a challenge for the nurse. Providing employee-requested programs on site, just before or after work hours or at lunchtime, is a strategy that can encourage and increase employee participation levels. Health education is more readily acceptable to clients when the programming meets their expressed interest and schedules and when information provided is appropriately matched to the client characteristics.

SCENARIO

You are the nurse in the health office of a moderate-sized corporation with access to multimedia resources. You provide a lending library of take-home videos, audiocassettes, and printed materials on various health-related topics such as "Self-Care

Management for Diabetics," "The Benefits of Low-Fat, High-Fiber Diet," and "Understanding Label Reading for Sodium, Fat, and Fiber Content." You provide a health "topic of the month" series; cancer awareness is the topic for the month. You have pamphlets on display in the lobby at the reception desk and an informational video playing in the health office waiting area on the topic. You provide several group teaching sessions for employees at various convenient times during the month. At these sessions, you demonstrate as well as provide opportunity for actual practice with models of breast self-examination for female employees, encouraging the women and men alike to share what they learned with their spouses or significant others. In addition, you have arranged with the local hospital to provide baseline mammograms for interested female employees.

In the non-health-care setting, the nurse as educator is free to select from a wide array of strategies that match the needs of the consumer for the achievement of behavioral outcomes. The instructional materials needed for support of educational efforts can be obtained through a variety of sources, such as health-care-related organizations that can provide up-to-date, reliable information. If the nurse is part of a health-care organization that has been contracted to provide the health education program, then that organization provides the resources. There is usually financial reimbursement by the non-health-care organization to the provider of health education when these programs are subcontracted. The learning needs can be anticipated when the population being served is known and the educational events are planned in advance. The difficulty in this type of setting is that health programming is often requested only sporadically when triggered by a news event about a health risk or by a variety of other motivating environment factors specific to each situation.

These settings lend themselves well to standardized prepackaged health education programming. A lending library of video- and audiotapes and a rack with printed materials are timesaving, cost-efficient, and motivating teaching strategies for a population with varied health information interests and needs.

SHARING RESOURCES AMONG SETTINGS

Professional nurses involved in client health education should use available opportunities to share resources among the three identified settings (Figure 13-1). Many already do this as printed or audiovisual materials are borrowed, rented, or purchased for small fees from area institutions, organizations, or agencies; nurse educators from health-care or health-care-related settings are contracted for or voluntarily provide health education programs to small and large groups in other health-care, health-care-related or non-health-care settings; and nurses from each category of setting collaborate on individual client situations or on major community health projects. The nurses from each of these settings can establish a health education committee in their community to coordinate health education programming, ensure effective use of all resources, and reduce duplication of efforts. The members of the committee can develop standardized health education content, delineate roles and services for each of the instructional settings, and share resources to provide a well-planned, comprehensive community program of health education for a wide client spectrum.

SUMMARY

Classification of instructional settings for client or patient education offers a method of analyzing the role of the nurse as educator and for selecting teaching strategies that best fit the organizational climate, the resources available, and the clientele served. Instructional settings are classified according to the purpose of the organization, institution, or agency that provides or sponsors health instruction. Health-care settings exist for the primary purpose of providing direct patient care with education as an integral part of health-care delivery services within the setting. A health-care-related setting consists of voluntary agencies whose purposes are advocacy, research, and educating the general public as well as professionals regarding specific health-care problems affecting society. A non-health-care setting includes institutions engaged in anything but health care as their operational purpose, but they may choose to provide health education or health-care services as a benefit to their membership or employees.

The factors that impact on instructional settings are directly related to the organization that provides the education, the environmental resources available, and the clientele who are serviced by the health education program. These factors need to be assessed prior to engaging in health education activities or selecting teaching strategies appropriate for the instructional setting. The learning needs and characteristics of the learners are the major determinants in choosing the teaching strategies to be used in any setting. These strategies are influenced to a lesser degree by the organizational and environmental factors of the particular setting. Teaching methods must be expanded to include multisensory, technologically advanced media to provide greater individualization and reach increasing numbers of clients. Even where organizational and environmental resources are limited, creative thinking and resourcefulness on the part of the nurse in the role of educator can expand the opportunities possible in any instructional setting to provide cost-effective client education that is well planned and comprehensive.

References

Blackwood, C., & White, B. (1991). Technology for teaching and learning improvement. In M.W. Galbraith (Ed.), *Facilitating adult learning: A transactional process* (pp. 135-165). Malabar, FL: Kreiger.

Breckon, D.J., Harvey, R.J., & Lancaster, R.B. (1985). *Community health education: Settings, roles and skills.* Rockville, MD: Aspen.

Bubela, N., Galloway, S., McCay, E., et al. (1990). Factors influencing patients' informational needs at time of hospital discharge. *Patient Education and Counseling, 16*(1), 21-28.

Cupples, S.A. (1991). Effects of timing & reenforcement of pre-operative education on knowledge & recovery of patients having coronary artery bypass graft surgery. *Heart and Lung, 20*(6), 654-660.

Davidhizar, R., & Rexroth, R. (1994). The benefits of triad communication in home health care. *Rehabilitation Nursing, 19*(6), 352-354.

DeMuth, J.S. (1989). Patient teaching in the ambulatory setting. *Nursing Clinics of North America, 24*(3), 645-654.

Graham, B.A., & Gleit, C.J. (1992). Teaching in selected settings. In N.I. Whitman, B.A. Grahman, C.J. Gleit, & M.D. Boyd (Eds.), *Teaching in nursing practice: A professional model,* 2nd ed. Norwalk, CT: Appleton-Lange.

Haggard, A. (1989). *Handbook of patient education.* Rockville, MD: Aspen.

Hiss, R.G., Frey, M.L., & Davis, W.K. (1986). Diabetes patient education in the office setting. *Diabetes Educator, 12*(3), 281-285.

Humphrey, C. (1988). The home as setting for care, clarifying the boundaries of practice. *Nursing Clinics of North America, 23*(2), 305-314.

Johnson, E.A., & Jackson, J. (1989). Teaching the home care client. *Nursing Clinics of North America, 24*(3), 687-692.

Knowles, M.S. (1964). The fields of operations in adult education. In G. Jensen, A.A. Liveright, & W. Hallenbeck (Eds.), *Adult education: Outlines of an emerging field of university study* (pp. 41-67). Washington, DC: Adult Education Association of the United States of America.

Knowles, M.S. (1983). How the media can make it or bust it in education. *Media and Adult Learning, 5*(2), 3-4.

Leckrone, L. (1991). Preparing your patient for surgery. *Nursing 91, 21*(7), 47-49.

Naylor, M.D., & Shaid, E.C. (1991). Content analysis of pre and post-discharge topics taught to hospitalized elderly by gerontological clinical nurse specialists. *Clinical Nurse Specialist, 5*(2), 111-116.

Opening the door to home care. (July 1995). *Report, 1, 4.*

Pesznecker, B.L., Zerwekh, J.V., & Horn, B.J. (1989). The mutual-participation relationship: Key to facilitating self-care practices in clients and families. *Public Health Nursing, 6*(4), 197-203.

Pruitt, R.H., Keller, L.S., & Hale, S.L. (1987). Mastering distractions that mar home visits. *Nursing and Health Care, 8*(6), 345-347.

Rankin, S., & Stallings, K.D. (1990). *Patient education: Issues, principles and practices,* 2nd ed. Philadelphia: Lippincott.

Redman, B.K. (1993). *The process of patient education,* 7th ed. St. Louis: Mosby–Year Book.

Rifas, E., Morris, R., & Grady, R. (1994). Innovative approach to patient education. *Nursing Outlook, 42*(5), 214-216.

Ruzicki, D.A. (1989). Realistically meeting the educational needs of hospitalized acute and short-stay patients. *Nursing Clinics of North America, 24*(3), 629-636.

Schroeder, W. (1980). Typology of adult learning systems. In J.M. Peters (Ed.), *Building an effective adult education enterprise* (pp. 41-77). San Francisco: Jossey-Bass.

Shendell-Falik, N. (1990). Creating self-care units in the acute care setting: A case study. *Patient Education and Counseling, 15*(1), 39-45.

Simonds, S.K. (March 1, 1973). President's committee on health education. *Hospitals, Journal of the American Hospital Association, 47,* 55-60.

Smith, L.F. (1986). New-parent teaching in the ambulatory care setting. *Maternal Child Nursing, 11*(4), 256-258.

Stulginsky, M.M. (1993a). Nurses' home health experience. Part I: The practice setting. *Nursing and Health Care, 14*(8), 402-407.

Stulginsky, M.M. (1993b). Nurses' home health experience. Part II: The unique demands of home visits. *Nursing and Health Care, 14*(9), 476-485.

Zarle, N.C. (1989). Continuity of care: Balancing care of elders between health care settings. *Nursing Clinics of North America, 24*(3), 697-705.

CHAPTER 14

Evaluation in Health-Care Education

Priscilla Sandford Worral

CHAPTER HIGHLIGHTS

Reporting Evaluation Results
    Be Audience Focused
    Stick to the Evaluation Purpose
    Stick to the Data

KEY TERMS

assessment	content evaluation
evaluation	evaluation research
formative evaluation	process evaluation
impact evaluation	program evaluation
summative evaluation	outcome evaluation

OBJECTIVES

After completing this chapter, the reader will be able to

1. Define the term *evaluation.*
2. Compare and contrast evaluation and assessment.
3. Identify purposes of evaluation.
4. Distinguish between five basic types of evaluation: process, content, outcome, impact, and program.
5. Discuss characteristics of various models of evaluation.
6. Describe similarities and differences between evaluation and research.
7. Assess barriers to evaluation.
8. Examine methods for conducting an evaluation.
9. Select appropriate instruments for various types of evaluative data.
10. Identify guidelines for reporting results of evaluation.

Evaluation is the process that can justify that what we do as nurses and as nurse educators makes a value-added difference in the care we provide. Early consideration of evaluation has never been more critical than in today's health-care environment. Crucial decisions regarding learners rest on the outcomes of learning. Can the patient go home? Can the nurse provide competent care? If education is to be justified as a value-added activity, the process of education must be measurably efficient and must be measurably linked to education outcomes. The outcomes of education, for the learner and for the organization, must be measurably effective.

Evaluation is a process within a process—a critical component of the nursing process, the decision-making process, and the education process.

Evaluation is the final component of each of these processes. Because these processes are cyclical, evaluation serves as the critical bridge at the end of one cycle that guides direction of the next cycle.

The sections of this chapter follow the steps in conducting an evaluation. These steps include determining the *focus* of the evaluation, including use of evaluation models; *designing* the evaluation; *conducting* the evaluation; determining methods of *analysis and interpretation* of data collected; *reporting* results of data collected; and *use* of evaluation results. Each aspect of the evaluation process is important, but all of them are meaningless if the results of evaluation are not used to guide future action in planning and carrying out educational interventions.

EVALUATION VERSUS ASSESSMENT

While assessment and evaluation are highly interrelated and are often used interchangeably as terms, they are not synonymous. The process of assessment is to gather, summarize, interpret, and use data to decide a direction for action. The process of evaluation is to gather, summarize, interpret, and use data to assess the extent to which an action was successful. The primary differences between the two terms are those of timing and purpose. For example, an education program begins with an assessment of learners' needs. From the perspective of systems theory, assessment data might be called the "input." While the program is being conducted, periodic evaluation lets the educator know whether the program and learners are proceeding as planned. After program completion, evaluation identifies whether and to what extent identified needs were met. Again from a systems theory perspective, these evaluative data might be called "intermediate output" and "output," respectively.

An important note of caution: Because you may *conduct* an evaluation at the end of your program, do not assume that you should *plan* it at this point in time. Evaluation as an afterthought is, at best, a poor idea and, at worst, a dangerous one. Data may be impossible to collect, be incomplete, or even be misleading. Assessment and evaluation planning ideally are concurrent activities. Where feasible, use the same data collection methods and instruments. This approach is especially appropriate for outcome and impact evaluations, as will be discussed later in this chapter. "If only. . ." is an all too frequent lament, which can be minimized by planning ahead.

DETERMINING THE FOCUS OF EVALUATION

In planning any evaluation, the first and most crucial step is to determine the focus of the evaluation. The focus then will guide evaluation design, conduct, data analysis, and reporting of results. The importance of a clear, specific, and realistic evaluation focus cannot be overemphasized. Usefulness

and accuracy of the results of an evaluation are heavily dependent on how well the evaluation is initially focused.

Evaluation focus includes five basic components: audience, purpose, questions, scope, and resources (Ruzicki, 1987). To determine these components, ask the following questions:

1. For whom is the evaluation being conducted?
2. Why is the evaluation being conducted?
3. What questions will be asked in the evaluation?
4. What is the scope of the evaluation?
5. What resources are available to conduct the evaluation?

The *audience* comprises the persons or groups for whom the evaluation is being conducted (Ruzicki, 1987). These individuals or groups include the primary audience, or the individual or group who requested the evaluation, and the general audience, or all those who will use evaluation results or who might benefit from the evaluation. The audience might include your patients, your peers, your supervisor, the nursing director, the staff development director, the chief executive officer of your institution, or a group of community leaders. When you report results of the evaluation, you will provide feedback to all members of the audience. In focusing the evaluation, however, first consider the primary audience. Giving priority to the individual or group who requested the evaluation will make focusing the evaluation easier, especially if results of an evaluation will be used by several groups representing diverse interests.

The *purpose* of the evaluation is the answer to the question "Why is the evaluation being conducted?" The purpose of an evaluation might be to decide whether to continue a particular education program or decide about effectiveness of the teaching process. If a particular individual or group has a primary interest in results of the evaluation, use input from that group to clarify the purpose.

An important note of caution: *Why* you are conducting an evaluation is not synonymous with *who* or *what* you are evaluating. For example, nursing literature on patient education commonly distinguishes among three types of evaluation: learner, teacher, and program. This distinction answers the question of *who* or *what* will be evaluated and is extremely useful for evaluation design and conduct. *Why* learner evaluation might be undertaken, for example, is answered by the reason or purpose for evaluating learner performance. Determining teaching or program effectiveness is another example of the purpose for undertaking evaluation.

An excellent rule of thumb in stating the purpose of an evaluation is: Keep it singular. In other words, state, "The purpose is. . . ," not "The purposes are. . . ." Keeping the purpose audience focused and singular will help avoid the all too frequent tendency to attempt too much in one evaluation.

Questions to be asked in the evaluation are directly related to the purpose for conducting the evaluation, are specific, and are measurable. Examples of questions are "To what extent are patients satisfied with the cardiac discharge teaching program?" and "How frequently do staff nurses use the diabetes teaching reference materials?" Asking the right questions is crucial if the evaluation is to serve the purpose intended. As will be discussed later in the chapter, delineation of evaluation questions is both the first step in selection of evaluation design and the basis for eventual data analysis.

The *scope* of an evaluation can be considered an answer to the question "How much will be evaluated?" "How much" includes "How many aspects of education will be evaluated?", "How many individuals or representative groups will be evaluated?", and "What time period is to be evaluated?" For example, will the evaluation focus on one class or on an entire program; on the learning experience for one patient or for all patients being taught a particular skill? Evaluation could be limited to the teaching process during a particular patient education class or could be expanded to encompass both the teaching process and related patient outcomes of learning. The scope of an evaluation is determined in part by the purpose for conducting the evaluation and in part by available resources. For example, an evaluation addressing learner satisfaction with faculty for all programs conducted by a staff development department in a given year is an evaluation that is broad and long-term in scope and will require expertise in data collection and analysis. An evaluation to determine whether a patient understands each step in a learning session on how to self-administer insulin injections is an example of an evaluation that in scope is narrow and at a point in time and will require expertise in clinical practice and observation.

Resources needed to conduct an evaluation include time, expertise, personnel, materials, equipment, and facilities. A realistic appraisal of what resources are accessible and available relative to what resources are required is crucial in focusing any evaluation. Remember to include the time and expertise required to collate, analyze, and interpret data and to prepare the report of evaluation results.

Evaluation can be classified into different types, or categories, based on one or more of the five components described above. The most common types of evaluation identified include process, content, outcome, impact, and program evaluation. A number of evaluation models have been developed that help to clarify differences among these evaluation types as well as how they relate to one another (Abruzzese, 1978; Haggard, 1989; Puetz, 1992; Rankin & Stallings, 1990).

EVALUATION MODELS

Abruzzese (1978) developed the Roberta Straessle Abruzzese (RSA) Evaluation Model for conceptualizing, or classifying, educational evaluation into different categories or levels. Although developed almost 20 years ago and from the perspective of staff development education, the RSA Model remains useful for conceptualizing types of evaluation from both staff development and patient education perspectives. The RSA Model pictorially places five basic types of evaluation in relation to one another based on purpose and related questions, scope, and resource components of evaluation focus (Figure 14–1). The five types of evaluation include process, content, outcome, impact, and program. Abruzzese describes the first four types as levels of evaluation leading from the simple, process evaluation, to the complex, impact evaluation. Total program evaluation encompasses and summarizes all four levels.

Process (Formative) Evaluation

The purpose of process or formative evaluation is to make adjustments in an educational activity as soon as they are needed, whether those adjustments be in personnel, materials, facilities, learning objectives, or even one's own attitude. Adjust-

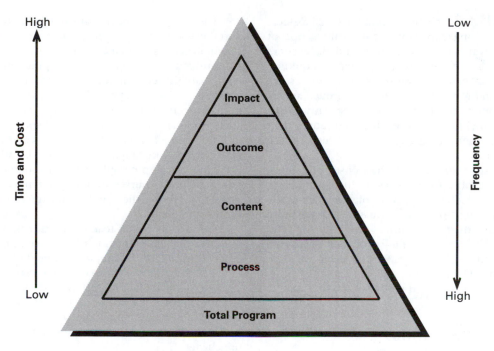

FIGURE 14–1. RSA Evaluation Model

Reprinted by permission of Roberta S. Abruzzese.

ments may need to be made after one class or session before the next is taught or even in the middle of a single learning experience. Consider, for example, evaluation of the process of teaching a newly diagnosed juvenile insulin-dependent diabetic and her parents how to administer insulin. Would you facilitate learning better by first injecting yourself with normal saline so they can see you maintain a calm expression? If you had planned to have the parent give the first injection, but the child seems less fearful, might you consider revising your teaching plan to let the child first perform self-injection?

Process evaluation, also called formative evaluation, is integral to the education process itself. In other words, process evaluation "forms" an educational activity because evaluation is an ongoing component of assessment, planning, and implementation (Boyd, 1992). As part of the education process, this ongoing evaluation helps the nurse anticipate and prevent problems before they occur or identify problems as they arise.

Consistent with the purpose of process evaluation, the guiding question is, "What can be done to better facilitate learning?" (Boyd, 1992). The nurse's teaching effectiveness, the teaching process, and the learner's responses are monitored on an ongoing basis. Abruzzese (1978) describes process evaluation as a "happiness index." While teaching and learning are ongoing, learners are asked their opinions about faculty, learning/course objectives, content, teaching and learning methods, physical facilities, and administration of the learning experience. Specific questions could include: Am I giving the patient time to ask questions? Is the information I am giving in class consistent with information included in the handouts? Does the patient look bored? Is the room too warm? Should I include more opportunities for return demonstration?

The scope of process evaluation generally is limited in breadth and time period to a specific learning experience such as a class or workshop, yet is sufficiently detailed to include as many aspects of the specific learning experience as possible while they occur. Learner behavior, teacher behavior, learner-teacher interaction, learner response to teaching materials and methods, and characteristics of the environment are all aspects of the learning experience within the scope of process evaluation. All learners and all teachers participating in a learning experience should be included in process evaluation. If resources are limited and a number of different groups are included among participants, a representative number of individuals from each group rather than everyone from each group may be included in the evaluation.

Resources usually are less costly and more readily available for process evaluation than for other types such as impact or total program evaluation. Although process evaluation occurs more frequently than any other type—during and throughout every learning experience—it occurs concurrently with teaching. The need for additional time, facilities, and dollars to conduct process evaluation is consequently decreased.

Content Evaluation

The purpose of content evaluation is to determine if learners have acquired the knowledge or skills taught during the learning experience. Abruzzese (1978) describes content evaluation as taking place immediately after the learning experience to answer the guiding question, "To what degree did the learners learn what was imparted?" or "To what degree did learners achieve specified objectives?" Asking a patient to give a return demonstration or asking participants to complete a cognitive test at the completion of a one-day seminar are common examples of content evaluation.

Content evaluation is depicted in the RSA Model as the level "in between" process and outcome evaluation levels. In other words, content evaluation can be considered as focusing on how the teaching-learning process affected immediate, short-term outcomes. To answer the question "Were specified objectives met *as a result of* teaching?" requires that the evaluation be designed differently from an evaluation to answer the question "Did learners achieve specified objectives?" Evaluation designs will be discussed in some detail later in this chapter. An important point to be made here, however, is that evaluation questions must be carefully considered and clearly stated because they dictate the basic framework for design and conduct.

The scope of content evaluation is limited to a specific learning experience and to specifically stated objectives for that experience. Content evaluation occurs at a circumscribed point in time, immediately after completion of teaching, but encompasses all teaching-learning activities included in that specific learning experience. Data are obtained from all learners targeted in a specific class or group. For example, if both parents and the juvenile diabetic are taught insulin administration, all three are asked to complete a return demonstration. Similarly, all nurses attending a workshop are asked to complete the cognitive posttest on workshop completion.

Resources used to teach content can also be used to carry out evaluation of how well that content was learned. For example, equipment included in teaching a patient how to change a dressing can be used by the patient to perform a return demonstration. In the same manner, a pretest used at the beginning of a continuing education seminar can be readministered at seminar completion to measure change.

Outcome (Summative) Evaluation

The purpose of outcome evaluation is to determine effects or outcomes of teaching efforts. Outcome evaluation is also referred to as summative evaluation because its intent is to "sum" what happened as a result of education. Guiding questions in outcome evaluation include, "Was teaching appropriate?", "Did the individual(s) learn?", "Were behavioral objectives met?", and "Did the patient who learned a skill before discharge use that skill correctly once home?" Just as process evaluation occurs concurrently with the teaching-learning experience, outcome evaluation occurs after teaching has been completed or after a program has been established.

Outcome evaluation measures changes occurring as a result of teaching and learning. Abruzzese (1978) differentiates outcome evaluation from content evaluation by focusing outcome evaluation on measuring more long-term change that "persists after the learning experience" (p. 243). Changes can include institution of a new process, habitual use of a new technique or behavior, or integration of a new value or attitude. Which changes you will measure usually will be dictated by the objectives established as a result of initial needs assessment.

The scope of outcome evaluation depends in part on the changes being measured, which, in turn, are dependent on objectives established for the educational activity. As has already been discussed, outcome evaluation focuses on a longer time period than does content evaluation. Whereas evaluating accuracy of a patient's return demonstration of a skill prior to discharge may be appropriate for content evaluation, outcome evaluation should include measuring a patient's competency with a skill in the home setting after discharge. Similarly, nurses' responses on a workshop posttest may be sufficient for content evaluation, but if the workshop objective states that nurses will be able to incorporate their knowledge into practice on the unit, outcome evaluation should include measuring nurses' knowledge or behavior some time after they have returned to the unit. Abruzzese (1978) suggests that outcome data be collected 6 months after baseline data to determine if a change has taken place.

Resources required for outcome evaluation are more costly and sophisticated than for process or content evaluation. Compared to resources required for the first two types of evaluation in the RSA Model, outcome evaluation requires greater expertise to develop measurement and data collection strategies, more time to conduct the evaluation, knowledge of baseline data establishment, and ability to conduct reliable and valid comparative data after the learning experience. Postage to mail surveys and time and personnel to carry out observation of nurses on the clinical unit or to complete patient/family telephone interviews are specific examples of resources that may be necessary to conduct an outcome evaluation.

Impact Evaluation

The purpose of impact evaluation is to determine the relative effects of education on the institution or the community. Put another way, the purpose of impact evaluation is to obtain information to decide whether continuing an educational activity is worth its cost. Examples of questions appropriate for impact evaluation include "What is the effect of

the education program on subsequent nursing staff turnover?" and "What is the effect of the cardiac discharge teaching program on long-term frequency of rehospitalization among patients who have completed the program?"

The scope of impact evaluation is broader, more complex, and usually more long-term than that of process, content, or outcome evaluation. Whereas outcome evaluation would focus on whether specific teaching resulted in achievement of specified outcomes, for example, impact evaluation would go beyond that to measure the effect or worth of those outcomes. Put another way, outcome evaluation would focus on a course objective, while impact evaluation would focus on a course goal. Consider, for example, a class on the use of body mechanics. The outcome objective is that the learner will demonstrate proper use of body mechanics in providing patient care. The goal is to decrease back injuries among the hospital's direct-care providers. This distinction between outcome and impact evaluation may seem subtle, but it is important to the appropriate design and conduct of an impact evaluation.

Resource requirements for conducting an impact evaluation are extensive and may be beyond the scope of an individual nurse educator. Literature on evaluation describes impact evaluation as most like evaluation research (Abruzzese, 1978; Hamilton, 1993; Waddell, 1992). Evaluation versus evaluation research will be addressed later in this chapter. The point to make here is that "good" science is rarely inexpensive and is never quick; good impact evaluation has the same characteristics. Resources needed to design and conduct an impact evaluation generally include reliable and valid instruments, trained data collectors, personnel with research and statistical expertise, equipment and materials necessary for data collection and analysis, and access to populations who may be culturally or geographically diverse. Because impact evaluation is so expensive and time-intensive, this type of evaluation should be targeted toward courses/programs where learning is critical to patient well-being or to safe, high-quality, cost-effective health-care delivery (Puetz, 1992).

Conducting an impact evaluation may seem a monumental task, but do not let that stop you from undertaking the effort. Rather, plan ahead, proceed carefully, and obtain the support and assistance of colleagues. Keeping in mind the purpose for conducting an impact evaluation should be helpful in maintaining the level of commitment needed throughout the process. The current managed-care environment requires justification for every health dollar spent. The value of patient and staff education may be intuitively evident, but the positive impact of education must be demonstrated if it is to be funded.

Program Evaluation

The purpose of program evaluation can be generically described as "designed and conducted to assist an audience to judge and improve the worth of some object" (Johnson & Olesinski, 1995, p. 53). The "object" in this case is an educational program. Using the framework of the RSA Model (Abruzzese, 1978), the purpose of total program evaluation is to determine the extent to which all activities for an entire department or program over a specified period of time meet or exceed goals originally established. Guiding questions appropriate for a total program evaluation from this perspective might be "To what extent did programs undertaken by members of the nursing staff development department during the year accomplish annual goals established by the department?" or "How well did patient education activities implemented throughout the year meet annual goals established for the institution's patient education program?"

The scope of program evaluation is broad, generally focusing on overall goals rather than on specific objectives. While the term *program* could be defined as an individual educational offering (Albanese and Gjerde, 1987), the resource requirements for conducting a program evaluation generally are too extensive to justify the effort on less than a broad scale. Abruzzese (1978) describes the scope of program evaluation as encompassing all aspects of educational activity (e.g., process, content, outcome, impact) with input from all the participants (e.g., learners, teachers, institutional representatives, community representatives). The time period over which data are collected may extend from several months to one or more years, depending on the time frame established for meeting the goals to be evaluated.

Resources required for program evaluation may include the sum of resources necessary to conduct process, content, outcome, and impact evaluations. A program evaluation may require significant expenditures for personnel if the evaluation is conducted by an individual or team external to the organization. Additional resources required include time, materials, equipment, and personnel necessary for data entry, analysis, and report generation.

As stated earlier, the RSA Model remains useful as a general framework for categorizing basic types of evaluation: process, content, outcome, impact, and program. As depicted in the model, differences between these types are, in large part, a matter of degree. For example, process evaluation occurs most frequently; impact evaluation occurs least frequently. Content evaluation focuses on immediate effects of teaching; outcome on more long-term effects of teaching. Conduct of process evaluation requires fewer resources compared with impact evaluation, which requires extensive resources for implementation. The RSA Model further illustrates one way that process, content, outcome, and impact evaluations can be considered together as components of total program evaluation.

Clinical examples of how different types of evaluation relate to one another can be found in Haggard's (1989) description of three dimensions in evaluating teaching effectiveness for the patient and in Rankin and Stallings's (1990) four levels of evaluation of patient learning. The three dimensions described by Haggard and four levels identified by Rankin and Stallings are consistent with the basic types of evaluation included in the RSA Model, as shown in Table 14-1.

As can be seen from Table 14-1, models developed from an education theory base, such as the RSA Model, have much in common with models developed from a patient care theory base, exemplified by the second two models. At least one important point about the difference between the RSA and other models needs to be mentioned, however. That difference is depicted in the learner evaluation model shown in Figure 14-2. This learner-focused model emphasizes the continuum of patient health/learner performance from needs assessment to patient health/learner performance once an adequate level of health status/performance has been regained or achieved. Both models have value in focusing and planning any type of evaluation but are especially important for impact and program evaluations.

TABLE 14–1.   Comparison of levels/types of evaluation across staff/patient
education evaluation models

Abruzzese (1978)	*Haggard (1989)*	*Rankin & Stallings (1990)*
Process	Patient assimilation of information during teaching	Patient-education intervention
Content	Patient information retention after teaching	Patient/family performance following learning
Outcome	Patient use of information in day-to-day life	Patient/family performance at home
Impact	N/A	Overall self-care and health maintenance
Program	N/A	N/A

DESIGNING THE EVALUATION

The design of an evaluation is created within the framework, or boundaries, already established by focusing the evaluation. In other words, the design must be consistent with the purpose, questions, and scope and must be realistic given available resources. Evaluation design includes at least three interrelated components: structure, methods, and instruments.

Designing Structure

An important question to be answered in designing an evaluation is "How rigorous should the evaluation be?" The obvious answer is that all evaluations should have some level of rigor. In other words, all evaluations should be systematic and carefully and thoroughly planned or structured before they are conducted. How rigor is translated into design structure depends on the questions to be answered by the evaluation, the complexity of the scope of the evaluation, and the expected use of evaluation results. The more the questions address cause and effect, the more complex the scope, and the more critical and broad-reaching the expected use of results, the more the evaluation design should be structured from a research perspective.

Evaluation Versus Research

Evaluation and research are neither synonymous nor mutually exclusive activities. The extent to which they are either very different or indistinguishable from one another depends on the type of evaluation and type of research considered. Ruzicki (1987, p. 234) makes the following distinction between the two:

> While both research and evaluation involve objective, systematic collection of data, evaluation is conducted to make decisions in a given setting. Research is designed so that it can be generalized to other settings and replicated in other settings. Furthermore, research seeks new knowledge, examines cause and effect relationships, tests hypotheses, whereas evaluation determines mission achievement, examines means-end processes, and assesses attainment of objectives.

This argument holds true when comparing "basic" research to process evaluation, for example. Basic research usually is defined as tightly controlled experimental studies of cause and effect conducted for the purpose of generating new knowledge. This new knowledge may or may not eventually influence practice. Process evaluation occurs concurrently with an educational intervention and is conducted in an uncontrolled or real-world setting for the purpose of making change as soon as the need for change is identified.

Differences between research and evaluation have become less distinct over the past several years with the advent of "applied" research, with the acceptance of qualitative measures and methods as legitimate research, and with the increasing

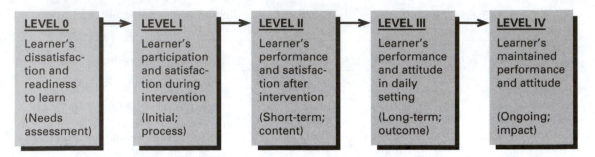

FIGURE 14–2. Five Levels of Learner Evaluation

SOURCE: Based on S.H. Rankin & K.D. Stallings (1990). *Patient education: Issues, principles, practices,* 2nd ed. Philadelphia: Lippincott.

importance given to results of outcome, impact, and program evaluations. The purpose for conducting applied research is to positively affect change in practice. There is little difference between this purpose and the purpose for conducting evaluation. Evaluation research, which is one type of applied research, can be defined as "a process of applying scientific procedures to accumulate reliable and valid data on the manner and extent to which specified activities produce outcomes or effects" (Hamilton, 1993, p. 148). Using this definition, Hamilton identifies program accreditation, program cost analysis, and outcome of treatment as appropriate for use of evaluation research designs and methods. Hamilton further describes impact evaluation as appropriate for use of quasi-experimental and experimental research design structures. A number of other authors support some use of research designs and data collection methods for outcome, impact, and program evaluations (Albanese & Gjerde, 1987; Berk & Rossi, 1990; Holzemer, 1992; Puetz, 1992; Waddell, 1992).

This does not mean that all outcome, impact, and program evaluations should be conducted as research studies. Some important differences do exist between evaluation and evaluation research. One of the most significant differences between evaluation and evaluation research is the influence of a primary audience. As was discussed earlier in this chapter, the primary audience, or the individual or group requesting the evaluation, is a major component in focusing an evaluation. The evaluator must design and conduct the evaluation consistent with the purpose and related questions identified by the primary audience. Evaluation research, on the other hand, does not have an identi-

fied primary audience. The researcher has autonomy to develop a protocol to answer a question posed by the researcher.

A second difference between evaluation and evaluation research is one of timing. The necessary timeline for usability of evaluation results may not be sufficient to prospectively develop a research proposal and obtain institutional review board approval prior to beginning data collection.

Given the discussion of evaluation versus evaluation research, how are decisions about level of rigor of an evaluation actually translated into an evaluation structure? The structure of an evaluation design depicts the number of groups to be included in the evaluation, the number of evaluations or periods of evaluation, and the time sequence between an educational intervention and evaluation of that intervention. A "group" can comprise one individual, as in the case of one-to-one nurse-patient teaching, or several individuals, as in the case of a nursing in-service program or workshop.

A process evaluation might be conducted during a single patient education activity where the educator observes patient behavior during instruction/demonstration and engages the patient in questions and answers upon completion of each new instruction. Because the purpose of process evaluation is to facilitate better learning while that learning is going on, education and evaluation occur concurrently.

Evaluation also may be conducted after an educational intervention. This is probably the most common structure used in conducting educational evaluations, although it is not necessarily the most appropriate. On completion of an educational activity, participants may be asked to complete a satisfaction survey to provide data for a process evaluation, or they may be given a cognitive test to provide data for a content evaluation. If the purpose for conducting a content evaluation is to determine whether learners know the content just taught, a cognitive posttest or immediate return demonstration is adequate. If the purpose for conducting the evaluation is to determine whether learners know after a class specific content that they did not know before attending that class, however, a structure that begins with collection of baseline data is more appropriate. Collection of baseline data, which can be compared with data collected at one or more points in time after learners have completed the educational activity, provides an opportunity to measure whether change has occurred. The ability to measure change in a particular skill or level of knowledge, for example, also requires that the same instruments be used for data collection at both points in time. Data collection will be discussed in more detail later in this chapter.

If the purpose for conducting an evaluation is to determine whether learners know content or can perform a skill *as a result of* an educational intervention, the most appropriate structure is one that includes at least two groups, one receiving education and one not receiving education. Both groups are evaluated at the same time even though only one group receives education. The group receiving the new education program is called the treatment or experimental group, while the group receiving standard care or the traditional education program is called the comparison or control group. The two groups may or may not be "equivalent." Equivalent groups are those with no known differences between them prior to some intervention, whereas nonequivalent groups may be different from one another in several ways. For example, patients on Nursing Unit A may receive an educational pamphlet to read prior to attending a class, while patients on Nursing Unit B attend the class without first reading the pamphlet. Because patients on the two units probably are different in many ways—age and diagnosis, for example—besides which educational intervention they received, they would be considered nonequivalent groups.

Use of the term *nonequivalent* is common to discussions of traditional research designs. Quasi-experimental designs, such as "nonequivalent control group" designs, should be among those considered in planning an outcome, impact, or program evaluation. Especially if the purpose of an evaluation is to demonstrate that an education program "caused" fewer patient returns to clinic or fewer nurses to leave the institution, for example, the evaluation structure must have the rigor of evaluation research.

Another type of quasi-experimental design, called a time-series design, might include only one group of learners from which evaluative data are collected at several points in time both before and after receiving an educational intervention. If data collected before the education consistently demonstrate lack of learner ability to comply with a treatment regimen, for example, and data collected after the education consistently demonstrate a significant improvement in patient compliance with that regimen, the evaluator could argue that the education was the reason for the improvement.

A detailed description of quasi-experimental designs is not the intent of this chapter. What is intended is to increase awareness of the value and usefulness of these designs, especially when the results of an evaluation will be used to make major financial or programmatic decisions. The literature on evaluation of nursing staff education and patient education has become an increasingly rich source of examples of how to conduct rigorous evaluation. A literature search that includes many or all of the following journals is a must for planning evaluation of health-care education in a cost-conscious and outcome-focused health-care environment: *Evaluation and the Health Professions, Journal of Continuing Education in Nursing, Adult Education Quarterly, Health Education Quarterly, Nurse Educator, Journal of Nursing Staff Development, Health Education Research, Nursing Management, Nursing Research,* and *Research in Nursing and Health.*

Evaluation Methods

Evaluation focus provides the basis for determining the evaluation design structure. The design structure, in turn, provides the basis for determining evaluation methods. Evaluation methods include those actions that are undertaken to carry out the evaluation according to the design structure. All evaluation methods deal in some way with data and data collection. Answers to the following questions will assist in selection of the most appropriate, feasible methods for conducting a particular evaluation in a particular setting and for a specified purpose:

1. What types of data will be collected?
2. From whom or what will data be collected?
3. How, when, and where will data be collected?
4. By whom will data be collected?

Types of Data to Collect

Evaluation of health-care education includes collection of data about people, about the educational program or activity, and about the environment in which the educational activity takes place. Process, outcome, impact, and program evaluations require data about all three: the people, the program, and the environment. Content evaluations may be limited to data about the people and the program, although this limitation is not necessary. Types of data that are collected about people can be classified as physical, cognitive, affective, or psychomotor (Redman 1993). Data that are collected about educational activities or programs generally include such program characteristics as cost, length, number of faculty required, amount and type of materials required, teaching-learning methods used, and so on. Data that are collected about the environment in which a program or activity is conducted generally include such environmental characteristics as temperature, lighting, location, layout, space, and noise level.

Given the possibility that an unlimited and overwhelming amount of data *could* be collected, how do you decide what data *should* be collected? The most straightforward answer to this question is that data should be collected that will answer evaluation questions posed in focusing the evaluation. The likelihood that you will collect the right amount of the right type of data to answer evaluation questions can be significantly improved, first, by remembering that any data you collect, you are obligated to use and, second, by using operational definitions.

An operational definition of a word or phrase is a definition that is written in measurement terms. Functional health status, for example, can be theoretically defined as an individual's ability to independently carry out activities of daily living

without self-perceived undue difficulty or discomfort. Functional health status can be operationally defined as an individual's composite score on the SF-36 survey instrument (Ware et al., 1978; Stewart et al., 1988). The SF-36, which has undergone years of extensive reliability and validity testing with a wide variety of patient populations and in several languages, is generally considered the "gold standard" for measuring functional health status from the individual's perspective. Similarly, patient compliance can be theoretically defined as the patient's regular and consistent adherence to a prescribed treatment regimen. For use in an outcome evaluation of a particular educational activity, patient compliance might be operationally defined as the patient's demonstration of unassisted and error-free completion of all steps in the sterile dressing change as observed in the patient's home on three separate occasions at 2-week time intervals. As you can see from these examples, an operational definition states exactly what data will be collected. In the first example, measurement of functional health status will require collection of patient survey data using a specific self-administered questionnaire. The second example provides even more information about data collection than does the first, by including where and how many times the patient's performance of the dressing change is to be observed, as well as stating that criteria for compliance include both unassisted and error-free performance on each occasion.

In addition to categorizing types of data as describing people, programs, or the environment, data can be categorized as quantitative or qualitative. Quantitative data are numeric and generally are expressed in statistics such as mean, median, ratio, F statistic, t statistic, or chi-square. Numbers can be used to answer questions of how much, how many, how often, and so on in terms that are commonly understood by the audience for the evaluation. Mathematical analysis can demonstrate with some level of precision and reliability whether a learner's knowledge or skill has changed since completing an educational program, for example, or how much improvement in a learner's knowledge or skill is the result of an educational program. Qualitative data include feelings, behaviors, words, and phrases and generally are expressed in themes or categories. Qualitative data can be described in quantitative terms, such as percentages or counts, but this eliminates the richness and insight that the use of qualitative data can offer. Qualitative data can be used as background to better interpret quantitative data, especially if the evaluation is intended to measure such value-laden or conceptual terms as satisfaction or quality.

Any evaluation will be strengthened by collecting both quantitative and qualitative data. For example, an evaluation to determine whether a stress reduction class resulted in decreased work stress for participants could include participants' qualitative expressions of how stressed they feel plus quantitative pulse and blood pressure readings.

From Whom or What to Collect Data

Data can be collected directly from the individuals whose behavior or knowledge is being evaluated, from surrogates or representatives of these individuals, or from documentation or databases already created. Whenever possible, plan to collect at least some data directly from individuals being evaluated. In the case of process evaluation, data should be collected from all learners and all educators participating in the educational activity. Content and outcome evaluations should include data from all learners. Because impact and program evaluations have a broader scope than do the first three types of evaluation, collecting data from all individuals who participated in an educational program over an extended period of time may be impossible due to the inability to locate participants or lack of sufficient resources to gather data from such a large number of people. When all participants cannot be counted or located, data may be collected from a subset, or sample, of participants who are considered to represent the entire group.

If an evaluation is planned to collect data from a sample of participants, be careful to include participants who are representative of the entire group. A random selection of participants from whom data will be collected will minimize bias in the sample but cannot guarantee representativeness. Consider the example of an impact evaluation conducted to determine whether a 5-year program supporting home-based health education actually improved general health status of individuals in the community served by the program. Suppose all members of the community could be counted. A random sample of community members could be generated by first listing and numbering all members' names, then drawing numbers using a random numbers table until a 10% sample is obtained. Such a method for selecting the sample of community members would eliminate intentional selection of those individuals who were the most active program participants and might have a better health status than does the community as a whole. At the same time, however, the 10% random sample could unintentionally include only those individuals who did not participate in the health education program. Data collected from this sample of nonparticipants would be equally as misleading as data collected from the first sample. A more representative sample for this evaluation should include both participants and nonparticipants, ideally in the same proportions in the sample as in the community.

Preexisting databases should never be used as the only source of evaluative data unless they were created for the purpose of that evaluation. Even though these data were collected for a different purpose, they may be helpful for providing additional information to the primary audience for the evaluation. Data already in existence generally are less expensive to obtain than are original data. The decision whether to use preexisting data depends on whether they were collected from people of interest in the current evaluation and whether they are consistent with operational definitions used in the current evaluation.

How, When, and Where to Collect Data

Methods for how data can be collected include observation, interview, questionnaire or written examination, record review, and secondary analysis of existing databases. Which method is selected depends, first, on the type of data being collected and, second, on available resources. Whenever possible, data should be collected using more than one method. Using multiple methods will provide the evaluator, and consequently the primary audience, with more complete information about the program or performance being evaluated than could be accomplished using a single method.

Observations can be conducted by the evaluator in person or can be videotaped for viewing at some later time. In the combined role of educator-evaluator, the nurse educator who is conducting a process evaluation can directly observe a learner's physical, verbal, psychomotor, and affective behaviors so that they can be responded to in a timely manner. Use of videotape or a non-participant observer also can be beneficial for picking up the educator's own behaviors of which the educator is unaware, but that might be influencing the learner.

The timing of data collection, or when data collection takes place, already has been addressed both in discussion of different types of evaluation and in descriptions of evaluation design structures. Process evaluation, for example, generally occurs during and immediately after an educational activity. Content evaluation takes place immediately after completion of education, while outcome evaluation occurs some time after completion of education, after learners have returned to the setting where they are expected to use new knowledge or perform a new skill. Impact evaluation generally is conducted from weeks to years after the educational program being evaluated because the purpose of impact evaluation is to determine what change has occurred within the community or institution as a whole as a result of an educational program.

Timing of data collection for program evaluation is less obvious than for other types of evaluation, in part because a number of different descriptions of what constitutes a program evaluation can be found both in the literature and in practice. As discussed earlier, Abruzzese (1978) describes data collection for program evaluation as occurring over a prolonged period because program evaluation is itself a culmination of process, content, outcome, and impact evaluations already conducted.

Where an evaluation is conducted can have a major impact on evaluation results. Be careful not to make the decision about where to collect data on the basis of convenience for the data collector. An appropriate setting for conducting a content evaluation may be in the classroom or skills laboratory where learners have just completed class instruction or training. An outcome evaluation to determine whether training has improved the nurse's ability to perform a skill with patients on the nursing unit, however, requires that data collection, in this case observation of the nurse's performance, be conducted on the nursing unit. Similarly, an outcome evaluation to determine whether discharge teaching in the hospital enabled the patient to provide self-care at home re-

quires that data collection, or observation of the patient's performance, be conducted in the home. What if available resources are insufficient to allow for home visits by the evaluator? To answer this question, keep in mind that the focus of the evaluation is on performance by the patient, not performance by the evaluator. Training a family member, a visiting nurse, or even the patient to observe and record patient performance at home is preferable to bringing the patient to a place of convenience for the evaluator.

By Whom Data Are Collected

Evaluative data are most commonly collected by the educator who is conducting the class or activity being evaluated because that educator is already present and interacting with learners. Combining the role of evaluator with that of educator is one appropriate method for conducting a process evaluation because evaluative data are integral to the teaching-learning process. Inviting another educator or a patient representative to observe a class can provide additional data from the perspective of someone who does not have to divide attention between teaching and evaluating. This second, and perhaps less biased, input can strengthen legitimacy and usefulness of evaluation results.

Data also can be collected by the learners themselves, by other colleagues within the department or institution, or by someone from outside the institution. Puetz's (1992) description of data collection using a participant evaluation team is an example of data collection that includes learners. The evaluation team is composed of a small number of randomly selected individuals who are scheduled to attend an educational program. Team members are introduced to other program participants at the beginning of the class, join other participants during the program, and collect data through self-report as well as through observation and interaction with others during breaks.

When selecting who will collect data, keep in mind that the individuals selected to complete this task become an extension of the evaluation instrument. If the data that are collected are to be reliable, unbiased, and accurate, the data collector must be unbiased and sufficiently expert at the task. Use of unbiased expert data collectors is especially important for collecting observation and interview data because these data are in part dependent on the subjective interpretation of the data collector. Other data also can be affected by who collects those data. For example, if staff nurses are asked to complete a job satisfaction survey and their head nurse is asked to collect the surveys for return to the evaluator, what problems do you think might occur? Might some staff nurses be hesitant to provide negative scores on certain items, even though they hold a negative opinion? Physiological data also can be altered, however unintentionally, by the data collector. Consider, for example, an outcome evaluation to determine whether a series of biofeedback classes given to young executives can reduce stress as measured by pulse and blood pressure. How might some executives' pulse and blood pressure results be affected by a data collector who is extremely physically attractive or outwardly angry?

Use of trained data collectors from an external agency is, in most cases, not a financially viable option. The potential for a data collector to bias data can be minimized using a number of less expensive alternatives, however. First, limit as much as possible the number of data collectors, as this automatically will decrease person-based variation. Ask individuals assisting you with data collection to wear similar neutral colors, to avoid cologne, and to speak in a moderate tone. Because "moderate tone," for example, may not be interpreted the same way by everyone, hold at least one practice session or "dry run" with all data collectors prior to actually conducting the evaluation. Whenever possible, ask for help with data collection from someone who has no vested interest in results and who will be perceived as unbiased and nonthreatening by those providing the data. Interview scripts to be read verbatim by the interviewer can ensure that all patients or staff being interviewed will be asked the same questions.

With the advent of continuous quality improvement as an expectation of daily activity in health-care organizations, health-care professionals are obligated to become more knowledgeable about principles of measurement and how to implement measurement techniques in their work setting (Joint Commission on Accreditation of Healthcare Organizations, 1995). One benefit this change in practice has for the nurse educator is that more people within the organization have some expertise in data collection and are moti-

vated to help with data collection activities. Another potential benefit is that data collection activities are likely to be already a part of practice. Not only might the nurse educator have readily available individuals to assist with data collection, but also the educator might have readily available and usable instruments and data.

Barriers to Evaluation

If evaluation is so crucial to health-care education, why is evaluation often an afterthought or even overlooked entirely? The reasons given for not conducting evaluations are many and varied but rarely, if ever, insurmountable. To overcome barriers to evaluation, they first must be identified and understood; then the evaluation must be designed and conducted in a way that will minimize or eliminate as many identified barriers as possible.

Barriers to conducting an evaluation can be classified into three broad categories:

1. Lack of clarity
2. Lack of ability
3. Fear of punishment or loss of self-esteem

Lack of Clarity

Lack of clarity most often is the result of an unclear, unstated, or ill-defined evaluation focus. Undertaking any action is difficult if the performer does not know the purpose for taking that action. Undertaking an evaluation certainly is no different. Often evaluations are attempted to determine the quality of an educational program or activity, yet quality is not defined beyond some vague sense of "goodness." What is goodness and from whose perspective will goodness be determined? Who or what has to demonstrate evidence of goodness? What will happen if goodness is or is not evident? Inability to answer these or similar questions creates a significant barrier to conducting an evaluation. Not knowing the purpose of an evaluation or what will be done with evaluation results, for example, can become a barrier for even the most seasoned evaluator.

Barriers in this category have the greatest potential for successful resolution because the best solution for lack of clarity is to provide clarity. You will recall that evaluation focus includes five components: audience, purpose, questions, scope, and resources. To overcome a potential lack of clarity, all five components must be identified and made available to those conducting the evaluation. A clearly stated purpose must include *why* the evaluation is being conducted. Part of the answer to why is a statement of what decisions will be made on the basis of evaluation results. Clear identification of who constitutes the primary audience is as important as a clear statement of purpose. It is from the perspective of the primary audience that terms such as *quality* should be defined and operationalized. While results of the evaluation will provide the information on which decisions will be made, the primary audience will actually make those decisions.

Lack of Ability

Lack of ability to conduct an evaluation most often is the result of insufficient knowledge of how to conduct the evaluation or the result of insufficient or inaccessible resources necessary to conduct the evaluation. Clarification of evaluation purpose, questions, and scope is often the responsibility of the primary audience. Clarification of resources, however, is the responsibility of both the primary audience and the individuals conducting the evaluation. The primary audience is accountable for providing the necessary resources—personnel, equipment, time, facilities, and so on—to conduct the evaluation they are requesting. Unless these individuals have some expertise in evaluation, they may not know what resources are necessary. The persons conducting the evaluation, therefore, must accept responsibility for knowing what resources are necessary and for providing that information to the primary audience. The person asked or expected to conduct the evaluation may be as uncertain about necessary resources as is the primary audience, however.

Lack of knowledge of what resources are necessary or lack of actual resources forms barriers to conducting an evaluation that can be difficult, although not impossible, to overcome. Lack of knowledge can be resolved or minimized by enlisting the assistance of individuals with needed expertise through consultation or contract, if funds are available, through collaboration, or indirectly through literature review. Lack of other resources—time, money, equipment, facilities, and so on—should be documented, justified, and pre-

sented to those requesting the evaluation. Alternative methods for conducting the evaluation, including the alternative of making decisions in the absence of any evaluation, also should be written and presented.

Fear of Punishment or Loss of Self-Esteem

Evaluation may be perceived as a judgment of personal worth. Those being evaluated may fear that anything less than a perfect performance will result in punishment or that their mistakes will be seen as evidence that they are somehow unworthy or incompetent as human beings. These fears form one of the greatest barriers to conducting an evaluation. Unfortunately, the fear of punishment or of being seen as unworthy may not easily be overcome, especially if the individual has had past negative experiences. Consider, for example, traditional quality assurance monitoring where results were used to correct deficiencies through punitive measures. To give another example, how many times has an educator interpreted learner dissatisfaction with a teaching style as learner dislike for the educator as a person? How many times have pediatric patients' parents said, "If you don't do it right, the doctor won't let you go home . . . and we will be very disappointed in you"? Every one of us probably has experienced "test anxiety" at some point in our own education.

The first step in overcoming this barrier is to realize that the potential for its existence may be close to 100%. Individuals whose performance or knowledge is being evaluated are not likely to say overtly that evaluation represents a threat to them. They are far more likely to demonstrate self-protective behaviors or attitudes that can range from failure to attend a class that has a posttest to providing socially desirable answers on a questionnaire to responding with hostility to evaluation questions. An individual may intentionally choose to "fail" an evaluation as a method for controlling the uncertainty of success.

The second step in overcoming the barrier of fear or threat is to remember that "the person is more important than the performance or the product" (Narrow, 1979, p. 185). If the purpose of an evaluation is to facilitate better learning, as in process evaluation, focus on the process. Consider the example of teaching a newly diagnosed diabetic how to administer insulin. The educator has carefully and thoroughly explained each step in the process of insulin administration, observing the patient's intent expression and frequent head nods during the explanation. When the patient tries to demonstrate the steps, however, he is unable to begin. Why? One answer may be that the use of an auditory teaching style does not match the patient's visual learning style. Another possibility might be that too many distractions are present in the immediate environment, making concentration on learning all but impossible.

A third step in overcoming the fear of punishment or threatened loss of self-esteem is to point out achievements, if they exist, or continue to encourage effort if learning has not been achieved. Give praise honestly, focusing on the task at hand.

Finally, and perhaps most importantly, use communication of information to prevent or minimize fear. Lack of clarity exists as a barrier for those who are the subjects of an evaluation as much as for those who will conduct the evaluation. If learners or educators know and understand the focus of an evaluation, they may be less fearful than if such information is left to their imaginations. Remember that failure to provide certain information may be unethical or even illegal. For example, any evaluative data about an individual that can be identified with that individual should only be collected with the individual's informed consent. The ethical and legal importance of informed consent as a protection of human rights is a central concern of institutional review boards. Institutional review board approval is a prerequisite to initiation of virtually every experimental medical intervention conducted on patients or families.

Evaluation Instruments

The intent of this chapter is to present key points to consider in selection, modification, or construction of evaluation instruments. Whenever possible, an evaluation should be conducted using existing instruments. Instrument development requires considerable expertise, time, and expenditure of resources. Construction of an original evaluation instrument, whether it is in the form of a questionnaire or a type of equipment, requires rigorous testing for reliability and validity. Timely provision of evaluative information for making decisions rarely allows the luxury of the several months to

several years needed to develop a reliable, valid instrument.

The first step in instrument selection is to conduct a literature search for evaluations similar to the evaluation being planned. A helpful place to begin is with the same journals listed earlier in this chapter. Instruments that have been used in more than one study should be given preference over an instrument developed for a single use because instruments used multiple times generally have been more thoroughly tested for reliability and validity. Once a number of potential instruments have been identified, each instrument must be carefully critiqued to determine whether it is, in fact, appropriate for the evaluation you are planning.

First, the instrument must measure the performance being evaluated exactly as that performance has been operationally defined for the evaluation. For example, if satisfaction with a continuing education program is operationally defined to include a score of 80% or higher on five specific program components, such as faculty responsiveness to questions, relevance of content, and so on, then the instrument selected to measure participant satisfaction with the program must include exactly those five components and must be able to be scored in percentages.

Second, an appropriate instrument should have documented evidence of reliability and validity with individuals who are as identical as possible to those from whom you will be collecting data. If you will be evaluating the ability of elderly patients to complete activities of daily living, for example, you would not want to use an instrument developed for evaluating the ability of young orthopedic patients to complete routine activities. Similarities in reading level and visual acuity also should exist if the instrument being evaluated is a questionnaire or scale that participants will complete themselves.

Existing instruments being considered for selection also must be affordable, must be feasible for use in the location planned for conducting data collection, and should require minimal training on the part of data collectors.

The evaluation instrument most likely to require modification from an existing tool or development of an entirely new instrument is a cognitive test. The primary reason for constructing a cognitive test is that the test must be consistent with content actually covered during the educational program or activity. The intent of a cognitive test is to be comprehensive and relevant and to fairly test the learner's knowledge of content covered. Use of a test blueprint is one of the most useful methods to ensure comprehensiveness and relevance of test questions because the blueprint enables the evaluator to be certain that each area of course content is included in the test and that content areas emphasized during instruction are similarly emphasized during testing.

CONDUCTING THE EVALUATION

To conduct an evaluation means to implement the evaluation design by using the instruments chosen or developed according to the methods selected. How smoothly an evaluation is implemented depends primarily on how carefully and thoroughly the evaluation was planned. Planning is not a complete guarantee of success, however. Three methods to minimize the impact of unexpected events that are likely to occur when carrying out an evaluation are (1) conduct a pilot test first, (2) include "extra" time, and (3) keep a sense of humor.

Conducting a pilot test of the evaluation means to try out the data collection methods, instruments, and plan for data analysis with a few individuals who are the same as or very similar to those who will be included in the full evaluation. A pilot test *must* be conducted if any newly developed instruments are planned for the evaluation to assess reliability, validity, interpretability, and feasibility of the new instruments. A pilot test *should* be conducted prior to implementing a full evaluation that will be expensive or time-consuming to conduct or on which major decisions will be made. Process evaluation generally is not amenable to pilot testing unless a new instrument will be used for data collection. Pilot testing should be considered prior to conducting outcome, impact, or program evaluations, however.

Including "extra" time during conduct of an evaluation means to leave room for the unexpected delays that almost invariably occur during evaluation planning, data collection, and translation of evaluation results into reports that will be meaningful and usable by the primary audience. Because those delays not only will occur but also are likely to occur at inconvenient times during

the evaluation, keeping a sense of humor is vitally important. An evaluator with a sense of humor also is more likely to maintain a realistic perspective in reporting results that include negative findings. An audience with a vested interest in positive evaluation results may blame the evaluator if results are lower than expected.

ANALYZING AND INTERPRETING DATA COLLECTED

The purposes for conducting data analysis are, first, to organize data so that they can provide meaningful information and, second, to provide answers to evaluation questions. *Data* and *information* are not synonymous terms. In other words, a mass of numbers or a mass of comments does not become information until that mass has been organized into coherent tables, graphs, or categories that are relevant to the purpose for conducting the evaluation.

Basic decisions about how data will be analyzed are dictated by the nature of the data and by the questions used to focus the evaluation. As described earlier, data can be quantitative or qualitative. Data also can be described as continuous or discrete. Age and level of anxiety are examples of continuous data; gender and diagnosis are examples of discrete data. Finally, data can be differentiated by level of measurement. All qualitative data are at the nominal level of measurement, meaning they are described in terms of categories such as "health focused" versus "illness focused." Quantitative data can be at the nominal, ordinal, interval, or ratio level of measurement. The level of measurement of the data determines what statistics can be used to analyze those data. A useful suggestion for deciding how data will be analyzed is to enlist the assistance of someone with experience in data analysis.

Analysis of data should be consistent with the type of data collected. In other words, all data analysis must be rigorous, but not all data analysis includes use of inferential statistics. For example, qualitative data, such as verbal comments obtained during interviews and written comments obtained from open-ended questionnaires, are summarized or "themed" into categories of similar comments. Each category or theme is qualitatively described by directly quoting one or more comments that are typical of that category. These categories then may be quantitatively described using descriptive statistics such as total counts and percentages.

Different qualitative methods for analyzing data are emerging as they gain legitimacy in a scientific environment once ruled by traditional experimental quantitative methods. One example of use of qualitative methods in evaluation is called fourth generation evaluation (Hamilton, 1993), or naturalistic or constructivist evaluation. Perhaps most useful in conducting a process evaluation, fourth generation evaluation focuses on teacher-learner interaction and observation of that interaction by the teachers and learners present. As the term *constructivist* might imply, evaluation is an integral component of the education process, that is, evaluation helps construct the education. Data collection, analysis, and use of results occur concurrently. Teacher and learner questions and responses are observed and recorded during an education program. These observations are summarized at the time of occurrence and throughout the program and are used to provide immediate feedback to participants in the educational activity.

The first step in analysis of quantitative data is organization and summarization using statistics such as frequencies and percentages that describe the sample or population from which the data were collected. A description of a population of learners, for example, might include such information as response rate and frequency of learner demographic characteristics. Table 14–2 presents an example of how such information might be displayed.

The next step in analysis of quantitative data is to select the statistical procedures appropriate for the type of data collected that will answer questions posed in planning the evaluation. Again, a good suggestion is to enlist the assistance of an expert.

REPORTING EVALUATION RESULTS

Results of an evaluation must be reported if the evaluation is to be of any use. Such a statement seems obvious, but how many times have you heard that an evaluation was being conducted and never heard anything more about it? How many times have you participated in an evaluation but have never seen the final report? How many times have you conducted an evaluation yourself but have not provided anyone with a report on findings? Almost all of us, if we are honest, would have to answer even the last question with a number greater than zero.

Reasons for not reporting evaluation results are diverse and numerous. Not knowing who should receive the results, belief that the results are not important or will not be used, inability to translate results into language useful for producing the report, and fear that results will be misused are four basic reasons for why evaluative data may never get from the spreadsheet to the customer.

A few guidelines established in planning an evaluation will significantly increase the likelihood that results of the evaluation will be reported to the appropriate individuals or groups, in a timely manner, and in usable form.

1. Be audience focused.
2. Stick to the evaluation purpose.
3. Stick to the data.

Be Audience Focused

The purpose for conducting an evaluation is to provide information for decision making by the primary audience. The report of evaluation results

TABLE 14–2. Demographic comparison of survey respondents to total course participants using group averages

Learner Demographics	Survey Respondents (n = 50)	All Course Participants (N = 55)
Age	25.5 years	27.5 years
Length of time employed	3.5 years	7.5 years
Years of post–high school education	2.0 years	2.0 years

must be consistent with that purpose. One rule of thumb to use: Always begin an evaluation report with an executive summary that is no longer than one page. No matter who the audience is, their time is important to them. A second important guideline is to present evaluation results in a format and language that the audience can use and understand without additional interpretation. This does not mean that technical information should be excluded from a report to a lay audience; it means that such information should be written using nontechnical terms. Graphs and charts generally are easier to understand than are tables of numbers, for example. If a secondary audience of technical experts also will receive a report of evaluation results, include in an appendix more detailed or technically specific information in which they might be interested. Third, make every effort to present results in person as well as in writing. A direct presentation provides an opportunity for the evaluator to answer questions and to assess whether the report meets the needs of the audience. Finally, include specific recommendations or suggestions for how evaluation results might be used.

Stick to the Evaluation Purpose

Keep the main body of an evaluation report focused on information that fulfills the purpose for conducting the evaluation. Provide answers to the questions asked. Include the main aspects of how the evaluation was conducted, but avoid a diary-like chronology of the activities of the evaluators.

Stick to the Data

Maintain consistency with actual data when reporting and interpreting findings. Keep in mind that a question not asked cannot be answered and data not collected cannot be interpreted. If you did not measure or observe a teacher's performance, for example, do not draw conclusions about adequacy of that performance. Similarly, if the only measures of patient performance were those conducted in the hospital, do not interpret successful inpatient performance as successful performance by the patient at home or at work. These examples may seem obvious; however, "conceptual leaps" from the data collected to the conclusions drawn from those data are a common occurrence. One suggestion that decreases the opportunity to over-

interpret data is to include evaluation results and interpretation of those results in separate sections of the report.

A discussion of any limitations of the evaluation is an important part of the evaluation report. For example, if several patients were unable to complete a questionnaire because they could not understand it or because they were too fatigued, say so. Knowing that evaluation results do not include data from patients below a certain educational level or physical status will help the audience realize that they cannot make decisions about those patients based on the evaluation. Discussion of limitations also will provide useful information for what not to do the next time a similar evaluation is conducted.

SUMMARY

The process of evaluation in health-care education is to gather, summarize, interpret, and use data to assess the extent to which an educational activity is efficient, effective, and useful for those who participate in that activity as learners, teachers, or sponsors. Five types of evaluation discussed in this chapter include process, content, outcome, impact, and program evaluations. Each of these types focuses on a specific purpose, scope, and questions to be asked of an educational activity or program to meet the needs of those who ask for the evaluation or who can benefit from its results. Each type of evaluation also requires some level of available resources for the evaluation to be conducted.

The number and variety of evaluation models, designs, methods, and instruments are experiencing an exponential growth as the importance of evaluation becomes more evident in today's health-care environment. A number of guidelines, rules of thumb, and suggestions have been included in the discussion of how a nurse educator might go about selecting the most appropriate model, design, methods, and instruments for a particular type of evaluation. Perhaps the most important point to remember, however, is one made at the beginning of this chapter: Each aspect of the evaluation process is important, but all of them are meaningless if the results of evaluation are not used to guide future action in planning and carrying out educational interventions.

References

Abruzzese, R.S. (1978). Evaluation in nursing staff development. In *Nursing staff development: Strategies for success.* St. Louis: Mosby–Year Book.

Albanese, M.A., & Gjerde, C.L. (1987). Evaluation. In H. VanHoozer et al. (Eds.), *The teaching process: Theory and practice in nursing.* Norwalk, CT: Appleton-Century-Crofts.

Berk, R.A., & Rossi, P.H. (1990). *Thinking about program evaluation.* Newbury Park, CA: SAGE.

Boyd, M. (1992). The teaching process. In N. Whitman et al. (Eds.), *Teaching in nursing practice: A professional model,* 2nd ed. Norwalk, CT: Appleton & Lange.

Haggard, A. (1989). Evaluating patient education. In *Handbook of patient education.* Rockville, MD: Aspen.

Hamilton, G. A. (1993). An overview of evaluation research methods with implications for nursing staff development. *Journal of Nursing Staff Development, 9*(3), 148-154.

Holzemer, W. (1992). Evaluation methods in continuing education. *Journal of Continuing Education in Nursing, 23*(4), 174-181.

Johnson, J.H., & Olesinski, N. (1995). Program evaluation: Key to success. *Journal of Nursing Administration, 25*(1), 53-60.

Joint Commission on Accreditation of Healthcare Organizations. (1995). *Accreditation manual for hospitals.* Oakbrook Terrace, IL: Joint Commission on Accreditation of Healthcare Organizations.

Narrow, B. (1979). *Patient teaching in nursing practice: A patient and family-centered approach.* New York: Wiley.

Puetz, B.E. (1992). Evaluation: Essential skill for the staff development specialist. In K.J. Kelly (Ed.), *Nursing staff development: Current competence, future focus.* Philadelphia: Lippincott.

Rankin, S.H., & Stallings, K.D. (1990). *Patient education: Issues, principles, practices,* 2nd ed. Philadelphia: Lippincott.

Redman, B.K. (1993). Evaluation of health teaching. In *The process of patient education,* 7th ed. St. Louis: Mosby–Year Book.

Ruzicki, D.A. (1987). Evaluating patient education—a vital part of the process. In C. E. Smith (Ed.), *Patient education: Nurses in partnership with other health professionals.* Orlando, FL: Grune & Stratton.

Stewart, A.L., Hays, R.D., & Ware, J.E. (1988). The MOS Short-Form General Health Survey: Reliability and validity in a patient population. *Medical Care, 26*(7), 724.

Waddell, D. (1992). The effects of continuing education on nursing practice: A meta-analysis. *Journal of Continuing Education in Nursing, 23*(4), 164-168.

Ware, J.E., Jr., Davies-Avery, A., & Donald, C.A. (1978). *Conceptualization and measurement of health for adults in the health insurance study: Vol. V, general health perceptions.* Santa Monica, CA: RAND Corp.

APPENDIX A

Readability and Comprehension Tests

How to Use the Spache Grade-Level Score Formula

1. For short passages, test the entire piece. For longer passages, test a minimum of three randomly selected samples of 100 words each. (If the 100-word mark in the sample falls after the midpoint of the sentence, count the sentence as a part of the sample.)

2. Average sentence length (a) can be determined by counting the number of words in the sample and dividing by the number of sentences. If a sentence is punctuated by a period, question mark, exclamation point, semicolon, or colon, count it as an independent sentence.

3. Count the number of words *not* on the Dale List (b) according to the following guidelines:

   - Count a word only once, even if it appears again or with variable endings later in the sample.
   - Do not count first names.
   - Do not count plurals or possessive endings of nouns.
   - Do not count regular verb forms (*-ing, -ed, -es*), but do count irregular verb forms.
   - Count adjective or adverb endings (*-ly, -er, -est*).
   - Count a group of words that consists of repetition of a single word (e.g., "oh, oh, oh"; "look, look, look") as a single sentence regardless of punctuation.
   - Do not count familiar letters like *A, B, C.*

4. Apply the formula:

$$GL = 0.141(a) + 0.086(b) + 0.839$$

   where GL is grade level, (a) is average sentence length, and (b) is the number of words not listed on Dale List.

   In other words, multiply the average sentence length in a sample of 100 words by 0.141. Then multiply the percent of words outside the Dale "Easy Word List" by 0.086.

To these figures, add a constant, 0.839. The sum represents the estimated reading difficulty of the book. This will be a figure such as 2.267, which, when rounded off as 2.3, designates a book equal in difficulty to readers of school textbooks commonly used in the third month of second grade. When using this formula, it is suggested that at least three samples from the reading material be scored and the results averaged for a more reliable estimate of reading difficulty (Spache, 1953; Spadero, 1983).

How to Use the Flesch Formula

1. To test a whole piece of writing, take three to five 100-word samples of an article or twenty-five to thirty 100-word samples of a book. For short pieces, test the entire selection. Do not pick "good" or "typical" samples, but choose every third paragraph or every other page. In a 100-word sample, find the sentence that ends nearest to the 100-word mark; that may be, for example, at the 94th or the 109th word. Start each sample at the beginning of a paragraph, but do not use an introductory paragraph as part of the sample. Count contractions and hyphenated words as one word; count numbers and letters separated by space as words.

2. Figure the average sentence length (SL) by counting the number of words and dividing by the number of sentences. In counting sentences, follow units of thought marked off by periods, colons, semicolons, question marks, or exclamation points.

3. Determine word length (WL) by counting the number of syllables in each word in the sample as they are normally read aloud (i.e., two syllables for $ ["dollars"] and four syllables for *1918* ["nineteen-eighteen"]. It helps to read silently aloud while counting. Divide the syllables by the number of words in the sample and multiply by 100.

4. Apply the formula:

$$RE = 206.835 - 0.846\,WL - 1.015\,SL$$

where RE is the reading ease score, WL is the average word length measured as syllables per 100 words, and SL is the average sentence length in words (Flesch, 1948; Spadero, 1983; and Spadero et al., 1980).

The reading ease score ranges from zero (practically unreadable) to 100 (very easy for any literate person) with interpretations in between (Table A-1).

TABLE A–1.   Reading ease scores

Reading Ease Score	Syllables per 100 Words	Average Sentence Length	Difficulty Level	Grade Level
0–30	192 or more	29 or more	Very difficult	College grad
30–50	167	25	Difficult	College
50–60	155	21	Fairly difficult	10–12
60–70	147	17	Standard	8–9
70–80	139	14	Fairly easy	7
80–90	131	11	Easy	6
90–100	123 or less	8 or less	Very easy	5

SOURCE: Adapted from Flesch, R. (1948). A new readability yardstick. *Journal of Applied Psychology, 32*(3), 230; and Spadero, D.C. (1983). Assessing readability of patient information materials. *Pediatric Nursing, 9*(4), 275.

How to Use the Fog Formula

1. Count 100 words in succession (W). If the selection is long, choose several samples of 100 words from the text, and average the results.

2. Count the number of complete sentences (S). If the 100th word falls past the midpoint of a sentence, include this sentence in the count.

3. Divide the words (W) by the number of sentences (S).

4. Count the number of words having three or more syllables (A), but do not count verbs ending in *-ed* or *-es* that make a word have a third syllable, do not count capitalized words, and do not count combinations of simple words, such as *butterfly*.

5. Apply the formula:

$$GL = (W/S + A) \times 0.4$$

In other words, to find the GL (grade level), divide the number of words (W) by the number of complete sentences (S) in the sample 100-word passage, add the number of words having three or more syllables (A), and multiply the result by a constant of 0.4 (Gunning, 1968; Spadero, 1983; Spadero et al., 1980).

How to Use the Fry Readability Graph

1. Select three 100-word sample passages from near the beginning, middle, and end of a book, article, pamphlet, or brochure. Skip all proper nouns as part of the 100-word count. Fewer than three samples and passages of less than 30 sentences can be used, but the user should be aware that there is necessarily a sacrifice in both reliability and validity.

2. Count the total number of sentences in each 100-word sample (estimating to the nearest tenth of a sentence for partial sentences).

3. Average the sentence counts of the three sample passages.

4. Count the total number of syllables in each 100-word sample. Count one syllable per vowel sound; for example, *cat* has one syllable, *blackbird* has two, and *continental* has four. Caution: Do not be fooled by word size (e.g., *polio* [three syllables], *through* [one syllable]). Endings such as *-y, -ed, -el,* or *-le* usually make a syllable (e.g., *ready* [two syllables], *bottle* [two syllables]). Graph users sometimes have trouble determining syllables. The clue is to believe what you hear (speech sounds), not what you see (e.g., *wanted* is a two-syllable word, but *stopped* is a one-syllable word). Count proper nouns, numerals, and initials or acronyms as words. A word is a symbol or group of symbols bounded by a blank space on either side. Thus, *1945, &,* and *IRS* are all words. Each symbol should receive a syllable count of one (i.e., the date *1945* is one word with four syllables, and the initials *IRS* is one word with three syllables).

5. Average the total number of syllables for the three samples.

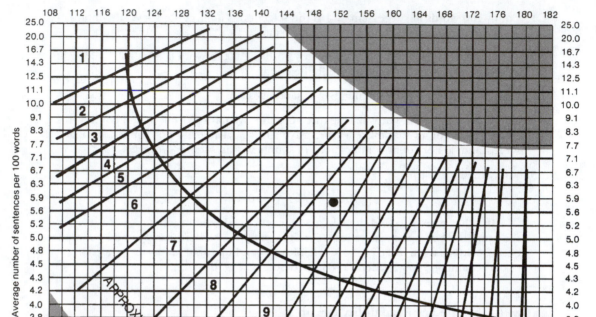

Average number of syllables per 100 words

FIGURE A–1.   Fry Readability Graph—Extended

SOURCE: Edward Fry, Rutgers University Reading Center, New Brunswick, NJ.

6. Plot on the graph the average sentence count and the average word count to determine the appropriate grade level of the material. For example,

	Number of Syllables	*Number of Sentences*
1st hundred words	153	6.3
2nd hundred words	161	5.9
3rd hundred words	139	5.2
Average count =	453 ÷ 3 = 151	17.4 ÷ 3 = 5.8

In the example, the average number of syllables is 151, and the average number of sentences is 5.8. When plotted on the graph (Figure A-1), the point falls within the approximate grade level of 9, which shows the materials to be at the ninth-grade readability level. If the point when plotted falls in the gray area, grade-level scores are invalid (Fry, 1968; Fry, 1977; Spadero et al., 1980).

How to Use the SMOG Formula

Passages Longer Than 30 Sentences

1. Count 10 consecutive sentences near the beginning, 10 consecutive sentences from the middle, and 10 consecutive sentences from the end of the selection to be assessed. A sentence is any independent unit of thought punctuated by a period, question mark, or exclamation point. If a sentence has a colon or semicolon, consider each part as a separate sentence.

2. From the 30 randomly selected sentences, count the words containing three or more syllables (polysyllabic), including repetitions. Abbreviated words should be read aloud to determine their syllable count (e.g., *Sept.* = *September* = three syllables). Letters or numerals in a string beginning or ending with a space or punctuation mark should be counted if, when read aloud in context, at least three syllables can be distinguished. Do not count words ending in *-ed* or *-es* if the ending makes the word have a third syllable. Hyphenated words are counted as one word. Proper nouns should be counted.

3. Approximate the reading grade level from the SMOG Conversion Table (Table A–2), or calculate the reading grade level by estimating the nearest perfect square root of the number of words with three or more syllables and then adding a constant of 3 to the square root. For example, if the total number of polysyllabic words was 53, the nearest perfect square would be 49. The square root of 49 would be 7. By adding a constant of 3, the reading level would be tenth grade.

TABLE A–2.   SMOG Conversion Table

Word Count	Grade Level
0–2	4
3–6	5
7–12	6
13–20	7
21–30	8
31–42	9
43–56	10
57–72	11
73–90	12
91–110	13
111–132	14
133–156	15
157–182	16
183–210	17
211–240	18

SOURCE: Developed by: Harold C. McGraw, Office of Educational Research, Baltimore County Public Schools, Towson, MD.

---

¹(Mastectomy:) **A Treatment for Breast Cancer**

²You've been (diagnosed) as having breast cancer and your doctor has (recommended) a (mastectomy.)

³If you're like most women, you (probably) have many concerns about this treatment for breast cancer.

⁴(Surgery) of any kind is a (frightening) (experience,) but (surgery) for breast cancer raises special concerns.

⁵You may be (wondering) if the (surgery) will cure your cancer, how you'll feel after (surgery) —and how you're going to look.

⁶It's not (unusual) to think about these things. ⁷More than (100,000) women in the United States will have (mastectomies) this year. ⁸Each of them will have (personal) concerns about the impact of the (surgery) on her life.

⁹This booklet is designed to ease some of your fears by letting you know what to expect—from the time you enter the (hospital) to your (recovery) at home. ¹⁰It may also help the special people in your life who are concerned about your (well-being.)

FIGURE A–2. Example of Counting Words with Three or More Syllables

Figure A–2 is an example of how to count all the words containing three or more syllables in a set of 10 sentences taken from one of the many pamphlets designed and distributed by the National Cancer Institute of the National Institutes of Health, Public Health Service, U.S. Department of Health and Human Services, entitled *Mastectomy: A Treatment for Breast Cancer* (1987, p. 1).

In Figure A–2, there are 20 words with three or more syllables. Note, the word *United* is not counted as a three-syllable word because only the *-ed* ending makes it polysyllabic (see rule 2). For this passage of 10 sentences, the grade level is eleventh grade.

Passages Shorter Than 30 Sentences

1. Count the number of sentences in the material and the number of words containing three or more syllables.

2. In the left-hand column of Table A–3, locate the number of sentences. Then in the column opposite, locate the conversion number.

3. Multiply the word count found in step 1 by the conversion number. Locate this number in Table A–2 to obtain the corresponding grade level.

   Example: If the material is 25 sentences long and 15 words of three or more syllables were counted in this material, the conversion number in Table A–3 for 25 sentences is 1.2. Multiply the word count of 15 by 1.2 to get 18. For the word count of 18, the grade level in Table A–2 is 7. Therefore, the material is at a seventh-grade reading level.

TABLE A–3. SMOG conversion for samples
with fewer than 30 sentences

Number of Sentences in Sample Material	Conversion Number
29	1.03
28	1.07
27	1.1
26	1.15
25	1.2
24	1.25
23	1.3
22	1.36
21	1.43
20	1.5
19	1.58
18	1.67
17	1.76
16	1.87
15	2.0
14	2.14
13	2.3
12	2.5
11	2.7
10	3

How to Use the Cloze Test

How to Construct a Cloze Test

1. Select a prose passage (one without reference to figures, tables, charts, or pictures) from printed education materials currently in use such as pamphlets, brochures, manuals, or instruction sheets. Be sure the material is typical of what is normally given to patients but has not been previously read by them. The chosen passage should include whole paragraphs so that readers benefit from complete units of thought.

2. Leave the first and last sentences intact, and delete every fifth word from the other sentences for a total of about 50 word deletions. Do not delete proper nouns, but delete the word following the proper noun. Replace all deleted words with a line or blank space, all of equal length.

How to Score a Cloze Test

1. Count as correct only those words that *exactly* replace the deleted words (synonyms are not to be counted as a correct answer).

2. Inappropriate word endings such as *-s, -ed, -er,* and *-ing* should be counted as incorrect.

3. The raw score is the number of exact word replacements.

High Blood Pressure

High blood pressure, also called hypertension, affects 37 million Americans—many of them older than 55. A dangerous, silent killer, __1__ can lead to stroke, __2__ attack and heart or __3__ failure. Yet, in most __4__, no one knows what __5__ high blood pressure. Body __6__, emotions, heredity, overweight, and __7__ high-sodium (salt) diet may __8__ something to do with __9__ blood pressure, but scientists __10__ uncertain. It has long __11__ recognized as a major __12__ factor in stroke and __13__ attack—cardiovascular diseases which __14__ nearly 1 million deaths __15__ year.

To understand high __16__ pressure, it is necessary __17__ know something about how __18__ heart and blood vessels __19__. Your heart is a __20__ that acts like a __21__. The left side of __22__ heart receives oxygen-rich blood __23__ the lungs and pumps __24__ through the arteries to __25__ parts of your body, __26__ it with nutrients and __27__. Blood that has distributed __28__ nutrients and oxygen returns __29__ the right side of __30__ heart which pumps it __31__ the pulmonary artery to __32__ lungs where it absorbs __33__, and then the process __34__ again.

The force exerted __35__ your blood flowing against __36__ walls of the blood __37__ is blood pressure. The __38__ action of your heart __39__ the force. Your blood __40__ varies from moment to __41__ depending upon the situations __42__ activities in which you __43__ involved. For example, when __44__ become excited, the small __45__ that nourish your tissues __46__. The heart must pump __47__ harder to force the __48__ through the arteries, causing __49__ blood pressure to rise. __50__ the blood pressure will __51__ to normal when you __52__. Because of these changes in blood pressure, the doctor will usually take several blood pressure readings over a period of time before making a diagnosis of high blood pressure.

FIGURE A–3. Sample Cloze Test

SOURCE: Adapted from American Heart Association (1983) *An older person's guide to cardiovascular health*, National Center, 7320 Greenville Avenue, Dallas, TX 75231. The information from this booklet is not current and is used for illustrative purposes only.

4. Divide the raw score by the total number of blank spaces to determine the percentage of correct responses. For example, if the passage has 50 blanks and the patient correctly filled in 25 blanks (10 were incorrect responses and 15 spaces were left blank), divide 25 by 50, and the percentage score would be 50%.

5. A score of 60% or above indicates the patient is fully capable of understanding the material. A score of 40% to 60% indicates the patient needs supplemental instruction. A score below 40% indicates that the material as written is too difficult for the patient to understand.

The following are the words that were deleted from the sample Cloze test in Figure A-3.

1. it	13. heart	25. all	37. vessels
2. heart	14. cause	26. supplying	38. pumping
3. kidney	15. a	27. oxygen	39. creates
4. cases	16. blood	28. its	40. pressure
5. causes	17. to	29. to	41. moment
6. chemistry	18. the	30. your	42. or
7. a	19. work	31. through	43. are
8. have	20. muscle	32. the	44. you
9. high	21. pump	33. oxygen	45. arteries
10. remain	22. your	34. begins	46. constrict
11. been	23. from	35. by	47. even
12. risk	24. it	36. the	48. blood

Note: Words are listed in missing order. Hyphenated words are counted as one word; words in parentheses are counted as a word.

Resources and Organizations for Special Populations

Blindness

National Diabetes Information Clearinghouse
Box NDIC
9000 Rockville Pike
Bethesda, MD 20892
(301) 468-2162

Resource Persons for Diabetes and Vision Impairment
VIP Special Interest Group
AADE
444 North Michigan Avenue
Suite 1240
Chicago, IL 60611-3901

Lists of members of American Association of Diabetes Educators (AADE) who possess specialized skills for working with visually impaired persons. List was compiled by the Visually Impaired Persons (VIP) Special Interest Group for the AADE and is available from that special interest group.

Resources for Visually Impaired Diabetics
Vision Foundation Inc.
818 Mt. Auburn Street
Watertown, MA 02172

The Vision Foundation publication is revised annually and is available for $4 prepaid for either large-print or cassette edition.

Deafness

The National Academy of Gallaudet College
Florida Avenue at 7th Street N.E.
Washington, DC 20002

Training programs; assistance in developing training programs; publications on working with deaf patients.

The National Center for Law and the Deaf
Gallaudet College
Florida Avenue at 7th Street N.E.
Washington, DC 20002

Guidelines for services for deaf patients; assistance in developing such guidelines.

The Registry of Interpreters for the Deaf
814 Thayer Avenue
Silver Spring, MD 20910

Information on interpreting and interpreters; referral to local agencies and state chapters of the Registry of Interpreters for the Deaf for assistance in locating interpreters.

Disability Services

Clearinghouse on Disability Information
U.S. Department of Education
Switzer Building
Room 3132
Washington, DC 20202
(202) 731-1241

Information Center for Individuals with Disabilities
Fort Point Place
First Floor
27–43 Wormwood Street
Boston, MA 02210-1606
(617) 727-5540

Library of Congress National Library Service for the Blind and Physically Handicapped
1291 Taylor Street NW
Washington, DC 20542
(202) 707-5100
(800) 424-9100
(TDD 202) 707-0744

Head Injury

National Head Injury Foundation
1776 Massachusetts Avenue NW
Suite 100
Washington, DC 20036
(202) 296-6443

Health-Care-Related Federal Agencies

National Institute on Disability and Rehabilitation Research
U.S. Department of Education
400 Maryland Avenue SW
Room 3060
Washington, DC 20202
(202) 732-1134

Rehabilitation Services Administration
Department of Human Services
605 G Street NW
Room 101M
Washington, DC 20001
(202) 727-3211

Learning Disabilities

A.D.D. Warehouse
300 Northwest 70th Avenue
Suite 102
Plantation, FL 33317
(305) 792-8944

Association for Children and Adults with Learning Disabilities
4156 Library Road
Pittsburgh, PA 15234
(412) 341-8077

Attention Disorders Association of Parents and Professionals Together (ADAPPT)
P.O. Box 293
Oak Forest, IL 60452
(312) 361-4330

Mental Health

Mental Health Law Project
1101 15th St. NW
Suite 1212
Washington, DC 20005

National Mental Health Association
1012 Prince Street
Alexandria, VA 22314-2971

Mental Retardation

Mental Retardation Association of America
211 East 300 South
Suite 212
Salt Lake City, UT 84111

National Association of Developmental Disabilities Councils
1234 Massachusetts Avenue NW
Suite 103
Washington, DC 20005

Neuromuscular Disorders

Amyotrophic Lateral Sclerosis Association
21021 Ventura Boulevard
Suite 321
Woodland Hills, CA 91364
(818) 990-2151

Epilepsy Foundation of America
4351 Garden City Drive
Landover, MD 20785
(301) 459-3700

Guillain-Barré Syndrome Foundation International
PO Box 262
Wynnewood, PA 19096
(215) 667-0131

Muscular Dystrophy Association
810 7th Avenue
New York, NY 10019
(212) 586-0808

Myasthenia Gravis Foundation, Inc.
53 W. Jackson Boulevard
Suite 660
Chicago, IL 60604
(312) 427-6252

National Ataxia Foundation
15500 Wayzata Boulevard
Suite 750
Wayzata, MN 55391
(612) 473-7666

National Multiple Sclerosis Society
205 E. 42nd Street
New York, NY 10017
(800) 624-8236

Parkinson's Disease Foundation
William Black Medical Research Building
Columbia Presbyterian Medical Center
650 W. 168th Street
New York, NY 10032
(800) 457-6676/(212) 923-4700

United Cerebral Palsy Foundation Associations
7 Penn Plaza, Suite 804
New York, NY 10001
(212) 268-6655

Spinal Cord

National Spinal Cord Injury Association
600 W. Cummings Park
Suite 2000
Woburn, MA 01801
(617) 935-2722

New England Paralyzed Veterans of America
1600 Providence Highway
Suite 101R
Walpole, MA 02081
(508) 660-1181

Paralyzed Veterans of America
801 18th Street NW
Washington, DC 20006
(202) 872-1300

Stroke

National Institute of Neurological and Communicative Disorders and Stroke
Building 31
Room 8A52
9000 Rockville Pike
Bethesda, MD 20892

National Stroke Association
300 E. Hampden Avenue
Suite 240
Englewood, CO 80110-2654
(303) 762-9922

Stroke Clubs International
805 12th Street
Galveston, TX 77550
(409) 762-1022

ADAPTIVE COMPUTERS

The following is a partial list of computer software and other adaptive equipment available to people with disabilities.

The Alliance for Technology Access (ATA), formerly called the National Special Education Alliance, is a growing network of nonprofit resource centers located around the country that specializes in using computers to help individuals with disabilities. For more information on the ATA contact:

Foundation for Technology Access
1307 Solano Avenue
Albany, CA 94706
(415) 528-0747

TSI/VTEK
455 N. Bernardo Avenue
Mountain View, CA 94039-7455
(800) 227-8418
Large Print Display Processor, Braille Display Processor, Optacon II

Blindness

Some Braille printers are able to print both Braille and standard text on the same page. This feature enables individuals who are blind to share their printed work with people who are sighted.

American Thermoform Corp.
2311 Travers Avenue
City of Commerce, CA 90040
(213) 723-9021
Ohtsuki Printer (Braille)

Enabling Technologies
3102 S.E. Jay Street
Stuart, FL 33497
(407) 283-4817
Romeo Brailler

Duxbury Systems, Inc.
435 King Street
P.O. Box 1504
Littleton, MA 01460
(508) 486-9766
Duxbury Braille Translator (software)

Head-Controlled Mouse

Prentke Romich Company
1022 Heyl Road
Wooster, OH 44691
(800) 642-8255
Headmaster Workstation

Pointer Systems, Inc.
One Mill Street
Burlington, VT 05401
(800) 537-1562
Freewheel

Outliners (Thought Processors)

In many instances, outlining software can be used in place of a word processor, and for people with learning disabilities, outlining software may be the best place to start almost any kind of writing.

Symmetry Corporation
761 E. University Drive, #C
Mesa, AZ 85203
(800) 624-2485
Acta Advantage

MECC
3490 Lexington Avenue North
St. Paul, MN 55126
(612) 481-3500
MECC Outliner

Computerized Speech Tools

**American Speech-Language and
Hearing Association**
10801 Rockville Pike
Rockville, MD 20852
(301) 897-5700

**United States Society for Augmentative
and Alternative Communication**
c/o Barkley Memorial Center
University of Nebraska
Lincoln, NE 68588
(402) 472-5463

Voice Recognition Systems

Voice recognition systems hold enormous potential for individuals with movement limitations; they effectively control the computer without any physical interaction taking place between the person and computer.

Articulate Systems, Inc.
2380 Ellsworth Street
Berkeley, CA 94720
(415) 549-1013
Voice Navigator

Voice Connection
17835 Skypark Circle
Suite C
Irvine, CA 92714
(714) 261-2366
IntroVoice

Newsletters and Magazines

Assistive Device News
Central Pennsylvania Special
    Education Regional Resource Center
150 South Progress Avenue
Harrisburg, PA 17109
(717) 367-1161

The Assistive Device News *is published by the Pennsylvania Assistive Device Center located at the Elizabethtown Hospital and Rehabilitation Center. The newsletter contains information about technology solutions for individuals with physical impairments.*

Augmentative Communication News
One Surf Way
Suite 215
Monterey, CA 93940
(408) 649-3050

The Augmentative Communication News *is a professional journal that focuses on augmentative communication, integration theory, technology, assessment, treatment, and the education of users who rely on augmentative communication systems.*

GLOSSARY

abstract conceptualization   A term used by Kolb as one of two ways of processing information; known as the "thinking" mode.

accommodator   One of the four learning style types according to Kolb's theory, combining the learning modes of concrete experience and active experimentation.

acculturation   Describes an individual's adaptation to the customs, values, beliefs, and behaviors of a new country or culture.

active experimentation   A term used by Kolb as one of two ways of processing information; known as the "doing" mode.

acuity   The degree of complexity of a patients' illness state, indicating a high level of required care.

adaptive computing   The professional services and the technology (both hardware and software) that make computing technology accessible for persons with disabilities.

adherence   Commitment or attachment to a prescribed, predetermined regimen.

affective domain   One of three domains in the taxonomy of educational objectives; deals with attitudes, values, and beliefs.

aids   See *instructional materials/tools.*

analogue   A type of model that uses analogy to explain something by comparing it to something else. The model performs like the real object, although its actual appearance may differ. A dialysis machine and the use of a description of a pump to explain how the kidneys and heart work respectivley are examples of analogues.

andragogy   The art and science of helping adults learn; a term coined by Malcolm Knowles to describe his theory of adult learning.

appearance   As an important feature of instructional tools, it is the way printed and display materials look to the reader. Appearance is a vital element in determining the effectiveness of media in capturing and holding the learner's attention through adequate use of white space, minimal use of words to convey the message, use of illustrations to break up blocks of print, and use of contrasts in color or shading.

assess   To gather, summarize, and interpret pertinent data about the learner to make a decision or plan.

assessment   The process of systematically collecting data to determine the relative magnitude, importance, or value of needs, problems, and strengths of the learner to decide a direction for action.

assessment phase   The first phase of the educational cycle, which provides the foundation for the rest of the educational process.

assimilator   One of the four learning style types according to Kolb's theory, combining the learning modes of abstract conceptualization and reflective observation.

attention deficit disorder (ADD)   A disorder of children with prominent attentional difficulties as demonstrated by inattention and impulsivity that are signs of developmentally inappropriate behavior.

audio learning resources   Instructional tools whose chief characteristic is exploitation of the learners' sense of hearing as a mechanism for teaching. Audiotapes and recorders are the best examples.

audiovisual materials   See *audiovisual tools*.

audiovisual tools   Nonprint instructional media that can influence all three domains of learning and stimulate the senses of hearing and/or sight to help convey the message to the learner. This category includes five major types: projected, audio, video, telecommunications, and computer formats.

autonomy   The right to self-determination.

behavioral objectives   Intended outcomes of the education process that are action oriented rather than content oriented and learner centered rather than teacher centered; also referred to as learning objectives.

behaviorist learning   One of the five major learning theories. According to behaviorists, the focus for learning is mainly on what is directly observable, and learning is viewed as the product of the stimulus conditions (S) and the responses (R) that follow. It is sometimes termed the S-R model of learning.

beneficence   The principle of doing good.

bodily-kinesthetic intelligence   A term used by Gardner to describe children who learn by processing knowledge through bodily sensations.

brain injury   Irreversible cerebral cell damage to neurons and axons resulting in degrees of difficulty with learning.

brain preference indicator (BPI)   A learning style instrument used to determine hemispheric dominance.

breach of contract   Failure, without legal excuse, to perform a promise (Lesnik & Anderson, 1962, p. 147). Violation of a binding agreement or obligation in the performance of professional duties.

chronic illness   A disease or disability that is permanent and can never be completely cured. It constitutes the number one medical malady of people in this country and affects the physical, psychosocial, economic, and spiritual aspects of an individual's life.

Cloze technique   A standardized test to measure comprehension of written materials (particularly recommended for health education literature) based on systematically deleting every fifth word from a portion of a text and having the reader fill in the blanks.

cognitive ability   The extent to which information can be processed, indicative of the level at which the learner is capable of learning; of major importance when designing instruction.

cognitive development   The process of acquiring more complex and adaptive ways of thinking as an individual grows from infancy to adulthood according to Piaget's four stages of cognitive maturation: sensorimotor, preoperational, concrete operations, and formal operations.

cognitive development perspective Focuses on the qualitative changes in perceiving, thinking, and reasoning as individuals grow and mature based on how external events are conceptualized, organized, and represented within each person's mental framework or schema.

cognitive domain One of three domains in the taxonomy of educational objectives; deals with aspects of behavior focusing on the way in which someone thinks in acquiring facts, concepts, principles, etc.

cognitive learning One of the five major learning theories. According to a cognitive theorist's perspective, in order to learn, individuals change as a result of the way they perceive, process, interpret, and organize information based on what is already known; the reorganization of information leads to new insights and understanding.

commercially prepared materials Predesigned, cost-effective printed educational materials that are widely available on a wide range of topics for purchase by educators as supplements to teaching-learning, such as brochures, pamphlets, books, posters, etc.

compliance Submission or yielding to predetermined goals through regimens prescribed or established by others.

comprehension The degree to which individuals understand what they have read or heard; the ability to grasp the meaning of a verbal or nonverbal message.

computer-assisted instruction (CAI) A nontraditional, individualized instructional method of self-study using the high technology of the computer to deliver an educational activity. The interactive capability of CAI holds enormous potential for reinforcing learning primarily in the cognitive domain, and its efficacy is dependent on programmatic software, hardware, and the learner's familiarity with and motivation to use this technology.

concrete experience A term used by Kolb to describe a dimension of perceiving; known as the "feeling" mode.

concrete operations period As defined by Piaget, this is the third stage in the cognitive development of children when the school-aged child (ages 7 to 11 years) is capable of logical thought processes and the ability to reason but the child is still incapable of abstract thinking.

concrete sequential A term used by Gregoric to describe learners who tend to operate in a highly structured, conservative manner. Details and time schedules are critical to these learners.

confidentiality A binding social contract or covenant; a professional obligation to respect privileged information between health professional and client.

content The actual information that is communicated to the learner through various teaching methods and tools (see *message*).

content evaluation A systematic assessment taking place immediately after the learning experience to determine the degree to which learners have acquired the knowledge or skills taught during a teaching/learning session.

converger One of the four learning style types according to Kolb's theory, combining the learning modes of abstract conceptualization and active experimentation.

corpus callosum The connector between the two hemispheres of the brain.

cosmopolitan orientation Persons with a worldly perspective on life who are receptive to new ideas and opportunities to learn new ways of doing things; a component of experiential readiness.

cost benefit   "Money well spent." Cost of services (e.g., education) insures return of satisfied clients and stability of the economic base of a health-care facility.

cost-benefit ratio   Relationship of program costs to economic benefits gained by the health-care institution.

cost recovery   Occurs when revenues generated are equal to or greater than expenditures.

cost savings   Monies realized through decreased use of expensive services, shortened length of stay, or fewer complications resulting from preventive services or patient education.

crystallized intelligence   The intellectual ability developed over a lifetime, which includes such elements as vocabulary, general information, understanding of social interactions, arithmetic reasoning, and capacity to evaluate experiences, which tends to increase over time as a person ages.

cultural assessment   An organized, systematic appraisal of beliefs, values, and practices of an individual or group to determine client needs as a basis for planning nursing care interventions.

cultural relativism   The values and behaviors every human group assigns to its conventions, which arise out of its own historical background and can only be accurately interpreted and understood in the light of that group's cultural world view.

culture   A complex concept that is an integral part of each person's life and includes knowledge, beliefs, values, morals, customs, traditions, and habits acquired by the members of a society.

culturological assessment   A systematic appraisal or examination of the cultural beliefs, values, and practices of individuals, groups, and communities to determine explicit needs and intervention practices within the cultural context of the people being evaluated.

delivery system   The physical form of instructional materials, including durable equipment used to present these materials, such as film and projectors, audiotapes and tape players, and computer programs and computers.

demonstration   A traditional instructional method by which the learner is shown by the teacher how to perform a particular skill, most frequently psychomotor in nature.

demonstration materials   Aids that stimulate the senses by combining sight with touch, smell, and sometimes even taste with the advantage of helping to teach cognitive and psychomotor skill development. Major forms of media in this category include many types of nonprint media, such as models, real equipment, diagrams, charts, posters, displays, photographs, and drawings.

desirable needs   Learning needs of the client that are not life dependent but related to well-being and can be met by the overall ability of nursing staff to provide quality care.

determinants of learning   Consist of learning needs, readiness to learn, and learning styles.

developmental disablility   A disorder that manifests itself during the developmental period when a child demonstrates subaverage general intellectual functioning with concurrent deficits in adaptive behaviors. Sometimes referred to as mental retardation or developmental delay.

developmental stages   Milestones marking changes in the physical, cognitive, and psychosocial growth of an individual over time from infancy to old age.

direct costs   Tangible, predictable costs associated with expenditures for personnel, equipment, etc.

disability   Inability to perform some key life functions; often used interchangeably with the term *functional limitation.*

discharge planning An interdisciplinary process, highly dependent on patient educational interventions for effectiveness, by which members of the health-care team (often led by nurses) plan and coordinate services for the purpose of providing continuity of care to patients and their families between various care settings.

displays Type of demonstration materials, frequently regarded as static, which may be permanently installed or portable. Included in this category are chalkboards, flip charts, and posters.

distance learning A telecommunications method of instruction using video technology to transmit live or taped messages directly from the instructor to the viewer.

diverger One of the four learning style types according to Kolb's theory, combining the learning modes of concrete experience and reflective observation.

domains of learning Cognitive, psychomotor, and affective are the three domains in which learning occurs.

Dunn and Dunn Learning Style Inventory A self-reporting instrument that is used in the identification of how individuals prefer to function, learn, concentrate, and perform in learning activities.

duty Responsibility, professional expectation.

dysarthria Difficulty with voluntary muscle control of speech due to damage to the central or peripheral nervous system that controls muscles essential to speaking and swallowing. Types of dysarthria include flaccid, spastic, ataxic, hypokinetic, or mixed. Persons with degenerative neurologic diseases often suffer with this disorder.

education An overall umbrella term used to describe the process, including the components of teaching and instruction, of producing observable or measurable behavioral changes (in knowledge, attitudes, and/or skills) in the learner through planned educational activities.

educational contract See *learning contract.*

education process A systematic, sequential, planned course of action that parallels the nursing process and consists of two interdependent operations, teaching and learning, which form a continuous cycle to include assessment of the learner, establishment of a teaching plan, implementation of teaching methods and tools, and evaluation of the learner, teacher, and education program.

educator role The teaching role a nurse assumes in supporting, encouraging, and assisting the learner to put learning of behaviors (knowledge, skills, and attitudes) into meaningful parts and wholes to reach an optimum potential of functioning.

embedded figures test (EFT) A test designed to measure how a person's perception of the environment (field independence/dependence) is influenced by the context in which it appears.

emotional readiness A state of psychological willingness to learn dependent on such factors as anxiety level, support system, motivation, risk-taking behavior, frame of mind, and psychosocial developmental stage.

ethical rights and duties A term that refers to the norms or standards of behavior of health-care professionals.

ethics Guiding principles of human behavior.

ethnicity A dynamic and complex concept referring to how members of a group perceive themselves and how, in turn, they are perceived by others in relation to the population subgroup's common heritage of customs, characteristics, language and history.

ethnocentrism   A concept in which the belief is held that one's own culture is superior and all other cultures are less sophisticated.

ethnomedical   A cultural orientation delineating the nature and consequences of illness problems and disease interventions rather than adhering to the biomedical orientation of defining diseases and illness interventions. In this context, the concept of illness incorporates the relationship of humans with their universe, bridging culture with a sensitivity toward the daily practices inherent within specific ethnic groups.

expressive aphasia   An absence or impairment of the ability to communicate through speech or writing due to a dysfunction of the Broca's area of the brain, which is the center of the cortex that controls motor abilities.

evaluate   To determine the significance of by careful appraisal or study; to reassess.

evaluation   A systematic and continuous process by which the significance of something is judged; the process of collecting and using information to determine what has been accomplished and how well it has been accomplished to guide decision making.

evaluation research   Scientific inquiry applied to a specific program or activity to assess processes, outcomes, and/or their relationship; "a process of applying scientific procedures to accumulate reliable and valid data on the manner and the extent to which specified activities produce outcomes or effects" (Hamilton, 1993, p. 148).

experiential readiness   A state of willingness to learn based on such factors as an individual's past experiences with learning, cultural background, previous coping mechanisms, and locus of control.

external locus of control   An individual's motivation to learn comes from outside oneself, attributing success or failure of an action to luck, the nature of the task, or to the efforts of someone else.

extraversion-introversion (EI)   Terms used to describe behavior that reflects an orientation to either the outside world of people or to the inner world of concepts and ideas; one of four dichotomous preference dimensions in the Myers-Briggs Type Indicator.

extrinsic feedback   A response provided by the teacher through the sharing of opinion or the conveying of a message through body language about how well a learner has performed; often used in relation to a psychomotor skill performance.

field dependence   One of two styles of learning in the cognitive domain identified by Witkin in which a person's perception of the environment is influenced by the surrounding field.

field independence   One of two styles of learning in the cognitive domain identified by Witkin in which a person's perception of the environment is separate from the surrounding field.

fixed costs   Predictable and controllable expenses that remain stable over time.

Flesch formula   An objective, statistical measurement tool for readability of written materials between fifth grade and college level, based on a count of the two basic language elements of average sentence length in words of selected samples and of average word length measured as syllables per 100 words of sample.

fluid intelligence   The intellectual capacity to perceive relationships, to reason, and to perform abstract thinking, which declines over time as degenerative changes occur with aging.

focus groups   Optimally 4 to 12 potential learners grouped together for the purpose of identifying points of view or knowledge about a certain topic. A facilitator leads the discussion by asking questions.

Fog formula   An index appropriate for use in determining readability of materials from fourth grade to college level based on average sentence length and the percentage of multisyllabic words in a 100-word passage.

formal operations period   As defined by Piaget, this is the fourth and final stage of cognitive development in which the adolescent (ages 12 to 18 years) is capable of abstract thought, internalization of ideas, complex logical reasoning, and understanding causality.

formal settings   Scheduled sessions in which teaching-learning takes place.

format   The general physical appearance of a book, pamphlet, or other printed materials, which includes such characteristics as the type face, the margins, the organization of information, the quality of the paper, etc.

formative evaluation   Systematic and continuous assessment of success of the teaching process made during the implementation of materials, methods, and activities to control, ensure, or improve the quality of performance in delivery of an educational program. Also referred to as process evaluation.

4MAT system   A learning style model based on Kolb's model combined with right/left brain research.

Fry formula   A measurement tool for testing the readability of materials (especially books, pamphlets, and brochures) at the level of first grade through college by using a graph to plot the number of syllables of words and the number of sentences in three 100-word samples.

functional illiteracy   The lack of fundamental education skills needed by adults to read, write, or comprehend information below the fifth-grade level of difficulty to function effectively in today's society; the inability to read well enough to understand and interpret written information for use as intended.

gaming   A nontraditional instructional method requiring the learner to participate in a competitive activity (which may or may not reflect reality) with preset rules.

Gardner's seven types of intelligence   A theory that describes the styles of learning in children.

gender differences   A comparison between the sexes as to how males and females act, react, and perform in situations affecting every sphere of life as a result of genetic and environmental influences on behavior.

gerogogy   The art and science of teaching the elderly.

Gestalt perspective   Emphasizes the importance of perception in learning, with a focus on the configuration or organization of a pattern of stimuli.

goal   A desirable outcome to be achieved by the learner at the end of the teaching-learning process; goals are global and more future oriented and long-term in nature than the specific, short-term objectives that lead step by step to the final achievement of a goal.

Gregorc Style Delineator   A self-analysis instrument designed to assess a person's learning style with respect to perceiving, ordering, processing, and relating information.

group discussion   A commonly employed, traditional method of instruction whereby a group of learners (ideally 3 to 20 people) gather together to exchange information, feelings, and opinions with each other and the teacher; the activity is learner centered and subject centered.

habilitation   Includes all the activities and interactions that enable individuals with a disability to develop new abilities to achieve their maximum potential.

hardware   Part of the delivery system for many types of media (e.g., computers, projectors, tape players).

Health Belief Model   A framework or paradigm used to explain or predict health behavior composed of the interaction between individual perceptions, modifying factors, and likelihood of action.

health-care-related setting   One of three classifications of instructional settings, in which health-care-related services are offered as a complementary function of a quasi-health agency. Examples: American Heart Association, American Cancer Society, Muscular Dystrophy Association, and Leukemia Society of America.

health-care setting   One of three classifications of instructional settings, in which the delivery of health care is the primary or sole function of an institution, organization, or agency. Examples: hospitals, visiting nurse associations, public health departments, outpatient clinics, physician offices, health maintenance organizations, extended-care facilities, and nurse-managed centers.

health-care team   A multidisciplinary group of health-care professionals and nonprofessionals who provide services to the patient and family members in an attempt to maximize optimal health and well-being of the client to whom their activities are directed.

health education   A participatory educational approach, often used interchangeably with the term *patient education* or *client education,* aimed at preventing disease, promoting positive health, and incorporating the physical, mental, and social aspects of learning needs.

Health Promotion Model   A framework that describes the interaction of health-promoting factors including cognitive perceptual factors, modifying factors, and likelihood of participation in health promoting behaviors.

hearing impairment   A complete loss or a reduction in sensitivity to sounds by persons who are deaf or hard of hearing.

hidden costs   Costs that cannot be predicted or accounted for until after the fact.

hierarchy of needs   Theory of human motivation based on integrated wholeness of the individual and levels of satisfaction of basic human needs organized by potency.

historically underrepresented groups   A more politically sensitive and correct term to substitute for the term *minority.*

humanistic learning   One of the five major learning theories, which views learning as being facilitated by curiosity, needs, a positive self-concept, and open situations where freedom of choice and individuality are promoted and respected.

illiteracy   The total inability of adults to read, write, or comprehend information.

illusionary representations   A category of instructional materials that depict realism, such as dimensionality. Examples are photographs, drawings, and audiotapes, which depend on imagination to fill in the gaps and offer the learner experiences that simulate reality.

impact evaluation   The process of assessing outcomes or effects of an educational activity that extend beyond the activity itself to address organizational and/or societal effects.

indirect costs   Costs that may be fixed but are not necessarily directly related to an educational activity (e.g., heating, electricity, housekeeping).

informal settings   Unplanned or spontaneous sessions in which teaching-learning takes place.

information processing perspective   Emphasizes the process of memory functioning in the way information is encountered, organized, stored, and retrieved.

input disability   A general category of learning disability that refers to the process of receiving and recording information in the brain, which includes visual, auditory, perceptual and integrative processing, such as dyslexia and short- and long-term memory disorders.

instruction   Often used interchangeably with teaching, it is in fact one aspect of teaching that involves the communicating of information about a specific skill in the cognitive, affective, or psychomotor domain with the objective of producing learning.

instructional materials/tools   The resources or vehicles used to help communicate information, which include both print and nonprint media, to aid teaching-learning by stimulating the various senses such as vision and hearing. These are intended to supplement, not replace, actual teaching. Synonymous terms are *educational aids* or *audio-visual materials*.

instructional method   A traditional or nontraditional technique or approach used by the teacher to bring the learner into contact with the content to be learned; a way or a process to communicate and share information with the learner.

instructional objectives   Intended outcomes of the education process that are in reference to an aspect of a program or a total program of study that are content oriented and teacher centered; also referred to as educational objectives.

instructional setting   A situation or area in which health teaching takes place as classified on the basis of what relationship health education has to the primary function of an organization, agency, or institution in which the teaching occurs.

instructional strategy   See *teaching strategy*.

internal locus of control   Individuals are motivated from within to learn, attributing success or failure to their own ability or effort.

interpersonal intelligence   A term used by Gardner to describe children who learn best in groups.

intrapersonal intelligence   A term used by Gardner to describe children who learn well with independent self-paced instruction.

intrinsic feedback   A response that is generated within the self, giving learners a sense of or a feel for how they have performed; often used in relation to a psychomotor skill performance.

judgment-perception (JP)   Terms used to describe behavior that reflects the way a person comes to a conclusion about something or becomes aware of something; one of four dichotomous preference dimensions in the Myers-Briggs Type Indicator.

justice   The equal distribution of benefits and burdens.

knowledge deficit   A gap in what a learner needs or wants to know; this category of nursing diagnosis can include learning needs in the cognitive, affective, and psychomotor domains.

knowledge readiness   A state of willingness to learn dependent on such factors as the learner's present knowledge base, the level of learning capability, and the preferred style of learning.

Knox Four-Step Appraisal   A systematic approach for assessing learning needs of caregivers and health-care organizations.

Kolb's Learning Style Inventory   An experiential learning model that includes four modes of learning reflecting the dimensions of perception and processing.

law   A clearly stated pronouncement of a binding custom, enforceable by a controlling body.

layout   The arrangement of printed and/or graphic information on a flat surface. Effective use of white space, graphics, and wording will depend heavily on this arrangement.

learner characteristics   One of the three major variables that refers to the learner's perceptual abilities, reading ability, self-direction, and learning style, which must be considered when making appropriate choices of instructional materials.

learning   A conscious or unconscious permanent change in behavior as a result of a lifelong, dynamic process by which individuals acquire new knowledge, skills, and/or attitudes that can be measured and can occur at anytime or in any place due to exposure to environmental stimuli.

learning contract   A mutually agreed on specific plan of action between the learner and educator clearly defining the specific behavioral objectives and predetermined goal to be achieved as a result of instruction. Also referred to as an educational contract.

learning disability (LD)   A generic term that refers to a heterogeneous group of disorders manifested by significant difficulties with learning. Inattention and impulsivity are signs indicating developmentally inappropriate behavior.

learning needs   Gaps in knowledge that exist between a desired level of performance and the actual level of performance (Healthcare Education Association, 1985).

learning styles   The way individuals perceive and then process information. Certain characteristics of style are biological in origin, whereas others are sociologically developed as a result of environmental influences.

lecture   The oldest, most commonly used, and most traditional instructional method by which the teacher verbally transmits information in a highly structured format directly to a group of learners.

legally blind   A person's vision is 20/200 or less in the better eye with correction, or if visual field limits in both eyes are within 20 degrees diameter.

legal rights and duties   A term that refers to rules governing behavior or conduct of health-care professionals that are enforceable under threat of punishment or penalty, such as a fine, imprisonment, or both.

linguistic intelligence   A term used by Gardner to describe children who have highly developed auditory skills and think in words.

Listening Test   A standardized test to measure comprehension using a selected passage from an instructional material written at approximately the fifth-grade level that is read aloud at a normal rate to determine what a person understands and remembers when listening.

literacy   The ability of adults to read, understand, and interpret information written at the eighth-grade level or above. An umbrella term used to describe socially required and expected reading and writing abilities; the relative ability of persons to use printed and written material commonly encountered in daily life.

locus of control   The location of control of behaviors as either self-directed or directed by others. Persons with internal or external locus of control differ particularly in the degree of responsibility taken for their own actions (see also *Internal Locus of Control* and *External Locus of Control*).

logical-math intelligence   A term used by Gardner to describe children who are strong in exploring patterns, categories, and relationships of objects.

low literacy   The ability of adults to read, write, and comprehend information between the fifth and the eighth-grade level of difficulty (also referred to as marginally literate or marginally illiterate).

malpractice   Failure to exercise an accepted degree of professional skill or learning by one rendering professional services that results in injury, loss, or damage to the recipient of those services.

mandatory needs   Requisites to be learned for survival or situations where the learner's life or safety is threatened.

media characteristics   One of the three major variables that refers to the form through which information will be communicated, which must be considered when making appropriate choices of instructional materials.

media/medium   The form in which information or ideas are conveyed to learners.

mental illness   A mental disability that may be acute or chronic, which affects a member or members of one in five families in the United States.

message   See *content*.

models   Three-dimensional instructional tools that allow the learner to immediately apply knowledge and psychomotor skills by observing, examining, manipulating, handling, assembling, and disassembling objects while the teacher provides feedback. Replicas, analogues, and symbols are all types of models that enhance instruction by means that range from concrete to abstract.

moral rights and duties   A term that refers to an internal value system, a certain "moral fabric," that is expressed externally in ethical behaviors of health-care professionals; often used interchangeably with the terms *morality* and *morals*.

morals   Synonymous with *ethics*; a value system.

motivation   A psychological force that moves a person in the direction of meeting a need or goal, evidenced by willingness or readiness to act.

motivational axioms   Premises on which an understanding of motivation is based, such as a state of optimum anxiety, learner readiness, realistic goal setting, learner satisfaction/success, and uncertainty-reducing or uncertainty-maintaining dialogue.

motivational incentives   Factors that influence motivation in the direction of the desired goal.

musical intelligence   A term used by Gardner to describe children who are talented in playing musical instruments, singing, dancing, and keeping rhythm and who often learn best with music playing in the background.

Myers-Briggs Type Indicator (MBTI)   A self-report inventory that uses forced-choice questions and word pairs to measure four dichotomous dimensions of behavior.

needs assessment   The process of determining through data collection what a person, group, organization, or community must learn and/or wants to learn to provide appropriate education programs to meet the required or desired needs of the learners.

negligence   Doing or nondoing of an act, pursuant to a duty, that a reasonable person in the same circumstances would or would not do and the acting or the nonacting is the proximate cause of injury to another person or property.

noncompliance   Nonsubmission or resistance of the individual to follow a prescribed, predetermined regimen.

non-health-care setting   One of three classifications of instructional settings, in which health care is an incidental or supportive function of an organization such as a business, industry, and school system.

nonmalfeasance   The notion of doing no harm.

nonprint instructional materials   Include the full range of audio and visual instructional materials, including demonstrations and displays.

numeracy   The degree of ability to read and interpret numbers.

nurse practice acts   Legal provisions of each state defining nursing and the standards of nursing practice, usually including patient teaching as a professional responsibility to protect the public from incompetent practitioners.

nursing process   A model for nursing practice using the problem-solving approach, which includes the phases of assessment, nursing diagnosis, planning, implementation, and evaluation of patient care (see the definition of *educational process* as it parallels the nursing process).

objectives (behavioral)   Statements defining specific health activities, quantitatively measurable and descriptive of the intended results (rather than the process) of instruction, to be competently achieved by the learner in a finite period of time. Well-stated objectives reflect the characteristic components of performance, conditions, and criteria.

one-to-one instruction   A common, traditional instructional method for exchange of information whereby the teacher delivers individual verbal instruction of learning activities in a format designed specifically to meet the needs of a particular learner.

operant conditioning   Focuses on the behavior of an organism as a result of a positive or negative reinforcer (stimulus or event) applied after a response that strengthens the probability that the response will be performed again; nonreinforcement and punishment decrease the likelihood that a response will continue to be performed.

outcome   The result of actions; may be intended (e.g., synonymous with stated goals) or unintended.

outcome evaluation   See *summative evaluation.*

output disability   A general category of learning disability that refers to orally responding and performing physical tasks, which include language and motor disorders.

parochial orientation   Persons who demonstrate close-mindedness in thinking, conservativeness, and less willingness to learn new material and who place trust in traditional authority figures; a component of experiential readiness.

patient education   A process of assisting consumers of health care to learn how to incorporate health-related behaviors (knowledge, skills, and/or attitudes) into everyday life with the purpose of achieving the goal of optimal health.

pedagogy   The art and science of helping children to learn.

PEMs   See *printed education materials*

physical maturation   Change in an individual's physical characteristics as a result of normal body growth and development during the aging process.

physical readiness   A state of willingness to learn dependent on such factors as measures of physical ability, complexity of task, health status, and gender.

possible needs   "Nice to know" information that is not essential at a given point in time or in situations in which learning is not directly related to daily activities.

posters   A type of display that combines print and nonprint media to help convey a message.

PRECEDE-PROCEED Model   A comprehensive epidemiological health promotion, planning, and evaluation model used in educational and environmental development.

preoperational period   As defined by Piaget, this is the second key milestone in the cognitive development of children when the child of the preschool age group (3 to 6 years) is acquiring language skills and gaining experience but thinking is precausal, animistic, egocentric, and intuitive, with only a vague understanding of relationships and multiple classifications of objects.

presentation   The form in which the message (content) is put forth, occurring along a continuum from real objects to symbols.

printed education materials (PEMs)   As the most common type of teaching tools, these include handouts, leaflets, books, pamphlets, brochures, and instruction sheets, which may be purchased or instructor developed. Also referred to as printed instructional materials.

process evaluation   See *formative evaluation.*

Productivity Environmental Preference Survey (PEPS)   The assessment tool used in the adult version of the Dunn and Dunn Learning Style Inventory.

program evaluation   A systematic assessment to determine the extent to which all activities for an entire department or program over a specified time period have accomplished the goals originally established.

programmed instruction   A type of self-study tool, usually printed or computerized, that takes the learner through the learning task step by step.

projected learning resources   Audiovisual instructional formats that depend primarily on the learners' sense of sight as the means through which messages are received. These resources require equipment to project images, usually in a darkened room, and include movies, slides, overhead transparencies, and others.

psychodynamic learning   One of the five major learning theories. Largely a theory of motivation stressing emotions rather than cognition and responses; this perspective emphasizes the importance of conscious and unconscious forces derived from earlier childhood experiences and conflicts that guide and change behavior.

psychoeducation   The education or training of a person with a psychiatric disorder with the goal of helping patients and their families independently manage mental illness to avoid frequent hospitalizations.

psychomotor domain   One of three domains in the taxonomy of educational objectives, which is concerned with the physical activities of the body, such as coordination, reaction time, and muscular control, related to the acquisition of a skill or task.

psychosocial development   The process of psychological and social adjustment as an individual grows from infancy to adulthood according to Erickson's eight stages of the psychological and social maturation of humans: trust versus mistrust; autonomy versus shame and doubt; initiative versus guilt; industry versus inferiority; identity versus role confusion; intimacy versus isolation; generativity versus self-absorption and stagnation; and ego integrity versus despair.

readability   The level of reading difficulty at which printed teaching tools are written. A measure of those elements in a given text of printed material that influence with what degree of success a group of readers will be able to read and understand the information; the ease, or conversely the difficulty, with which a person can understand or comprehend the style of writing of a selected printed passage.

readiness to learn   The time when the learner is receptive to learning and is willing and able to participate in the learning process; preparedness or willingness to learn.

realia   The most concrete form of stimuli that can be used to deliver information. Example: a real person or a model being used to demonstrate a procedure such as breast self-examination.

REALM (Rapid Estimate of Adult Literacy in Medicine)   A reading skills test to measure a patient's ability to read medical and health-related vocabulary.

receptive aphasia An absence or impairment of the ability to comprehend what is read or heard due to a dysfunction of the Wernicke's area of the brain, which controls sensory abilities. Although hearing is unimpaired, the person is unable to understand the significance of the spoken word and is unable to communicate verbally.

reflective observation A term used by Kolb to describe a dimension of perceiving; known as the "watching" mode.

rehabilitation The relearning of previous skills, which often requires an adjustment to altered functional abilities and altered lifestyle.

replicas A facsimile constructed to scale that resembles the features or substance of the original object. It may be examined or manipulated by the learner to get an idea of how something works. Example: resuscitation dolls.

respondeat superior Master-servant rule; "let the master respond and answer" (Lesnik & Anderson, 1962, p. 200).

respondent conditioning Emphasizes the importance of stimulus conditions and the associations formed in the learning process whereby, without thought or awareness, learning takes place when a newly conditioned stimulus (CS) becomes associated with a conditioned response (CR); also termed classical or Pavlovian conditioning.

return demonstration A traditional instructional method by which the learner attempts to perform a skill, most frequently psychomotor in nature, with cues or prompting as needed from the teacher.

role-modeling The use of self as a role model, often overlooked as an instructional method, whereby the learner acquires new behaviors and social roles by identification with the role model.

role-playing A nontraditional method of instruction by which learners participate in an unrehearsed dramatization, acting out an assigned part of a character as they think the character would act in reality.

SAM (Suitability Assessment of Materials) An evaluation instrument designed to measure the appropriateness of print materials, illustrations, and video- and audiotaped instructions for a given patient population.

selective attention The process of recognizing and selecting appropriate and inappropriate stimuli.

self-composed instructional materials Printed instructional materials composed by individual instructors for the purposes of supplementing teaching.

Self-Efficacy Theory A framework that describes the belief that one is capable of accomplishing a specific behavior.

self-instruction A nontraditional method of instruction used by a teacher to provide or design teaching materials and activities that guide the learner in independently achieving the objectives of learning.

self-study materials Written materials that are designed to allow the learner to independently master understanding of concepts or tasks.

sensing-intuition (SN) Describes how individuals perceive the world, either directly through the five senses or indirectly by way of the unconscious; one of four dichotomous preference dimensions in the Myers-Briggs Type Indicator.

sensorimotor period As defined by Piaget, this is the first key milestone in the cognitive development of children in the age group of infancy to toddlerhood when learning is enhanced through movement and manipulation of objects in the environment via visual, auditory, tactile, olfactory, taste, and motor stimulation.

sensory deficits   A category of common physical disabilities that includes, in particular, hearing and visual impairments.

simulation   A nontraditional method of instruction whereby an artificial or hypothetical experience is created that engages the learner in an activity reflecting real-life conditions but without the risk-taking consequences of an actual situation.

simulation laboratories   A type of learning laboratory that contains real equipment in a lifelike setting, but that allows the learner to practice manipulating and using this equipment as a prelude to performing a task in a real-life situation. Frequently used to supplement the learning of psychomotor skills.

SMOG formula   A relatively easy to use, popular, valid test of readability based on 100% comprehension of printed material from grade 4 to college level.

social cognition perspective   An aspect of cognitive theory that highlights the influence of social factors on perception, thought, motivation, and behaviors.

social learning   One of five major learning theories, this theory is seen as a mixture of behaviorist, cognitive, and psychodynamic influences; much of learning is a social process that occurs by observation and watching other people's behavior to see what happens to them. Role-modeling is a central concept of this theory, with cognitive or psychodynamic aspects of internal processing and motivation sometimes considered in the learning process.

socioeconomic differences   Variation in health status, health behavior, or learning abilities among individuals of different social and economic levels.

software   Computer programs and other instructional materials such as videotapes and overhead transparencies.

Spache Grade-Level Score   A readability formula specifically designed to judge materials written for children at grade levels below the fourth grade (elementary grades first through third).

spatial intelligence   A term used by Gardner to describe children who learn by images and pictures.

spinal cord injury   Traumatic insult to the spinal cord resulting in alterations or complete disruption of normal motor, sensory, and autonomic functions.

staff education   A process of assisting nursing staff personnel to acquire knowledge, skills, or attitudes regarding nursing practice for the purpose of maintaining or improving their ability to deliver optimal care to the consumer.

summative evaluation   Systematic assessment of the degree to which individuals have learned or objectives have been met as a result of education intervention; also referred to as outcome evaluation.

support system   Resources and significant others, such as family and friends, on whom the patient relies or is dependent for information or assistance in managing activities of daily living and who may serve as a positive or negative influence on teaching efforts.

symbolic models   See *symbols.*

symbols   A type of model that conveys a message to the learner through the use of abstract constructs, like words, that stand for the real thing. Cartoons and printed materials are examples of symbolic forms of a message.

task characteristics   One of the three major variables defined by the behavioral objectives in the cognitive, affective, and psychomotor domains of learning, which must be considered when making appropriate choices of instructional materials.

taxonomic hierarchy   See *taxonomy.*

taxonomy   A form of hierarchical classification of cognitive, affective, and psychomotor domains of behaviors according to their degree or level of complexity.

teachable moment   As defined by Havighurst, that point in time when the learner is most receptive to a teaching situation; it can occur at any hour that a patient, family member, staff member, or nursing student has a question or needs information.

teaching   As one component of the educational process, it is a deliberate, intentional act of communicating information to the learner in response to identified learning needs with the objective of producing learning to achieve desired behavioral outcomes.

teaching plan   Overall blueprint or outline for instruction clearly defining the relationship between the essential components of behavioral objectives, instructional content, teaching methods and tools, time frame for teaching, and methods of evaluation that fit together in a logical pattern of flow to achieve a predetermined goal.

teaching strategy   An overall plan of action for instruction that anticipates barriers and resources of the learning experience to achieve specific educational objectives.

telecommunications   Technological devices for the deaf (TDD).

telecommunications learning resources   Instructional tools used to help convey information via electrical energy from one place to another such as telephones, televisions, and computers.

Theory of Reasoned Action   A framework that is concerned with prediction and understanding of human behavior within a social context.

Therapeutic Alliance Model   An interpersonal provider-patient model that addresses the continuum of compliance, adherence, and collaboration in therapeutic relationships.

thinking-feeling (TF)   An approach used by individuals to arrive at judgments through impersonal, logical, subjective, or empathetic processes; one of four dichotomous preference dimensions in the Myers-Briggs Type Inventory.

tools   See *instructional materials/tools.*

transcultural nursing   A formal area of study and practice comparing and analyzing different cultures and subcultures with respect to cultural care, health practices, and illness beliefs with the goal of using these insights to provide culture-specific and culture-universal care to diverse groups of people.

transfer of learning   The effects of learning one skill on the subsequent performance of another related skill.

triad communication   A technique of involving a third person, such as a family member, significant other, or caregiver, in the communication pattern of the nurse and the client to serve as a listener and learner in the teaching situation for the purpose of assisting the client in understanding content, encouraging family or caregiver involvement and support, and enhancing client compliance with treatment regimens.

variable costs   Not predictable, volume-related expenses.

veracity   Truth telling; honesty.

visual impairment   A reduction or complete loss of vision due to infection, accident, poisoning, or congenital degeneration of the eye(s). See *legally blind.*

WRAT (Wide Range Achievement Test) technique   A word recognition screening test used to assess a person's ability to recognize and pronounce a list of words out of context as a criterion for measuring comprehension of written materials. Level I test is designed for children ages 5 to 12 years; level II is intended to test persons over 12 years of age.

INDEX